eureka

Neurology & Neurosurgery

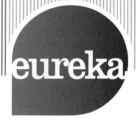

Neurology & Neurosurgery

Dawn R Collins BSc PhD
Principal Teaching Fellow
Warwick Medical School, University of
Warwick
Coventry, UK

John A Goodfellow BSc (Hons) BM
BCh MRCP PhD
Honorary Clinical Academic Fellow
University of Glasgow
Specialty Registrar in Neurology
and Associate Clinical Director
Neuroimmunology Laboratory
Institute of Neurological Sciences
Glasgow, UK

Adikarige Haritha Dulanka Silva
MA (Hons) MBBChir MPhil (Cantab)
MRCS (Eng)
Specialty Registrar in Neurosurgery
Queen Elizabeth Hospital, University
Hospitals Birmingham NHS Foundation
Trust
Birmingham, UK

Ronan Dardis MBBCh MSc MPhil
MMedSci FRCS FRCSI (Neuro Surg)
Consultant Neurosurgeon and Clinical
Lead for Neurosurgery
University Hospitals Coventry and
Warwickshire NHS Trust
Coventry, UK

Sanjoy Nagaraja MD MRCS(Edin)
MRCS(Lon) FRCR
Clinical Director of Radiology
Consultant Interventional
Neuroradiologist
University Hospitals Coventry and
Warwickshire NHS Trust
Coventry, UK

Series Editors

Janine Henderson MRCPsych
MClinEd
MB BS Programme Director
Hull York Medical School
York, UK

David Oliveira PhD FRCP
Professor of Renal Medicine
St George's, University of London
London, UK

Stephen Parker BSc MS DipMedEd
FRCS
Consultant Breast and General
Paediatric Surgeon
St Mary's Hospital
Newport, UK

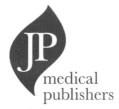

JP
medical
publishers

London • Philadelphia • New Delhi • Panama City

© 2016 JP Medical Ltd.

Published by JP Medical Ltd, 83 Victoria Street, London, SW1H 0HW, UK

Tel: +44 (0)20 3170 8910   Fax: +44 (0)20 3008 6180

Email: info@jpmedpub.com   www.jpmedpub.com, www.eurekamedicine.com

ISBN: 978-1-907816-74-1

British Library Cataloguing in Publication Data
A catalogue record for this book is available from the British Library

Library of Congress Cataloging in Publication Data
A catalog record for this book is available from the Library of Congress

Publisher:	Richard Furn
Development Editors:	Thomas Fletcher, Paul Mayhew, Alison Whitehouse
Editorial Assistants:	Sophie Woolven, Katie Pattullo
Copy Editor:	Kim Howell
Graphic narratives:	James Pollitt
Cover design:	Forbes Design
Page design:	Designers Collective Ltd

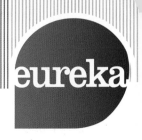

Series Editors' Foreword

Today's medical students need to know a great deal to be effective as tomorrow's doctors. This knowledge includes core science and clinical skills, from understanding biochemical pathways to communicating with patients. Modern medical school curricula integrate this teaching, thereby emphasising how learning in one area can support and reinforce another. At the same time students must acquire sound clinical reasoning skills, working with complex information to understand each individual's unique medical problems.

The *Eureka* series is designed to cover all aspects of today's medical curricula and reinforce this integrated approach. Each book can be used from first year through to qualification. Core biomedical principles are introduced but given relevant clinical context: the authors have always asked themselves, 'why does the aspiring clinician need to know this'?

Each clinical title in the series is grounded in the relevant core science, which is introduced at the start of each book. Each core science title integrates and emphasises clinical relevance throughout. Medical and surgical approaches are included to provide a complete and integrated view of the patient management options available to the clinician. Clinical insights highlight key facts and principles drawn from medical practice. Cases featuring unique graphic narratives are presented with clear explanations that show how experienced clinicians think, enabling students to develop their own clinical reasoning and decision making. Clinical SBAs help with exam revision while starter questions are a unique learning tool designed to stimulate interest in the subject.

Having biomedical principles and clinical applications together in one book will make their connections more explicit and easier to remember. Alongside repeated exposure to patients and practice of clinical and communication skills, we hope *Eureka* will equip medical students for a lifetime of successful clinical practice.

Janine Henderson, David Oliveira, Stephen Parker

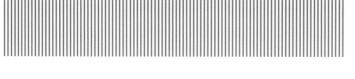

About the Series Editors

Janine Henderson is the MB BS undergraduate Programme Director at Hull York Medical School (HYMS). After medical school at the University of Oxford and clinical training in psychiatry, she combined her work as a Consultant Psychiatrist with postgraduate teaching roles, moving to the new Hull York Medical School in 2004. She has a particular interest in modern educational methods, curriculum design and clinical reasoning.

David Oliveira is Professor of Renal Medicine at St George's, University of London (SGUL), where he served as the MBBS Course Director between 2007 and 2013. Having trained at Cambridge University and the Westminster Hospital he obtained a PhD in cellular immunology and worked as a renal physician before being appointed as Foundation Chair of Renal Medicine at SGUL.

Stephen Parker is a Consultant Breast and General Paediatric Surgeon at St Mary's Hospital, Isle of Wight. He trained at St George's, University of London, and after service in the Royal Navy was appointed as Consultant Surgeon at University Hospital Coventry. He has a particular interest in e-learning and the use of multimedia platforms in medical education.

About the Authors

Dawn Collins is a Principal Teaching Fellow at Warwick Medical School. She has been teaching neurobiology and neuropharmacology to medical students for over 10 years, and currently leads teaching on brain and behaviour. Her research time is spent studying fear and anxiety, and developing learning aids for students.

John Goodfellow is a Specialty Registrar in neurology. He enjoys teaching medical students and PACES candidates, and has written a number of undergraduate medical textbooks and a clinical skills DVD. He has a clinical and research interest in neuroimmunology.

Adikarige Haritha Dulanka Silva is a Specialty Registrar in neurosurgery. He qualified from Cambridge University and has been a clinical supervisor teaching medical students and junior doctors in pathology, physiology, anatomy, clinical medicine and surgery throughout his undergraduate, foundation and specialty registrar training. His clinical interest is in neuro-oncology and spinal surgery.

Ronan Dardis is a Consultant Neurosurgeon. He was previously Honorary Associate Clinical Professor at the University of Warwick, where he delivered part of the preclinical and clinical neuroscience teaching. He is particularly interested in brain trauma, neuro-oncology and spinal conditions.

Sanjoy Nagaraja is a Consultant Interventional Neuroradiologist and Clinical Director of Radiology. He has been a consultant for the past 6 years after finishing his training in neuroradiology at the John Radcliffe Hospital, Oxford.

Preface

Neurology and neurosurgery inspire a mixture of fear and fascination in most medical students due to the perceived complexity of the nervous system. *Eureka Neurology & Neurosurgery* demystifies the nervous system, and the diagnosis and management of neurological disorders, by integrating the core neuroscience and clinical knowledge in an accessible way.

Chapter 1 covers core neuroscience: the structural framework that underpins clinical practice. Chapter 2 lays out the tools required to apply this knowledge when evaluating and managing neurological patients. Subsequent chapters describe the spectrum of neurological and neurosurgical disorders, from infections to traumatic injury. Clinical cases are brought to life using graphic narratives and neuroradiological imaging, while figures and boxes simplify key concepts and provide clinical correlates. Dedicated chapters cover emergency presentations and the integrated management of patients with chronic neurological conditions. Finally, clinical SBAs provide a useful revision aid.

We hope you enjoy this book and that it provides you with confidence when approaching patients with neurological disorders.

Dawn Collins
John Goodfellow
Dulanka Silva
Ronan Dardis
Sanjoy Nagaraja
January 2016

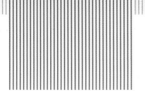

Contents

Chapter 13 Motor neurone and genetic neurodegenerative diseases

Chapter 14 Dementia

Chapter 15 Congenital and hereditary conditions

Chapter 16 Peripheral neurological disease

Chapter 17 Emergencies

Chapter 18 Integrated care

Chapter 19 Self-assessment

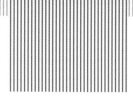

Glossary

ABCDE	Airway, Breathing, Circulation, Disability, Exposure		MPTP	1-methyl-4-phenyl-1,2,3,6-tetrahydropyridine
ACE	angiotensin-converting enzyme		MR	magnetic resonance
ADC	apparent diffusion coefficient		MRI	magnetic resonance imaging
AIDS	acquired immunodeficiency syndrome		MS	multiple sclerosis
AMA	antimitochondrial antibody		NMDA	N-methyl-D-aspartate
AMPLE	Allergies, Medications, Past medical history, Last meal, Events surrounding injury		NSAID	non-steroidal anti-inflammatory drug
ANA	antinuclear autoantibody		OCB	oligoclonal band
ANCA	antineutrophil cytoplasmic antibody		PCR	polymerase chain reaction
anti-dsDNA	anti-double-stranded DNA autoantibody		PET	positron emission tomography
			PNS	parasympathetic nervous system
ATLS	Advanced trauma life support			
AVM	arteriovenous malformation		SNS	sympathetic nervous system
AZT	azidothymidine		SPECT	single-photon emission computerised tomography
BOLD	blood oxygenation level-dependent		STIR	short tau inversion recovery
BP	blood pressure		SUDEP	sudden unexpected death in epilepsy
			SUNCT	short-lasting, unilateral, neuralgiform headache attacks with conjunctival injection and tearing
CN	cranial nerve			
CSF	cerebrospinal fluid			
CT	computerised tomography		UMN	upper motor neurone
DMPK	dystrophia myotonica protein kinase		V	volume
DWI	diffusion-weighted imaging		V_{blood}	volume of blood
			V_{brain}	volume of brain
EEG	electroencephalogram or encephalography		$V_{cerebrospinal\ fluid}$	volume of cerebrospinal fluid
			$V_{extra\ mass}$	volume of extra mass
FLAIR	fluid-attenuated inversion recovery		V_{total}	total intracranial volume
HAART	highly active antiretroviral therapy		WHO	World Health Organization
HIV	human immunodeficiency virus			
ICHD	International Classification of Headache Disorders			
ICP	intracranial pressure			
LMN	lower motor neurone			

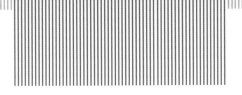

Acknowledgements

Thanks to the following medical students for their help reviewing chapters: Jessica Dunlop, Aliza Imam, Roxanne McVittie, Daniel Roberts and Joseph Suich.

The publisher thanks the following authors for the use of a number of published figures:

Figure 3.1 is reproduced from Chopdar A, Aung T. Multimodal Retinal Imaging. London: JP Medical Ltd, 2014.

Figure 8.8 is reproduced from Inamadar AC, Palit A, Ragunatha S. Textbook of Pediatric Dermatology, 2nd Edition. New Delhi: Jaypee Brothers, 2014.

Figure 12.1 is reproduced from Craythorne E, Day ML. Pocket Tutor Dermatology. London: JP Medical Ltd, 2015.

Figures 12.4a–b, 12.5 are reproduced from Sharma Om P, Mihailovic-Vucinic Violeta. Lesions of Sarcoidosis: A Problem Solving Approach. New Delhi: Jaypee Brothers, 2014.

Figures 15.5a, 15.5c are reproduced from Verma A, Kunju PAM, Kanhere S, Maheshwari N. IAP Textbook of Pediatric Neurology. New Delhi: Jaypee Brothers, 2014.

Figure 15.5b, 16.8 is reproduced from Chattopadhyay BSP. Common Skin Diseases: A Clinical Approach. New Delhi: Jaypee Brothers, 2014.

We would like to thank all of our family, friends and colleagues for their support during the writing of this book, and to everyone at JP Medical for making this possible.

DC, JG, DS, RD, SN

Thanks to Dr Terence Jones for his contribution to the radiology section in chapter 2 and to Dr Praveen Varra for his work on the radiological images.

SN

Chapter 1
First principles

Starter questions

Answers to the following questions are on page 115.

1. Does having a bigger brain make a person more intelligent?
2. The nervous system controls the body, but what controls the nervous system?
3. What is the dominant side of the brain?

Overview of the nervous system

The nervous system controls every aspect of bodily function from homeostasis to thought processing, and both conscious and unconscious behaviours. It detects changes in the external and internal environments, integrates and interprets this information and generates appropriate responses. The complex nature of the nervous system means that even small changes have wide-ranging effects on both physical and mental health.

Despite this complexity, patterns are apparent at both the structural and the functional level. These patterns are clinically useful; they enable location of damage to the nervous system, as well as recognition and

prediction of its effects. The ability to correlate a patient's signs and symptoms with the physiology, biochemistry and anatomy of their nervous system, and to express this knowledge and understanding fluently and clearly, are essential skills.

Organisation of the nervous system

The nervous system is considered in terms of divisions, starting with the cells that make up the system and then in terms of the system-wide anatomical and functional divisions.

Cellular components of the nervous system

The nervous system consists of two types of cell.

- **Neurones** are the functional units, responsible for processing information and communicating between cells and regions of the nervous system
- **Glia** provide structural and functional support, maintaining the environment within the nervous system so that it is optimal for neuronal function

A neurone communicates chemically and electrically along its axon. This is a projection from its cell body to its terminals. At these terminals, it synapses with, i.e. has specialised junctions with, other neurones (**Figure 1.1**). Disruption to this communication produces neurological disorders. For example, brain damage from stroke can cause loss of movement, and excessive neuronal activity results in epilepsy.

Knowledge of how and where changes in neuronal communication occur within the nervous system is key to the diagnosis of neurological disorders.

Anatomical divisions: the central and peripheral nervous systems

The nervous system has two main anatomical divisions: the central nervous system and the peripheral nervous system (**Figure 1.2**):

- The **central nervous system**, which comprises the brain and the spinal cord
- The **peripheral nervous system**, which is the neural tissue outside the brain and spinal cord:
  - **spinal nerves**
  - **cranial nerves**
  - **autonomic nerves**
  - **associated ganglia** (clusters of neuronal cell bodies)

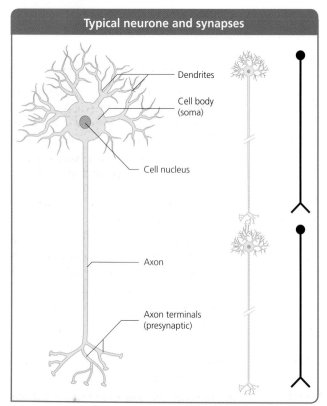

Typical neurone and synapses

Dendrites

Cell body (soma)

Cell nucleus

Axon

Axon terminals (presynaptic)

Figure 1.1 Neurones and synapses. A typical neurone is shown on its own and synapsing with another neurone; the convention used for depicting synapses in simplified form is also shown.

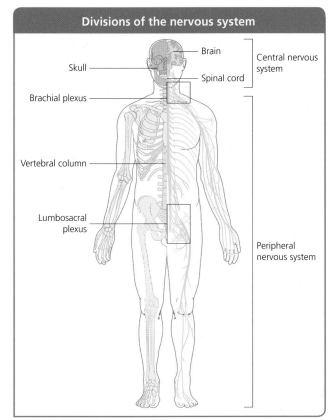

Divisions of the nervous system

- Brain
- Skull
- Spinal cord
- Brachial plexus
- Central nervous system
- Vertebral column
- Lumbosacral plexus
- Peripheral nervous system

Figure 1.2 Divisions of the nervous system.

Functional divisions: the somatic and autonomic nervous systems

Functionally, the nervous system is divided into somatic and autonomic systems. The two systems link the central and peripheral systems, enabling the body to respond appropriately to changes in both the internal and external environments.

The somatic nervous system

The somatic nervous system controls conscious and unconscious sensation as well as voluntary movement. It has two types of neuronal pathways:

- afferent pathways carrying sensory input from the body to the brain
- efferent pathways conveying motor output from the brain to muscles

These act synergistically to elicit the appropriate responses to stimuli.

The autonomic nervous system

This division of the efferent (motor) system provides automatic and unconscious control of the viscera and homeostasis. The autonomic nervous system has two divisions.

- The **sympathetic nervous system** is best known for its role in the fight-or-flight response
- The **parasympathetic nervous system** maintains steady state behaviours

These two systems usually act in opposition to maintain homeostasis by adjusting bodily functions in response to internal and external stimuli (**Table 1.1**).

Orientation

Three major axes, or planes, are used to describe relative position in the nervous system (**Figure 1.3**).

- The **coronal axis** divides the front from the back; in the context of the brain, this axis

Functions of the autonomic nervous system		
Function	Sympathetic nervous system	Parasympathetic nervous system
Heart function	Increased heart rate	Decreased heart rate
Bloody supply	Increased blood pressure	Decreased blood pressure
	Vasoconstriction	None
	Direction of blood to voluntary muscles	Direction of blood to the gut
Lung function	Bronchorelaxation	Bronchoconstriction
Gut function	Decreased gut motility	Increased gut motility
	Decreased ingestion and excretion	Excretion of ingested food
Pupillary reflex	Dilation of pupils	Constriction of pupils
Salivary gland function	Inhibition of salivation	Stimulation of salivation
Nasolacrimal duct function	Inhibition of lacrimation	Stimulation of lacrimation
Bladder function	Relaxation	Constriction
	Reduced micturition	Increased micturition

Table 1.1 Functions of the autonomic nervous system

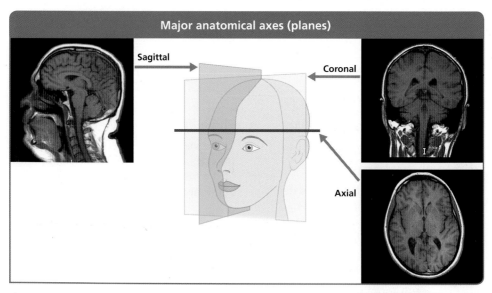

Figure 1.3 Visualising the three major anatomical axes (planes) through the brain: MRI images and their corresponding locations on a three-dimensional view of the head.

can be visualised by thinking about how headphones are worn
- The **sagittal axis** divides lengthwise; a **mid-sagittal** line divides the brain into left and right halves
- The **axial axis** cuts across the body; this axis is also termed horizontal or transverse

(imagine a slice going through the head to the horizon)

Other axes are:

- rostral or cranial (anterior or head end)
- caudal (posterior or 'tail' end)
- dorsal (back or posterior) and ventral (front or anterior)

- superior (above or upper) and inferior (lower or below)
- medial (closer to the midline) and lateral (towards the outer edges of the tissue)

The central nervous system

The central nervous system comprises the brain and the spinal cord.

The brain

The brain is subdivided into the cerebrum (the cerebral hemispheres), the diencephalon, the brainstem and the cerebellum (**Figure 1.4**).

The cerebrum

Most of the brain is cerebrum. The cerebrum controls the flow of information, from acquisition, integration and association (see page 42) to decision making and expression of responses (see page 43).

Cerebral hemispheres and lobes of the brain

The cerebrum comprises two cerebral hemispheres, which are each subdivided into four main lobes (**Figure 1.5**):

- The **frontal lobe** is primarily associated with motor function and higher cognition (thought processing)

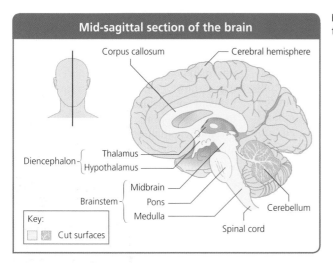

Mid-sagittal section of the brain

Corpus callosum
Cerebral hemisphere

Diencephalon { Thalamus
Hypothalamus

Brainstem { Midbrain
Pons
Medulla

Cerebellum

Spinal cord

Key:
Cut surfaces

Figure 1.4 Mid-sagittal section of the brain.

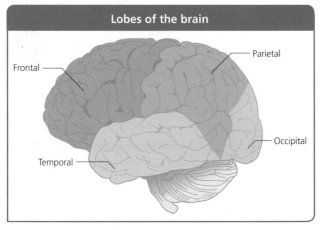

Lobes of the brain

Frontal
Parietal
Temporal
Occipital

Figure 1.5 Lobes of the brain.

- The **parietal lobe** is home to sensory function
- The **temporal lobe** is responsible for language, learning, memory and emotional interpretation, as well as audition (hearing), olfaction (smell) and gustation (taste)
- The **occipital lobe** is dedicated to interpretation of visual stimuli

The limbic system, which used to be called the limbic lobe, lies deep within the cerebral hemispheres. It is a functional group of interlinked regions. Its functions include learning and memory formation, spatial perception and emotional control.

A hidden lobe, the insula, which lies behind the lateral sulcus and the frontal and temporal lobes also regulates emotions (see page 48).

Structural organisation of the cerebrum

The cerebral hemispheres comprise grey matter and white matter.

Grey matter The outermost layer of the cerebrum – the cortex – is composed of grey matter and contains the cell bodies of the cerebral neurones and glia. Within grey matter the neurones are further organised into layers and the 'columns' (see page 42).

White matter The inner region of each cerebral hemisphere – its subcortical layer – is composed of white matter. This contains the axonal projections from the neurones; these axons connect the cortex to the rest of the central nervous system. The axons are wrapped in layers of myelin (see page 14), giving the matter its white colour.

Within the subcortical pathways of the white matter lie the deep cortical nuclei, including the basal ganglia and forebrain nuclei (see pages 43–48). Nuclei are clusters of functionally related neurones.

Primary, secondary and association cortices

Cortical areas with one specific function are called primary or secondary cortices, for example the primary motor cortex and the secondary visual cortex. These areas account for about 20% of the total surface volume of the cerebral hemispheres.

The remaining areas are association cortices (see page 48). These integrate different types of information derived from different sources, for example combining visual input with information on emotional status.

Brodmann areas

The cerebral cortex is generally mapped by function. However, it has also been mapped and divided into numbered areas according to histological composition: Brodmann areas. Some of these are synonymous with specific functions; for example, area 17 is the primary visual cortex and area 4 the primary motor cortex. Neurologists and neurosurgeons most often refer to areas according to their function or location, but Brodmann area numbers are also used interchangeably.

Diencephalon

The thalamus and hypothalamus comprise the diencephalon (**Figure 1.4**). They have pivotal roles in homeostasis and consciousness.

The thalamus integrates and transmits information on sensation and movement, acting as a hub for incoming activity from the spinal cord and brainstem and outgoing activity from the cerebrum.

The hypothalmus is the hub for all the autonomic functions that keep the body within optimal physiological ranges, including thermoregulation, appetite and thirst. It receives information about the body's internal environment from the nervous system and from substances circulating in the blood and cerebrospinal fluid (see page 53). It transmits information to the brainstem and spinal cord to control the activity of the organs. The hypothalamus also drives rapid survival mechanisms such as the fight-or-flight response.

Brainstem

Caudal to the diencephalon is the brainstem, which is divided into the midbrain, pons and medulla (see **Figure 1.34**) and:

- is the site of major control centres for bodily functions such as respiration and circulation
- contains the nuclei of most of the cranial nerves, which control the head and neck
- is the main site of production for several neurotransmitters (see page 62)

The brainstem has a vital role in controlling the flow of information to and from the cerebrum. It is also responsible for maintaining consciousness and arousal levels.

The brainstem and cerebellum are the oldest parts of the brain, both developmentally and evolutionarily.

Cerebellum

The cerebellum lies superior to the brainstem and inferior to the posterior portion of the cerebral lobes (**Figure 1.4**). It consists of highly folded layers of grey and white matter, and is connected to the brainstem by three pairs of cerebellar peduncles; these are stalks comprising large bundles of axons.

In collaboration with the basal ganglia (see page 48) and thalamus, the cerebellum coordinates and fine-tunes movement. It also has a role in procedural memory, i.e. the memory needed to perform complex motor skills such as riding a bike or driving a car.

Damage to the cerebellum results in an inability to coordinate motor function. This is commonly apparent as changes in speech (slurring) or gait.

Spinal cord

The spinal cord is a long, thin, tube-like extension of the central nervous system. It starts at the base of the brainstem, then travels down within the vertebral column to carry information between the brain and periphery, and vice versa. The cord is not simply a conduit, as once thought, but actively modifies and integrates the information that passes through it.

The cord is formed of 31 segments named according to the region of the vertebral column from which they arise during development (pages 25 and 71). These regions are shown in **Figure 1.6** and are:

- cervical (in the neck region)
- thoracic (in the thorax, i.e. upper trunk)
- lumbar (in the abdomen, i.e. lower trunk)
- sacral (in the strong, triangular bony section at the base of the vertebral column)

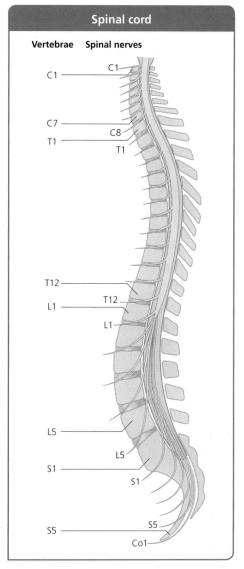

Figure 1.6 Spinal cord, spinal nerves and spinal segments from which they are derived. See also Figure 1.7.

- coccygeal (in the coccyx or tail bone region)

For example, the thoracic cord has 12 segments, T1–T12. The spinal cord bulges in both the cervical and the lumbar areas. These contain the nerves innervating the arms and legs, which require greater control than that needed for the trunk.

The peripheral nervous system

The peripheral nervous system comprises 43 pairs of nerves: 31 pairs of spinal nerves and 12 pairs of cranial nerves. Spinal nerves originate within the spinal cord and exit from the spine to innervate regions of the body. Cranial nerves originate in the brainstem within the cranium (hence their name), and exit through several foramina (openings) in the cranium to innervate the head and neck (see **Figures 1.58–1.60** and **Table 1.8**).

Spinal nerves

The spinal nerves innervate the entire body. Each spinal nerve has both sensory and motor components and is named according to the spinal level at which it and exits the spinal cord; for example, nerve T3 arises from the third thoracic level of the spinal cord. On exiting the vertebral column they are often called peripheral nerves.

Each pair of spinal nerves arises from one spinal segment (**Figure 1.7**) and exits the spinal cord.

Dermatomes The sensory organisation of the skin maps to the segmental organisation of the cord and nerves: each nerve receives input from a specific region of the skin called a dermatome (see **Figure 1.47**).

Myotomes Spinal nerves also innervate muscles. However, because each nerve may innervate a number of muscles the muscle map (myotome) uses groups of nerves to indicated innervation for simplicity.

Nerve plexuses

A nerve plexus is a network of branching and interconnecting nerves. After exiting the spinal column, peripheral nerves C5–T1 form a plexus, the brachial plexus, on each side of the body; similarly, L1–S4 form a lumbar plexus on each side (**Table 1.2**; see **Figures 1.2** and **1.45**).

These plexuses branch into the major motor nerves that control limb function. They also

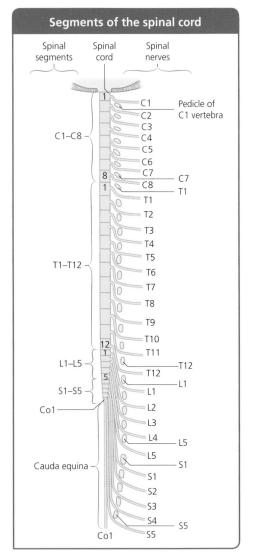

Figure 1.7 Segments of the spinal cord: each spinal nerve exits the spinal canal via an intervertebral foramen between the pedicles of adjacent vertebrae: the further down the spine the more inferior the nerve's exit with respect to the location of its spinal segment. Nerves exit on both sides but for simplicity only one side is shown and enlargements of the cord, which are at C5–T1 and L1–S3 levels, are not shown.

receive sensory information via cutaneous (skin) branches. Because there are differences in the branching patterns of motor and sensory nerves, the myotomal (motor) and dermatomal (sensory) maps are not the same.

Major plexuses and corresponding spinal and peripheral nerves			
Plexus	Spinal nerves	Peripheral nerves	Components of nerve
Brachial	C5–T1	Radial	C5–C8
		Median	C6–T1
		Ulnar	C7–T1
		Axillary	C5–C6
		Musculocutaneous	C5–C7
Lumbosacral	L1–S4	Sciatic	L4–S2
		Tibial	L4–S2
		Common peroneal	L4–S1
		Femoral	L1–L4
		Obturator	L2–L4

Table 1.2 Derivation of the main peripheral nerves from the plexuses and their spinal nerves

Cranial nerves

The 12 pairs of cranial nerves carry sensory, motor and parasympathetic information. They are named in two ways (see pages 100–106 and **Table 1.36**):

■ according to the information that they carry, i.e. their major innervation; for example, the oculomotor nerve controls eye (ocular) movement (motor)
■ by Roman numerals, i.e. I–XII, according to their anatomical position from rostral to caudal

Cranial nerves are clinically important, because they pass through several areas of the brain and skull that are prone to damage, making the location of internal injury sites easily identifiable.

Protection of the central nervous system

Skeletal protection

The entire central nervous system is encased in bone: the brain and brainstem by the skull, and the spinal cord by the vertebral column. These strong 'boxes' isolate and protect the delicate neural tissue.

Meninges

Between the central nervous system and the bone that protects it are membranes called the meninges. These consist of three layers (see page 27 and **Figure 1.19**):

■ the pia mater
■ the arachnoid mater and
■ the dura mater

The meninges envelop the neural tissue and the cerebrospinal fluid that supports it, which circulates in the space between the pia mater and the arachnoid mater – the subarachnoid space (see page 29).

> **Damage to meningeal** tissue or its bony casing, for example as a result of meningeal inflammation or compression by a bony outgrowth of vertebral bone, can produce neurological disturbance.

The ventricular system

The ventricular system is a network of fluid-filled spaces in the central nervous system (**Figure 1.8**). The cerebrospinal fluid they contain passes from the fourth ventricle into the subarachnoid space between meningeal layers surrounding the brain and spinal cord. The fluid acts as a shock absorber, cushioning and thereby protecting the brain and spinal cord (see page 30). It also helps maintain physiological stability by removing waste products, and it facilitates communication

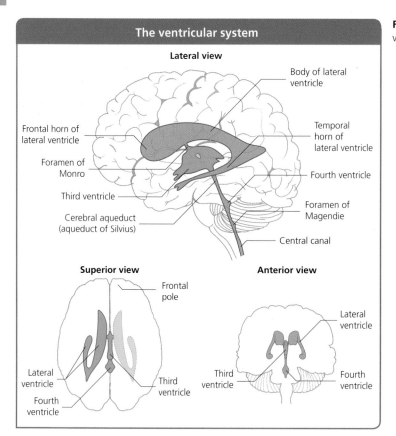

The ventricular system

Lateral view

Body of lateral ventricle

Frontal horn of lateral ventricle

Temporal horn of lateral ventricle

Foramen of Monro

Fourth ventricle

Third ventricle

Foramen of Magendie

Cerebral aqueduct (aqueduct of Silvius)

Central canal

Superior view

Frontal pole

Anterior view

Lateral ventricle

Lateral ventricle

Third ventricle

Third ventricle

Fourth ventricle

Fourth ventricle

Figure 1.8 The ventricular system.

by transporting substances such as neuro-modulators and hormones.

Vasculature of the nervous system

A complex network of blood vessels supplies the central nervous system. Maintenance of a constant supply of blood to all regions at all times is vital to keep the system working efficiently and even small changes in supply can cause potentially life-threatening failure of the nervous system.

Arterial supply

The two internal carotid arteries and two vertebral arteries supply blood to the brain (**Figure 1.9**). These are linked by the circle of Willis, a loop of anastomotic (communicating) vessels situated at the base of the brain (see **Figures 1.9** and **1.23**). All major cerebral arteries arise from the circle of Willis. The brainstem and cerebellar regions are also supplied by branches of the circle of Willis, as well as being supplied directly by the vertebral arteries.

The spinal cord is supplied by spinal arteries arising from the vertebral arteries. It also receives supply from arteries that arise from the aorta and follow the nerve root to radiate around each segment of the cord (see page 72).

Venous drainage

Blood leaves the brain via a complex system of major veins and sinuses, i.e. channels between the dura mater to reach the internal jugular veins (see **Figure 1.26** and page 37).

Venous drainage from the spinal cord is via Batson's plexus, a network of valveless veins in the epidural space, the space between the dura mater and the vertebral bones. These veins return blood to the systemic circulation.

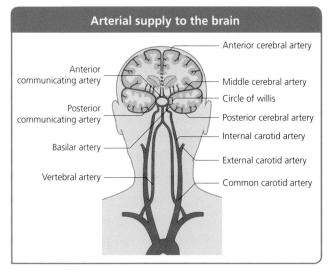

Arterial supply to the brain

- Anterior cerebral artery
- Anterior communicating artery
- Middle cerebral artery
- Circle of willis
- Posterior communicating artery
- Posterior cerebral artery
- Internal carotid artery
- Basilar artery
- External carotid artery
- Vertebral artery
- Common carotid artery

Figure 1.9 Arterial supply to the brain arises from the carotid arteries, supplying the brain's anterior circulation, and the vertebral arteries, supplying the brain's posterior circulation. The anterior and posterior circulations are linked by the circle of Willis; this is a loop of vessels from which all the main arteries supplying the cerebrum and brainstem arise.

Cells and signalling

Starter questions

Answers to the following questions are on page 115.

4. What is the language code of the nervous system?
5. Why are there so many different types of neurotransmitter?

Several types of neurone and glia (**Table 1.3**) have evolved to enable and support rapid and effective communication throughout the nervous system and the periphery to control both mind and body. Even small changes in the structure and function of these cells have a major impact on how the body works. Knowing which elements have changed, and how, may be crucial for determining the best therapeutic approach.

Structure of neurones and glia

Neurones

Neurones are classified by their structure and function. All types of neurone have the following features in common (**Figure 1.1**).

- A **cell body (soma)**: the metabolic hub of the cell
- **Dendrites**: processes that extend outwards from the cell body and receive signals from other cells
- An **axon**: a process that projects towards the target cell
- **Synapses**: junctions between a neurone and other cells (either neurones or other cell types). These enable communication between the two synapsing cells

Neurones are classified as either principal cells or interneurones, depending on their function. Many are also defined by their structure. For example, pyramidal cells in the cortex have triangular cell bodies, and basket cells have dendrites that form a basket shape around the cell body.

Principal cells

These are the neurones that communicate information throughout the nervous system. Principal cells are responsible for information acquisition (e.g. sensory input), integration (e.g. linking sensation to mood) and deposition (storage, e.g. memory formation).

Principal cells generally use glutamate as a neurotransmitter (see page 17). Glutamate excites target cells to rapidly propagate information.

Principal cells are classified into three types according to the number of inputs the cell body receives.

- **Multipolar neurones** have many dendrites and one axon entering the cell body, and are the most common type of cell in the central nervous system
- **Bipolar neurones** have two main processes and are located in specialised sensory organs (see page 107)
- **Unipolar neurones** have one process and are usually sensory cells, the cell bodies of which are grouped into ganglia

Interneurones

These are neurones that transmit information between other neurones. Using this definition, > 90% of neurones are 'interneurones'. However, in practice this term is reserved for the smaller interneurones in a specific region. These interneurones are generally inhibitory and use γ-aminobutyric acid (GABA) as a neurotransmitter.

Inhibitory interneuronal networks regulate patterns of activity in cortical areas. They do this by reducing the excitatory activity of principal cells flowing through the region.

Cells of the nervous system				
Cell type	Structure	Feature(s)	Function(s)	Location(s)
PRINCIPAL CELLS				
Multipolar neurone		Multiple processes on the cell body	Principal cell: communication	Principal and interneuronal cells in central nervous system
Bipolar neurone		Cell body with two principal processes	Principal cell: communication	Organs of special senses, for example retinal cells (in the eye) and olfactory cells (in the nose)
Unipolar neurone		Cell body with one process	Principal cell: communication	Often sensory cells
GLIA				
Astrocytes		Large and star-shaped, with multiple processes	Glial cell: structure, homeostasis and neurovascular communication	Ubiquitous, and the major glial cell in the central nervous system
Ependyma		Cuboid, ciliated epithelial cell	Glial cell: production and movement of cerebrospinal fluid	Lining the ventricular system
Microglia		Small, with multiple processes	Glial cell: immune response	Anywhere (triggered by trauma)
Oligodendroglia		Large, with broad processes	Glial cell: structure, providing myelin for axons	Central nervous system
Schwann cells		Large, with broad processes	Glial cell: structure, providing myelin for axons, and homeostasis	Peripheral nervous system

Table 1.3 Cells of the nervous system

Glia

Glial ('glue') cells have pivotal roles in the control of neuronal growth, as well as in the regeneration of damaged tissue, by providing structural and chemical signals to direct and orient growth. Most primary tumours of the brain are formed by glia, which makes these cells of particular interest clinically. There are five types of glia (see **Table 1.3**).

- Astrocytes
- Ependymal cells
- Microglia
- Oligodendroglia
- Schwann cells

Astrocytes

These are star-shaped cells that form a bridging layer between neurones and blood vessels. One of their vital roles is maintenance of the blood–brain barrier, a structural barrier that isolates and protects the brain from the rest of the body (see page 32). Astrocytes also modulate neuronal transmission through endocytosis (internalisation) of substances released by, or in the vicinity of, the neurone.

Ependymal cells

These are simple, ciliated, cuboid cells that form the sheets of membrane lining the ventricular system. They produce and transport cerebrospinal fluid (see page 31). A subgroup of ependymal cells, tanycytes, also transport substances between the cerebrospinal fluid and the blood and neural tissue.

Microglia

These are small glia that are activated by trauma. They are the central nervous system version of macrophages; they function as part of the immune response. Microglia are rapidly activated by insults to the nervous system that cause inflammation, including trauma, infections and neurodegenerative disorders. Once activated, they remove foreign material and cellular debris through phagocytosis (ingestion).

Oligodendroglia, Schwann cells and the myelin sheath

These cells produce the myelin sheath that forms a protective covering for the axons of neurones around axons (**Figure 1.10**). The sheath is a fatty coating that acts like insulation on an electrical wire, which is essential for the movement of signals along axons (see page 16), improving the accuracy and rate of axonal conduction and synaptic transmission along the axon. An axon with myelin covering is known as a fibre.

Oligodendroglia produce the myelin around the axons of the central nervous system. Schwann cells produce myelin for axons in the peripheral nervous system.

To form the myelin sheath, oligodendroglia wrap somal projections called foot processes around the axon. In contrast, peripheral myelin is formed when whole Schwann cells wrap around the axon.

Nervous system tumours are named according to the type of glial cell from which they originate.

- ■ Astrocytomas are growths of astrocytes and can develop throughout the central nervous system
- ■ Ependymomas are formed by ependymal cells and are located in the ventricular system
- ■ Schwannomas form in the peripheral nervous system and impinge on peripheral nerves

---

Repair and regeneration

As a general rule neogenesis, the production of new cells, is limited to a few regions of the brain, occurring primarily in the limbic system and temporal lobes (see page 45). In most of the nervous system, damaged neuronal tissue is unlikely to repair itself except when:

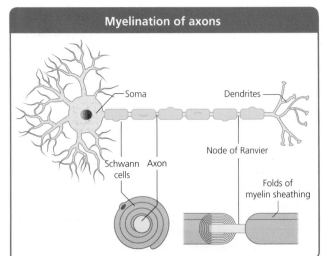

Myelination of axons

Soma

Dendrites

Node of Ranvier

Schwann cells

Axon

Folds of myelin sheathing

Figure 1.10 Myelination of axons. The nodes of Ranvier are unmyelinated regions between Schwann cells; their existence is vital to the rapid transmission of signals along the axon (see page 16).

- the amount of local damage is not extensive
- the cell body remains intact despite the damage
- viable glia are present (Schwann cells in the peripheral nervous system, or oligo-dendroglia in the central nervous system), which provide chemical and structural cues to guide regrowth
- electrical guidance cues from surrounding tissue are present

Communication by neurones

Rapid communication along and between neurones is achieved by action potentials. An action potential is a transient change in electrical charge within the cell; it occurs when the neurone is activated ('fires'). The pattern of action potentials encodes the information transmitted by neurones, in a similar way to Morse code.

The action potential

Differences in the concentration of sodium ions (Na^+) and potassium ions (K^+) on the inside and outside of a neurone result in an electrical charge or potential across its membrane, the membrane potential. Rapid changes in this charge generate an action potential (**Figure 1.11**). The action potential travels along the cell membrane, just like electricity passing through a cable, to the synapse. At the synapse, the action potential is transmitted to the next neurone in the pathway.

Generation of an action potential requires a sequence of changes in the membrane potential of the neurone.

Resting potential

At rest, the membrane potential is held at a set voltage: typically 70 mV. The value for the resting potential is negative because differences in the intracellular and extracellular concentrations of K^+ and Na^+ ions mean that the inside of the cell has a negative charge compared with the outside of the cell, i.e. the membrane is hyperpolarised.

The resting potential is maintained by constant movement of ions across the membrane through ion channels (see page 19). This movement is driven by electrical potential and differences in chemical concentration across the membrane (the ionic gradient). The concentration of K^+ is higher inside the cell than outside the cell; conversely, Na^+ concentration is higher outside the cell than inside it.

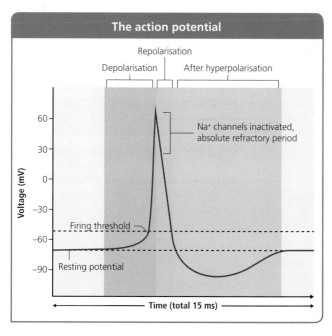

The action potential

Repolarisation

Depolarisation | After hyperpolarisation

Na^+ channels inactivated, absolute refractory period

Firing threshold

Resting potential

Voltage (mV): 60, 30, 0, −30, −60, −90

Time (total 15 ms)

Figure 1.11 Depolarisation is caused primarily by an influx of Na^+ ions through Na^+ channels. An action potential is generated at the firing threshold, which triggers the opening of all Na^+ channels and a surge in Na^+ influx, resulting in a rapid upswing in membrane potential. Underlying repolarisation is the inactivation of Na^+ channels, preventing further Na^+ influx, as well as K^+ efflux through activated K^+ channels. The absolute refractory period is the period during which it is not possible to generate another action potential. After hyperpolarisation there is a brief decrease in membrane potential past the resting potential as a consequence of K^+ efflux, before the original concentration gradients for Na^+ and K^+ ions, and therefore the resting potential, are restored.

The movement of K$^+$ and Na$^+$ down their concentration gradients depends on membrane permeability. The membrane is more permeable to K$^+$ ions than to Na$^+$ ions. The concentration gradient for K$^+$ drives 'leakage' of K$^+$ ions from the cell, but this efflux is balanced by the import of K$^+$ ions. The relative impermeability of the membrane to Na$^+$ ions means they remain outside the cell, and are unable to move down their concentration gradient.

Depolarisation

When a stimulus from another neurone or another point on the membrane of the neurone causes K$^+$ efflux to increase, the membrane potential becomes less negative, i.e it depolarises. This depolarisation causes voltage-sensitive Na$^+$ channels to open. The subsequent movement of Na$^+$ ions into the cell triggers the opening of more Na$^+$ channels until the net influx of Na$^+$ is greater than the efflux of K$^+$.

Firing of an action potential

An action potential is fired when the membrane potential reaches a certain voltage: the firing threshold. The firing threshold acts like the sound of the starter gun at a race; it triggers the rapid opening of all Na$^+$ channels. This causes an inward surge of Na$^+$ ions, which is responsible for the firing element (spike) of the action potential. The size and duration of this spike depends on the number of Na$^+$ channels present and the length of time they are open.

The open Na$^+$ channels then begin a brief period of inactivation, during which they are open but ion movement is blocked. The channels then close completely.

Many drugs alter neuronal activity by opening and closing ion channels directly, but some act indirectly. Benzodiazepines, including diazepam, work with GABA to enhance the GABA channel activity. However, these drugs have no effect on channel activity if GABA is not present.

Repolarisation

As the Na$^+$ channels close, K$^+$ efflux continues and the cell begins to repolarise. As the cell reaches resting membrane potential, rectifying channels enable the influx of K$^+$ ions to restore the original ionic gradient and the resting membrane potential.

Refractory period

During repolarisation, there is a refractory period when most Na$^+$ channels are inactivated and K$^+$ efflux is greatest, making it impossible to trigger another action potential. This limits the firing ability of the neurone to protect it from overactivation and death.

After hyperpolarisation

Some K$^+$ channels remain open past the point at which resting membrane potential is reached. The K$^+$ movement through these channels results in a brief period of hyperpolarisation before the ionic movement normalises and resting potential is fully restored.

Propagation of the action potential

Generation of an action potential across one section of an axonal membrane alters the ionic gradient in the adjacent section. This triggers the opening of voltage-gated Na$^+$ channels in the adjacent section, which depolarises in consequence. This process continues along the axon, propagating the impulse (the action potential) throughout the neurone.

Rapid transmission is enhanced by the structure of the myelin sheath (see page 17). The axon has multiple small myelin-free sections, nodes of Ranvier, along its length; these are the spaces between myelinating glial cells. Na$^+$ influx at one node of Ranvier triggers Na$^+$ influx at the next, with current 'jumping' between the nodes. This type of conduction is termed saltatory (Latin: saltare, 'to leap'), and it increases the speed at which the action potential travels along the axon (**Figure 1.12**).

The action potential reaches the terminal end of the axon, where it triggers the release of either a chemical or an ionic signal that crosses the synapse and triggers an action potential in the next neurone, as described below. In this way, signals cross the synapse and transmission of information continues.

Prolonged depolarisation of cortical neurones can trigger spreading depression, a transient wave of inactivity that spreads outwards across the cortex. These waves can occur spontaneously and are associated with problems such as migraine and trauma.

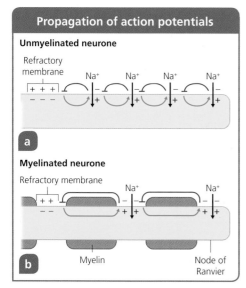

Propagation of action potentials

Unmyelinated neurone

Refractory membrane

a

Myelinated neurone

Refractory membrane

Myelin   Node of Ranvier

b

Figure 1.12 In the axon of an unmyelinated neurone (a) generation of an action potential (AP) across one region of membrane triggers opening of voltage-gated Na+ channels in the adjacent region, which depolarises and thus triggers opening of Na+ channels in the next region, and so on. Thus the AP travels like a wave down the axon. Because myelin is an electrical insulator, in the axon of a myelinated neurone (b) depolarisation is restricted to the unmyelinated regions – the nodes of Ranvier. Na+ influx at one node creates an electrical current along the length of myelinated axon between it and the next node almost instantaneously; hence conduction of the AP is far faster than it would be via the several cycles of channel opening and depolarisation that would be required to travel the same length of unmyelinated axon. This saltatory conduction is about six times faster than conduction in unmyelinated axons. In both types of conduction, the AP cannot travel backwards, because rearward areas of the membrane are in the refractory period.

Chemical and electrical synaptic transmission

Cell–cell communication occurs at the synapse between the presynaptic neurone and the postsynaptic neurone. There are two forms of synapse: chemical and electrical (**Figure 1.13**). A network of neurones consists of neurones linked by synapses of one or both forms.

Chemical communication

At chemical synapses, neurotransmitters and neuromodulators (see page 19) are released from the presynaptic terminal. These substances bind to receptors on the postsynaptic terminal to initiate ionic movement and generate an action potential.

> **Synaptic plasticity is the ability of synapses to alter the way they respond to stimulation.** This is key for learning and the formation of memories. It allows neurones to produce enhanced or reduced responses to similar stimuli. The hippocampus, a key region for learning and memory, has high levels of plasticity (see page 47).

Neurotransmitters

Neurotransmitters are produced by neurones for cell-to-cell communication, to transmit a signal from one cell to the next. They are stored in vesicles in the presynaptic terminal and released when the terminal is depolarised during an action potential. Neurotransmitter diffuses across the synaptic cleft to activate receptors on the postsynaptic terminal. Activation of these receptors generates an action potential, activates intracellular signalling cascades or does both in the postsynaptic cell. Intracellular signalling cascades are biochemical pathways that control cellular function and structure.

Types of neurotransmitter

A wide range of small molecules act as neurotransmitters and neuromodulators. These include amino acids, peptides and gases (**Table 1.4**).

- In the central nervous system, the major excitatory neurotransmitter is glutamate and the major inhibitory neurotransmitter is GABA. Neurones using glutamate as a transmitter are glutamatergic; those using GABA are GABAergic.
- In the peripheral nervous system, the major neurotransmitters are acetylcholine (in cholinergic neurones), for both somatic and autonomic transmission, and noradrenaline (norepinephrine, in adrenergic neurones), for autonomic transmission only (see page 95)

Imbalances of specific neurotransmitters are associated with many different disorders (**Table 1.5**).

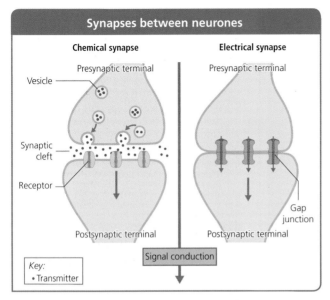

Figure 1.13 Synapses between neurones. At a chemical synapse, neurotransmitters carry a signal across the cleft. At an electrical synapse, gap junctions allow charge to pass from one cell to the next.

Production and metabolism of neurotransmitters

Many neurotransmitters are by-products of metabolic pathways. For example, glutamate (glutamic acid) is a by-product of the citric acid cycle (the tricarboxylic acid cycle or Krebs). Some neurotransmitters share a chemical precursor. For example, adrenaline (epinephrine) is a breakdown product of noradrenaline (norepinephrine), which is itself a metabolite of dopamine.

Neurotransmitter–receptor interactions

Each neurotransmitter binds selectively to specific receptors. These are named according to the neurotransmitter for which they have most affinity, for example 'glutamate receptors' and 'GABA receptors'.

Receptors for a specific neurotransmitter may be divided into structurally and functionally different subtypes. For example, there are two subtypes of acetylcholine receptor: muscarinic receptors and nicotinic receptors. They are particularly responsive to muscarine and nicotine, respectively.

The effect of a neurotransmitter depends on the receptors available for it to bind to (see page 19). For example, dopamine has excitatory or inhibitory effects depending on the type of dopamine receptor expressed on the neurone: D_1 or D_2, respectively.

Therapeutically, using the precursor of a neurotransmitter, instead of the neurotransmitter itself, often bypasses problems of drug metabolism and accessibility. For example, dopamine reverses the symptoms of Parkinson's disease, but it does not cross the blood–brain barrier and is rapidly metabolised. In contrast, the dopamine precursor levodopa crosses the blood–brain barrier and is then metabolised to dopamine and reaches the target site.

Neurotransmitter–pathway interactions

The complexity of networks often means that changes in the levels of one neurotransmitter affect the levels of another. For example, the release of noradrenaline (norepinephrine) affects the way that serotonin-containing cells fire because these cells often express receptors for noradrenaline. Receptors for a specific neurotransmitter may be divided into structurally and functionally different subtypes. For example, there are two subtypes of acetylcholine receptor: muscarinic receptors and nicotinic receptors. They are particularly responsive to muscarine and nicotine, respectively.

Similar interactions occur between serotonin, dopamine and acetylcholine pathways.

This means that drugs affecting one of these neurotransmitters has effects both up- and downstream of the desired target.

Neuromodulators

Neuromodulators (see **Table 1.4**) are substances that change neuronal activity indirectly, without altering neurotransmitter–receptor binding. Clinically, they are used to produce more subtle changes in neurotransmission than those achieved with the use of neurotransmitters, or their precursors, as drugs.

Neuromodulators are often found in vesicles, colocalised with the main neurotransmitter. They generally act via G-protein–coupled receptors (see page 20) to adjust receptor sensitivity to neurotransmitters.

Receptors

Receptors for neurotransmitter are classified into two types (**Figure 1.14**).
- **Ionotropic receptors** facilitate the movement of ions
- **G-protein–coupled receptors** use G-proteins to activate intracellular signalling cascades

Both are activated by binding of a neurotransmitter or neuromodulator.

Receptor activation

The activation of ionotropic receptors opens ion channels. In contrast, activated G-protein–coupled receptors trigger cellular signalling cascades that modulate cellular activity.

N-methyl-D-aspartate (NMDA) receptors are ionotropic. Activation of NMDA receptors

Principal neurotransmitters and neuromodulators	
Substance	Main roles
NEUROTRANSMITTERS	
Glutamate	Excitatory
GABA	Inhibitory
Aspartate	Excitatory
Glycine	Inhibitory
Acetylcholine	Signal transmission at neuromuscular junctions
Adrenaline (epinephrine)	Stress and arousal
Noradrenaline (norepinephrine)	Stress and arousal
Dopamine	Motivation and motor function
Serotonin	Homeostasis arousal and mood
Histamine	Arousal
NEUROMODULATORS	
Neuropeptide Y	Appetite
Substance P	Pain
Vasopressin	Osmoregulation
Somatostatin	Growth
Anandamide	Pain and arousal
OTHERS	
Nitric oxide	Modulation (not found in vesicles)
Carbon dioxide	
Adenosine	
Adenosine triphosphate	
GABA, γ-aminobutyric acid.	

Table 1.4 Principal neurotransmitters and neuromodulators

Common disorders associated with neurotransmitter imbalance		
Disorder type	Disorder	Neurotransmitter imbalance
Motor	Parkinson's disease	Decreased dopamine production
	Huntington's disease	Decreased GABA and acetylcholine levels
	Myasthenia gravis	Decreased acetylcholine receptivity
Sensory	Migraine	Increased serotonin levels
	Fibromyalgia	Increased substance P or serotonin levels
Cognitive	Alzheimer's disease	Reduced acetylcholine production
	Schizophrenia	Increased dopamine production
	Depression	Reduced serotonin or noradrenaline (norepinephrine) levels
	Epilepsy	Decreased GABA levels
GABA, γ-aminobutyric acid.		

Table 1.5 Common disorders associated with imbalance of specific types of neurotransmitter

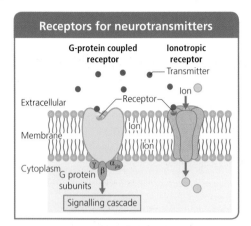

Receptors for neurotransmitters

Figure 1.14 The two types of receptors in the nervous system.

by glutamate opens channels for cations (Na⁺ ions and calcium ions, Ca^{2+}). Activation of ionotropic receptors tends to be rapid and short-lasting. However, it may trigger longer-term changes because Ca^{2+} influx activates intracellular signalling cascades.

Metabotropic glutamate receptors are G-protein–coupled receptors. Their activation triggers intracellular signalling cascades using second messengers such as cyclic AMP and adenylate cyclase to regulate channel opening, gene transcription and gene expression. These receptors have slower effects on neuronal activity because of the nature of the cascades.

> Changes in the function of ionotropic and G-protein–coupled receptors are associated with some genetic and autoimmune disorders. Some genetic mutations, such as those that cause neonatal epilepsies, change the structure of ionotropic receptors, thereby altering ion channel function and preventing normal transmission. In the autoimmune disorder myasthenia gravis, antibodies develop that bind to acetylcholine receptors, thereby preventing normal transmission.

Receptor specificity

Like neurotransmitters, many drugs act at specific receptors. Knowledge of how each neurotransmitter and drug acts at the receptor enables physicians to understand why and how these drugs exert their beneficial and adverse effects. A drug may act as an agonist or antagonist at a specific receptor, and accordingly excite or inhibit the receptor. For example, triptans relieve the symptoms of migraine by acting as agonists at serotonin receptors. They specifically target 5-HT$_{1B}$ and 5-HT$_{1D}$ serotonin receptors, which are present on cranial blood vessels. Activation of these receptors causes the vessels to narrow, thereby reversing the vasodilation that occurs during a migraine headache.

Electrical communication

The two neurones sharing an electrical synapse are in direct physical contact; unlike neurones at a chemical synapse, they are not separated by a synaptic cleft (see **Figure 1.13**). Ions and other small molecules pass through specialised pores in the adjacent neuronal membranes. The passive movement of ions through these gap junctions transmits electrical signal from the presynaptic to the postsynaptic cell. Alone, this signal is usually insufficient to generate an action potential in the postsynaptic cell, but it can increase the likelihood of generation of an action potential. In this way, electrical synapses enable adjacent cells to coordinate and synchronise their activity.

Neuronal activity patterning and synchrony

Neurones carry information in a similar way to Morse code: patterns of activity convey the message. The synchronous firing of a group of interconnected neurones creates a strong signal that can be transmitted effectively over long distances making communication more reliable.

Disruption of neuronal activity patterning is common in many disorders. For example, epilepsy is linked to a breakdown in synchrony, which allows larger numbers of neurones to fire rapidly and randomly. Migraine is associated with vasospasm in blood vessels, which is caused by a breakdown in coordination of the sympathetic activity controlling the smooth muscles of the vasculature.

Development of the nervous system

Starter questions

Answers to the following questions are on page 116.

6. Why do some brain regions maintain the ability to produce new cells and change their structure?
7. How does the brain know when to stop folding?

Development of the nervous system starts 3 weeks after conception and continues throughout gestation and beyond. It was thought that in adulthood once the nervous system was formed, no new neurones could be produced. However, it is now known that new neurones are produced in certain regions of the brain throughout life.

Development: gastrulation to neurulation

Development of the central nervous system begins with gastrulation, a period of rapid growth, multiplication and differentiation of cells. Gastrulation is followed by neurulation, the formation of the closed neural tube, which occurs in the fourth week.

Development of the dermal layers

Gastrulation produces the three main cellular layers that form in the embryo by day 16 after conception (**Figure 1.15**). Each of these dermal layers has a different destiny:

- The **endoderm** forms most of the viscera
- The **mesoderm** forms the vascular system, musculature and connective tissue
- The **ectoderm** forms the nervous system

Formation of the neural tube

Neurulation is the formation of the neural tube, which is the precursor of the entire central nervous system. This process is the thickening and infolding of the ectodermal tissue, which lies above the notochord, a rod-like

formation of mesoderm that secretes factors that determine the fate and position of surrounding tissue.

The thickened ectoderm first forms the neural plate, a flat, pear-shaped structure. Its wider end becomes the cranial tissue. As the plate develops, a groove appears along its midline. As the tissue expands and broadens, it folds inwards along the groove to create the neural tube (see Day 24, **Figure 1.15**).

Mesoderm located on either side of the neural tube expands to form somites, the precursors to bones, including the skull and vertebral column, as well as the musculature that at this stage surrounds the nervous system. The musculature receives its innervation from cells of the neural crest.

The neural crests

As the neural plate folds inwards to create the neural tube, the tops of the two folds, the neural crests, are also internalised. Cells from each crest migrate laterally to lie either side of the tube.

Neural crest cells differentiate into the various cell types of the peripheral nervous system, including:

- unipolar neurones of the sensory system
- sympathetic neurones
- Schwann (neurolemmal) cells

Closure of the neural tube

The neural tube fuses dorsally along its length, starting in the middle and extending cranially and caudally. The tube openings, the anterior (cranial) and posterior (caudal) neuropores, are in contact with the amniotic

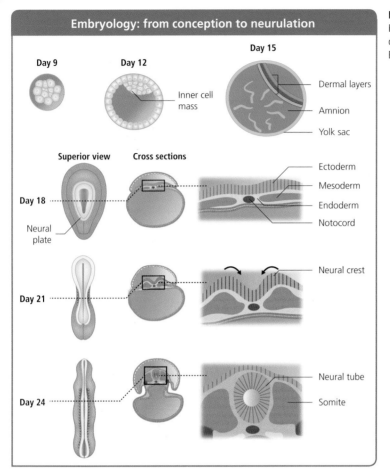

Figure 1.15
Embryological development from Day 9 to neurulation.

fluid until they close. Closure of the neuropores isolates the neural tube from the exterior. The anterior neuropore closes around day 26, the posterior neuropore around day 28. Common defects in neuropore closure are shown in **Table 1.6**.

> **Neural tube defects are among the most common birth defects, affecting about 1 in 1000 conceptions.** They are associated with insufficient maternal levels of folate, which is required for new cell growth and for DNA and RNA synthesis. Neural tube defects occur when one or both neuropores fail to close. Defects are classified as 'open', if the neural tissue is exposed to the exterior, or 'closed', if it is covered by skin and fatty deposits.

Development of the brainstem, midbrain and cerebral hemispheres

Cellular proliferation at the cranial end of the neural tube leads to further growth and the formation of three distinct portions (**Table 1.7** and **Figure 1.16**):

■ prosencephalon (forebrain)
■ mesencephalon (midbrain)
■ rhombencephalon (hindbrain)

As these structures expand, they start to fold in certain locations. These folds are called flexures.

■ The cervical flexure marks the division between spinal cord and brainstem

	Common neural tube defects		
Condition	Neuropore(s) affected and clinical deficit	Deficiency	
Spina bifida occulta	Posterior neuropore Missing vertebral arch		
Meningomyelocele	Posterior neuropore Extrusion of meninges and spinal cord		
Meningocele	Posterior or anterior neuropore Extrusion of meninges		
Myelocele	Posterior and anterior neuropores		
Meningoencephalocele	Anterior neuropore Extrusion of brain and meninges through skull		
Anencephaly	Anterior neuropore No formation of skull vault or brain		

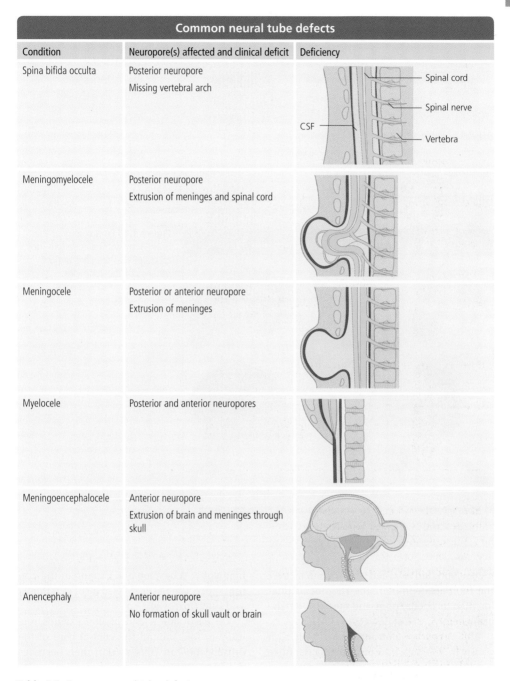

Table 1.6 Common neural tube defects

- The mesencephalic flexure marks the transition from midbrain to cerebrum

The delineation of regions of the nervous system occurs early in development, as they arise from the elongation and enlargement of the neural tube.

Development of the brainstem and cerebellum

Further expansion and folding of the rhombencephalon produces the pontine flexure. As this fold deepens, a lip of tissue called the

Regions of the nervous system			
General	Embryo	Region	Adult
Forebrain (prosencephalon)	Telencephalon	Cerebrum	Cerebral hemispheres
	Diencephalon	Diencephalon	Thalamus and hypothalamus
Midbrain (mesencephalon)	Mesencephalon	Brainstem	Midbrain
Hindbrain (rhombencephalon)	Metencephalon		Pons and cerebellum
	Myelencephalon		Medulla
Spinal cord	Spinal cord	Spinal cord	Spinal cord

Table 1.7 Development of different regions of the nervous system

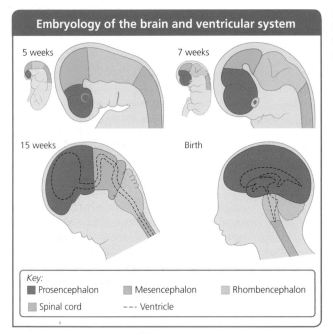

Figure 1.16 Embryology of the brain and ventricular system (not to scale). Dashed lines are the outlines of the ventricles.

metencephalon is forced outwards to lie over the rhombencephalon. The rhombencephalon then forms the pons and medulla, i.e. the brainstem.

The metencephalon folds repeatedly as it grows. In this way, it forms the folia (leaf-like structure) of the cerebellum.

Development of the cerebrum

During expansion, the prosencephalon forms two large lateral protrusions: the telencephalon. These expand upwards and laterally to produce the two cerebral hemispheres. As the hemispheres develop and expand in the cranial space, the tissue folds to form gyri (folds) and sulci (furrows).

On each side telencephalon extends rostrally to fold around the central core of the prosencephalon. This section then becomes the diencephalon.

Development of the ventricular system

As the brain develops its lobular shape, the cranial end of the neural tube grows and expands to form interconnected fluid-filled spaces which become the ventricular system:

- The caudal end of the neural tube becomes the central canal of the spinal cord (**Figure 1.16**)
- The telencephalon spaces form the lateral ventricles
- The diencephalon space forms the third ventricle
- The gap between the rhombencephalon and the metencephalon forms the fourth ventricle

Development of the spinal cord

The caudal end of the neural tube remains small in diameter. It elongates to form the spinal cord.

> **In lumbar puncture,** a needle and syringe are used to extract cerebrospinal fluid from the subarachnoid space around the spinal cord. In adults, it is carried out at the L3–L4 or L4–L5 level to avoid damaging the spinal cord; the spinal nerves forming the cauda equina (horse's tail) move out of the way of the incoming needle. In children, lumbar puncture must be done at L4–L5 or below.

In the early stages of development, the growth rate of the cord parallels that of the vertebral column, as shown in **Figure 1.17**.

However, towards the end of the 2nd month the growth of the vertebral column starts to accelerate, leading to disparity between the length of the cord and that of the vertebral column. At birth, the spinal cord terminates at vertebral level L3 (the third lumbar level). By adulthood, the spinal cord ends at about the L1–2 level.

Myelination and development

Schwann cells, which are derived from neurolemmal neural crest cells, provide the myelin coating on peripheral neurones by wrapping around their axons (see **Figure 1.10**; see page 14).

Myelination of nerves begins about 6 months into fetal development. The descending pathways controlling motor function are among the last to become fully myelinated; myelination of these nerves takes up to 2 years after birth. During this period, a child is unable to exert conscious control over the spinal reflex pathways that are already developed in the spinal cord, for example those involved in limb movement and bladder function (see page 91). As a result, the reflexes occur spontaneously and are uninhibited; this is why babies kick their legs as if running when lifted, and cannot control their bladders. As myelination progresses, the child slowly gains control of these behaviours.

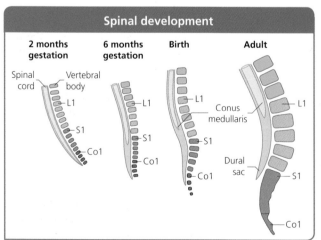

Figure 1.17 Development of the spine, spinal cord and vertebral column.

Spinal development

2 months gestation · 6 months gestation · Birth · Adult

Spinal cord · Vertebral body · L1 · S1 · Co1 · L1 · S1 · Co1 · L1 · Conus medullaris · S1 · Co1 · Dural sac · L1 · S1 · Co1

The environment of the brain

Starter questions

Answers to the following questions are on page 116.

8. Is the skull always a rigid, fixed box?
9. Do we really need meninges?

Protection of the brain and maintenance of the environment surrounding it are vital for life.

The skull

The skull houses and protects the brain and organs of the head. It lies underneath the skin and subcutaneous layers of the scalp, and comprises the cranium (calvaria) and bones of the face. The brain housed within a large cavity formed by the bones of the cranium and the base of the skull, which form the vault and floor of the cavity, respectively.

> Skull fractures are first described as 'cranial' or 'base of skull', and then according to the degree of bone displacement. For example, in linear fractures the full thickness of the bone is broken but it is immobile. In contrast, in depressed fractures the bone is shifted inwards, potentially damaging the underlying tissue.

The cranium

The superior aspect of the cranium comprises four large plates of bone:

- the frontal bone
- two parietal bones
- the occipital bone

There are three sutures (specialised joints) between these bones.

- The coronal suture between the frontal and parietal bones
- The sagittal suture between the two parietal bones

- The lambdoid suture between the parietal bones and the occipital bone

The front part of the skull includes the orbital bones comprising the eye sockets, the nasal bone, and the maxilla and mandible, i.e. the upper and lower jawbones, respectively. On either side of the skull is a temporal bone. Each temporal bone is fused along the squamous suture to the ipsilateral parietal bone, i.e. the parietal bone on the same side. It is also fused with the occipital bone and the ipsilateral greater wing of the sphenoid bone and zygomatic bone (cheekbone). The external auditory meatus forms the ear canal.

> The pterion is an 'H' shape marking the junction between the frontal, parietal, temporal and sphenoid bones. It is a weak point in the skull. The anterior middle meningeal arteries, which supplies the dura mater, lies underneath the pterion and is often ruptured when it is damaged. The result is an extradural haemorrhage (see page 200).

Foramina

There are many foramina (openings) in the skull base, allowing the passage of blood vessels and nerves. The largest is the foramen magnum, through which the brainstem passes, becoming the spinal cord as it exits (**Table 1.8** and **Figure 1.18**; for other foramina, see **Figure 1.59**).

Fossae

The inner surface of the skull base is divided into three pairs of compartments, the fossae (singular, fossa) (**Figure 1.15**). The anterior

Skull foramina	
Locations and foramina	**Contents**
ANTERIOR FOSSA	
Cribriform plate	CN I
Optic canal	CN II
	Ophthalmic artery
MIDDLE FOSSA	
Superior orbital fissure	CN III
	CN IV
	CN V$_1$
	CN VI
	Ophthalmic vein
	Sympathetic fibres
Foramen rotundum	CN V2
Foramen ovale	CN V3
	Accessory meningeal artery
Foramen spinosum	Middle meningeal artery
Foramen lacerum (connects to carotid foramen)	Internal carotid artery
	Pterygoid artery
POSTERIOR FOSSA	
Internal auditory meatus [connects to external auditory meatus (CN VIII) and stylomastoid foramen (CN VII and stylomastoid artery)]	CN VII
	CN VIII
	Labyrinthine artery
Jugular foramen	CN IX
	CN X
	CN XI
	Internal jugular vein
	Inferior petrosal sinus
	Sigmoid sinus
Hypoglossal foramen	CN XII
Foramen magnum	Medulla
	CN XI (ascending)
	Anterior and posterior spinal arteries
	Vertebral arteries
	Venous plexus of vertebral canal
CN, cranial nerve.	

Table 1.8 Skull foramina (openings)

fossae hold the frontal lobes of the brain and the middle fossae hold the temporal lobes. The cerebellum rests in the posterior fossae.

Meninges

Three layers of membranous tissue, the meninges, surround the brain and spinal cord (**Figure 1.19**):

- the **dura mater** ('tough mother')
- the **arachnoid mater** ('spider-like mother')
- the **pia mater** ('tender mother')

The principal function of the meninges is to protect the brain and spinal cord.

The dura mater is the outermost layer; it adheres to the interior wall of the skull. The dura mater has two tough, inflexible layers: the outer periosteal layer, next to the bone and the inner meningeal layer, next to the arachnoid mater. Dura mater at certain points forms folds called fibrous septa .

The arachnoid mater is the middle layer and adheres to the inside of the meningeal layer of the dura mater. It projects web-like fibres (arachnoid trabeculae) inwards to the pia mater. The resulting space between the arachnoid mater and pia mater, the subarachnoid space, contains the cerebral arteries, major veins and cerebrospinal fluid.

The pia mater is the innermost layer of tissue. This is a thin layer of epithelial cells adhering to the surface of the brain and following its contours closely.

Fibrous septa

The two layers of dura mater separate at specific sites to form the rigid fibrous septa between brain structures (**Figure 1.20**). The septa protect the brain by limiting its movement, including rotation, within the cranial cavity. They ease pressure on the cerebellum, midbrain and brainstem by lifting the cerebrum. The septa also act as a barrier to prevent the spread of infection. The gaps created by infolding of the meningeal layer of the dura mater form the major venous sinuses (see page 28).

The skull fossae and foramen magnum

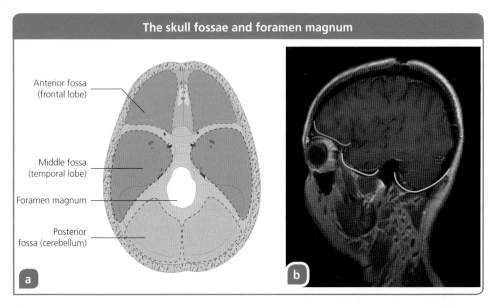

Anterior fossa
(frontal lobe)

Middle fossa
(temporal lobe)

Foramen magnum

Posterior
fossa (cerebellum)

a

b

Figure 1.18 The fossae and principle foramen of the skull.In part (b) a sagittal MRI shows the position of the lobes of the brain within the fossae: frontal lobe in the anterior cranial fossa (red line), temporal lobe in the middle cranial fossa (green line), cerebellum in the posterior cranial fossa (orange line).

Scalp, skull and meningeal layers protecting the brain

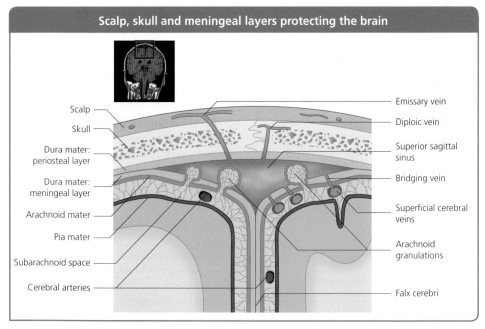

Scalp

Skull

Dura mater:
periosteal layer

Dura mater:
meningeal layer

Arachnoid mater

Pia mater

Subarachnoid space

Cerebral arteries

Emissary vein

Diploic vein

Superior sagittal
sinus

Bridging vein

Superficial cerebral
veins

Arachnoid
granulations

Falx cerebri

Figure 1.19 Protection of the brain: the scalp, skull and meningeal layers. Cerebrospinal fluid circulates within the subarachnoid space and, via arachnoid granulations, drains into the sinus, into which veins also drain from the brain, skull and scalp.

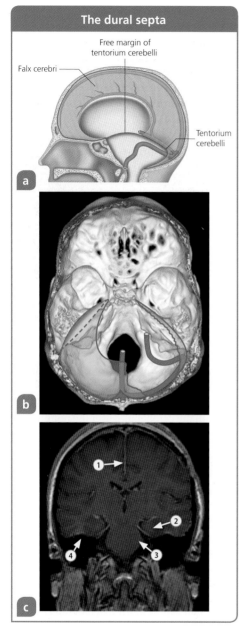

The dural septa

Free margin of
tentorium cerebelli

Falx cerebri

Tentorium
cerebelli

a

b

c

Figure 1.20 The dural septa. (a) Location of the falx cerebri and tentorium cerebelli within the skull. (b) (c) Coronal MRI showing the location of the septa and noting the position of the uncus and midbrain, two regions that can be involved in brain herniation. Note: the falx cerebelli ① which divides the cerebellum is not shown in part b. ② Uncus of temporal lobe. ③ Midbrain. ④ Tentorium cerebelli.

The three septa are the:

- falx cerebri
- tentorium cerebelli
- falx cerebelli

The falx cerebri separates the left and right cerebral hemispheres. It contains the superior and inferior sagittal sinuses (see page 37).

The tentorium cerebelli separates the cerebral hemispheres from the cerebellum and joins the falx cerebri at the posterior midline. The midbrain passes through a gap in the septum: the tentorial notch. The tentorium cerebelli contains the transverse, straight and superior petrosal sinuses.

The falx cerebelli separates the two hemispheres of the cerebellum and contains the occipital sinus.

When the pressure in the cranial vault (intracranial pressure) increases, parts of the brain may be forced around these septa. This effect is called herniation and damages and compresses vital brain structures (see page 192).

Meningeal spaces

Between and around the meningeal layers are true or potential spaces. A true meningeal space is visible in the absence of pathology. In contrast, a potential meningeal space becomes visible only when expanded by pathological conditions such as bleeding.

The three meningeal spaces are:

- **the subarachnoid space**, a true space between the arachnoid and pia mater, which contains cerebrospinal fluid and vasculature (see page 28)
- **the extradural space** (Latin, 'outside the dura'), the potential space between the bones of the cranial vault and the outer, periosteal layer of the dura mater
- **the subdural space**, the potential space between the inner, meningeal layer of the dura mater and the arachnoid mater

Termination of meninges

The periosteal layer of the dura mater is present only in the cranial cavity, whereas the meningeal layer extends through the foramen magnum to form the dura mater of the spinal cord. This means that the cord has only one dural layer, which terminates at the S2 vertebral level.

The arachnoid mater, like the dura mater, extends along the spinal cord. At the termination of the cord (L1–L2), the arachnoid membrane remains attached to the meningeal layer and extends to the S2 vertebral layer, creating a large subarachnoid space between L1 or L2 and S2: the lumbar cistern.

Beyond the termination of the dura mater, the pia mater continues as a single filamentous strand: the filum terminale. The pia mater eventually attaches to the last vertebra, the coccyx.

Cisterns

Cisterns are expanded subarachnoid spaces, filled with cerebrospinal fluid, where the arachnoid mater and pia mater are widely separated (**Figure 1.21**). The major cisterns are:

- **the lumbar cistern**, between L1 and S2, from which cerebrospinal fluid is extracted during a lumbar puncture
- **the cisterna magna**, also known as the cerebellomedullary cistern
- **the pontine cisterns**, comprising the prepontine and pontomedullary cisterns
- **the perimesencephalic cisterns**, comprising the interpeduncular, quadrigeminal and ambient cisterns

> **The size and position of the cisterns in radiological images of the brain and spinal cord are clinically informative.** Reduction in size or displacement of the cisterns indicates increased intracranial pressure.

The ventricular system

The ventricular system has its origins in the neural tube (see page 24) and comprises (**Figure 1.21**).

- The two lateral ventricles, which lie in the lobes of the cerebrum
- The third ventricle, which lies in the thalamic and hypothalamic area
- The fourth ventricle, which lies underneath the cerebellum, over the pons and medulla

These structures are connected by the following foramina:

- The interventricular foramen (foramen of Monro) connects the lateral ventricles with the third ventricle
- The cerebral aqueduct (of Sylvius) connects the third and fourth ventricles
- The median aperture (foramen of Magendie) connects the fourth ventricle to the central canal of the spinal cord
- The two lateral apertures (foramina of Luschka) connect the fourth ventricle to the subarachnoid spaces of the cisterna magna

The ventricles are lined with the choroid plexus, the highly vascularised tissue that produces cerebrospinal fluid (see page 31). The rest of the ventricular system is lined with ciliated ependymal cells (see page 14), which move the cerebrospinal fluid through the system.

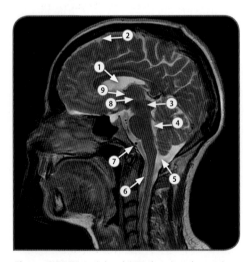

Figure 1.21 T2-weighted MRI showing the main features of the ventricular system and cisterns. Cerebrospinal fluid appears white in this scan. ① Body of lateral ventricle. ② Cerebrospinal fluid in cranial subarachnoid space. ③ Cerebral aqueduct. ④ Fourth ventricle. ⑤ Cisterna magna. ⑥ Spinal subarachnoid space. ⑦ Pontine cistern. ⑧ Third ventricle under diencephalon. ⑨ Foramen of Munro.

Cerebrospinal fluid

Cerebrospinal fluid is the fluid that fills the ventricular system and bathes the brain and spinal cord. It has multiple functions (**Table 1.9**), which contribute to maintenance of the optimal environment for central nervous system function. The constituents of cerebrospinal fluid are listed in **Table 1.10**.

> **Changes in the composition of the cerebrospinal fluid usually indicate pathology.** For example, in bacterial meningitis the cerebrospinal fluid can look yellow and cloudy, and its glucose concentration is lower and white blood cell count higher than in normal cerebrospinal fluid.

Production of cerebrospinal fluid

Cerebrospinal fluid is produced predominantly in the choroid plexus. The choroid plexus is a collection of frond-like villi (projections), which protrude into the cavities of the lateral, third and fourth ventricles. It is formed by infiltration of the local vasculature into the surrounding tissue and pia mater during development.

A small amount of cerebrospinal fluid is also produced by ventricular ependymal cells (glia; see page 14) and the pia mater.

As blood passes through the blood vessels in the choroid plexus, plasma leaks into the surrounding tissue. The plasma is then filtered through the choroid epithelial cells and exuded into the ventricle at a rate of about 20–25 mL/h. The filtrate contains a mix of salts, sugars and proteins, which help maintain homeostasis and support metabolism in the central nervous system. An adult has approximately 140 mL of cerebrospinal fluid in circulation: 40 mL in the ventricles, 25 mL in the cranial subarachnoid space and 75 mL in the spinal subarachnoid space.

Circulation of cerebrospinal fluid

Cerebrospinal fluid circulates through the lateral, third and fourth ventricles; the central canal of the spinal cord; and the cerebral and vertebral subarachnoid spaces. The ciliated ependymal cells work with the pulsatile movements generated by the cerebral vasculature to move the fluid throughout the system before it is reabsorbed.

Absorption of cerebrospinal fluid

Most cerebrospinal fluid is absorbed into the venous drainage via the arachnoid villi and arachnoid granulations (see **Figure 1.19**). Arachnoid villi are thickened out-pouchings of arachnoid membrane, which protrude through the inner meningeal layer of dura mater to enter the venous drainage. Arachnoid granulations are clusters of arachnoid villi.

Absorption is passive and depends on the gradient between the pressure in the skull and vertebral column and the pressure of venous blood in the sinuses. A very small proportion of cerebrospinal fluid is absorbed by the lymphatic system via lymph nodes.

Functions of cerebrospinal fluid	
Function	Benefit
Shock absorption and cushioning	Separates brain and spinal cord from bony structures (skull, vertebral column)
	Dissipates force of trauma
Buoyancy	Supports brain, reducing its effective weight (from 1500 g in air to 50 g in cerebrospinal fluid)
Homeostasis	Maintains stable ionic environment (e.g. acid–base balance)
Communication	Carries neurotransmitters and hormones around CNS
Nutrition	Transports vital nutrients around CNS
Excretion	Removes waste products

Table 1.9 Functions of cerebrospinal fluid

Composition of cerebrospinal fluid					
Profile	Normal value or range	Bacterial meningitis	Viral meningitis	Haemorrhage	Multiple sclerosis
Volume (mL)	125–150	–	–	–	–
Rate mL/h	20	–	–	–	–
Appearance	Clear and colourless	Cloudy and turbid	–	Red and cloudy	–
pH	7.28–7.32	–	–	–	–
Pressure (mmHg)	7–15	↑	↑	↑	–
Red blood cell concentration	0	–	·	↑	·
White blood cell concentration cells/mm^3	< 5	↑	↑	↑	·
Glucose (CSF:serum ratio)	≥ 60%	↓	·	↓	·
Protein (g/L)	0.2–0.4	↑	↑	–	–
Lactate ((mmol/L)	< 2.8	↑	–	↑	–
Bacterial DNA	Absent	Present	–	–	–
Viral DNA	Absent	–	Present	–	–
Antibodies	Absent	Present	Present	–	Present
Oligoclonal bands	Absent	–	–	–	Present

–, normal value; ↑, increased; ↓, decreased.

Table 1.10 Composition of cerebrospinal fluid, and changes associated with common disorders

Hydrocephalus ('water on the brain'; see page 204) results from accumulation of cerebrospinal fluid.

- Non-communicating hydrocephalus occurs when the flow of cerebrospinal fluid is blocked, for example by a tumour compressing the interventricular foramen
- Communicating hydrocephalus develops through overproduction of cerebrospinal fluid or prevention of its reabsorption, for example when exudate blocks the arachnoid villi and granulations in cases of bacterial meningitis

The blood–brain barrier

The blood–brain barrier is a 'wall' formed between the blood vessels and the brain parenchyma (the tissue of the brain) (**Figure 1.22**). It is essential for maintaining the integrity of the nervous system and has two principal functions that make the brain a 'privileged site':

- It restricts movement of hydrophilic, water-soluble substances and other large molecules, thereby maintaining a stable environment for optimal functioning
- It prevents most immune cells from entering the brain and potentially causing inflammatory damage

The blood–brain barrier is formed by the epithelial layers of the vasculature, brain tissue and epithelial layers of the ventricular system. These layers have:

- no fenestrations, i.e. none of the 'windows' that are present on most capillaries and allow the passage of small molecules and proteins
- tight junctions, which prevent movement of water and solutes
- a continuous basement membrane, which is a high-density layer of cells strengthened by collagen

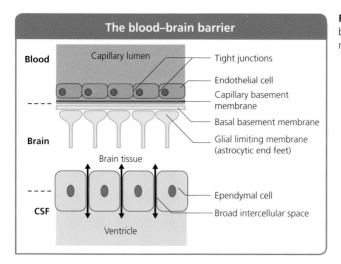

Figure 1.22 The blood–brain barrier. Its layers isolate the nervous system from the exterior.

- many mitochondria, which provide energy for active transport mechanisms

The tissue surrounding the vessels consists mainly of astrocytes (glia), the foot processes of which line the basement membrane of the vessels. This arrangement further reduces the likelihood of substances crossing the membrane.

The blood–brain barrier is highly permeable to water, gases such as carbon dioxide and oxygen, and lipophilic (fat-based) substances; it also allows the movement of some electrolytes. However, it is impermeable to larger hydrophilic (water-based) molecules and proteins. Transport processes, including diffusion, active transport and special carrier-mediated transport, enable movement of essential substances such as glucose and amino acids.

Loss of blood–brain barrier integrity

The blood–brain barrier is compromised at two main sites in the brain:

- the choroid plexus
- the circumventricular organs, the regions surrounding the ventricles, including the hypothalamic median eminence (see page 53) and area postrema (see page 61) in the medulla

The reduced integrity of the blood–brain barrier in these regions exposes them to circulating factors such as hormones or drugs. This makes the circumventricular organs ideally situated to control various survival mechanisms, including control of appetite, thirst, circadian rhythms (physiological process showing a rhythmic daily pattern) and seasonality.

Unlike the blood–brain barrier, the capillary endothelial cells at the circumventricular organs have fenestrations and lack tight junctions. These features create a leaky barrier, which allows substances to pass easily between the blood and the brain.

However, tight junctions are present on the ependymal cells of the ventricular system at the circumventricular organs, reducing the free flow of substances between the cerebrospinal fluid and the brain. This creates a directional flow from blood to cerebrospinal fluid: the blood/brain–cerebrospinal fluid barrier.

Cerebral blood supply

Knowledge of the brain's vascular supply is vital for correlating neurological symptoms with certain types of damage to structures in the brain.

The a vascular supply of the brain is divided into two circulations.

- **The anterior circulation** supplies the anterior and middle regions of the cerebrum; it originates from the internal carotid arteries, which are branches of the common carotid arteries, which supply the head and neck (see **Figure 1.9**)

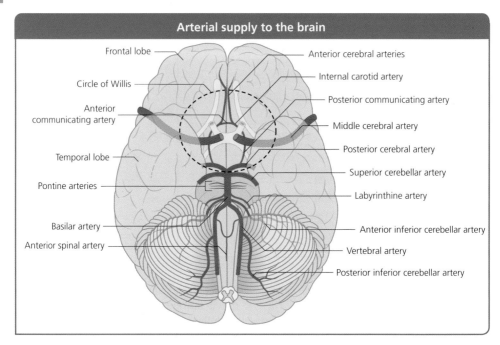

Arterial supply to the brain

Frontal lobe
Anterior cerebral arteries
Circle of Willis
Internal carotid artery
Anterior communicating artery
Posterior communicating artery
Middle cerebral artery
Temporal lobe
Posterior cerebral artery
Pontine arteries
Superior cerebellar artery
Labyrinthine artery
Basilar artery
Anterior inferior cerebellar artery
Anterior spinal artery
Vertebral artery
Posterior inferior cerebellar artery

Figure 1.23 Figure 1.20 Arterial supply to the brain (inferior view).

■ **The posterior circulation** supplies the posterior regions of the cerebrum, cerebellum and brainstem; it originates from the vertebral arteries, which are branches of the subclavian arteries, which supply the head, thorax and arms

The anterior and posterior circulations are linked by an anastomotic ring formed by connecting arterial branches: the circle of Willis.

The circle of Willis

The circle of Willis (**Figures 1.23 and 1.24**) lies at the basal surface of the brain and comprises:

■ the internal carotid arteries, which become the middle cerebral arteries
■ the anterior cerebral arteries, which form the anterior circulation with the middle cerebral arteries
■ the anterior communicating artery, which connects the anterior cerebral arteries to complete the anterior portion of the circle
■ the basilar artery, which is formed by fusion of the vertebral arteries and bifurcates (divides into two branches) to form the posterior cerebral arteries

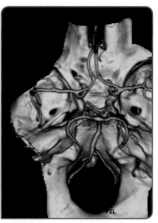

Figure 1.24 Appearance of the circle of Willis and skull base in a 3D reconstruction from a CT angiogram.

■ the posterior cerebral arteries, which form the posterior circulation with the basilar artery
■ the posterior communicating arteries, which connect the anterior and posterior portions of the circle

Vascular territories

Each pair of cerebral arteries supply distinct regions of the central nervous system (**Table 1.11** and **Figure 1.25**).

Blood supply to the nervous system			
Region	Major vascular division	Major arteries	Sites supplied
Cerebrum	Anterior circulation	Anterior cerebral arteries	Medial frontal and parietal lobes
		Middle cerebral arteries	Most lateral frontal, parietal and temporal lobes
	Posterior circulation	Posterior cerebral arteries	Inferior part of and medial temporal lobe
			Occipital lobe
Brainstem	Posterior circulation	Posterior cerebral arteries	Midbrain
		Basilar arteries	■ Anterior: branches of posterior cerebral arteries
		Vertebral arteries	■ Posterior: branches of superior cerebellar arteries
		Superior cerebellar arteries	
		Anterior inferior cerebellar arteries	Pons
			■ Anterior: branches of basilar artery
		Posterior inferior cerebellar arteries	■ Posterior: anterior inferior cerebellar arteries
		Anterior spinal arteries	Medulla
			■ Medial third: vertebral arteries and anterior spinal arteries
			■ Middle third: anterior inferior cerebellar arteries
			■ Lateral and posterior third: posterior inferior cerebellar arteries
Cerebellum	Posterior circulation	Superior cerebellar arteries	Superior half of cerebellum
			Superior cerebellar peduncle
		Anterior inferior cerebellar arteries	Anterior inferior half of cerebellum
			Middle cerebellar peduncle
		Posterior inferior cerebellar arteries	Posterior inferior half of cerebellum
			Inferior cerebellar peduncle
Spinal cord	Posterior circulation	Anterior spinal arteries	Anterior two thirds of spinal cord
		Posterior spinal arteries	Posterior third of spinal cord

Table 1.11 Blood supply to the major regions of the nervous system

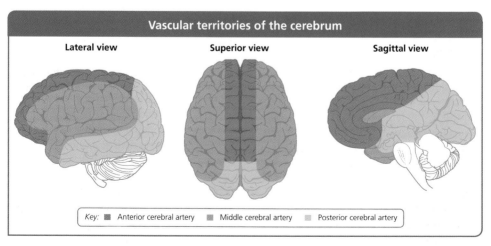

Figure 1.25 Vascular territories of the cerebrum.

In cases of neurovascular insult such as stroke, rapid identification of the vessel involved is imperative because rapid treatment is required to limit the extent of damage; as neurologists say, 'time is brain' (see page 244).

The main arterial supply to the cerebrum consists of vessels that run over the surface of the brain and along the furrows (fissures and sulci, page 41) between folds of brain tissue on its surface. Only the perforating vessels penetrate the tissue itself; these are very small, so minor changes in blood flow can dramatically affect the tissue they supply.

Territory supplied by the anterior cerebral arteries

The anterior cerebral arteries arise from the internal carotid arteries and run anteriorly along the longitudinal fissure, the deep groove between the cerebral hemispheres (see page 34), to supply the medial aspects of the frontal and parietal lobes. Lateral projections of these arteries supply a strip of tissue running along the medial edge of the cerebral hemispheres (**Figure 1.25**).

Deep branches of the anterior cerebral arteries supply the anterior portions of the basal ganglia and thalamus (see page 36). The anterior communicating artery connects the two anterior cerebral arteries and supplies the caudate nucleus (one of the basal ganglia nuclei, see page 48) and a portion of the internal capsule (a band of white matter within the cerebrum, see page 48).

Territory supplied by the middle cerebral arteries

The middle cerebral arteries are the longest branches of the internal carotid arteries and supply the lateral aspect of the cerebral hemisphere (**Figure 1.25**). Each middle cerebral artery originates from the ipsilateral internal carotid artery and travels through the lateral sulcus. Superior branches supply the middle and inferior regions of the frontal and parietal lobes, and inferior branches supply the superior and middle aspects of the temporal lobes.

Deep branches of the middle cerebral arteries known as the lenticulostriate arteries supply regions of the basal ganglia, thalamus and internal capsule, through which the main pathways for motor and sensory function pass.

Loss of blood supply from the lenticulostriate arteries can have devastating effects, such as loss of movement and sensation on one side of the body. This is because these arteries supply the main motor and sensory fibres that pass through the internal capsule.

Each anterior choroidal artery arises directly from the ipsilateral internal carotid artery and supplies the basal ganglia and thalamic territories immediately inferior to the lenticulostriate arteries.

Territory supplied by the posterior cerebral arteries

The posterior cerebral arteries are formed by bifurcation of the basilar artery and reach around the midbrain before projecting along the longitudinal fissure and calcarine sulcus (a sulcus that divides the occipital lobe into superior and inferior regions), in each occipital lobe, to supply the posterior portions of the cerebral hemispheres: the occipital lobes and the posterior parietal and inferior regions of the temporal lobes (**Figure 1.25**). On the medial surface, it supplies the entire temporal and occipital lobes. Deep branches supply posterior aspects of the thalamus and basal ganglia.

'Watershed areas'

These are the parts of the brain where vascular territories overlap. A watershed area receives its supply only from the fine, most distal branches of two arteries. Compared with areas supplied by the larger proximal branches, it is therefore more susceptible to damage if there is a reduction in blood flow. As a result, a 'watershed stroke' can occur if there is a general decrease in blood supply to the brain or if a major vessel supplying both territories becomes occluded. The main watershed zones are:

- anterior cerebral and middle cerebral arteries (both are fed by the carotid arteries)
- the middle cerebral and posterior cerebral arteries

Cerebral venous drainage

Most blood is drained from the brain via the dural venous sinuses (**Figure 1.26**) and ultimately into the jugular veins. The sinuses are valveless channels that allow free communication between venous branches. There are upper and lower groups.

Upper group

- The superior sagittal sinus, which runs along the midline between the hemispheres and lies in the superior aspect of the falx cerebri
- The inferior sagittal sinus, which runs along the midline above the diencephalon, in the inferior aspect of the falx cerebri
- The straight sinus, which drains the inferior sagittal sinus and runs along the midline where the falx cerebri connects to the tentorium cerebelli

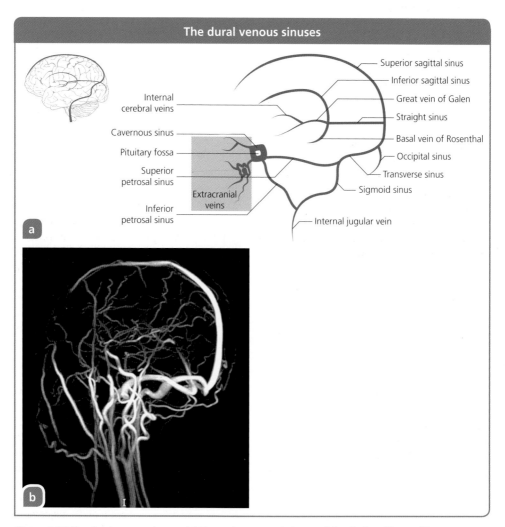

The dural venous sinuses

- Internal cerebral veins
- Cavernous sinus
- Pituitary fossa
- Superior petrosal sinus
- Extracranial veins
- Inferior petrosal sinus
- Superior sagittal sinus
- Inferior sagittal sinus
- Great vein of Galen
- Straight sinus
- Basal vein of Rosenthal
- Occipital sinus
- Transverse sinus
- Sigmoid sinus
- Internal jugular vein

a

b

Figure 1.26 The dural venous sinuses. (a) The main venous drainage of the skull and brain. (b) 3D MR venogram reconstruction of the sagittal view of the dural venous sinuses.

- The transverse sinuses, which run horizontally along the edge of the occipital bone in the tentorium cerebelli
- Sigmoid sinuses, which are 'S'-shaped sinuses formed from the anterior portions of the tentorium cerebelli, and connect to the jugular veins in the skull base

The superior sagittal sinus and straight sinus drain into the confluence of sinuses before proceeding, via the transverse and sigmoid sinuses, to the jugular veins.

Lower group

- **Cavernous sinuses**, large venous formations covered by dura mater in the base of skull and formed by multiple veins
- **Anterior and posterior intercavernous sinuses**, which join with the cavernous sinuses and form a venous loop around the pituitary fossa, a hollow in the skull base that contains the pituitary gland

Cavernous sinuses are unique because major arteries, the internal carotids, and multiple cranial nerves (IV, VI, V_1 and V_2) travel through them. The optic nerve and pituitary gland also lie nearby. Damage to the cavernous sinuses, from tumours, thrombotic clots or infection, results in severe headache and the loss of vision, eye movement and facial sensation.

Intracranial veins

Intracranial veins drain into the venous sinuses and are divided into superficial and deep cerebral veins.

Superficial cerebral veins

These lie at the surface of the brain and drain into the sinuses via a network of bridging veins. They include the superficial middle cerebral (Sylvian) vein, which lies along the lateral sulcus and drains into the superior sagittal sinus.

Deep cerebral veins

These communicate with superficial cerebral veins or drain directly into the venous sinuses. The deep cerebral veins include the internal cerebral veins and the basal vein (vein of Rosenthal), which join to form the great cerebral vein of Galen.

The great vein of Galen unites with the inferior sagittal sinus. This forms the straight sinus (**Figure 1.26**).

Extracranial veins

These drain the skull and facial regions. The extracranial veins include the emissary and diploic veins, which drain the scalp and cranial vault, respectively.

Control of cerebral blood volume and flow

The brain requires a constant supply of energy, in the form of glucose and oxygen, to function effectively. It uses 15–20% of total cardiac output and 20% of oxygen intake, despite accounting for only 2% of total body weight.

Deficits in cerebral blood volume, i.e. the amount of blood in the cerebrum, and cerebral blood flow, i.e. the rate at which blood travels through the cerebral vasculature, reduce the brain's ability to function. Therefore, if not corrected swiftly, these deficits can lead rapidly to deterioration in tissue function and death.

Understanding cerebral blood volume and flow is vital for the treatment of neurosurgical and neurological disorders, because the threshold for ischaemia and neurological dysfunction is lower in the injured brain than in the normal brain (**Table 1.12**).

Three critical factors determine cerebral blood volume and flow.

- **Cerebral vascular resistance**, the diameter of the cerebral arteries
- **Cerebral perfusion pressure**, the pressure gradient controlling cerebral blood flow, calculated as cerebral perfusion pressure = mean arterial pressure – intracranial pressure
- **Cerebral metabolic rate**, the rate of cerebral oxygen consumption

Cerebral autoregulation

Cerebral autoregulation maintains cerebral blood flow at an optimal level by decreasing

Cerebral blood flow thresholds for ischaemia and neurological dysfunction		
Status of brain	Flow threshold (mL/100 g tissue/min)	Effects
Normal	50	Normal function, with grey matter receiving more cerebrospinal fluid than white matter does
	24–30	Transient neurological deficits
	8–23	Reversible neurological dysfunction
	< 8	Irreversible neurological dysfunction
Abnormal or injured	15–20	Reversible neurological dysfunction
	10–15	Irreversible neurological dysfunction

Table 1.12 Cerebral blood flow thresholds for ischaemia and neurological dysfunction in the normal and injured brain

cerebral blood volume to offset the effect of increased cerebral vascular resistance, and vice versa. Cerebral autoregulation encompasses several physiological processes, principally constriction and dilation of arterioles and adjustments in mean arterial pressure. Through these mechanisms, blood flow is kept constant over a wide range of cerebral perfusion pressures (50–150 mmHg); this effect is known as the autoregulatory plateau (**Figure 1.27**).

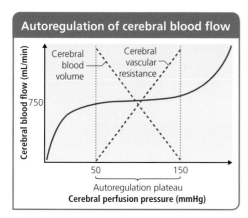

Autoregulation of cerebral blood flow

Cerebral blood volume

Cerebral vascular resistance

Cerebral blood flow (mL/min)

750

50   150

Autoregulation plateau
Cerebral perfusion pressure (mmHg)

Figure 1.27 Autoregulation of cerebral blood flow. The relationship between cerebral perfusion pressure and blood flow has an autoregulation plateau where changes in either can be compensated, maintaining cerebral blood flow at an optimal 750 mL/min. Within this range, when perfusion pressure rises there is a compensatory increase in vascular resistance and decrease in blood volume to maintain flow. Compensation does not occur outside this range.

Outside the limits of autoregulation, i.e. cerebral perfusion pressure < 50 or > 150 mmHg, these mechanisms are disrupted.

■ At severely low cerebral perfusion pressure, there is insufficient pressure to push blood through the arterioles; consequently, cerebral blood volume and flow decrease, resulting in global cerebral hypoxia and ischaemia
■ Excessively high cerebral perfusion pressure stretches arterioles, which damages the vascular endothelium and disrupts the blood–brain barrier; this results in bleeding, oedema or both, and a rapid increase in intracranial pressure and cerebral dysfunction

Intracranial pressure

This is the pressure in the cranial vault. Intracranial pressure is related to the amount of tissue and fluid present in the brain at any one time. The total intracranial volume (V_{total}) is the sum of the elements found in the rigid compartment of the skull:

$$V_{total} = V_{brain} + V_{blood} + V_{cerebrospinal\ fluid} + V_{extra\ mass}$$

The rigid cranial vault cannot expand or contract, so V_{total} is unchangeable; this is known as the Monro–Kellie doctrine. If one of the constituent volumes of V_{total} increases, for example V_{blood}, as a result of haemorrhage, the others must adjust to compensate for the change and thereby prevent an increase in intracranial pressure.

Mechanisms preventing increases in intracranial pressure

Two principal compensatory mechanisms enable small increases in volume to be accommodated so that there is little change in intracranial pressure (**Figure 1.28**):

- movement of cerebrospinal fluid out of the subarachnoid space, ventricles and skull cisterns and into the lumbar cistern
- movement of venous blood out of the dural sinuses and into the internal jugular veins

However, the effects of these mechanisms are limited. Once the compensatory threshold is reached, intracranial pressure increases rapidly and exponentially (**Figure 1.28**), often with devastating results, for example herniation and coning.

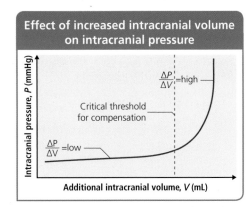

Figure 1.28 The effect of increased intracranial volume on intracranial pressure. Compensatory mechanisms accommodate volume changes with little or no increase in intracranial pressure until the critical threshold, maximum compensatory limit, is reached; after which point pressure rises exponentially with further volume changes.

Control of intracranial pressure is a key management principle when treating neurological disorders. This is particularly true in neurosurgery.

Cerebrum

Starter questions

Answers to the following questions are on page 116.

10. Can people survive without a cortex?
11. How much of the brain is actually used?

The cerebrum forms the bulk of the brain. It is the processing centre where information is stored, integrated and understood and, where conscious and unconscious decisions about appropriate responses are made.

Gross anatomy of the cerebrum

The adult cerebrum is about the size of a small honeydew melon, about 15 cm in length and 1350 g in weight. It comprises a left and a right hemisphere. The two hemispheres are physically joined by the corpus callosum, an area that links corresponding regions of the two hemispheres (**Figure 1.29c**). The surface of each hemisphere is highly folded; this allows a higher density of cells and connections to be concentrated into the limited volume available for the brain within the skull cavity.

Gyri

The cerebral surface is moulded into folds called gyri (singular, gyrus). Several of these gyri are useful landmarks when localising different regions of the cerebrum. Two of the most functionally significant are the precentral gyrus and the postcentral gyrus, which house the primary motor cortex and the primary sensory cortex, respectively (**Figure 1.29**; see pages 43–45).

Sulci and fissures

The spaces or furrows between the folds are called sulci (singular, sulcus). Large sulci are called fissures; the largest is the longitudinal fissure between the left and right hemispheres (**Figure 1.29**).

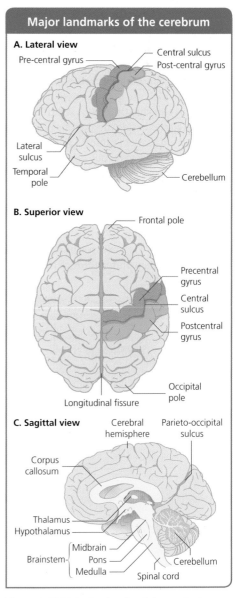

Major landmarks of the cerebrum

A. Lateral view
Pre-central gyrus — Central sulcus — Post-central gyrus — Lateral sulcus — Temporal pole — Cerebellum

B. Superior view
Frontal pole — Precentral gyrus — Central sulcus — Postcentral gyrus — Occipital pole — Longitudinal fissure

C. Sagittal view
Cerebral hemisphere — Parieto-occipital sulcus — Corpus callosum — Thalamus — Hypothalamus — Brainstem {Midbrain — Pons — Medulla} — Cerebellum — Spinal cord

Figure 1.29 Major landmarks of the cerebral hemispheres, and their spatial relationship to the brainstem and cerebellum

Larger sulci are useful anatomical landmarks. They form the boundaries of the lobes, for example the central sulcus separates the frontal and parietal lobes (see page 43).

Neuronal activity in grey matter is metabolically incredibly demanding. The brain requires 20% of the body's total oxygen intake, 90–95% of this is used by grey matter.

Structural division of the cerebrum

The cerebrum consists of an outermost layer of grey matter (the cortex), with white matter lying beneath. This is the opposite of the arrangement in the spinal cord, where white matter surrounds grey.

Grey matter

Grey matter contains the cell bodies of the neurones, which are grey because they have no fatty myelin sheathing. It is stratified into six layers named after the dominant type of cell within each layer (**Table 1.13**). Most of the cortex has all six layers, but primary cortices (see page 6) have between three and five.

The different cell types present in grey matter have various properties, such as short projections linking cells in the same layer, or long projections spanning all layers. These differences determine the ways in which activity is integrated and transmitted through the cortex.

White matter

The white matter contains the axons of the cortical neurons. Its silvery white colour is the colour of the myelin sheaths around the axons. The axons group to form tracts, large bundles of axon fibres, the physical wiring of neural pathways connecting different regions of the central nervous system. They vary dramatically in size, from the short association fibres, which range from micrometres to centimetres in length and connect different regions of the cortex, to the long corticospinal motor tracts, which run up to a metre in length through the brain and down the spinal cord (see page 88).

Functional division of the cerebral hemispheres

The two hemispheres have separate and combined functions, for example motor

Histological layers of the cerebral cortex			
Layer		Name	Contents
I		Molecular	Few neurones
II		External granular	Granule cells (granular appearance)
			Stellate cells (star-shaped)
III		External pyramidal	Pyramidal cells (small)
IV		Internal granular	Granule cells
			Stellate cells
V		Internal pyramidal	Pyramidal cells (large)
VI		Multiform	Granule cells
			Stellate cells
			Pyramidal cells
			Fusiform cells (spindle-shaped)

Table 1.13 Histological layers of the grey matter in the cerebral cortex

control is bilateral whereas language control is unilateral. This division of function underlies the concept of cerebral dominance.

Cerebral dominance

The term cerebral dominance is used to describe the lateralisation of brain functions, i.e. when activity associated with certain behaviours, such as speech, is located in one hemisphere only. This phenomenon is an essential consideration in clinical situations, for example when localising a lesion or surgically removing a tumour.

The dominant hemisphere is responsible for logical and analytical aspects of perception, including:

- language: it contains Broca's and Wernicke's areas, vital for speech production and the understanding of language, respectively; see page 49 and **Figure 1.32**)
- mathematical processing
- writing

The non-dominant hemisphere governs more artistic and representational aspects of perception, such as:

- the interpretation of emotional salience and tonality of language, i.e. the characteristics of speech (prosody)
- spatial recognition
- musical interpretation

> The size of an individual's corpus callosum, which connects the left and right hemispheres, often correlates with certain behavioural predispositions, e.g. the ability to multitask. Increased connectivity between the hemispheres allows rapid cross-coordination of dominant and non-dominant behaviours, e.g. musicians link the analytical (dominant) in controlling pace and timing with the artistic (non-dominant) in regulating tonality and conveying emotion, to produce music.

Cerebral lobes

Each of the two cerebral hemispheres has four principal lobes: the frontal, temporal, parietal and occipital lobes (**see Figure 1.5**). The lobes are divided by sulci and imaginary lines:

- The central sulcus divides the frontal lobe from the parietal lobe (**Figure 1.29a**)
- The lateral sulcus divides the frontal lobe from the temporal lobe (**Figure 1.29a**)
- The parieto-occipital sulcus separates the parietal lobe from the occipital lobe, and is visible only in a mid-sagittal view (**Figure 1.29c**)
- An imaginary line running horizontally from the lateral sulcus to the occipital–parietal boundary separates the temporal lobe from the parietal lobe, and another imaginary line runs from the meeting point of the horizontal and occipital-parietal boundary point to the midbrain, marking the boundary of the temporal and occipital lobes

The frontal lobe

The frontal lobe is associated primarily with motor function (see page 84) and higher cognition, i.e. thought processing, reasoning and intelligence (**Table 1.14**). Damage to this region commonly results in motor deficits and behavioural changes, including alterations in personality. The frontal lobe has two zones:

- The vertical zone, where the gyri lie vertically next to the central sulcus, contains the principal areas controlling motor function
- The horizontal zone, where the gyri lie horizontally, contains the prefrontal areas (all cortical areas in front of the motor control area), which contains centres responsible for higher cognition and speech

Function in the frontal lobe

The frontal lobes can be thought of as the lobes of expression. This is because they control both motor function, required for behavioural expression, and higher cognition, which underlies the expression of personality and intellect.

Motor control

Immediately anterior to the central sulcus is the precentral gyrus (see **Figure 1.29**). This

The frontal lobe		
General function	Specific function(s)	Region(s)
Motor	Executive motor function	Primary motor cortex
	Planning of motor function	Premotor cortex
	Head and trunk turning	Supplemental motor area
	Eye movement towards opposite (contralateral) side	Frontal eye fields
Association	Gait	Prefrontal cortex
	Conscious bladder control	
	Cognition	
	Behavioural control	
Language	Speech production	Broca's area

Table 1.14 Regions and functions of the frontal lobe

contains the primary motor cortex, which produces movement (see pages 84-89). The premotor and supplementary motor areas are anterior to the precentral gyrus. They are involved in planning and rehearsal of movement.

In the prefrontal cortex is another motor area, which lies anterior to the voluntary motor areas on the medial aspect of the frontal lobe: the frontal eye fields. This area controls visual attention, for example that given to moving objects, as well as saccadic eye movement, an involuntary fast scanning movement that helps build mental images of scenes.

Areas involved in the conscious control of urination and defecation are also situated in the anterior prefrontal cortex.

The area responsible for motor control of speech production, Broca's area, is situated on the inferior frontal gyrus in the prefrontal area, close to the premotor cortex (see page 50 and **Figure 1.32**).

Higher cognition

The prefrontal areas, which are rostral to the motor area of the lobe, consist mainly of association cortices (see page 48). These regions integrate and assimilate information arising from all aspects of the nervous system, i.e. motor, sensory and homeostatic.

The prefrontal areas are responsible for decision making and higher processing. They determine intellect and personality, so damage to these regions has a serious impact on both, often reducing patients to 'animalistic' versions of themselves.

Before the advent of antipsychotic drugs, removal of the prefrontal areas of the frontal lobe (lobotomy) was sometimes carried out in an attempt to address severe chronic psychotic behaviours. Lobotomy was controversial: it had a calming effect (without affecting intelligence), but it induced permanent extreme apathy in many patients, often to the point of making independent life impossible, and sometimes it resulted in catastrophic brain damage and death.

The parietal lobe

The parietal lobe is the main centre for sensory processing and assimilation (integration of information) to form mental images of objects (**Table 1.15**). Damage to this region changes perception and the ability to make associations. The parietal lobe has two zones:

- the vertical zone contains the principal areas controlling sensation
- the horizontal zone contains association cortex that integrates multimodal information

The parietal lobe		
General function	Specific function(s)	Region(s)
Sensory	Primary centre for sensation	Primary sensory cortex
	Secondary centre	Secondary sensory cortex
Association	Integration of sensory input	Superior parietal lobule
	Visual, auditory and spatial processing	Inferior parietal lobule
	Language	
Vision	Fibres for lower quadrant visual field	Optic radiation

Table 1.15 Parietal lobe regions and function

> **Damage to the non-dominant parietal lobe often results in hemispatial neglect.** The patient ignores the side of the body opposite, i.e. contralateral to, the side on which the parietal lobe has sustained damage. This is an example of sensory inattention.

Function in the parietal lobe

The parietal lobes can be thought of as the lobes of perception, because they contain the sensory centres and the largest expanses of cortex dedicated to integration of information.

Sensation

The postcentral gyrus lies immediately behind the central sulcus and contains the main centre for sensory perception: the primary sensory cortex. The secondary somatosensory cortex is an arbitrary region located posterior to the postcentral gyrus.

Association

Behind the primary and secondary sensory cortices lie two horizontal zones, the superior and inferior parietal lobules. The superior lobule forms the posterior parietal association cortex, which integrates information about sensation with input from other areas, for example integrating visual input with information about emotional status (see page 48). This process enables specific sensations to be understood in the context of an individual's general experience.

The occipital lobe

The occipital lobe is the processing centre for visual information. Three concentric rings of cortical tissue make up the lobe:

- the primary visual cortex, which is the primary centre for all visual afferent information
- the secondary visual cortex
- the tertiary visual cortex, the visual association area

Each of these areas process visual information with varying degrees of complexity. For example, the primary visual cortex is responsible for depth perception, object recognition and spatial location, but further interpretation of visual information requires higher-order processing in the association cortices.

Damage to the occipital lobe results in characteristic visual deficits. However, because the pathways and areas involved in vision are well understood, lesions sites can be readily identified (see page 109).

The temporal lobe

The temporal lobe has many functions (**Table 1.16**), the principal one being language (see page 49). Damage to this region commonly causes and problems with language.

The lobe also contains the primary centres for hearing, smell and taste, as well as tracts supplying visual information. Consequently,

The temporal lobe		
General function	**Specific function(s)**	**Region(s)**
Hearing	Primary centre for auditory input	Primary auditory cortex
	Secondary centre	Secondary auditory cortex
Association	Perception	Parieto-occipitotemporal association cortex
	Visual, auditory and spatial processing	
	Language	
Language	Interpretation of both written and spoken language	Wernicke's area
		Auditory association cortex
Vision	Fibres for upper quadrant visual field	Optic radiation
Memory and emotion	Long- and short-term memory	Limbic system
	Emotional salience	
	Recognition	

Table 1.16 Temporal lobe regions and function

damage to the temporal lobe can cause deficits in sensation for almost all the primary senses.

Function in the temporal lobe

The temporal lobe has a role in the understanding of language and the processing of information relating to the special senses of smell, taste and vision (see page 107). It is also considered the lobe of remembrance, because it contains centres for learning, memory and emotions.

Language

The temporal lobe has, on its superior aspect, the interpretational centre for both spoken and written language: Wernicke's area (see **Figure 1.32** and page 49). This area receives, integrates and assimilates information obtained by reading or hearing words. Wernicke's area is also responsible for decision making regarding responses to written or spoken language. Damage to this area results in an inability to understand language.

Special senses

The temporal lobes primary and secondary auditory cortices lie adjacent to Wernicke's area, in the superior part of the temporal lobe.

Centres for olfaction (smell) are located in the amygdala, which forms part of the limbic system. Centres for gustation (taste) cross the medial aspect of the lobe and into the insula.

The temporal lobe also contains fibres of the optic radiation, a fibre bundle that travels from the thalamus to the visual cortices (see page 109).

Learning, memory and emotions

In addition to its other functions, the temporal lobe is involved in learning, memory and emotional perception. This is primarily because it houses a significant proportion of the limbic system, which has a primary role in these functions.

The limbic system

The limbic system was originally called a lobe, but it is now called a system because it comprises interlinked cortical and subcortical structures that share functions. The system spans the medial aspects of the frontal and parietal lobes but most of it is situated in the medial regions of the temporal lobe (**Figure 1.30**). It has four main functions:

■ memory
■ learning
■ perception (emotional and spatial)
■ motivation

Most structures in the limbic system are situated immediately below the cortex, wrapping around the diencephalon. They include regions of the frontal, parietal and temporal lobes. The limbic system has high levels of synaptic plasticity, which is key to its function in learning and memory.

Areas of the brain with greater plasticity are more susceptible to hyperactivity. For example, epilepsy is often associated with the temporal and limbic regions. Localised hyperactivity often generates signs and symptoms specific to the area, with seizures originating in the hippocampus often preceded by feelings of déjà vu, and those originating in the amygdala by anxiety or olfactory hallucinations.

of plasticity in this region are ideal for integrating and embedding information to form memories.

The extent of amnesia (memory loss) is a good indicator of the severity of damage caused in trauma. Amnesia has two forms:

- anterograde: new memories cannot be formed

- retrograde: previous memories are lost

Unilateral hippocampal lesions generally do not affect memory as compensation for the loss occurs in the undamaged side. However, bilateral lesions can result in patients being unable to remember both distant and recent events, making every day seem like a new life.

The hippocampus

The hippocampus, so called because it is shaped like a seahorse, is a key region in spatial perception, learning and memory. It has folded and stratified cortical tissue that receives information from and projects information to a wide range of areas, including the frontal lobe and hypothalamus, to control behaviour.

In the hippocampus, neurones form interconnected loops, which enable information to be repeatedly recycled. The large network of interconnected neurones and high levels

The amygdala

This structure, named after its almond shape, is situated in the uncus, a hook-like protrusion of tissue lying on the medial aspect of the temporal lobe (see **Figure 1.30**). The amygdala controls negative emotions such as fear and anxiety, and expression of learned behaviours. It has a large two-way connection to the frontal lobe, which controls more positive emotions such as reward. Interplay between the two areas controls mood.

The amygdala is involved in the recognition of faces, particularly facial expressions, and

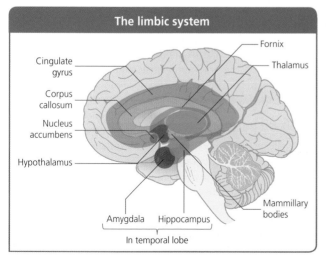

The limbic system

Cingulate gyrus

Corpus callosum

Nucleus accumbens

Hypothalamus

Fornix

Thalamus

Mammillary bodies

Amygdala   Hippocampus

In temporal lobe

Figure 1.30 Regions of the limbic system and the location of its inner and outer arcs.

also has a role in olfaction, because it contains the primary olfactory area (see page 111).

> **Bilateral lesions of the amygdala, usually caused by infection (e.g. herpes simplex encephalitis), can cause Klüver–Bucy syndrome,** which classically presents with:
>
> - Hyperorality: putting objects in the mouth
> - Dietary changes: often overeating due to hyperorality
> - Emotional blunting: placidity or lack of emotional expression
> - Visual agnosia: deficits in recognising objects, particularly faces

The insula

The insula, or insular cortex, is located in the recess of the lateral sulcus and bridges the region between the frontal and temporal lobes. It contains the primary gustatory cortex and is also involved in perception of the internal environment, from emotional status to homeostatic control.

The basal ganglia

The basal ganglia lie deep within the white matter of the cerebrum, midbrain and brainstem (**Figure 1.31**). They are group of interconnected subcortical nuclei that help fine-tune and coordinate motor function:

- caudate nucleus
- putamen
- globus pallidus (divided into external and internal segments)
- subthalamic nuclei (part of the diencephalon)

> **Damage to** basal ganglia regions is implicated in many common movement disorders, including Parkinson's disease.

The caudate nucleus and putamen are known collectively as the striatum; they work together to control motor activity. These two regions are divided by the internal capsule, a region of white matter containing motor and sensory fibres.

The putamen and globus pallidus are lateral to the caudate nucleus and thalamus. They form a lens-shaped structure: the lentiform nucleus.

The substantia nigra, which is located in the brainstem, not the cerebrum, is usually grouped alongside the basal ganglia because of its role in motor function. It modulates activity in the network (see **Figure 1.55** and page 89).

Association cortices

The three association cortices (**Table 1.17**) link and integrate the functions of the lobes and are named after their location.

- **The parieto-occipitotemporal association cortex** interacts with the primary sensory and motor cortices and is involved in most sensorimotor processing, interpretation and evaluation
- **The limbic association cortex** is involved in learning and memory formation, spatial perception, motivation and emotional processing
- **The prefrontal association cortex** is involved in higher cognition, reasoning, rationale, motivation and mood, and is the region that determines 'who we are'; damage to this area often results in patients reverting to more 'animalistic' or instinctive forms of behaviour

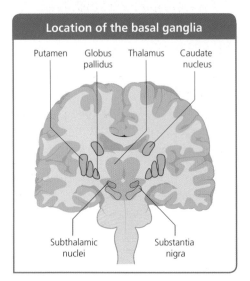

Location of the basal ganglia

Putamen   Globus pallidus   Thalamus   Caudate nucleus

Subthalamic nuclei   Substantia nigra

Figure 1.31 Location of the basal ganglia deep in the cerebrum.

Cortical association areas		
Lobe	Association area(s)	Function(s)
Frontal	Prefrontal association cortex	Gait
		Sphincter control
		Higher cognition
		Behaviour
Temporal	Parieto-occipitotemporal association cortices	Audiovisual processing
	Auditory association cortex	Spatial and motor processing
	Wernicke's area	Language
Parietal	Limbic association cortex	Higher cognition, learning and memory, behaviour and spacial processing
	Parieto-occipitotemporal association cortices	Audiovisual processing
		Spatial and motor processing
		Higher-order sensory processing
Occipital	Visual association cortex (tertiary visual cortex)	Higher-order visual processing

Table 1.17 Cortical association areas and their functions

Association fibres

Two groups of association fibres increase the speed of communication between association cortices.

- **Commissural pathways** are tracts connecting the left and right hemispheres
- **Association fibres** connect within (short fibres) and between (fasciculi) lobes

The corpus callosum is the largest commissural pathway; it lies under the falx cerebri in the longitudinal fissure. Another interhemispheric pathway, the anterior commissure, is located in the anterior aspect of the brain.

Short association fibres connect the gyri within a lobe. Long tracts, the superior and inferior longitudinal fasciculi, run through the cerebrum, connecting the frontal to the parietal lobe and the temporal to the occipital lobe, respectively. The arcuate fasciculus connects the temporal and frontal lobes and is primarily involved in language.

Disconnection syndromes are caused by damage to association fibre pathways. The most severe, interhemispheric disconnection, is caused by damage to the corpus callosum. Commonly known as 'split brain', it causes mismatched behaviours. For example, if a patient is shown two objects, one in each visual field, and asked to name the object and point to a picture of it, the patient will name the right visual field object and point to the one on the left.

Language

Verbal and written communication is one of humanity's defining features and a key 'higher' function. Language skills are easy to test and the pathways involved are well understood. Accordingly, deficits in language production can help in identifying possible lesion sites.

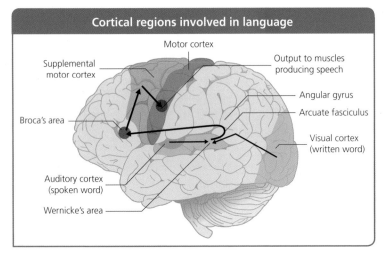

Figure 1.32 Cortical regions and pathways involved in the interpretation of language (blue) and the control of production of speech (red) are shown.

Understanding language

The understanding of spoken and written language involves a sequence of events (**Figure 1.32**):

1. Information from the visual cortex (for writing) or the auditory cortex (for speech) is transmitted to Wernicke's area, the main hub for understanding language, for processing
2. Language information is combined with input from other areas, for example sensory information about the external and internal environments and memory, to add context to the linguistic information
3. Wernicke's area interprets and integrates the information and decides what responses are appropriate
4. Decisions are then transferred to the motor regions for speech production or other actions

Speech disorders are divided into three categories.

■ Dysphasias are language abnormalities caused by damage to cerebral language centres or connections (aphasia is absence of speech)

■ Dysarthrias are disorders of articulation caused by damage to motor pathways or structures producing speech

■ Dysphonias are problems with volume, tonality and accuracy

Speech production

To produce speech, the sequence of events is as follows.

1. Information detailing the speech required is carried by the arcuate fasciculus from Wernicke's area to Broca's area in the frontal lobe
2. Broca's area decides what motor patterns are required to produce the correct movements of mouth, lips, tongue, pharynx and larynx, and how breathing should be controlled
3. These decisions are passed to the supplemental motor areas, where the movements are mentally rehearsed, fine-tuned and modified (see page 84)
4. The final information about the pattern of movements required for speech is sent to the primary motor cortex
5. Information is transmitted from the primary motor cortex to the spinal cord via the descending (motor) tracts
6. The descending tracts modify the activity of the spinal motor neurones, which control the musculature of the larynx and tongue, as well as respiration (see page 88)
7. As speech is produced, sensory information about the speech is fed back to the speech centres, enabling corrections for characteristics such as accuracy, tonality and volume to be made

Dysphasias and localisation of damage			
Type	Region	Features with damage	Additional features
Broca's (motor)	Frontal lobe	Expressive dysphasia ■ Comprehension normal ■ Expression (speech delivery) poor (dysarthria or non-fluent) ■ Repetition poor ■ Naming poor	Motor problems, including contralateral (i.e. right) hemiparesis (weakness), often in face and arms
Wernicke's (sensory)	Temporal lobe	Receptive dysphasia ■ Comprehension poor ■ Expression normal ■ Speech meaningless or irrelevant ■ Repetition poor ■ Naming poor	Visual field changes because of the proximity of optic radiation
Conduction	Arcuate fasciculus	Conduction dysphasia ■ Comprehension normal ■ Expression normal ■ Repetition poor	Deficits associated with damage to frontal lobe region, temporal lobe region, or both
Global	Lateral sulcus (Wernicke's and Broca's areas affected)	Mixed deficit: expressive and receptive dysphasia ■ Comprehension poor ■ Expression poor ■ Repetition poor ■ Naming poor	Deficits associated with damage to frontal lobe region, temporal lobe region, or both

Table 1.18 Dysphasias associated with damage to language regions in the cerebrum

Projections to other structures ensure that appropriate behaviours accompany the speech, for example maintenance of eye contact and correct posture and gesticulations.

Interruption to the flow of information at any point in these pathways produces an alteration in the pattern of speech, i.e. a dysphasia, which is specific to the area of injury (**Table 1.18**). Therefore knowledge of the type of dysphasia can be used clinically to localise damage to the cerebrum.

Thalamus and hypothalamus

The thalamus and hypothalamus are situated directly beneath the cerebrum, and together form the diencephalon (**Figure 1.33**). The two structures act as hubs, integrating information and transmitting it to and from the cortex. They also maintain the body's internal environment within optimal, homeostatic, ranges. The thalamus regulates conscious behaviours, whereas the hypothalamus controls automatic survival behaviours.

The thalamus

The thalamus (Greek, 'inner chamber') is a walnut-sized structure that acts as the hub connecting the cerebrum and the brainstem. It was originally thought to be a simple relay station, because most of the sensory and motor pathways pass through it. However, it is now understood to actively participate in the control of certain functions, including

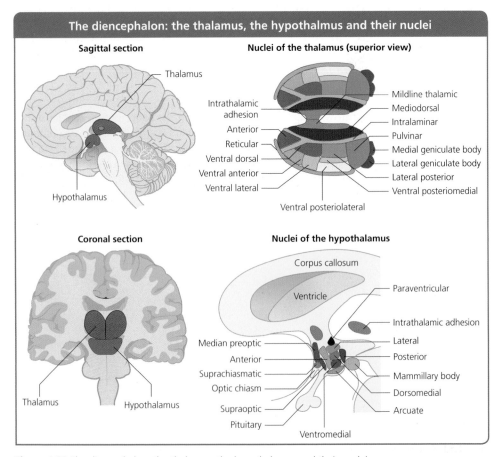

The diencephalon: the thalamus, the hypothalmus and their nuclei

Sagittal section

Thalamus

Hypothalamus

Nuclei of the thalamus (superior view)

Intrathalamic adhesion
Anterior
Reticular
Ventral dorsal
Ventral anterior
Ventral lateral

Mildline thalamic
Mediodorsal
Intralaminar
Pulvinar
Medial geniculate body
Lateral geniculate body
Lateral posterior
Ventral posteriomedial

Ventral posteriolateral

Coronal section

Thalamus   Hypothalamus

Nuclei of the hypothalamus

Corpus callosum

Ventricle

Median preoptic
Anterior
Suprachiasmatic
Optic chiasm
Supraoptic
Pituitary

Ventromedial

Paraventricular
Intrathalamic adhesion
Lateral
Posterior
Mammillary body
Dorsomedial
Arcuate

Figure 1.33 The diencephalon: the thalamus, the hypothalamus and their nuclei.

memory formation, arousal and consciousness (see page 60).

The two hemispheres of the thalamus are
linked by the intrathalamic adhesion. This is a
band of tissue containing neurones and axon
fibres (**Figure 1.33**).

Anatomical divisions

The thalamus has 12 nuclei (**Table 1.19** and
Figure 1.33). Nine of these are separated anatomically into three main groups of nuclei.

- The **anterior nuclei** regulate learning,
  memory and alertness, and communicates
  with the limbic system
- The **medial nuclei** are linked to emotion
  and cognition; they communicate with the
  limbic system and frontal lobes
- The **lateral nuclei** provide sensorimotor
  information to the cortex

The remaining three nuclei form sheet-like
structures separating the nuclear groups.

Functional divisions

Functionally, the nuclei are divided into
three groups (see **Table 1.19**):

- **Relay nuclei** control motivation and
  provide sensorimotor information to the
  cortical regions

- Intralaminar nuclei regulate motor function
  and consciousness; they relay motor
  information to the basal ganglia and
  sensory information to the cortex
- The **reticular nucleus** controls consciousness and sleep; it links the reticular formation to the thalamic nuclei

> Focal (localised) epileptic activity
> can rapidly turn into generalised
> (global) epilepsy once it reaches the
> **thalamus**. This is because the thalamus's
> connections to the rest of the cortex are
> so extensive.

The hypothalamus

The hypothalamus is the 'homeostatic hub',
maintaining the endocrine and autonomic
set points that allow the body to function
optimally. It is an almond-sized structure
located ventral to the thalamus; the two
structures are separated by the hypothalamic sulcus. The hypothalamus comprises
13 nuclei (**Table 1.20** and **Figure 1.33**).

Anatomical divisions

The nuclei are grouped according to their
proximity to the ventricle.

Thalamic nuclei and their functions			
Functional division	Nucleus	Anatomical division	Function
Relay nuclei	Anterior nucleus	Anterior	Emotion and cognition
	Ventral anterior	Lateral	Motor relay
	Ventral posterior lateral	Lateral	Sensory relay (body)
	Ventral posteriomedial	Lateral	Sensory relay (head and neck)
	Ventrolateral	Lateral	Motor relay
	Mediodorsal	Medial	Emotion and cognition
	Medial geniculate	Lateral	Auditory relay
	Lateral geniculate	Lateral	Visual relay
	Midline thalamic	Medial	Emotion and cognition
	Pulvinar	Lateral	Visual orientation
Intralaminar nuclei	Intralaminar		Arousal and motor relay
Reticular nucleus	Reticular		Arousal

Table 1.19 Thalamic nuclei and their functions

Hypothalmic nuclei and their functions		
Anatomical division	Nucleus	Function
Anterior (parasympathetic)	Preoptic	Blood pressure regulation, sexual function and arousal
	Supraoptic	Osmoregulation
	Suprachiasmatic	Control of diurnal rhythm
	Paraventricular	Stress responses, appetite regulation and autonomic control
	Anterior	Thermoregulation
Middle	Arcuate	Appetite and growth regulation
	Dorsomedial	Cardiovascular and gastrointestinal function
	Ventromedial	Appetite regulation and mood
	Lateral	Thirst (zona incerta) and mood
Posterior (sympathetic)	Posterior	Blood pressure regulation and thermoregulation
	Dorsal	Control of diurnal rhythm
	Mamillary	Memory
	Tuberomammillary	Sleep–wake cycle

Table 1.20 Hypothalamic nuclei and their functions

- The **periventricular nuclei** are the peri- and paraventricular nuclei and the arcuate nucleus
- The **medial nuclei** are the dorsal and ventral medial nuclei
- The **lateral nuclei** are the lateral nucleus and the medial forebrain bundle

Periventricular nuclei are next to the cerebrospinal fluid-filled ventricles, which are regions with reduced integrity blood–brain barrier (see page 32). Therefore the periventricular nuclei have easy access to circulating substances, which enables them to respond rapidly to changes in the internal environment.

Hypothalamic connections to and from the limbic and frontal regions allow higher functions, such as mood and memory, to influence homeostasis. This is why a person can consciously learn to blush less, and how yogis can control their heart rate during meditation.

Functional divisions

The nuclei can be divided into three functional groups (see **Table 1.20**):

- The **anterior (supraoptic) nuclei** primarily control parasympathetic function
- The **middle (tuberal) nuclei** control thirst and feeding behaviours
- The **posterior (mammillary) nuclei** control sympathetic function

Damage to the ventromedial hypothalamus and lateral nucleus have opposing effects.

- Damage to the ventromedial hypothalamus, the 'satiety centre', often leads to overeating and obesity
- Damage to the lateral nucleus, the 'hunger centre', causes reduced food intake

Hypothalamic axes

The hypothalamic axes are pathways that control specific survival behaviours. There are three main axes (**Table 1.21**).

- The **hypothalamic–pituitary–adrenal axis** regulates stress responses
- The **hypothalamic–pituitary–thyroid axis** regulates general metabolic rate
- The **hypothalamic–pituitary–gonadal (or ovarian) axis** controls reproduction

Hypothalmic axes: hormones and functions				
Axis	Hypothalamic hormones	Pituitary hormones	Targets	Functions regulated
Hypothalamic–pituitary–adrenal	Corticotrophin-releasing hormone Vasopressin	Adrenocorticotrophic hormone	Adrenal gland ■ Glucocorticoid ■ Cortisol	Stress Digestion Immunity
Hypothalamic–pituitary–thyroid	Thyrotrophin-releasing hormone	Thyroid-stimulating hormone	Thyroid gland ■ Thyroxine ■ Tri-iodothyronine	Metabolism Growth Development
Hypothalamic–pituitary–gonadal (or ovarian)	Gonadotrophin-releasing hormone	Luteinising hormone Follicle-stimulating hormone	Gonads ■ Oestrogen ■ Testosterone	Menstrual cycles Ovarian cycles Spermatogenesis

Table 1.21 Hypothalamic axes: hormones and functions

The hypothalamus is connected to the pea-sized pituitary gland by the infundibulum, a stalk made up of axonal fibres. The main fibre pathway in the infundibulum is the hypothalamohypophyseal pathway.

The hypothalamohypophyseal pathway innervates the pituitary gland.

■ Signals to the anterior pituitary gland stimulate the release of hormones into the hypothalamic circulation, the hypophyseal portal system
■ Signals to the posterior pituitary gland stimulate the release of the hormones vasopressin and oxytocin directly into the systemic circulation

Once hormones are released into the circulation by the pituitary gland, they act on specific target organs to mediate behavioural changes.

Autonomic regulation

The hypothalamus controls the autonomic nervous system directly by acting on the sympathetic and parasympathetic pre-ganglionic neurones in the brainstem and spinal cord. It also indirectly influences the system by interacting with the brainstem nuclei that control organ function (see page 98). Therefore the hypothalamus has wide-ranging effects on the activity of the autonomic nervous system; these are vital for maintaining body function within optimal ranges.

Brainstem

Starter questions

Answers to the following questions are on page 116.

13. Why are the essential physiological functions controlled by the brainstem?
14. Why does sleep deprivation impair memory?

Originally described as the conduit between the brain and spinal cord, the brainstem is now known to be vital for survival. Minute areas of damage in the brainstem can have a devastating effect, because many of the key nuclei involved in the regulation of homeostasis and consciousness are located here. The brainstem also contains the nuclei of the cranial nerves and production sites for five of the main neurotransmitters.

- **the pons**, which is the middle, bulbous section of the brainstem
- **the medulla**, the funnel-shaped caudal section of the brainstem that extends to the spinal cord

The brainstem is connected to the cerebellum by peduncles (see page 64). The cavity between the brainstem and cerebellum forms the fourth ventricle, which terminates caudally at the obex (Latin, 'barrier').

Gross anatomy of the brainstem

The brainstem is situated in the posterior fossa of the skull, and connects the thalamus and the spinal cord. It has three parts (**Figure 1.34**). Rostral to caudal, these are:

- **the midbrain**, which lies directly underneath the thalamus and the third ventricle

Functional anatomy of the brainstem

The brainstem has a high concentration of functional centres that directly regulate various behaviours from respiration to bladder activity. It is the location of the nuclei of most of the cranial nerves, the functions of which include carrying sensory information and

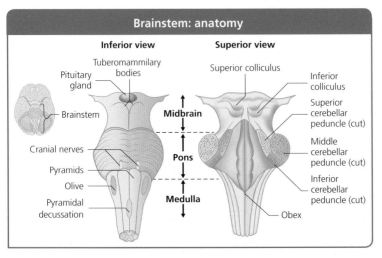

Brainstem: anatomy

Inferior view   Superior view

Tuberomammilary bodies — Pituitary gland — Brainstem — Cranial nerves — Pyramids — Olive — Pyramidal decussation — **Midbrain** — **Pons** — **Medulla**

Superior colliculus — Inferior colliculus — Superior cerebellar peduncle (cut) — Middle cerebellar peduncle (cut) — Inferior cerebellar peduncle (cut) — Obex

Figure 1.34 Anatomy of the brainstem.

controlling the muscles of the head and neck (see **Table 1.22** and page 100). Ascending sensory and descending motor tracts for the rest of the body pass through the brainstem, making this the most multifunctional area of the central nervous system.

Midbrain

The midbrain controls the visual and auditory reflexes. The two pairs of bumps on its ventral surface are the superior and inferior colliculi (**Figure 1.34**).

- **The superior colliculus** controls head movement towards visual stimuli
- **The inferior colliculus** controls head movement towards sounds

The midbrain has roles in eye movement and facial sensation. It contains the nuclei for cranial nerves III and IV, which help control eye movement, and part of the sensory nuclei of cranial nerve V (**Figure 1.35**; see page 103).

Damage to the midbrain often causes miosis (pinpoint pupils). Damage to cranial nerve III means that the parasympathetic signals that pass through this nerve are no longer able to dilate the pupils. In coma patients, pupil size indicates the physical level at which the brainstem has been damaged.

The midbrain also contains the red nucleus, from which the rubrospinal tracts arise (see page 88). These tracts control movement and muscle tone.

The substantia nigra (Latin, 'black substance') lies in the rostral midbrain. Because of its connections to the basal ganglia, it is a key area in the fine-tuning of motor control (see page 89). The substantia nigra appears black because it contains many dopaminergic neurones, which contain a dark pigment called neuromelanin.

Nuclei located in the brainstem		
Brainstem region	Nuclei [nerves]	Functions
Midbrain	Oculomotor [CN III]	■ Motor and autonomic control
	Accessory oculomotor (Edinger–Westphal) [CN III]	
	Trochlear [CN IV]	
	Trigeminal [CN V]	
	Red nucleus	
Pons	Trigeminal [CN V]	■ Motor and sensory control
	Abducens [CN VI]	■ Hearing and balance
	Facial [CN VII]	
	Vestibular [CN VIII]	
	Cochlear [CN VIII]	
Medulla	Trigeminal [CNV]	■ Motor, autonomic and sensory control
	Vestibular [CN VIII]	■ Hearing and balance
	Cochlear [CN VIII]	
	Nucleus ambiguus [CN IX, X]	
	Dorsal motor nucleus of vagus [CN X]	
	Hypoglossal [CN XII]	
Reticular formation within midbrain, pons and medulla	Raphe nuclei	■ Arousal and consciousness
	Locus coeruleus	■ Motivation
	Cuneiform nuclei	■ Integration
	Pedunculopontine nucleus	■ Motor and autonomic control

Table 1.22 Nuclei located within regions of the brainstem

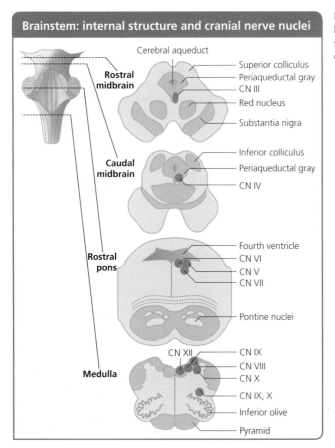

Brainstem: internal structure and cranial nerve nuclei

Cerebral aqueduct

Rostral midbrain
- Superior colliculus
- Periaqueductal gray
- CN III
- Red nucleus
- Substantia nigra

Caudal midbrain
- Inferior colliculus
- Periaqueductal gray
- CN IV

Rostral pons
- Fourth ventricle
- CN VI
- CN V
- CN VII
- Pontine nuclei

Medulla
- CN XII
- CN IX
- CN VIII
- CN X
- CN IX, X
- Inferior olive
- Pyramid

Figure 1.35 Cross sections of the brainstem showing its internal structure and and the locations of cranial nerve nuclei.

Pons

The pons contains the peduncles, three pairs of fibre bundles that connect the brainstem to the cerebellum (**Figure 1.34**; see page 64). The pons and cerebellum coordinate unconscious proprioception, i.e. the sense of the position and movement of the body, via these structures (see page 83).

The pons also has roles in facial sensation and eye movement, via activity in the nuclei for cranial nerves V and VI, respectively (**Figure 1.35**). It also houses the nuclei for cranial nerve VII, which controls facial movement, and cranial nerve VIII, which controls hearing and balance.

Medulla and medullary pyramids

The medulla contains paired regions called the pyramids (**Figure 1.34**). This is where many sensory and motor tracts decussate, i.e. cross from one side to the other. If there is damage to the motor and sensory tracts above the decussation, this causes deficits on the contralateral side of the body. This knowledge is helpful in identifying the site of motor and sensory lesions.

Dorsolateral to the pyramids are two olive-shaped prominences: the inferior olivary nuclei (see **Figure 1.34**). These nuclei are involved in motor control (see page 65) and hearing (see page 114).

On the dorsal aspect of the medulla, the sensory dorsal columns (large, long bundles of fibres that resemble columns) (see page 80) appear as two pairs of folds, the gracile and cuneate tubercles, running either side of the midline below the obex.

The nuclei for cranial nerves IX, X, XI, XII, and for parts of cranial nerves V, VII and VIII are in the medulla (**Figure 1.35**), making it a hub for the control of movement of the head and neck (see page 100).

The medulla also houses major nuclei controlling vital homeostasic functions, including respiration and cardiac control (see page 98).

Blood supply to the brainstem

The brainstem receives most of its blood supply via five arteries:

- **Two posterior cerebral arteries** supply the dorsal and lateral midbrain
- **The basilar artery** supplies the ventral and lateral midbrain and the medial pons
- **Two vertebral arteries** supply the ventral medulla

The cerebellar arteries supply the dorsal and lateral midbrain, pons and medulla. The anterior spinal arteries supply the medial medulla.

The brainstem is supplied by perforating vessels that penetrate the deep tissue.

> **Lacunar (lake-like) infarcts are small areas of infarction caused by blockage of the narrow perforating vessels supplying the brain.** Lacunar infarcts in the brainstem often have serious consequences, including coma and death, because of damage to the vital centres it contains.

Upper and lower regions of the brainstem differ in their venous drainage.

- The upper regions drain either into the basal vein and then to the great cerebral vein of Galen, or into the venous sinuses
- The lower regions drain into spinal veins or the venous sinuses

Each of these vessels feed into the jugular veins to carry blood from the brainstem back into the systemic circulation.

The reticular formation

The reticular formation is a collection of cells, nuclei and networks that lies in the brainstem and extends to the upper cervical regions of the spinal cord (**Figure 1.36**). The main nuclei of the reticular formation, and their functions, are listed in **Table 1.22**. It is not well defined structurally, but functionally it regulates arousal, alertness and consciousness.

It contains two main tracts.

- **The ascending reticular activating system** is poorly understood but contains tracts that control arousal, i.e. consciousness and the sleep-wake cycle, and alertness
- **The descending reticulospinal** tracts are well understood pathways that control movement (see page 59)

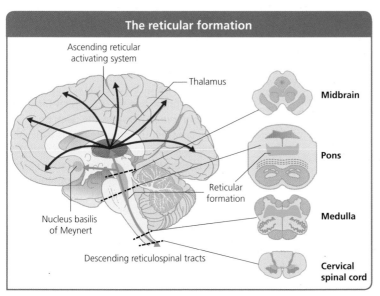

The reticular formation

Ascending reticular activating system

Thalamus

Midbrain

Pons

Reticular formation

Nucleus basilis of Meynert

Medulla

Descending reticulospinal tracts

Cervical spinal cord

Figure 1.36 The reticular formation. Sagittal view of the brain and cross sections of the brainstem showing the reticular formation and ascending and descending reticular tracts.

Control of the sleep–wake cycle

One of the main functions of the reticular formation is control of the normal daily pattern of sleep and wakefulness: the sleep–wake cycle.

Two neurotransmitters, histamine and acetylcholine, play major roles in control of the sleep–wake cycle. Histamine triggers activity in cholinergic neurones that project to the thalamus, thereby enhancing the activity of the glutamatergic neurones within it. This increases transmission through the thalamus to the cortex. The resulting free flow of information to the cortex results in consciousness, i.e. a high level of arousal and awareness of surroundings, and the ability to respond to them.

Histamine levels decrease during sleep. Lower levels of histamine mean that there is less activation of cholinergic neurones, and consequently less activation of glutamatergic neurones in the thalamus. This reduces the flow of information to the cortex, thereby reducing the level of consciousness.

In paradoxical sleep, also called REM sleep after the rapid eye movements that characterise it, further decreases in histamine levels will also reduce activity in serotonergic and noradrenergic (norepinephrinergic) neurones in the reticular formation, which normally dampen (inhibit) cholinergic activity. As a result, cholinergic input to the thalamus increases, triggering the cortical activity that produces REM sleep and dreams.

> Histamine has a major role in maintaining arousal as well as activating inflammatory responses. Therefore antihistamine treatments for allergies often cause drowsiness.

Functional centres of the brainstem

In evolutionary terms, the brainstem is one of the oldest regions of the central nervous system. It is vital for life because it contains nuclei that control respiration, cardiovascular function, bladder function, nausea and vomiting, and responses to pain.

Respiration

The main sites for the generation of respiratory patterns are in the medulla. Two main groups of nuclei are responsible.

- **The rostral medullary group** contains inspiratory neurones, which trigger inhalation
- **The ventral medullary group** contains inspiratory and expiratory neurones (the latter inhibit inspiratory neurones and are used only during forced exhalation, with normal exhalation being passive, resulting from relaxation of the intercostal muscles)
- This group of nuclei also includes the **pre-Bötzinger complex**, the main pacemakers (a group of cells that generates a rhythmic pattern of activity) for respiration, which activate inspiratory neurones

The pace and depth of respiration are controlled by two regions in the pons.

- **The pneumotaxic centre** (nucleus parabrachialis) in the rostral pons limits inspiratory volume by switching off inspiratory neurones in the medulla, enables forced exhalation by activating expiratory neurones in the medulla, and sets the respiratory rate
- **The apneustic centre** in the caudal pons increases activity in inspiratory neurones, thereby prolonging inspiration

Control of respiration

Inspiratory neurones activated by afferent input from cranial nerves IX and X send information to C3–C5 which form the phrenic nerve (a nerve in the neck and thorax), to contract the diaphragm, as well as to T3–T6, to contract the intercostal muscles. These movements result in inspiration.

Expansion of the lungs by inspiration triggers stretch receptors, signals from which are carried by cranial nerve X to the medulla. Here, the signals excite expiratory neurones and inhibit inspiratory neurones, thereby causing forced exhalation.

In normal exhalation, the pneumotaxic centre inhibits the apneustic centre. This stops the activation of inspiratory neurons, thereby terminating inspiration and relaxing the intercostal muscles.

Cardiovascular function

The heart has its own pacemakers to maintain constant activity, but it also relies on brainstem reflexes to adjust the vasculature to control blood pressure, and the autonomic nervous system to fine-tune the pace and strength of the heartbeat (see page 96).

The medulla has two main regions responsible for cardiovascular control.

■ The nucleus of the solitary tract regulates parasympathetic control of heart rate, via cranial nerve X, and adjusts activity descending to the spinal sympathetic preganglionic neurones
■ The rostral ventrolateral medulla contains groups of **cells known as presympathetic neurones**, which control the spinal sympathetic preganglionic neurones to maintain blood pressure

The nucleus of the solitary tract sends cardiorespiratory information to the hypothalamus via ascending reticular tracts. Next, this information is integrated with forebrain and limbic system information to link heart rate and respiratory rate to cognitive and emotional state. Output from the hypothalamus then adjusts heart and respiratory rate via the brainstem centres.

Bladder function

One of the main centres of bladder control is in the pons: the pontine micturition centre. This controls the spinal circuits and muscle tone of the sphincters that regulate bladder activity (see page 96). Its activity can be altered by the frontal micturition centre in the frontal lobe, which provides conscious control of bladder function.

The frontal micturition centre decides whether urination is appropriate and sends information to the motor cortex to control the external sphincters. Relaxation of these sphincters allows urination, while the frontal micturition centre simultaneously sends signals to the pontine micturation centre to initiate the bladder reflex, i.e. contraction of the bladder muscle to expel urine.

Defecation

Defecation, like bladder function, is controlled by centres in both the frontal lobe and the brainstem. The defecation centres lie adjacent to the bladder control centres.

Movement of faeces from the colon to the rectum activates the defecation reflex, i.e. relaxation of the internal rectal sphincter to enable defecation. Faecal movement also triggers a spontaneous contraction of the external sphincter, which is under conscious control from the frontal defecation centre.

Once the decision that it is appropriate to defecate is made, signals are sent from the frontal defecation centre to the brainstem defecation centre, which controls the spinal circuits underlying the defecation reflex. The rectal musculature responds by relaxing further and straightening to ease the passage of the faeces.

The frontal centre then signals to the motor cortex to relax the external sphincter. Relaxation enables the waves of peristalsis to push the faeces out of the body.

Nausea and vomiting

The area postrema is a region of the medulla; it is next to the fourth ventricle. Here, the blood–brain barrier is incomplete, so it can detect changes in circulating substances (see page 32). The area postrema contains the chemoreceptor trigger zone, which is sensitive to toxins and drugs circulating in the blood and cerebrospinal fluid. Detection of such substances activates the vomit centre to trigger nausea and vomiting reflexes.

Activation of the vomiting reflex causes the gut to contract forcibly. Thus the gut contents, and the potentially toxic substances it contains, are expelled from the body to prevent damage.

Pain

The brainstem contains areas that control pain sensations, including the:

- periaqueductal grey
- rostral ventral medulla
- locus coeruleus

The periaqueductal grey, a region of grey matter around the cerebral aqueduct in the midbrain, receives information from cortical and limbic regions. It controls behavioural responses to pain by increasing activity in the descending tracts that inhibits pain sensation in the spinal cord, as well as by increasing reflex motor activity to facilitate a rapid escape from the painful situation.

The rostral ventral medulla contains raphe nuclei (Greek: raphe, 'seam') (**Figure 1.37**). These nuclei send signals along their descending serotonin- and opioid-containing projections to inhibit pain transmission in the spinal cord.

The locus coeruleus sends descending noradrenergic projections to the spinal cord. Their activation inhibits pain sensation.

The periaqueductal grey and raphe nuclei contain high numbers of opioid receptors. Therefore these areas are the probable targets for analgesics such as codeine and morphine.

Neurotransmitter production

Five key neurotransmitters have their main sites of production in the brainstem (**Figure 1.37**).

- **Serotonin** is produced in raphe nuclei throughout the brainstem, and regulate emotions and mood, appetite, and arousal and alertness
- **Dopamine** is produced in the midbrain, in the substantia nigra and ventral tegmental area, a broad region of the brainstem (**Figure 1.37**), and regulates cognition, reward, motivation, attention and motor control
- **Noradrenaline (norepinephrine)** is produced in the pons and medulla, in the locus coeruleus and lateral tegmental area, respectively, and regulates arousal, mood and motor activity
- **Acetylcholine** is produced in the pedunculopontine tegmental nuclei and laterodorsal tegmental nuclei, on the midbrain–pons border, and regulates arousal and motor function; the nucleus basilis of Meynert in the forebrain supplies acetylcholine to the cortex

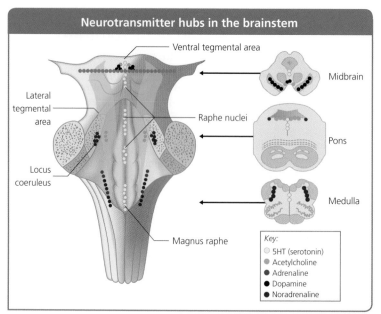

Neurotransmitter hubs in the brainstem

Ventral tegmental area

Midbrain

Lateral tegmental area

Raphe nuclei

Pons

Locus coeruleus

Medulla

Magnus raphe

Key:
- 5HT (serotonin)
- Acetylcholine
- Adrenaline
- Dopamine
- Noradrenaline

Figure 1.37
Major sites of neurotransmitter production in the brainstem (neurotransmitter hubs), shown in a superior view and cross sections.

- **Histamine** is produced by many cells found across the brainstem in the reticular formation, which controls alertness and arousal; it is also produced by the tuberomammillary bodies (see **Table 1.20**) of the hypothalamus

Axons carry neurotransmitters to higher cortical, cerebellar and spinal areas, where they are released to produce specific effects.

Cerebellum

Starter questions

Answers to the following questions are on page 116.

15. Why does the cerebellum have so many folds?
16. Why does alcohol cause staggering, slurred speech and personality changes?

The cerebellum (Latin, 'little brain') maintains the body's balance and position. This is achieved by integrating motor control, proprioception and motor learning.

Gross anatomy of the cerebellum

The cerebellum sits in the posterior fossa. It is separated from the cerebrum by the tentorium cerebelli, the tough septa formed by folding of the dura mater (see page 27).

It is attached to the dorsal brainstem by three pairs of peduncles: superior, middle and inferior. The peduncles are large bundles of fibres running to and from the cerebellum.

> **The cerebellum is only a tenth the size of the cerebrum**. However, it contains more neurones than the rest of the brain.

Like the cerebrum, the cerebellum has many folds, called folia because they are leaf-shaped in cross-section (**Figure 1.38**). However, compared with the cerebral gyri the cerebellar folds are thinner and more compressed; these features enable greater folding. This enables a huge number of cells to be compacted into a very small space; this close proximity allows the rapid processing and integration of neuronal activity needed to enable movements to be rapidly altered while being performed.

The cerebellum is separated into two hemispheres along its midline. The division is marked by a structure called the vermis (Latin, 'worm'), which controls balance and the position of the trunk. The cerebral

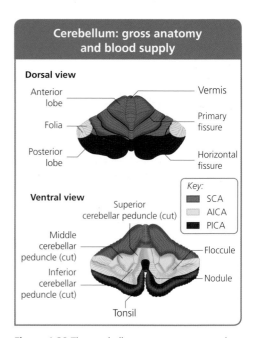

Cerebellum: gross anatomy and blood supply

Dorsal view

Anterior lobe — — Vermis

Folia — — Primary fissure

Posterior lobe — — Horizontal fissure

Key:
- SCA
- AICA
- PICA

Ventral view

Superior cerebellar peduncle (cut)

Middle cerebellar peduncle (cut) — — Floccule

Inferior cerebellar peduncle (cut) — — Nodule

Tonsil

Figure 1.38 The cerebellum: gross anatomy and blood supply. SCA, superior cerebellar arteries; AICA, anterior inferior cerebellar arteries; PICA, posterior inferior cerebellar arteries.

hemispheres are divided into anterior and posterior lobes. These are separated structurally by a large fold, the primary fissure, and nominally into lateral and medial aspects (**Figure 1.38**).

The anterior aspect of the cerebellum contains the tonsils and flocculonodular lobe (**Figure 1.38**). The tonsils are vestigial, functionally redundant, organs. The flocculonodular lobe , comprising the floccule and nodule, has roles in balance and the vestibulo-ocular reflex (see page 114).

Excessive intracranial pressure can force the tonsils through the foramen magnum. This tonsillar herniation can compress vital cardiorespiratory centres in the medulla, and without rapid treatment usually leads to death.

Structural organisation of the cerebellum

The cerebellum consists of cortical grey matter and subcortical white matter, in which the deep cerebellar nuclei are embedded (**Figure 1.39**).

The cerebellar cortex

The cerebellar cortex comprises three layers of grey matter.

- The molecular layer is outermost and contains many inhibitory interneurones as well as neurones called parallel fibres, which communicate with the dendrites of another type of neurone, Purkinje cells
- The **Purkinje layer**, in the middle, contains mostly Purkinje bodies, and is the main site of integration in the cerebellum; the cells send projections to the deep cerebellar nuclei
- The **granule cell layer**, which is innermost, contains granule cells, the projections of which ascend to the molecular layer and then run horizontally through this layer, forming the parallel fibres

Cerebellar white matter

The cortex receives input via two types of fibre in the white matter (**Figure 1.39**):

- **mossy fibres**, so named because they resemble moss, enter the cerebellum from the spinal cord and brainstem, then communicate with the deep cerebellar nuclei and granule cells

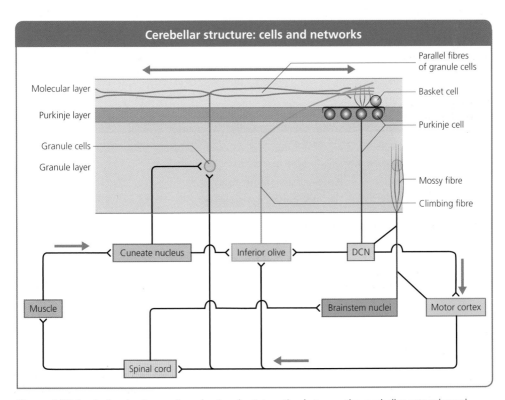

Figure 1.39 Cerebellar structure: cells and networks. Interaction between the cerebellar networks and brainstem nuclei modifies activity from the motor cortex to fine-tune movement. Arrows denote direction of travel through network. DCN: deep cerebellar nuclei.

- **climbing fibres**, so named because they ascend through the layers using other fibres and cells as scaffolding, like climbing plants, arise in the olivary nuclei in the brainstem and contact communicate with the Purkinje cell dendrites in the molecular layer

The cells and fibres form networks allowing rapid integration and processing of information, and they generate output that passes via the white matter to the deep cerebellar nuclei (**Figure 1.39**).

Deep cerebellar nuclei

The deep cerebellar nuclei send information from the cerebellar cortex to areas that contribute to motor control to fine-tune movement. There are four groups of deep cerebellar nuclei.

- **The dentate nuclei** receive input from lateral cerebellar regions, and their output adjusts voluntary motor control
- **The emboliform nuclei** receive input from intermediate regions, and their output adjusts voluntary motor control
- **The fastigial nuclei** receive input from the vermis, and their output adjusts balance and body position

- **The globose nuclei** receive input from intermediate regions, and their output adjusts voluntary motor control

Functional organisation of the cerebellum

The functional organisation of the cerebellum, like that of the cerebrum, has been mapped: specific areas control certain regions of the body, somatotopic organisation. However, the maps of the cerebellum are duplicated and distorted across the cerebellar surface; they are fractured somatotopic maps.

The cerebellar maps show that:

- the anterior and posterior cerebellar lobes control distal limb and head movements
- the anterior portions of the posterior lobes integrate vestibular information, thereby controlling balance
- the vermis controls movement of the trunk and proximal limbs

Clinically, damage to the right side of the cerebellum affects the right side of the body, because the tracts enter the cerebellum on the ipsilateral (same) side.

Cerebellar signs and symptoms		
Mnemonic	Sign or symptom	Feature
D	Dysdiadochokinesia	Abnormal rapid-alternating movement
	Dysmetria	Past-pointing or overshooting
	Dysrhythmia	Abnormal timing of movement
A	Ataxia	Appendicular: abnormal movement in extremities
		Truncal ataxia: wide-based gait and unsteadiness
N	Nystagmus	Variable nystagmus (may change direction)
	Nausea and vomiting	Indicates vestibular instability
I	Intention tremor	Slow tremor increased with activity or posture maintenance
S	Slurred speech	Slow, uncoordinated speech, like that in cases of alcohol intoxication
	Scanning dysarthria	Irregular rate and volume of speech
H	Hypotonia	Decreased tone, often with pendular (swinging) reflexes
	Heel–shin test	Test of coordination for ataxia
	'Head spin'	Feeling of rotational movement indicates vertigo

Table 1.23 Signs and symptoms of damage to the cerebellum

Cerebellar damage causes various characteristic symptoms and signs (**Table 1.23**), which relate to the structural organisation of the area. For example, damage to the vermis produces truncal ataxia, a wide-based staggering gait, whereas impaired balance, postural instability and uncontrolled eye movements develop if the flocculonodular lobe is damaged (see page 64).

Blood supply to the cerebellum

The cerebellum is supplied by three pairs of arteries (**Figure 1.38**).

■ The superior cerebellar arteries branch from the basilar artery
■ The anterior inferior cerebellar arteries branch from the basilar artery
■ The posterior inferior cerebellar arteries branch from the vertebral arteries

> **Insufficiency in the vertebral and basilar arteries**, from which the cerebellar arteries arise, accounts for a quarter of strokes.

Role of the cerebellum in motor control

Information about body position, muscle tone and dynamics, terminates in the cerebellum. Here, it is used to fine-tune coordination and correct errors during movement. The cerebellum also receives input from the following (see page 65):

■ spinal cord via the spinocerebellar tracts
■ cortex via the pontocerebellar tracts
■ vestibular organs via the vestibular nuclei in the brainstem

Together with the basal ganglia, the cerebellum modifies the patterns of cortical activity that control movement; this is done via a system of re-entrant loops (see page 89). Information from the motor cortex passes through the cerebellar circuitry (see page 65), where it is adjusted in response to proprioceptive information arriving at the cerebellum.

Once modified, the information is returned to the motor cortex for delivery to the muscle groups producing the specific movement.

Error correction

Error correction is the adjustment of motor function to ensure accurate movements, for example by preventing over-reaching or stopping short when trying to touch something. The cerebellum acts as a comparator, comparing the planned activity to the actual movement being produced, and rapidly corrects any errors.

■ Information regarding the planned motor activity arrives from the motor cortices via the mossy fibres
■ Information about the actual motor activity being produced is carried to the cerebellum by the climbing fibres
■ Both mossy and climbing fibres communicate with the Purkinje cells, the patterns of motor activity are compared, and information regarding any adjustments required is sent to the motor cortex

> **Alcohol intoxication decreases blood flow to the cerebellum, reducing its function.** This results in a staggering gait, exaggerated gesticulations and slurred speech.

Procedural learning

The cerebellum controls procedural (or motor) learning: this occurs when repetition of motor patterns leads to improved performance over time, as when learning to ride a bicycle. Procedural learning is achieved by gradually eliminating errors and fine-tuning activity patterns by comparing required and actual behaviours. Eventually, recall of the correct motor pattern is so rapid and efficient that little further adjustment is required and the movement appears automatic.

One way that procedural learning can occur is via a type of synaptic plasticity in which long-term depression of neuronal activity in incorrect or inefficient pathways makes it more likely that activation of correct or efficient pathways will occur.

Vertebral column and spinal cord

Starter questions

Answers to the following questions are on page 117.

17. Does the spinal cord only transmit impulses?
18. Where do upper and lower motor neurones meet?

The vertebral column (colloquially the 'spine' or 'backbone'):

■ encases the spinal cord
■ supports and maintains head and body movement
■ forms the attachment and articulation (movement) points for the ribs and pelvic girdle

The spinal cord (pages 71–76) is a column of neural tracts. These carry sensory and motor information into and out of the central nervous system, so the spinal cord functions as the interface between brain and body.

Vertebral column

The vertebral column is about 70 cm long in men and 60 cm long in women. It consists of 33 vertebrae (**Figure 1.40**):

■ 7 cervical vertebrae, articulating joints in the neck region
■ 12 thoracic vertebrae, articulating joints in the thorax
■ 5 lumbar vertebrae, articulating joints in the abdominal region
■ 5 sacral vertebrae, fused to form the sacrum in the pelvic region
■ 4 coccygeal vertebrae, fused to form the coccyx or tailbone

The vertebrae are held together by a complex arrangement of ligaments and musculature (see page 71). This arrangement gives the column flexibility to move, rotate and pivot around the cord without damaging it.

Four natural curvatures produce the column's characteristic 'S' shape.

Viewed laterally, the cervical and lumbar regions are concave posteriorly, and the thoracic and sacral regions are convex laterally (see **Figure 1.40**). Deformities in spinal curvature include:

■ **Kyphosis**: an exaggerated outward curvature, usually thoracic and leading to a hunched back
■ **Lordosis** (swayback): an exaggerated inward curvature, mainly in the lumbar region
■ **Scoliosis**: a lateral curvature, resulting in a sideways 'S' or 'C' shape

The vertebrae

Every vertebral bone comprises a vertebral body and a vertebral arch (**Figure 1.40**). However, there are differences in the detailed structure of vertebrae at different spinal levels (**Figure 1.41**).

The vertebral body is a disc-shaped bony formation in the anterior portion of the spine. The vertebral bodies are stacked in a column, with a cartilaginous disc between each body and the next (see below). Together, the vertebral bodies are the spine's main weight-bearing component. The vertebral arch is formed from two pedicles (left and right), which connect the body to two laminae (left and right), flat sections of bone that join to form the apex of the arch.

The vertebral foramen is formed by the body and arch, and contains the spinal cord. The spinal nerves exit underneath the pedicle on either side, through the gap between adjacent vertebrae, i.e. the intervertebral foramen (see **Figure 1.42**).

Vertebral processes

The vertebral bones have a number of processes. These are bony structures projecting outwards from the vertebrae, and increase the stability of joints and support their articulation (**Figures 1.40** and **1.41**).

- **The spinous process** is formed by fusion of the laminae, and serves as an attachment point for musculature; cervical vertebrae have bifid (two-point) spinous processes, whereas lumbar vertebrae are large and strong with stumpy processes (**Table 1.24**)
- **Two transverse processes** arise at the point of fusion of the laminae and pedicles, and are attachment points for musculature
- **Two superior articulating processes** form joints with the vertebra immediately above
- **Two inferior articulating processes** form joints with the vertebra immediately below

> The pars interarticularis, or pars, is the region of bone between the inferior and superior articular processes. Hangman's fracture is a bilateral fracture of the pars in the cervical vertebrae. Stress fractures (spondylolysis) of the pars are common sports injuries. They are especially associated with sports requiring repetitive rotation, compression or extension, such as shot-put, javelin and weightlifting.

Facets

The facets are small articular surfaces on the vertebral bones. They are covered in cartilage, enabling smooth rotational movement at the joints. The facet on the superior articular process of one vertebra faces the facet on the inferior articular process of the vertebra above, forming a facet joint called the zygapophyseal joint (**Figure 1.41**). Thoracic vertebrae also have facets on their vertebral bodies and transverse processes; these articulate with the ribs.

Intervertebral discs

The intervertebral discs lie between the bodies of adjacent vertebrae. They are elastic, flexible and compressible discs of cartilage that allow multidirectional movement of the column and act as shock absorbers.

Each disc comprises an outer ring, called the

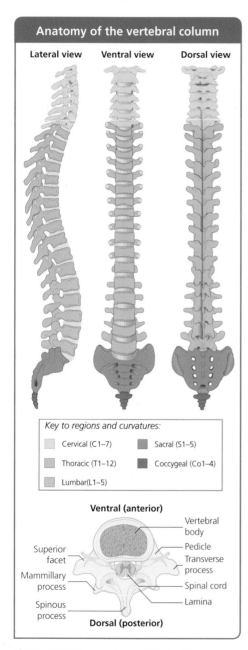

Anatomy of the vertebral column

Lateral view Ventral view Dorsal view

Key to regions and curvatures:

- Cervical (C1–7)
- Thoracic (T1–12)
- Lumbar(L1–5)
- Sacral (S1–5)
- Coccygeal (Co1–4)

Ventral (anterior)

Vertebral body
Pedicle
Transverse process
Spinal cord
Lamina

Superior facet
Mammillary process
Spinous process

Dorsal (posterior)

Figure 1.40 Gross anatomy of the vertebral column. The spinal cord runs down the spinal column within the vertebral foramen, as shown in the superior view of a lumbar vertebra in the lower part of the figure.

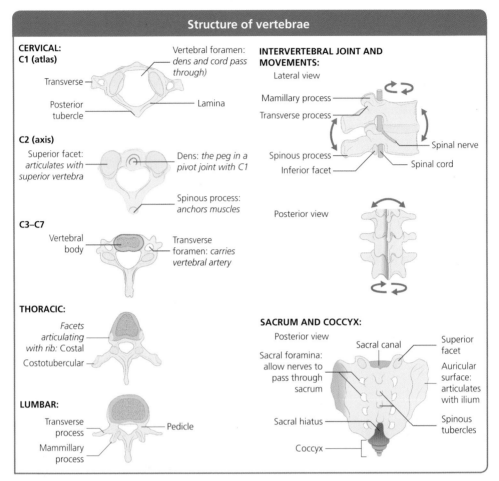

Structure of vertebrae

CERVICAL:
C1 (atlas)

Transverse

Posterior tubercle

Vertebral foramen: dens and cord pass through)

Lamina

C2 (axis)

Superior facet: articulates with superior vertebra

Dens: *the peg in a pivot joint with C1*

Spinous process: *anchors muscles*

C3–C7

Vertebral body

Transverse foramen: *carries vertebral artery*

THORACIC:

Facets articulating with rib: Costal

Costotubercular

LUMBAR:

Transverse process

Pedicle

Mammillary process

INTERVERTEBRAL JOINT AND MOVEMENTS:
Lateral view

Mamillary process

Transverse process

Spinous process

Inferior facet

Spinal nerve

Spinal cord

Posterior view

SACRUM AND COCCYX:

Posterior view

Sacral foramina: allow nerves to pass through sacrum

Sacral canal

Superior facet

Auricular surface: articulates with ilium

Sacral hiatus

Spinous tubercles

Coccyx

Figure 1.41 The vertebrae. The superior views (left) show the differences in structure at the different spinal levels. The structure of the vertebrae, intervertebral disc and intervertebral facet joints allows spinal movement in three axes, shown for lumbar vertebrae here (right). See also Figure 11.9, showing facet joints on CT.

Vertebral characteristics

Feature	Cervical vertebrae	Thoracic vertebrae	Lumbar vertebrae
Number of vertebrae	7	12	5
Vertebral body	Small	Medium	Large
Intervertebral discs	Thick	Thin	Very thick
Spinous process	Thin and bifid	Long and thick	Short and stumpy
		Project anteriorly	Project posteriorly
Transverse process	Small	Large	Large and stumpy
Foramina	Vertebral and 2 transverse	Vertebral	Vertebral

Table 1.24 Vertebral characteristics

annulus fibrosus, and a pulpy centre, known as the nucleus pulposus.

- the annulus fibrosus is made of tough fibrocartilage
- the nucleus pulposus consists of a highly elastic, soft, gel-like substance containing collagen

A herniated disc, colloquially known as a slipped disc, occurs when the annulus fibrosis ruptures and the nucleus pulposis it contains is pushed through the opening. Disk herniation compresses spinal nerves roots (see page 157).

Musculature

Muscles of the vertebral column are classified into three main groups with overlapping functions.

- The splenius muscles (splenius capitis and splenius cervicis) move the head at the neck
- The erector spinae group (iliocostalis, longissimus and spinalis) are the main extensor muscles
- The transversospinalis muscle group (semispinalis capitis, semispinalis cervicis, semispinalis thoracis, multifidus and rotators) rotate and extend the vertebral column

Ligaments

Tough but flexible ligaments connect the vertebral bones to stabilise and control vertebral movement by limiting extension, flexion and rotation.

- The anterior longitudinal ligament runs the length of the column along the anterior aspect of the vertebral column
- The posterior longitudinal and supraspinous ligaments run the length of the column along the posterior aspect of the vertebral bodies and spinous processes
- The ligamentum flavum connects the laminae of adjacent vertebrae
- Interspinous ligaments connect the spinous processes of adjacent vertebrae
- Intertransverse ligaments connect the transverse processes of adjacent vertebrae

Additional small ligaments connect the bones at the zygapophyseal joint.

Spinal fractures generally result from excessive extension, flexion or rotation of the column. Compression fractures result from collapse of the weight-bearing vertebral body; they commonly occur in patients with osteoporosis.

Spinal cord

The spinal cord commences at the caudal end of the medulla. It projects through the foramen magnum and runs for 40–50 cm down within the vertebral column. In adults, the cord terminates at the L1–L2 vertebral level (see page 25), in children it terminates at the L3-L4 level.

The cord has five regions, the first four of which are each subdivided into a number of segments (see **Figure 1.7**):

- cervical: C1–C8
- thoracic: T1–T12
- lumbar: L1–L5
- sacral: S1–S5
- conus medullaris: Co1

Each segment houses one pair of peripheral (spinal) nerves. The terminal segment, the conus medullaris, contains a further pair, the coccygeal nerves.

The spinal cord is shorter than the vertebral column. The spinal cord has two regions of enlargement: the cervical enlargement (C5–T1) and the lumbosacral enlargement (L1–S3). These contain nerves to the limbs, which require increased sensory and motor innervation compared with the trunk.

The spinal cord is shorter than the vertebral column. Despite this discrepancy, the paired spinal nerves originating from each segment exit at the vertebral level from which they originated during development (see page 25).

Nerves travelling to lower lumbar levels and below form the cauda equina (Latin, 'horse's tail') as each one courses within the subarachnoid space from the cord segment from which it originates to the vertebral level at which it exits from the spine.

Environment of the spinal cord

A stable local environment is provided by the cerebrospinal fluid and vasculature, with physical protection supplied by the vertebral column.

Meninges and cerebrospinal fluid

The cord is surrounded by the three meningeal layers: the dura mater, the arachnoid mater and the pia mater (see page 27). The dura mater is separated from the vertebral column by layers of fat and connective tissue. These form the epidural space (**Figure 1.42**), which is commonly used as an injection site for delivering pain-relieving drugs and administering local anaesthetic to the lower half of the body.

> **Epidural injections are carried out at higher spinal levels (L1–L2) than lumbar puncture (L3–L4 or below).** This is because epidural injections do not cross the dura mater and are less likely than lumbar puncture to damage the spinal cord and nerves.

The spinal cord terminates at the L1–L2 level, but the dura mater and arachnoid mater extend to the S2–S3 level. Cerebrospinal fluid flows in the subarachnoid space, between the arachnoid mater and the pia mater, accumulating in the lumbar cistern (see page 30). The lumbar cistern is accessed during lumbar puncture.

In the meningeal sac (the fluid-filled cavity formed by the subarachnoid space), the spinal cord is suspended in the cerebrospinal fluid by segmental denticulate ligaments projecting from the pia mater to the dura mater.

The cord is tethered from the conus medullaris to the coccyx by the filum terminale, an extension of the pia mater.

Blood supply

The bulk of the spinal cord, i.e. its ventral (anterior) and lateral regions, are supplied by perforating vessels originating from the anterior spinal artery, which itself arises from the vertebral arteries (**Figure 1.43**). At the cervical to upper thoracic levels, the anterior spinal artery is supplied by branches of the vertebral arteries; at the lower thoracic and lumbar levels, it is supplied by radicular branches arising from the descending aorta.

The cord between the dorsal roots and down to the central canal is supplied by the two posterior spinal arteries, which arise from the vertebral and posterior inferior cerebellar arteries.

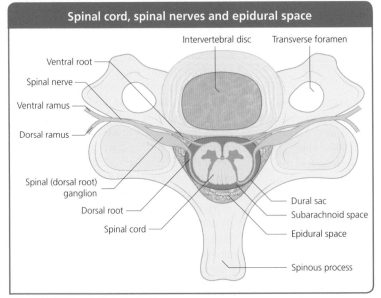

Spinal cord, spinal nerves and epidural space

- Intervertebral disc
- Transverse foramen
- Ventral root
- Spinal nerve
- Ventral ramus
- Dorsal ramus
- Spinal (dorsal root) ganglion
- Dorsal root
- Spinal cord
- Dural sac
- Subarachnoid space
- Epidural space
- Spinous process

Figure 1.42 The environment of the spinal cord, showing a superior view of the spinal nerves and the epidural space. The presence of transverse foramina make this instantly recognisable as a cervical cervical vertebra.

Blood supply of the spinal cord

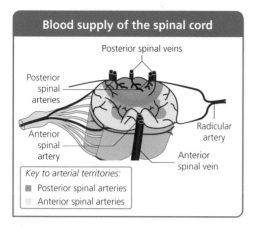

Figure 1.43 Blood supply of the spinal cord.

Ventral and dorsal supplies form a network around the cord.

The radicular arteries that supply the lower regions of the spinal cord are segmental medullary arteries. Segmental medullary arteries arise from the aorta and enter the vertebral column to supply the spinal meninges and supplement the supply to the spinal cord. The radicular arteries include the:

- thoracic radicular artery
- great radicular artery (of Adamkiewicz)
- ascending sacral arteries

Internal structure of the spinal cord

The cord in cross-section is 1.0–1.5 cm in diameter and comprises grey matter surrounded by white matter (**Figure 1.44**). The white matter contains the axons of the ascending and descending tracts. Grey matter contains the neuronal cell bodies and intrinsic spinal circuitry. The grey matter is butterfly-shaped and divided into three pairs of function-specific horns (**Table 1.25** and **Figure 1.44**).

- The dorsal, or posterior, horns carry information on sensation
- The ventral, or anterior, horns carry motor output
- The lateral horns, or intermediolateral columns, carry autonomic output

> **Immediately after severe trauma involving the spinal cord there is often spinal shock, a complete loss of function below the spinal level affected.** The cord recovers gradually, over days to months, and then shows the characteristic patterns of dysfunction depending on the region of damage (see page 450).

Laminae of the spinal cord

Region	Lamina(e)	Nucleus or nuclei	Function(s)
Dorsal horn	I	Marginal zone*	Sensory (mixed)
	II	Substantia gelatinosa	Sensory (mixed)
	III and IV	Nucleus proprius	Sensory (mixed)
	V	Neck of dorsal horn	Proprioception
	VI	Ventral dorsal horn	Proprioception
	VII	Nucleus dorsalis and intermediolateral column	Autonomic
Anterior horn	VIII	Medial (motor neurones) and spinal commissural cells	Motor
	IX	Motor neurones	Motor
Central zone	X	Substantia grisea centralis	Sensory

*The substantia gelatinosa often includes lamina I cells, because of difficulties distinguishing myelinated lamina I regions from dorsal root inputs.

Table 1.25 Laminae of the spinal cord

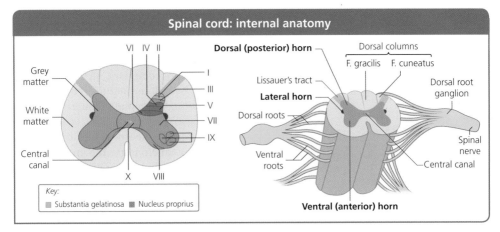

Figure 1.44 Internal anatomy of the spinal cord. The grey matter comprises three 'horns': the dorsal (posterior) horn carrying sensory fibres, the ventral (anterior) horn carrying motor fibres and the lateral horn carrying fibres of the sympathetic division of the autonomic nervous system.

Regional organisation

Grey matter and white matter differ in their distribution through the cord, which reflects the different sensory, motor and autonomic requirements at each spinal level.

The cervical and lumbar enlargements contain a substantial amount of grey matter in both dorsal and anterior horns, because of the large amount of input and output required to control the limbs.

In thoracic regions, the lateral horns are pronounced because the bulk of the sympathetic innervation arises here, whereas the anterior horns, containing motor neurones, are greatly reduced.

Grey matter dominates the sacral regions, because minimal input ascends from these levels. However, cervical regions have a large proportion of white matter, including ascending tracks from the body and descending tracks to the lower levels of the cord.

Laminar organisation

The grey matter of the cord is divided into functional nuclei. These divisions parallel an older classification, Rexed's laminae, which identifies layers I–X according to cyto-architectural composition. The names are used interchangeably (see **Table 1.25** and **Figure 1.44**).

Interneurones located in the laminae play a huge role in shaping activity as it travels through the grey matter. For example, inhibitory interneurones in laminae I and II, i.e. the substantia gelatinosa, can reduce pain sensation by preventing transmission of pain signals to the brain.

Spinal nerves

Spinal nerves are mixed; they carry different types of information. Sensory information is carried to sensory neurones in each dorsal horn via projections into the ipsilateral dorsal root, and motor output is carried from motor neurones in each anterior horn via projections into the ipsilateral ventral root (**Figure 1.42**). Signals from each lateral horn exit the cord via autonomic nerves in the ipsilateral anterior horn (see page 95).

The cell bodies of the sensory neurones form a cluster, the dorsal root ganglion, just before the afferent nerves enter the spinal cord at the dorsal horn on each side.

Each spinal segment, for example T2, provides one pair of spinal nerves. These cross the subarachnoid space and exit the vertebral column through the intervertebral foramen as peripheral nerves.

Nerve plexuses

On exiting the vertebral column, most peripheral nerves branch and join with surrounding nerves to form plexuses (**Figure 1.45**). The exceptions are the thoracic

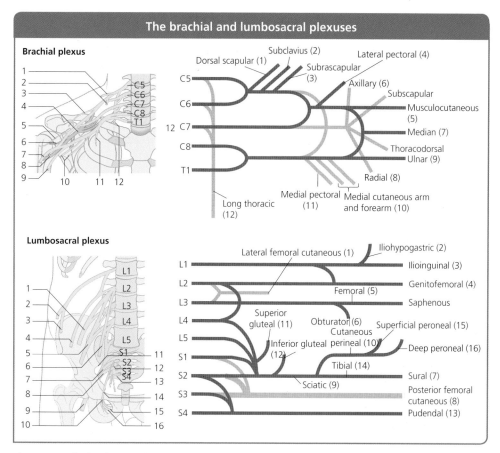

Figure 1.45 The brachial and lumbosacral plexuses.

nerves, T2–T11, i.e. the intercostal nerves. The two largest plexuses are the brachial and lumbosacral plexuses.

- **The brachial plexus** contains nerves C5–T1 and innervates the neck, shoulders, arms and upper trunk
- **The lumbosacral plexus** contains nerves L1–S4 and innervates the lower back and abdomen, genitals and legs

Functions of the spinal cord

The spinal cord is not only a conduit that links the brain and periphery. It is actively involved in many processes, including reflexes, motor coordination and sensation.

Reflex generation

Intrinsic spinal circuitry generates reflex activity. This ranges from classic deep tendon reflexes (see page 91) to autonomic reflexes (see page 92).

Intrinsic pattern generation

Coordination of activity in the spinal cord may generate patterns of activity strong enough to drive functional circuits. For example, experiments show that in some animals spinal circuits generate walking movements in the legs even in the absence of a head.

Network synchronisation

To coordinate activity, neuronal activity in networks often occurs in patterns, with synchronised firing. Synchronised activity in the spinal cord can be adjusted by cells within it, for example inhibitory interneurones. This ability indicates a level of plasticity and control independent of input from higher control centres. One example is the crossed extensor reflexes (see page 91), in which coordination of excitatory and inhibitory motor output in both spinal hemispheres is required to produce counterbalancing and complementary activity in the legs.

Control of spinal function

Spinal nerve activity, including reflexes, is modified by various factors, including input from higher centres. An example of this phenomenon is inhibition of the reflexes by the descending tracts (see page 88).

Crosstalk between afferent inputs to the spinal cord, in which activity in one neurone is detected by and responded to by another, like crossed wires, can also modify neuronal activity. For example, referred pain results from crosstalk between autonomic and somatic input (see page 79).

Somatosensory system

Starter questions

The answer to the following question is on page 117.

19. Why do people feel pain?

The ability to sense change in the internal and external environments is vital for survival. The sensory system enables the rapid detection, transmission and interpretation of such changes.

Organisation of sensation

Sensation is divided into two categories.

- **Somatic sensation** (Greek: soma, 'body') is the general sensation of pain, temperature, touch, pressure, vibration and proprioceptive information
- **Special senses** require specialised sensory organs to detect specific modalities (see page 107)

Sensory receptors

Sensation is detected by sensory receptors, which transduce (transform) physical signals into electrical signals for transmission through the nervous system (**Figure 1.46**). The four main groups for somatic sensation are:

- **mechanoreceptors**, which detect tactile sensation, i.e. touch and pressure
- **thermoreceptors**, which detect temperature changes
- **nociceptors**, which detect painful (noxious) stimuli
- **proprioceptors**, which detect changes in the position and movement of the body

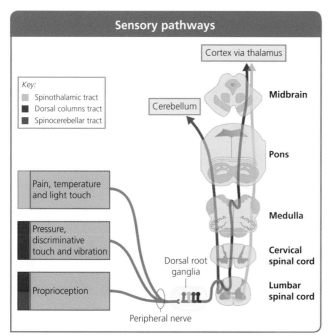

Figure 1.46 Sensory pathways, showing the route travelled by sensory input, from the periphery to the brain. Lower limb sensory input enters the spinal cord at the lumbar level.

Sensory receptors can be classified by structure (**Table 1.26**). The most well-defined types are as follows.

- Free nerve endings: the simplest type of sensory receptor exists as a group of fine branches at the end of a nerve
- Encapsulated nerve endings: the branches at the end of the nerve are enclosed in a capsule of connective tissue
- Specialised receptors: receptors for a special sense have a complex structure for detecting a specific type of sensation (see page 107); the nerve endings are neither free nor encapsulated

Most mechanoreceptors are encapsulated nerve endings. Proprioceptors are specalised receptors.

Transmission of sensation

All sensory pathways follow the same general route: the afferent pathway (see page 77).

When a sensory receptor is activated, the information is received by a first-order neurone, the primary sensory neurone. This carries the information via an afferent projection within a peripheral nerve to the central nervous system, where it is communicated to a second-order neurone. A projection from the second order neurone then carries the information to the brain, often via a third order neurone in the thalamus before reaching the cortex for processing.

The cell bodies of somatosensory neurones are located in clusters outside the vertebral column: the dorsal root ganglia, one on each side (see **Figure 1.42**). Their afferent projections enter the cord at the dorsal horns, where the communication through the central nervous system begins.

Dermatomes

Each spinal segment and nerve provides sensory innervation for a specific cutaneous

Sensory receptors				
Group	Receptor names	Type(s)	Modality or modalities	Location(s)
Mechanoreceptors	Tactile (Meissner) corpuscles	Encapsulated	Touch and vibration	Hairless skin
	Hair follicle receptors	Free nerve ending (plexuses)	Movement and touch	Hair root
	Pacinian corpuscles	Encapsulated	Pressure and vibration	Skin, joints, tendons, muscle and some viscera
	Tactile (Merkel) cells	Free nerve ending	Light touch	Skin
	Bulbous (Ruffini) corpuscles	Encapsulated	Stretch and pressure	Skin, ligaments and tendons
	Free nerve endings	Free nerve ending	Touch, pressure and stretch	Everywhere
Thermoreceptors		Free nerve ending	Temperature: cold (10–40°C) and warm (32–48°C)	Skin
Nociceptors		Free nerve ending	Pain: acute and chronic, and hot and cold	Everywhere
Proprioceptors	Nuclear bag fibres	Specialised	Stretch (dynamic)	Muscle: part of muscle spindle
	Nuclear chain fibres	Specialised	Stretch (sensitive to static tone)	Muscle: part of muscle spindle
	Golgi tendon organs	Specialised	Tension	Tendons
	Ruffini endings	Specialised	Stretch and angle change	Deep layers of skin, ligaments and tendons

Table 1.26 Sensory receptors

Dermatomes

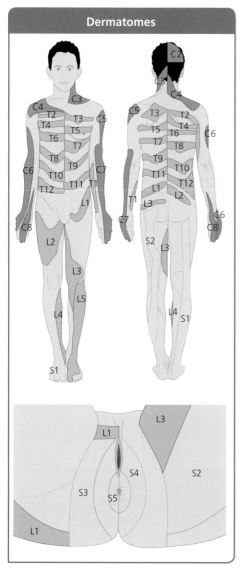

Figure 1.47 An evidence-based dermatone map. A dermatome is a skin region making sensory input to a specific spinal segment; for simplicity, in the top diagrams each dermatome is shown on only the left or the right side of the body.

Referred pain

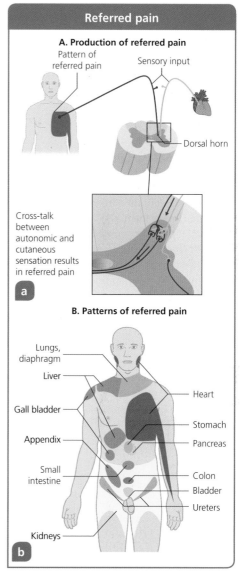

Figure 1.48 Referred pain. Convergence of pain sensation from the viscera and sensory information from the skin results in pain from the viscera being felt in the skin.

region called a dermatome (**Figure 1.47**). The dermatomal map is a clinically useful tool for identifying the level of a spinal lesion.

Referred pain

Overlap between visceral and cutaneous sensory information results in referred sensation. Visceral pain is carried by neurones that run alongside the sympathetic innervation to the organ, entering the spinal cord at the same level and converging with cutaneous sensory input (**Figure 1.48a**). Consequently, pain is felt in the cutaneous region from which the sympathetic neurones for that organ arise. For example, cardiac pain is felt in the chest and radiates along the arm (**Figure 1.48b**), consistent with the dermatomal map for the cutaneous innervations T1–T5.

Phantom limb pain is pain that is perceived when no limb, or painful stimulus, is present. It results from inappropriate activation of neurones that transmit false pain sensation to the cortex, which still contains sensory areas for the missing limb, giving a conscious sensation of pain.

The sensory (ascending) tracts

Axonal projections from the second-order neurones form the ascending tracts (**Table 1.27**). These project from the cord to either the thalamus, via the spinothalamic tracts and dorsal columns, or the cerebellum, via the spinocerebellar tracts (**Figure 1.41**).

- Axons of the spinothalamic and dorsal column reach the thalamus, where they communicate with third-order neurones projecting to the cortex; here, the signals give rise to an awareness of the feeling, i.e. conscious sensation (see page 82)
- Spinocerebellar pathways never reach the cortex, so the signals they carry generate no conscious awareness of the feeling; this is known as unconscious sensation

Location in cord

The ascending tracts are grouped in specific regions of the spinal cord (**Figure 1.49**).

Spinothalamic tracts are ventrolateral to the anterior horn, and the spinocerebellar tracts are in the lateral aspects between the dorsal and ventral roots. The dorsal columns are contained within the white matter between the dorsal roots.

Conscious sensation

The ascending tracts that carry conscious sensation are the:

- spinothalamic tracts
- dorsal columns

Spinothalamic tracts

The two spinothalamic tracts are:

- the **lateral spinothalamic tract**, which conveys information on pain and temperature
- the **anterior spinothalamic tract**, which transmits crude touch and pressure

The ascending sensory tracts					
Type	Sensation(s)	Tracts	Decussations	Routes	Terminations
Conscious	Pain and temperature	Lateral spinothalamic	Spinal cord	Lateral lemniscus	Cortex
	Pressure and crude touch	Anterior spinothalamic	Spinal cord	Lateral lemniscus	Cortex
	Proprioception, vibration and discrimination	Dorsal column	Brainstem	Medial lemniscus	Cortex
Unconscious	Proprioception	Anterior spinocerebellar (ventral)	Spinal cord and cerebellum		Cerebellum
		Posterior spinocerebellar (dorsal)	None		Cerebellum
		Cuneocerebellar	None		Cerebellum
		Rostral spinocerebellar	Unknown		Cerebellum

Table 1.27 The ascending sensory tracts

Spinal locations of the ascending (sensory) tracts

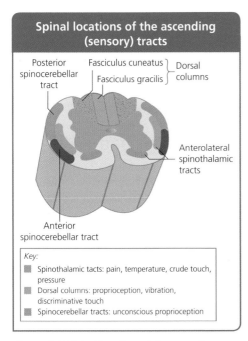

Posterior spinocerebellar tract

Fasciculus cuneatus ⎤ Dorsal
Fasciculus gracilis ⎦ columns

Anterolateral spinothalamic tracts

Anterior spinocerebellar tract

Key:
- ▣ Spinothalamic tacts: pain, temperature, crude touch, pressure
- ▣ Dorsal columns: proprioception, vibration, discriminative touch
- ▣ Spinocerebellar tracts: unconscious proprioception

Figure 1.49 Spinal locations of the ascending (sensory) tracts.

These tracts overlap and are often grouped together as the anterolateral spinothalamic tract.

Sensory afferents enter the cord via the dorsolateral (Lissauer's) tract, a small region of white matter running between the dorsal roots and grey matter of the cord, and project to the dorsal horn, where they communicate with second-order neurones in laminae I and II, i.e. the substantia gelatinosa, of the grey matter (see page 73). As they enter the cord, some fibres ascend the cord slightly in the dorsolateral tracts (see **Figure 1.44**), so they do not always enter the cord at the segmental level to which they project.

Aδ- and C-fibres are types of nerves that carry pain information. C-fibres are unmyelinated and have a slower response than myelinated Aδ-fibres. Aδ-fibres give rise to acute, sharp, 'ouch' pain, whereas C-fibres are associated with more chronic, dull, 'groan' pain.

Spinothalamic tracts decussate in the spinal cord, i.e. they cross over to the contralateral side of the cord. The fibres run across the grey matter, under the central canal, and join the ascending tracts of the contralateral cord. The fibres often ascend as they cross the cord, causing a discrepancy between their point of entry at the cord and the end point of decussation. Clinically, this ascension can cause discrepancies when mapping the dermatomes to lesion sites (see page 156).

Fibres ascend in the spinothalamic tract in the spinal cord, and within the lateral lemniscus, a bundle of fibres in the brainstem, to the thalamus, where they communicate with third-order neurones. The third-order neurones then transmit the information to the primary sensory cortex in the postcentral gyrus.

The dorsal columns

These carry proprioceptive, vibration and discriminative touch information. Afferent fibres enter the cord and travel to the dorsal column. The column comprises two pathways separated by a thin membrane, the septum:

- **The fasciculus gracilis pathway** runs the length of the spinal cord, and carries proprioceptive information from the legs and trunk (remember: the gracilis travels up from the ground)
- **The fasciculus cuneatus pathway** emerges in the upper thoracic levels of the cord, and carries information from the arms, chest and neck

Fibres ascend in the fasciculus gracilis and fasciculus cuneatus to the nucleus gracilis and nucleus cuneatus, respectively, in the medulla, where they communicate with second-order neurones. Second-order projections decussate at this level and ascend within the medial lemniscus pathway in the brainstem to the thalamus, where they communicate with third-order neurones that project to the sensory cortex.

A number of fibres also project to the cerebellum via the cuneocerebellar tract. This tract conveys proprioceptive information that the cerebellum integrates with unconscious sensation (see page 67).

All sensory and motor tracts pass to and from the cortex via the internal capsule, a band of white matter separating the thalamus from the basal ganglia. Consequently, even minor damage to this area, as is commonly present in stroke patients, can cause significant loss of sensory and motor function.

Cortical processing of sensation

Awareness of a sensation occurs when information reaches the higher processing centres in the brain, where information is interpreted and integrated and decisions are made.

The ascending tracts project to the sensory regions of the parietal lobe. The postcentral gyrus, also known as the sensory strip, contains the primary sensory cortex, which is responsible for perception of sensation.

All spinal tracts decussate (cross) by the level of the medulla, so projections to the thalamus and cortex contain sensory information from the contralateral side of the body. This is why stroke-related damage to one side of the brain affects the opposite side of the body.

Integration of sensation with other modalities and memory occurs in the parietal association cortices. Many fascinating disorders arise when this area is damaged. These include neglect, in which the contralateral body and environment are ignored, and astereognosis, in which objects are recognised visually but not by touch (see page 149).

Cortical mapping of sensation

Organisation of the postcentral gyrus is represented by a somatotopic map of the body, showing how activity in specific regions of the cortex correspond to sensation in particular areas of the body.

The sensory homunculus (Latin, 'little man') graphically depicts this mind–body relationship (**Figure 1.50**). The homunculus arrangement shows that certain body parts, for example fingers and lips, have a larger cortical representation than others. These areas have a greater concentration of nerve endings and are therefore highly sensitive. Areas with low sensitivity require less cortical space.

Unconscious pathways

Unconscious pathways carry muscle and joint sensation directly to the cerebellum, where it is used to adjust and fine-tune motor control and body position (see page 67). First-order afferents enter the dorsal horn and project to the nucleus dorsalis (Clarke's column or Clarke's nucleus) in the intermediate spinal cord, where they synapse with second-order neurones. These second-order neurones project to the cerebellum via a number of tracts (see page 67).

■ Anterior and posterior cerebellar tracts carry information from the lower limbs and trunk
■ Rostral and cuneocerebellar tracts carry information from the upper body

Other tracts are also involved in unconscious sensation and are linked to the

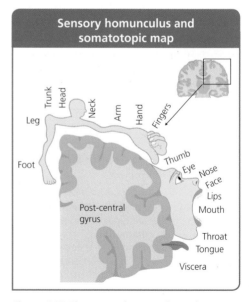

Figure 1.50 The sensory homunculus and a somatotopic map of the postcentral gyrus showing regional distribution of sensory input.

control of arousal and movement of the body in response to changing sensation. For example, the spinotectal tract controls body movement in response to visual stimuli.

Sensory pathways in the face and head

Sensory output from the head and neck is carried by the trigeminal nerve, cranial nerve V (**Table 1.28**; see page 103).

Conscious sensation

As in the spinal cord, three pathways carry conscious sensation:

- the **ventral trigeminal tract** for pain and temperature
- the **dorsal trigeminal tract** for crude touch and pressure
- the **mesencephalic trigeminal tract** for proprioception, vibration and discrimination

Cell bodies of neurones in the dorsal and ventral trigeminal tracts lie in the trigeminal ganglion. Cell bodies of neurones in the mesencephalic trigeminal tract are located in the mesencephalic trigeminal nucleus; this is the only pathway in the central nervous system that contains the cell bodies of peripheral sensory afferents.

Sensory fibres enter the brainstem at the pons. They enter the trigeminal nucleus to communicate with second-order neurones.

The trigeminal tracts project to specific regions of the trigeminal nucleus.

- The ventral trigeminal tract descends to the medullary portion
- The dorsal trigeminal tract descends to the pontine
- The mesencephalic trigeminal tract ascends to the mesencephalic trigeminal nucleus

Damage to individual regions results in characteristic patterns of sensory loss. For example, in lateral medullary syndrome, also known as Wallenberg's syndrome, pain and temperature sensation is lost on the ipsilateral (same) side of the face and the contralateral side of the body; however, facial touch and proprioception are unaffected.

The second-order neurones decussate as they exit the trigeminal nucleus and ascend to the cortex via the thalamus.

Some of the proprioceptive branches of the mesencephalic trigeminal tract descend to influence motor activity originating in the trigeminal motor nucleus in the pons (see page 102). This proprioceptive input forms the afferent branch of the monosynapatic jaw jerk reflex (see **Table 1.35**).

Unconscious sensation

Propriceptive information to the cerebellum travels ipsilaterally in the mesencephalic trigeminal tracts (see **Table 1.28**).

Trigeminal sensory tracts				
Sensation	Tract	Decussation	Route	Termination
Pain and temperature	Ventral trigeminal	Brainstem	Trigeminal lemniscus	Cortex
Pressure and crude touch	Dorsal trigeminal	Brainstem	Trigeminal lemniscus	Cortex
Proprioception, vibration and discrimination	Mesencephalic trigeminal	Brainstem	Trigeminal lemniscus	Cortex
Unconscious proprioception	Mesencephalic trigeminal	None		Cerebellum

Table 1.28 The trigeminal sensory tracts

Somatic motor

Starter questions

Answers to the following questions are on page 117.

20. Why does the brain constantly inhibit movement?
21. How can an athlete start moving quicker than an impulse can travel from the brain to muscle?

The somatic motor system comprises the neural pathways that generate controlled, smooth and fluid voluntary movements of the muscles of the body. Movement relies on intact communication between three components of the motor system:

- motor cortices
- descending tracts
- motor units

Signals arise in the motor cortex and travel via descending tracts to motor units, which communicate with muscles fibres to stimulate movement. This activity is adjusted and fine-tuned by the basal ganglia and cerebellum (see page 89).

Motor cortex

The primary motor cortex, also known as the motor strip, is located in the precentral gyrus of the frontal lobe (**Figure 1.51**; see also **Figure 1.29**). The motor neurones here produce the patterns of activity that execute motor function. Some are called Betz cells (or giant pyramidal cells) and are the largest neurones in the nervous system; their axons form part of the descending corticospinal tracts, which control voluntary movement.

The primary motor cortex is organised topographically, with regions of cortex corresponding to specific body areas. The results of cortical mapping, summarised by the motor homunculus (**Figure 1.51a**), show the heavier representation of regions such as the fingers and lips, which require greater innervation to control the fine, skilled movements needed for delicate manipulations and speech.

Cortical maps can be altered by intensive skills training. For example, elite musicians have larger cortical areas devoted to controlling hand and finger movement and sensation than those of novices.

Cortical generation of movement

Initial planning of movement involves obtaining a detailed mental body image and plan of the movement required. A mental body image is generated by the parietal lobes through integration of sensorimotor, proprioceptive and higher cognitive information.

Information regarding planned movement is generated in the supplemental and premotor areas in the frontal lobes. Theses areas also integrate information about body position to enable accurate production of the required movement.

Functional magnetic resonance imaging shows cortical activity levels in real time (see page 170). During specific patterns of movement, the brain shows high levels of sequential activity in the supplemental, premotor and motor cortices. When the movement is thought about but not performed, only the supplemental and premotor cortices are active.

Final decisions about the speed and sequence of movement execution are generated in the premotor and supplementary motor areas. These areas also mentally

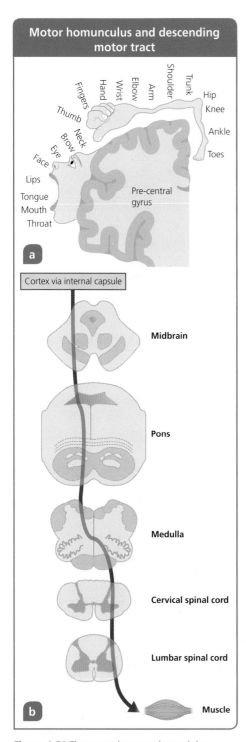

Motor homunculus and descending motor tract

Thumb, Fingers, Hand, Wrist, Elbow, Arm, Shoulder, Trunk

Neck, Brow, Eye, Face

Hip, Knee, Ankle, Toes

Lips
Tongue
Mouth
Throat

Pre-central gyrus

a

Cortex via internal capsule

Midbrain

Pons

Medulla

Cervical spinal cord

Lumbar spinal cord

Muscle

b

Figure 1.51 The motor homunculus and the descending corticospinal tract.

rehearse and modify the actions required before sending this information to the primary motor cortex. The information is then transmitted to the muscles via the descending tracts (**Table 1.29**; see page 88), which control activity in the motor units.

Motor units

Movement occurs when motor units are activated. Each motor unit comprises a motor neurone and the multiple muscle fibres with which it communicates. This component of the motor system is called the 'final common pathway', because it is the final stage before activation of muscle.

The cell body of the motor neurone, located in one of the anterior horns of the grey matter of the spinal cord, sends an axonal projection towards the muscle it innervates (**Figure 1.52**). The projection exits the cord via the anterior horn and ventral roots as part of the spinal nerve, and travels to the muscle within a peripheral nerve. On reaching the muscle, the nerve branches to activate multiple muscle fibres to cause their contraction.

Motor units also form the efferent branch of the spinal reflex arcs, which are activated in response to input from sensory afferents (see page 91).

There are two types of motor neurone (**Table 1.30**).

■ **α-Motor neurones** have large, myelinated axons that transmit information rapidly to muscle fibres to activate muscle contraction via the neuromuscular junction
■ **γ-Motor neurones** have smaller, myelinated axons that adjust the sensitivity of the muscle spindles, stretch receptors that regulate muscle tone and power (see page 89)

The neuromuscular junction

Communication between motor nerves and muscle fibres occurs at the neuromuscular junction. It is here that nerve signals

The descending tracts					
Group	Tract	Motor functions	Origins	Decussations	Terminations
Pyramidal	Lateral corticospinal	Rapid, skilled, voluntary limb movements	Cortex	Medulla	Spinal cord (cervical and lumbar enlargements)
	Anterior corticospinal	Proximal limb and trunk	Cortex	None	Cervical and thoracic cord
Extrapyramidal	Rubrospinal	Tone of limb muscles	Red nucleus	Midbrain	Cervical cord
	Reticulospinal	Posture, gait and autonomic	Reticular formation	None	Spinal cord
	Tectospinal	Eye and head position in response to visual stimulus	Superior colliculus	None	Cervical cord
	Vestibulospinal	Head and neck position, and balance	Vestibular nuclei	Midbrain	Spinal cord

Table 1.29 The descending tracts

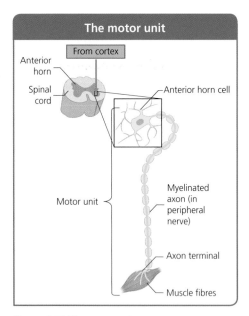

The motor unit

Anterior horn · From cortex · Spinal cord · Anterior horn cell · Motor unit · Myelinated axon (in peripheral nerve) · Axon terminal · Muscle fibres

Figure 1.52 The motor unit.

are converted into muscular contractions (**Figure 1.53**).

1. Action potentials arrive at the presynaptic terminal of the neuromuscular junction
2. Depolarisation opens voltage-gated Ca^{2+} channels, allowing Ca^{2+} to enter the presynaptic terminal
3. The Ca^{2+} influx triggers fusion of acetylcholine-containing vesicles with the presynaptic membrane and the consequent release of acetylcholine into the synaptic cleft
4. Acetylcholine binds to receptors on the motor end plate, the contact point for the axon terminal, formed in a depression on the muscle fibre surface, thereby stimulating muscle contraction

In myaesthenia gravis (see page 438), circulating autoantibodies reduce acetylcholine binding at the neuromuscular junction by blocking cholinergic receptors. In this way, the autoantibodies slow muscle activity and reduce tone, effects that manifest as progressive muscle fatigue and weakness. Drug therapy prevents acetylcholine breakdown, increasing the amount of acetylcholine available at the neuromuscular junction.

Upper and lower motor neurones

Motor neurones are divided into two groups.

- **Upper motor neurones** include all neurones of the motor cortex, including those in the basal ganglia and cerebellar motor circuits, and the descending tracts

Nerve fibres and functions				
Fibre	Myelin	Diameter (μm)	Conduction (m/s)	Function
Motor				
α	✓	12–20	70–120	Control of skeletal muscle
γ	✓	3–6	10–50	Control of muscle spindle length
β	✓	< 3	3–15	Control of autonomic function
Sensory				
Aα	✓	12–20	70–120	Proprioception
Aβ	✓	5–12	70–120	Mechanoreception
Aδ	✓	2–5	6–30	Pain and temperature reception
C	×	0.4–1.2	0.5–2.0	Pain, temperature and itch reception
β	✓	< 3	3–15	Carries sensation from internal organs

✓, present; ×, absent.

Table 1.30 Nerve fibres and function

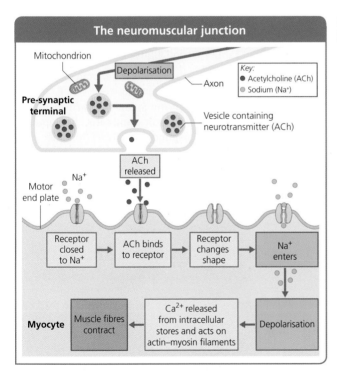

Figure 1.53 The neuromuscular junction.

- **Lower motor neurones** are the motor neurones located in the anterior horn and their axons that project to the musculature in the peripheral nerve

Lesions to upper or lower motor neurones generate clinically distinct signs and symptoms (see page 136).

> Motor neurone disease is a group of degenerative disorders that arise from damage to cells of the motor system (see page 378). Depending on the location of the neural damage, patients present with:
>
> - only upper motor neurone signs, e.g. pseudobulbar palsy
> - only lower motor neurone signs, e.g. progressive bulbar palsy
> - both upper and lower motor neurone signs, e.g. amylotrophic lateral sclerosis

Descending tracts

There are two groups of descending tracts.

- **Corticospinal (pyramidal) tracts** arise in the cortex and control the activity of all voluntary muscles, enabling rapid and skilled movements (see **Figure 1.51**)
- **Extrapyramidal tracts** arise in the brainstem and adjust muscle tone, balance and posture; they are also involved in basic voluntary movements that require non-complex coordination

Corticospinal tracts

Most fibres of the corticospinal tract decussate at the level of the medullary pyramid (hence the alternative name), forming the lateral corticospinal tracts in the spinal cord (**Figure 1.54**). These travel down the lateral funiculus, a column of fibres located in the lateral area of the spinal cord white matter, of the spinal cord to control activity of the lower motor neurones in the anterior horn.

The uncrossed corticospinal fibres mostly form the anterior corticospinal tracts and travel ipsilaterally down the medial aspect of spinal cord, decussating at the level at which they communicate with the anterior horn cells.

The few remaining uncrossed fibres travel ipsilaterally in the lateral corticospinal tracts.

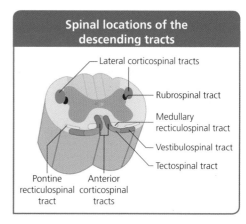

Spinal locations of the descending tracts

- Lateral corticospinal tracts
- Rubrospinal tract
- Medullary recticulospinal tract
- Vestibulospinal tract
- Tectospinal tract
- Pontine recticulospinal tract
- Anterior corticospinal tracts

Figure 1.54 Spinal locations of the descending tracts. The term pyramidal is used to describe the corticospinal tracts, which decussate at the medullary pyramids. All other tracts are classed as extrapyramidal.

Extrapyramidal tracts

These modulate the activity of neurones in the anterior horns in reponse to changes in sensory and proprioceptive input. The extrapyramidal tracts arise in the brainstem (see **Table 1.29** and **Figure 1.54**).

- **Rubrospinal tracts** travel from the midbrain red nucleus to the spinal cord to modulate motor neurone activity in reponse to cortical and cerebellar input
- **Reticulospinal tracts** travel from the reticular formation to the spinal cord and modulate voluntary and reflex activity in response to cortical, thalamic and cerebellar inputs
- **Tectospinal tracts** travel between the superior colliculus to the spinal cord and adjusts head movement and posture in response to visual stimulation
- **Vestibulospinal tracts** travel from the vestibular nuclei to the spinal cord and adjusts movement and posture in response to changes in balance

> Clinically, extrapyramidal signs are associated with damage to the basal ganglia, the extrapyramidal tracts, or both. The signs include those in Parkinson's disease, i.e. tremor, shaking and stiffness, which are caused by increased muscle tone and reduced motor activity (see page 313).

Descending inhibition

The descending tracts control muscle function by inhibiting activity in the reflex arcs in the spinal cord. Damage to these tracts, i.e. in cases of an upper motor neurone lesion, leads to a loss of this inhibition, causing characteristic signs including hyper-reflexia, increased in the strength of reflex responses and changes in muscle tone and power (see page 136).

Muscle tone and power

Muscle tone is the tension in a muscle, and muscle power is the strength of a muscle. Both are controlled by a combination of specialised sensory and motor components: Golgi tendon organs, muscle spindles and both α- and γ-motor neurones.

Muscle power depends on the number of motor units recruited at any time; more power requires more motor units to be active. Motor units act in rotation to maintain a constant level of muscle power.

Muscle tension is detected by specialised sensory receptors: the Golgi tendon organs located at the tendon–muscle border. Afferents from the Golgi tendon organ enter the spinal cord and inhibit α-motor neurones, thereby reducing contraction and protecting the muscle from damage.

Muscle spindles are clusters of stretch receptors that detect changes in the length of a muscle. They comprise modified muscle fibres, known as intrafusal fibres, embedded in the muscle, i.e. the extrafusal fibres. Afferent input from the spindle activates:

- α-motor neurones, causing contraction of the muscle
- γ-motor neurones, which adjust the length of the spindle, enabling it to respond rapidly to additional changes in muscle stretch, if needed

Activation of muscle spindles causes the muscles to contract, thereby protecting them from overstretching and tearing.

Fine-tuning of motor control

Motor output from the cortex is adjusted and corrected by two circuits of neurones known as re-entrant loops, which involve the basal ganglia and cerebellum. These receive motor output from the cortex and pass it to the basal ganglia or cerebellum, where it is adjusted and corrected before being transmitted via the thalamus back to the motor cortex and out to the periphery (**Figure 1.55**).

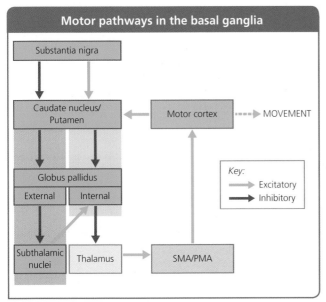

Motor pathways in the basal ganglia

Substantia nigra → Caudate nucleus/Putamen ← Motor cortex ┄┄► MOVEMENT

Globus pallidus (External / Internal)

Subthalamic nuclei / Thalamus → SMA/PMA

Key:
→ Excitatory
➔ Inhibitory

Figure 1.55 Direct and indirect pathways between the basal ganglia control the fine tuning of movement. Colours used here correlate with those in Figure 1.48a. SMA/PMA, supplementary motor areas/premotor areas.

> The basal ganglia and cerebellum do not directly influence the motor output in the corticospinal tracts; they fine-tune it. Therefore they are considered part of the extrapyramidal system.

Role of the basal ganglia in movement

The basal ganglia influence motor control through two circuits or pathways (**Figure 1.55**).

- **The direct (excitatory)** pathway enhances cortical motor output as it passes via the striatum and globus pallidus, the internal section, to the thalamus and back to the cortex

- **The indirect (inhibitory)** pathway inhibits motor outflow as it passes via the striatum to the globus pallidus through the subthalamic nuclei and back to the cortex via the thalamus

The substantia nigra acts on both pathways to modulate information passing through the striatum. Interplay between the pathways facilitates or suppresses motor activity, and damage to them underlies a number of common disorders (**Table 1.31**).

> In Parkinson's disease, loss of dopaminergic cells in the substantia nigra leads to reduced excitation in the direct pathway and enhanced inhibition in the indirect pathway. These effects result in bradykinesia (reduced motor activity).

Basal ganglia disorders

Disorder	Cause(s)	Area affected	Motor effects	Other features or notes
Parkinson's disease	Idiopathic and iatrogenic	Substantia nigra	Bradykinesia (slow and hard to initiate) Tremor (resting) Rigidity (lead pipe: slow, smooth movement; cogwheel: stiff, step-like movement)	Festinating gait (small steps that speed up over distance) Lack of facial expression Micrographia No weakness Normal reflexes
Huntington's disease	Genetic	Striatum	Choreiform (jerky, involuntary movement) Clumsy, unsteady gait Difficulty with speech and swallowing	Cognitive changes
Sydenham's chorea	Infection	Striatum	Choreiform	Generally affects limbs, face and trunk Self-resolving
Hemiballismus	Vascular	Subthalamic nuclei	Involuntary unilateral large-amplitude flinging movements	Mainly of proximal limb muscles
Dystonias	Primary: genetic Secondary: unclear	Unclear	Twisting muscle spasms	Often focal conditions: writer's cramp
Athetosis	Degenerative	Striatum	Snake-like writhing movements	
Wilson's disease (hepatolenticular)	Genetic	Striatum	Choreoathetotic	Dementia and liver cirrhosis

Table 1.31 Basal ganglia disorders

Reflexes

Starter questions

Answers to the following questions are on page 117.

22. Why do we need reflexes?
23. Do reflexes change over time?

Reflexes are stereotypic involuntary movements triggered by activation of a reflex arc, a functional input–output circuit made up of sensory and motor pathways. Most reflexes, for example lifting the foot immediately after stepping on a sharp object, evolved as survival mechanisms.

The three main groups of reflexes are:

- deep tendon reflexes
- flexor reflexes
- other reflexes, including superficial and primitive reflexes

The pathways involved in the deep tendon and flexor reflexes are well understood. The results of tests of these reflexes indicate the integrity of the nervous system at specific levels of the spinal cord.

Deep tendon reflexes

A deep tendon, or proprioceptive, reflex is activated by stretching the tendon. In the clinic this is usually done by tapping the tendon with a reflex hammer.

The monosynaptic reflex arc, also called the myotatic or stretch reflex, is the simplest reflex; it has only one synapse (**Figure 1.56**). Sensory input activates motor neurones directly to produce muscle contraction. The spinal levels for these reflexes are shown in **Table 1.32**; changes in response indicate lesion type and location (see page 156).

The inverse myotatic reflex, or inverse stretch reflex, is activated by increased muscle tension and protects muscles from damage from over-contraction. In this reflex, activation of an inhibitory interneurone by sensory input reduces motor neurone activity, thereby relaxing the muscle.

Reciprocal innervation, in which sensory input to one arc also activates that of the opposing muscle to contract or relax it, enables muscle groups to work in synchrony throughout the reflex response (**Figure 1.56**).

> **Reflexes can be artifically enhanced (reinforced) by using Jendrassik's manoeuvre.** The patient performs a movement, usually firmly clasping both hands together, as a distraction from the reflex testing and thereby reduces the conscious control of muscle movements.

Flexor reflexes

In flexor reflexes, two reflex arcs work together to withdraw a limb from a painful stimulus (**Figure 1.56**).

- The **flexor withdrawal reflex** activates the flexor muscle and simultaneously inhibits the extensor muscle, triggering withdrawal of the limb
- In the **crossed extensor reflex**, sensory information crosses the spinal cord to activate the extensor and inhibit the flexor in the contralateral limb, thereby counterbalancing withdrawal of the limb

Other reflexes

Other reflexes generally involve complex interactions between sensory input and motor output, and have networks that span many levels of the central nervous system. Therefore many of them are not clinically demonstrable. However, some can be useful indicators of the integrity of the nervous

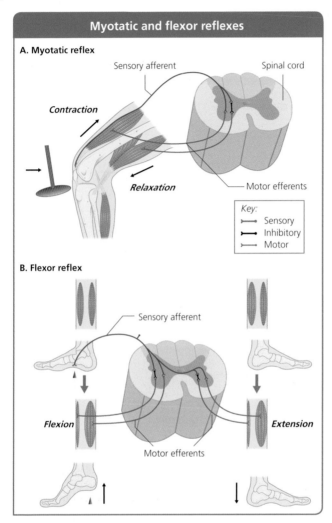

Myotatic and flexor reflexes

A. Myotatic reflex

Sensory afferent

Spinal cord

Contraction

Relaxation

Motor efferents

Key:
Sensory
Inhibitory
Motor

B. Flexor reflex

Sensory afferent

Flexion

Extension

Motor efferents

Figure 1.56 Myotatic and flexor reflexes. (a) Myotatic (stretch) reflex and reciprocal innervation. Tapping the patellar tendon stretches the quadriceps tendon causing reflex contration of the quadriceps muscle and relaxation of the hamstrings (b). Flexor reflexes. Standing on a sharp object triggers the flexor reflex to raise the same leg; the crossed extensor reflex counterbalances the shift in weight by extension of the contralateral limb.

system and accordingly are briefly described here.

Superficial reflexes

Superficial, or cutaneous, reflexes are those in which tactile stimulation triggers muscle contraction. These reflexes are generally polysynaptic, i.e. they involve many synapses, and their circuitry spans multiple spinal levels (**Table 1.33**).

Postural reflexes

Postural reflexes involve numerous brainstem regions and control movement of the body, head or both in reponse to three main sensory inputs:

- **proprioceptive information** about the position and movement of the body
- **vestibular information** about the position and movement of the head
- **visual information** about position of the body relative to the surrounding environment

Autonomic reflexes

Autonomic reflexes control visceral responses to stimuli, such as increasing peristaltic activity of the gut in response to

Deep tendon reflexes	
Reflex	Spinal level
Biceps	C5-C6
Triceps	C7-C8
Brachioradialis (supinator)	C5-C6
Extensor digitorum*	C6-C7
Flexor digitorum profundis (finger flexor)†	C6–T1
Patellar (knee jerk)	L3-L4
Achilles (ankle jerk)	S1–S2

*Extension of fingers on contraction of extensor digitorum is normal

†Hoffmann's sign is flexion and adduction of thumb in response to finger flexion; Mayer's and Trömner's reflexes are variants of finger flexor reflex; Mayer's is the most sensitive of the three

Table 1.32 Deep tendon reflexes

Superficial reflexes		
Reflex	Spinal level	Notes
Abdominal	T6-L1	Contraction of abdominal muscles on tactile stimulation of skin above (T6–T10) and below (T10-L1) the umbilicus
Cremasteric	L1-L2	Tactile stimulation of the inner thigh causes elevation of the testicles
Anocutaneous	S2–S4	Contraction of the anal sphincter on perianal stimulation ('anal wink')
Plantar response	L5–S1	Extensor plantar (raised, fanned toes) is Babinski's sign; 'negative Babinski' does not exist

Table 1.33 Superficial reflexes

ingestion of toxic substances to speed expulsion of the toxin. In this type of reflex, sensory input modulates parasympathetic and sympathetic activity affecting the smooth muscle of organs. Responses to autonomic reflexes are generally slower than those to somatic reflexes.

Primitive reflexes

Primitive reflexes are important for infant survival because they enable infants to suckle and encourage parental bonding. They include the following.

- **The suckling reflex** is a sucking motion in response to an object touching the roof of the mouth
- **The (palmar) grasp reflex** is the grasping of any object that strokes the palm
- **The rooting reflex** is the turning of the head towards an object touching the cheek or mouth
- **The startle reflex (Moro's reflex)** is rapid head and leg extension, abduction and adduction of the arms and crying in response to sudden loss of support
- **The snout reflex** is pouting in response to tapping of the lips

> **Primitive reflexes elicited past infancy are an upper motor neurone sign linked to certain conditions.** These include cerebral palsy and some frontal lobe disorders, including autism and dementia.

Cranial nerve reflexes

Reflexes in the head and neck are controlled by the cranial nerves. They include deep tendon, superficial and postural reflexes (**Table 1.34**).

Cranial nerve reflexes			
Reflex	Type	Afferent branch	Efferent branch
Jaw jerk	Deep tendon	CN V	CN V
Corneal (blink)	Superficial	CN V	CN VII
Gag	Superficial	CN IX	CN X
Pupillary (light)	Autonomic	CN II	CN III
Accomodation	Autonomic	CN II	CN III
Vestibuloocular	Postural	CN VIII	CNs III, IV and VI

Table 1.34 Cranial nerve (CN) reflexes

Autonomic nervous system

Starter questions

Answers to the following questions are on page 117.

24. Can the autonomic nervous system be controlled consciously?
25. Why does the nervous supply to the gastrointestinal system have its own division?

The autonomic nervous system controls the unconscious, involuntary bodily functions, including breathing, swallowing, sweating and the activity of all internal organs. It is a motor system that, like the somatic motor system, comprises reflex loops and motor units controlled by descending inputs from the brain.

The autonomic nervous system has two synergistic divisions (**Figure 1.57**).

- The **sympathetic nervous system** primes the body for stressful situations

- The **parasympathetic nervous system** maintains the body during more placid states

These divisions control automatic responses to changes in the internal and external environments (**Table 1.35**). Both are made up of two types of cell:

- **preganglionic neurones** located in the brainstem and spinal cord, which send projections to the postganglionic neurones
- **postganglionic neurones** located in ganglia, which send projections to the target organ, for example the heart or sweat glands

Sympathetic nervous system

The sympathetic nervous system produces a state of heightened arousal combined with a readiness for action by initiating the fight-or-flight response. In this way, it prepares the body for escape from danger.

The sympathetic preganglionic neurones are located in the lateral horns, of the thoracolumbar (T1–L2/L3) spinal cord. Their projections are short; they leave the cord via the anterior horn and branch from the spinal nerve to form the white ramus communicans (Latin: ramus, 'branch'; communicans, 'communicating'). On exiting the vertebral column, they connect with the string of 21–23 pairs of ganglia running along the ventral aspect of the column. These are the paravertebral or sympathetic chain ganglia, formed by the cell bodies of the postganglionic neurones.

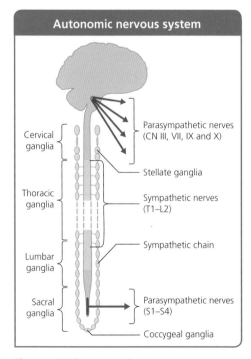

Autonomic nervous system

Cervical ganglia

Thoracic ganglia

Lumbar ganglia

Sacral ganglia

Parasympathetic nerves (CN III, VII, IX and X)

Stellate ganglia

Sympathetic nerves (T1–L2)

Sympathetic chain

Parasympathetic nerves (S1–S4)

Coccygeal ganglia

Figure 1.57 The autonomic nervous system.

Autonomic nervous system: innervation and function					
Organ	SNS effects	Origin	PNS effects	Origin	Lesions*
Eye	Pupil dilation	T1	Pupil constriction Raising of eyelid ↑ Lacrimation	CN III	SNS: miosis, ptosis and enopthalmos PNS: pupil dilation, full ptosis and dry eye
Mouth	↓ Salivation	T1	↑ Salivation	CN III and CN VII	SNS: drooling PNS: dry mouth
Skin	↑ Sweat secretion Vasoconstriction Contraction of erector pili muscles	T1–L3			SNS: dry, flushed regions of skin
Heart	↑ Force of contraction	T1–T5	↓ Force of contraction	CN X	Compensated: local pacemaker drives heart
Lungs	Dilation of bronchi Constriction of arteries	T1–T4	Constriction of bronchi ↑ Secretions Dilation of arteries	CN X	Damage to spinal cord can alter pace Damage to higher centres alters respiratory pattern and depth
Liver	↑ Glycolysis	T5–T12			Unlikely
Gastrointestinal tract	↓ Peristalstis ↓ Secretions Contraction of sphincters	T5–L2	↑ Peristalsis ↑ Secretions Relaxation of sphincters Defecation	CN X S2–S4	Compensated: local pacemaker provides drive
Kidney	↓ Output Adrenal stimulation	T5–T12		CN X	Unlikely
Bladder	Relaxation of detrusor Contraction of sphincter vesicae	T11–L2	Contraction of detrusor Relaxation of sphincter	S2–S4	Neurogenic bladder (bladder dysfunction caused by neuronal damage) Upper motor neurone: hyper-reflexic, dysnergic bladder Lower motor neurone: flaccid, acontractile bladder
Genitals	Orgasm and/or ejaculation and detumescence	L1–L2 in males T12–L1 in females	Erection ↑ Seminal and vaginal secretions	S2–S4	SNS: priapism (painful and persistent erection)

↑, Increased; ↓, decreased; CN, cranial nerve; PNS, parasympathetic nervous system; SNS, sympathetic nervous system.

*Because of bilateral innervation, unilateral lesions are generally compensated; innervations to the eye and skin are the exception.

Table 1.35 The autonomic nervous system: innervation and function

In mutiple systems atrophy, the lateral horns of the spinal cord are often damaged. This degenerative disorder is similar to Parkinson's disease but presents with additional autonomic dysfunction, including hypotension, incontinence and impotence.

The paravertebral ganglia supply organs above the diaphragm, which receive innervation from the cervical to mid-thoracic spinal sympathetic levels (**Figure 1.57**). Organs below the diaphragm, incuding the genitalia, bladder and rectum, are innervated by autonomic projections from the mid-thoracic to lumbar spinal cord. These travel via the three prevertebral ganglia, which are external to the sympathetic chain: the coeliac, superior and inferior mesenteric ganglia.

Axonal projections from the postganglionic neurones reach their target organ by wrapping around the vasculature travelling towards it. In the sympathetic system, postganglionic neurone projections are long because the sympathetic ganglia are located far from their target organs. In the parasympathetic system, the ganglia are located near the target organs.

The adrenal gland differs from other sympathetic innervations, because the cells of the postganglionic neurones form the gland. Activated postganglionic neurones release noradrenaline (norepinephrine) and adrenaline (epinephrine) directly into the bloodstream to act as hormones.

Parasympathetic nervous system

In the absence of a stressful situation, the parasympathetic nervous system dominates the output of the autonomic nervous system. It controls behaviours associated with relaxed states, including lower respiratory rate and blood pressure, digestion and sexual arousal.

The preganglionic neurones of the parasympathetic nervous system are located in the craniosacral regions of the central nervous system: the brainstem nuclei for cranial nerves III, VII, IX and X, and the lateral horn of the S2–S4 region of the spinal cord sacrally (**Figure 1.57**).

Preganglionic axons travel with either the cranial nerves or the vasculature and synapse with postganglionic neurones in terminal ganglia located close to their target organ.

Projections from cranial postganglionic neurones innervate the head, thoracic organs and upper gastrointestinal tract. Sacral innervations control lower regions of the gastrointestinal tract and excretory and reproductive organs (see **Table 1.35**).

The following are the main cranial parasympathetic nervous system ganglia:

- The **ciliary ganglion**, associated with cranial nerve III, innervates the iris (eye) to control pupil size
- The **pterygopalatine ganglion**, associated with cranial nerve VII, innervates the lacrimal gland
- The **submandibular ganglion**, associated with cranial nerve VII, innervates the salivary glands
- The **otic ganglion**, associated with cranial nerve IX, innervates the parotid salivary gland

Ganglia for cranial nerve X and the sacral parasympathetic nervous system are located in the following plexuses:

- the **cardiac plexus**, which innervates the heart
- the **pulmonary plexus**, which innervates the lungs
- the **intermural plexus**, which innervates the gastrointestinal tract
- the **hypogastric plexus**, which innervates the excretory and reproductive organs

Autonomic neurotransmitters

Acetylcholine is the neurotransmitter used by preganglionic neurones of both the sympathetic and parasympathetic nervous systems. Acetylcholine binds to nicotinic cholinergic receptors, which are activated rapidly to enable fast onward transmission to the organ.

Postganglionic neurones of the sympathetic nervous system generally release noradrenaline (norepinephrine), which binds to adrenergic receptors on the target organ. There are two main types of adrenergic receptor, α and β, with various subtypes. As a result, sympathetic activity can have a range of effects on the organ.

In contrast, postganglionic neurones of the parasympathetic nervous system release acetylcholine, which binds to muscarinic cholinergic receptors in the organ. These take longer than nicotinic receptors to produce their effects, so stimulation of the organ is gradual.

The postganglionic neurones of the sympathetic nervous system that innervate the sweat glands seem to be unique, because they release acetylcholine instead of noradrenaline. This occurs because of interactions between the neurones and the target sweat gland during development leads to selection of neurones with cholinergic function.

Many drugs produce their beneficial effects by influencing autonomic function through interactions with neurotransmitters. However, many adverse effects also result from these interactions.

> **Botulinum toxin type A blocks acetylcholine release at the neuromuscular junction.** Therefore injections are used to reduce muscle spasm. This property is exploited in treatment of incontinence, excessive sweating, pain and migraine.

Autonomic reflexes

The activity of the autonomic nervous system, like that of the somatic motor system, can be altered by sensory pathways in the spinal cord. Sensory information from the organs is transmitted via nerves situated alongside the autonomic innervation to the organ.

Sensory information enters the spinal cord via the dorsal horns. Here, projections from sensory neurones synapse with neurones carrying autonomic output, thereby creating a reflex arc similar to those of the somatic motor system.

Autonomic reflexes are slower than somatic motor reflexes, because the fibres involved are unmyelinated or only slightly myelinated. The conduction rate for autonomic reflexes is 0.5–30 m/s, which contrasts with 80–120 m/s in somatic motor neurones.

Crosstalk between autonomic and somatic sensory pathways causes pain to be felt in the cutaneous regions innervated by these levels; this phenomenon is called referred pain (see **Figure 1.48**).

> **Information on visceral pain is carried by fibres situated alongside the sympathetic innervation.** Therefore knowledge of the origin of sympathetic nerves for specific organs enables the pattern of referred pain to be predicted.

Like the motor system, autonomic reflexes are modified by descending pathways. Damage to these descending tracts results in hyper-reflexia, similar to the effects of upper motor neurone lesions (see page 142).

Unilateral damage to peripheral innervation is often compensated for. However, bilateral damage results in lower motor neurone–type effects (see **Table 1.35**).

Higher control of the autonomic nervous system

The hypothalamus maintains autonomic nervous system activity within a discrete range by controlling homeostatic set points. Hypothalamic activity is modified by input from even higher centres, for example emotional input from the frontal and temporal lobes. Modification of hypothalamic activity by higher centres underlies the potential voluntary control of autonomic activity, as when people learn to override fear responses.

The hypothalamus modulates motor output to the autonomic nervous system via descending input to visceromotor centres in the brainstem. These centres are groups of cells that regulate the activity of specific organs. An example is the respiratory centre, which controls the depth and rate of respiration (see page 60). The visceromotor centres then send signals via descending tracts to control activity in the circuitry underlying autonomic reflexes.

Enteric nervous system

The enteric nervous system is distinct from the central, peripheral and autonomic nervous systems. It controls the gastrointestinal system and consists of two intramural plexuses, so called because they are in the walls of the gastrointestinal tract.

- The **myenteric (Auerbach's) plexus** controls the longitudinal muscles of the gut wall
- The **submucosal (Meissner's) plexus** controls its circular muscles

These plexuses are networks of sympathetic and parasympathetic neurones that function independent of the autonomic nervous system. The neurones work synergistially to control peristalsis, the wave-like muscular contractions that move boluses of food through the gastrointestinal tract.

Damage to the autonomic nervous system cannot extinguish enteric nervous system activity, because pacemaker cells located in the plexuses initiate peristalsis. Innervation from the sympathetic and parasympathetic nervous systems can only modulate the activity of the enteric nervous system.

Cranial nerves

Starter questions

The answer to the following question is on page 117.

26. What is emotional incontinence?

The cranial nerves form part of the peripheral nervous system. However, they are generally considered separately because of their specialised roles in the head and neck region.

There are 12 pairs of cranial nerves (**Figure 1.58, Table 1.36**), so called because they pass through a number of cranial foramina (**Figure 1.59**). They carry sensory, motor and parasympathetic information (**Table 1.36**). All the cranial nerves also carry proprioceptive information to the central nervous system.

Functional organisation

Cranial nerves are classified into the following functional groups:

- **General somatic afferent**: cranial nerves that receive general sensory information, including cutaneous sensation
- **Special somatic afferent**: the nerves that sense vision, hearing and balance
- **General visceral afferent**: the nerves responsible for sensation from glands and internal organs
- **Special visceral afferent**: the nerves for gustation and olfaction
- **General somatic efferent**: Cranial nerves that control the voluntary muscles in the eye and tongue
- **General visceral efferent**: the nerves that control smooth muscles and glands
- **Somatic visceral efferent**: the nerves that control the voluntary movements in facial expression, mastication and speech

Most cranial nerves have nuclei located in the brainstem (**Figure 1.60**). The exceptions are cranial nerves I and II.

Cranial nerve I: the olfactory nerve

Cranial nerve I is purely sensory and its activity confers the sense of smell. Odour is detected by sensory cells located in the nasal mucosa. The sensory information is then transmitted along the fine unmyelinated axons of cranial nerve I, which travel through the cribriform plate and into the skull (**Figure 1.59**). Here, the unmyelinated axonal fibres communicate with neurones in the olfactory bulb. Axons from these neurones form the olfactory tract, and project to the olfactory cortices, where the information is processed (see page 111).

Cranial nerve I is the shortest cranial nerve, comprising only the sensory projections that travel a few millimetres through the cribriform plate to the olfactory bulb. Although the olfactory tract is often regarded as cranial nerve I, it is actually part of the central nervous system.

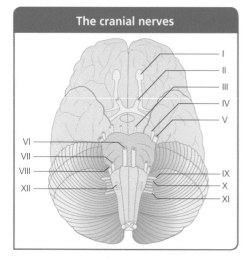

The cranial nerves

I
II
III
IV
V
VI
VII
VIII
IX
X
XI
XII

Figure 1.58 The cranial nerves.

Cranial nerve II: the optic nerve

Cranial nerve II is purely sensory; it is responsible for vision. Sensory receptors called rods and cones located in the retina transmit visual information to the visual cortex via a well-understood pathway (see page 109).

This nerve develops from the forebrain and is actually part of the central nervous system, though is classed as peripheral due to it's location outside of the brain and spinal cord.

Cranial nerves: foramina and functions			
Number (name)	Entry or exit foramen	Information carried	Function
I (olfactory)	Cribriform plate	Sensory	Olfaction
II (optic)	Optic canal	Sensory	Vision
III (oculomotor)	Superior orbital fissure	Motor	Eye movement
		Parasympathetic	Pupillary movement
IV (trochlear)	Superior orbital fissure	Motor	Eye movement
V (trigeminal)	V_1: superior orbital fissure V_2: foramen rotundum	Sensory	Sensation: face, mouth, anterior two thirds of tongue, sinuses and supratentorial meninges
	V_3: foramen ovale	Motor	Mastication and sound attenuation
VI (abducens)	Superior orbital fissure	Motor	Eye movement
VII (facial)	Auditory canal (stylomastoid foramen)	Sensory	Sensation: external auditory meatus
			Gustation: anterior two thirds of tongue
		Motor	Facial expression, sound and mouth opening
		Parasympathetic	Lacrimal and salivary glands (except parotid)
VIII (vestibulocochlear)	Auditory canal	Sensory	Audition and proprioception
IX (glossopharyngeal)	Jugular foramen	Sensory	Sensation: external auditory meatus, middle ear, pharynx and posterior third of tongue
			Gustation: posterior third of tongue
			Other: chemoreceptor and baroreceptor information from carotid bodies
		Motor	Swallowing
		Parasympathetic	Parotid gland
X (vagus)	Jugular foramen	Sensory	Sensation: pharynx, infratentorial meninges and external auditory meatus
			Gustation: epiglottis and pharynx
			Other: chemoreceptor and baroreceptor information from aortic arch
		Motor	Swallowing and speech
		Parasympathetic	Heart, lungs and gastric system, (upper two thirds)
XI (spinal accessory)	Jugular foramen (ascending spinal fibres enter via the foramen magnum)	Motor	Shoulder and head movement
XII (hypoglossal)	Hypoglossal canal	Motor	Tongue movement

Table 1.36 Cranial nerves (CN): foramina and functions

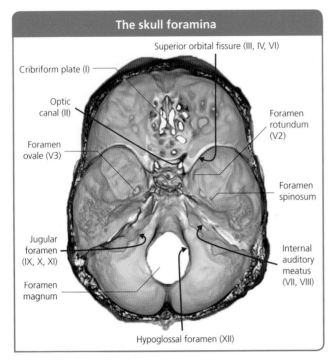

The skull foramina

Superior orbital fissure (III, IV, VI)

Cribriform plate (I)

Optic canal (II)

Foramen rotundum (V2)

Foramen ovale (V3)

Foramen spinosum

Jugular foramen (IX, X, XI)

Internal auditory meatus (VII, VIII)

Foramen magnum

Hypoglossal foramen (XII)

Figure 1.59 The skull foramina.

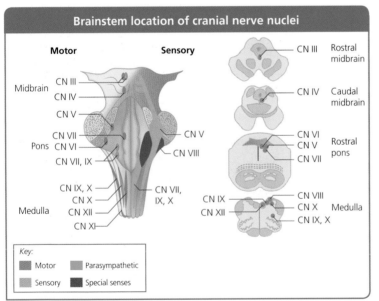

Brainstem location of cranial nerve nuclei

Motor

Sensory

Midbrain
CN III
CN IV
CN V

Pons
CN VII
CN VI
CN VII, IX

CN V
CN VIII

Medulla
CN IX, X
CN X
CN XII
CN XI

CN VII, IX, X

CN III   Rostral midbrain

CN IV   Caudal midbrain

CN VI
CN V   Rostral pons
CN VII

CN IX
CN XII

CN VIII
CN X   Medulla
CN IX, X

Key:
Motor   Parasympathetic
Sensory   Special senses

Figure 1.60 Brainstem location of cranial nerve nuclei.

The axons of cranial nerve II are myelinated by oligodendrocytes, whereas Schwann cells myelinate peripheral nerves. Furthermore, cranial nerve II is wrapped in meninges, which surround the central, not the peripheral, nervous system , though is classes as peripheral due to it's location outside of the brain and spinal cord.

Cranial nerve III: oculomotor

Cranial nerve III is a mixed nerve with motor and parasympathetic components. Together with cranial nerves IV and VI, it controls eye movement. The motor component of cranial nerve III originates in the midbrain oculomotor nuclei and elevates the eyelid by activating the action of the levator palpebrae superioris muscle. It also generates eye movement by activating the superior, inferior and medial rectus and the inferior oblique muscles (**Figure 1.61**).

Parasympathetic supply arising in the Edinger–Westphal nucleus causes pupil constriction by activating the sphincter pupillae muscle and accomodation by activating the ciliary muscles (see page 107).

Cranial nerve IV: trochlear

Cranial nerve IV is a pure motor nerve. The cell bodies of the motor neurones are located in the midbrain trochlear nuclei. They innervate the superior oblique muscle, which cause intorsion (inward rotation) and depression of the eyeball (**Figure 1.61**).

Cranial nerve IV is the only cranial nerve that decussates.

Cranial nerve V: trigeminal nerve

Cranial nerve V is a mixed nerve; it carries both sensory and motor information. Information for general facial sensation is carried by three trigeminal branches, which innervate specific regions (**Figure 1.62**).

- V_1 is the ophthalmic branch
- V_2 is the maxillary branch
- V_3 is the mandibular branch

Sensory information from the back of the head and neck is carried by cervical spinal nerves C2 and C3.

Sensory cell bodies are located in the trigeminal ganglion. Their projections terminate in the trigeminal nucleus, which runs throughout the brainstem to the upper cervical spinal levels. The trigeminal tracts carry sensory information to the cortex (see page 83).

The motor neurones of cranial nerve V originate in the trigeminal motor nucleus and run alongside the sensory pathways to the musculature. Lower motor neurones receive bilateral innervation from upper motor neurones and supply the following muscles:

- the muscles of mastication, i.e. masseter, pterygoids and temporalis, for chewing

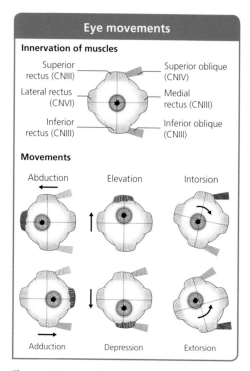

Figure 1.61 Cranial innervation of eye muscles and eye movements. The tendon of the superior oblique muscle loops through the trochlear nerve, changing the direction of muscle movement. As a result activation of the superior oblique rotates the pupil inward toward the nose and downward (intorsion). The inferior oblique rotates the pupil outward and upward (extorsion).

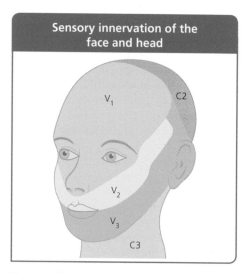

Figure 1.62 Sensory innervation of the face and head by cervical nerves C2 and 3 and three branches of CN V (trigeminal nerve).

- the mylohyoid, which opens the mouth for swallowing and speech
- the anterior belly of the digastric, which works with the mylohyoid to open the mouth
- the tensor palati, which tenses the palate during swallowing
- the tensor tympani, which tenses the tympanic membrane in the ear to reduce vibrations

Cranial nerve V also receives sensory input from part of the meninges, and carries parasympathetic input to the salivary glands for cranial nerve VII as it approaches the gland.

Cranial nerve VI: abducens nerve

Cranial nerve VI is a purely motor nerve. It innervates the lateral rectus, which abducts the eyeball, i.e. moves it laterally (**Figure 1.61**).

Motor neurones originate in the abducens nuclei in the pons. From here, the nerve leaves the brainstem, passes through the cavernous sinus (see page 37) and enters the orbit via the superior orbital fissure.

Cranial nerve VII: facial nerve

Cranial nerve VII is a mixed nerve, carrying sensory, motor and parasympathetic information. It provides sensory input, on taste, from the anterior two thirds of the tongue, and somatic sensation from the external auditory meatus. Motor neurones control the muscles of facial expression.

Information on taste is carried by the lingual nerve and chorda tympani to the gustatory region of the brainstem: the nucleus of the solitary tract. Somatic sensation from the external auditory meatus projects to the spinal trigeminal nucleus. Sensory cell bodies are located in the geniculate ganglion.

Motor output originates in the pontine facial motor nuclei (see **Figure 1.60**). On exiting the stylomastoid foramen, an aperture in the base of the skull cranial nerve VII divides into five branches (**Figure 1.63**):

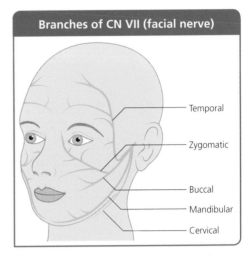

Branches of CN VII (facial nerve)

- Temporal
- Zygomatic
- Buccal
- Mandibular
- Cervical

Figure 1.63 Branches of CN VII (facial nerve).

- temporal
- zygomatic
- buccal
- mandibular
- cervical

Forehead sparing is a characteristic of upper motor neurone lesions of cranial nerve VII. The muscles of the forehead receive input from both sides of the cortex. In cases of unilateral damage, the input that remains intact allows movement of the forehead to be retained. Lower motor neurone lesions of cranial nerve VII paralyse all the muscles of the face (**Figure 1.64**).

A small motor branch innervates the stapedius muscle in the middle ear, one of the muscles that enable hearing (see page 112). Another small branch innervates the digastric muscle in the jaw.

Parasympathetic innervation arises in the superior salivatory nucleus, in the pons (see **Figure 1.60**). Branches of cranial nerve VII travel via:

- the chorda tympani to the submandibular ganglion to innervate the salivary glands
- the greater petrosal nerve to the sphenopalatine ganglion to innervate the lacrimal glands

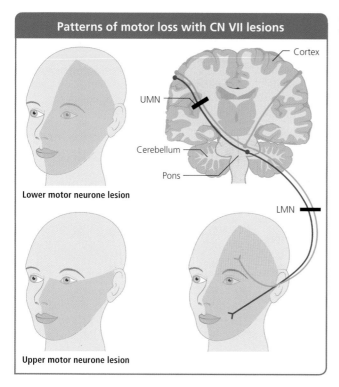

Patterns of motor loss with CN VII lesions

Cortex

UMN

Cerebellum

Pons

Lower motor neurone lesion

LMN

Upper motor neurone lesion

Figure 1.64 Patterns of motor loss with CN VII (facial nerve) lesions.

The largest salivary gland, the parotid, is innervated by cranial nerve IX.

Cranial nerve VIII: vestibulocochlear nerve

Cranial nerve VIII is purely sensory, responsible for hearing and balance. It divides into two branches.

- **The cochlear branch** carries information about sounds, and the cochlear cell bodies form the spiral ganglia
- **The vestibular branch** carries information about the position and movement of the head, and the vestibular cell bodies form the superior and inferior vestibular ganglia

The two branches fuse as they exit the auditory canal to form cranial nerve VIII, which passes through the internal auditory meatus to the pons, where they communicate with cells in the cochlear and vestibular nuclei (**Figure 1.60**). Information is then carried into the central nervous system for higher processing (see page 113).

Cranial nerve IX: glossopharyngeal nerve

Cranial nerve IX is a mixed nerve. Sensory input carries information on taste from the posterior third of the tongue, somatic sensation from the external auditory meatus and pharynx, chemoreceptor information about blood composition from the carotid bodies, and baroreceptor information about blood pressure from the carotid sinus. Motor fibres innervate the stylopharyngeus muscle, which raise the larynx and pharynx to aid swallowing and parasympathetic innervation is supplied to the parotid gland.

Brainstem nuclei for cranial nerve IX include (**Figure 1.60**):

- **the nucleus ambiguus**, where the motor innervation arises
- **the inferior salivatory nucleus**, which contains the parasympathetic component
- **the nucleus of the solitary tract**, which receives taste, chemoreceptor and baroreceptor information

- **the spinal trigeminal nucleus**, which receives information for somatic sensation from the external auditory meatus

Cranial nerve IX exits the medulla below the pontomedullary junction, crosses the subarachnoid space and exits through the jugular foramen, an aperture in the base of the skull.

Cranial nerve X: vagus nerve

Cranial nerve X is a mixed nerve. It is called the vagus (Latin, 'vagrant' or 'wanderer') because its branches follow a meandering path around the body. It carries information on sensation from the pharynx, meninges and external auditory meatus, and on taste from the epiglottis and pharynx. Cranial nerve X also carries some of the chemoreceptor and baroreceptor information for cranial nerve IX.

Cranial nerve X controls motor function for swallowing and speech by activating the pharyngeal and laryngeal muscles, respectively. It also provides parasympathetic innervation to the heart, lungs, abdominal organs and upper gastrointestinal tract (see page 97).

Motor innervation originates in two nuclei (**Figure 1.60**).

- The dorsal motor nucleus of the vagus contains the parasympathetic supply
- The nucleus ambiguus innervates the muscles of the pharynx, larynx and upper oesophagus

Sensory innervation projects to two areas (**Figure 1.60**):

- the nucleus of the solitary tract, which receives information for taste and visceral sensation
- the spinal trigeminal nucleus, which receives information for somatic sensation from the external auditory meatus and meninges

Cranial nerve X exits the brainstem as several rootlets, which cross the subarachnoid space and leave the cranial cavity through the jugular foramen.

The recurrent laryngeal nerve, a branch of cranial nerve X, travels down to the thorax before ascending to innervate the larynx. This route means that the nerve is often trapped in patients with apical lung cancer, resulting in vocal cord paralysis and a hoarse, rasping voice.

Cranial nerve XI: spinal accessory nerve

Cranial nerve X I is a motor nerve that innervates the sternocleidomastoid muscle, which rotates and flexes the neck. It also innervates the upper parts of the trapezius (the lower parts are innervated by C3 and C4).

Cranial nerve XI is not a true cranial nerve, because its main nuclei are located not in the brain but in the upper cervical spinal cord. Its efferents exit the cord and ascend through the foramen magnum to the intracranial cavity, then exit through the jugular foramen to innervate the muscles.

The cranial part of the accessory nerve arises in the nucleus ambiguus of the medulla (**Figure 1.60**), and is considered part of cranial nerve X.

Cranial nerve XII: hypoglossal

Cranial nerve XII is purely motor. It controls tongue movement, because it innervates all tongue muscles except the palatoglossus, which is innervated by cranial nerve X. The hypoglossal nucleus is in the medulla (**Figure 1.60**) and receives bilateral innervation from upper motor neurones.

Lower motor neurone damage to cranial nerve XII results in typical motor signs in the tongue. These include wasting and fasciculations, a rapid flickering of muscle activity and deviation towards the lesion side when 'stuck out'.

Cranial nerve XII exits the skull through the hypoglossal canal. It descends to the lower portion of the digastric muscles before ascending to the submandibular region.

Special senses

The 'special senses' are vision, smell, taste, hearing and balance. The sensations are detected by specialised sensory receptors detecting light, chemicals (for smell and taste), sound vibration and movement, respectively. Each of these organs is innervated by a specific cranial nerve.

Vision

Vision is the perception of the surrounding environment from information carried by light waves. The organ of vision is the eye. It receives information carried by light waves and transmits it via the visual pathway to the visual cortex of each occipital lobe (see page 45).

Gross anatomy of the eye

The eye has a tough exterior comprising sclera and cornea (**Figure 1.65**).

- **The sclera** is the tough, fibrous 'white' of the eye, consisting of the connective tissues collagen and elastin
- **The cornea** is the transparent exterior; it is composed of collagen and proteins, including albumin, surrounded by a layer of epithelial cells

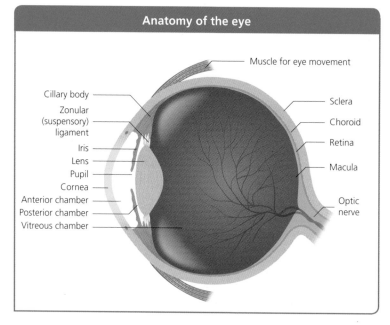

Anatomy of the eye

Muscle for eye movement

Cillary body
Zonular (suspensory) ligament
Iris
Lens
Pupil
Cornea
Anterior chamber
Posterior chamber
Vitreous chamber

Sclera
Choroid
Retina
Macula
Optic nerve

Figure 1.65 Anatomy of the eye.

Internally, the eye has three chambers.

- **The anterior chamber** contains fluid aqueous humour
- **The posterior chamber** contains the lens and its supporting structures (see page 107)
- **The vitreous chamber** contains gel-like vitreous humour

The iris is the coloured muscular ring in the sclera. The pupil functions like the aperture of a camera. Pupil size is under autonomic control: sympathetic action dilates it (mydriasis) and parasympathetic action constricts it (miosis) (see page 57).

The lens is a tough, clear, crystalline structure that focuses light rays on the back of the eyeball (see page 107). It is biconvex, i.e. curved outwards on both sides, and has three parts.

- **Capsule:** the elastic outermost layer of the lens, made of smooth, transparent collagen
- **Epithelium:** a layer of cuboidal epithelial cells that control homeostasis of the lens
- **Fibres:** transparent, tightly packed fibres composed of crystallin

The lens is suspended in the eye from the zonula fibres, which are connected to the ciliary muscles. These muscles are used to produce the accommodation reflex (see page 109).

Extraocular muscles inserted in the sclera and skull are controlled by cranial nerves III, IV and VI (see page 103).

> **Damage to the extraocular muscles, or the nerves that control them, often causes diplopia (double vision).** Developmental misalignment, known as 'squint' (strabismus), does not cause diplopia, because discrepancies are compensated for in this condition.

The retina

The lens focuses light on to the retina (**Figure 1.66**), a multilayered structure containing sensory photoreceptors.

- **Rods** are used when light is scarce, such as at night
- **Cones** are used in daylight and other bright conditions

Cones are concentrated in the macula and fovea, the centrepoint of the retina where light is focussed; their density determines visual acuity (clarity of vision). Rods are

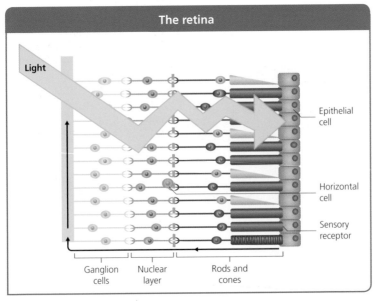

The retina

Light

Epithelial cell

Horizontal cell

Sensory receptor

Ganglion cells   Nuclear layer   Rods and cones

Figure 1.66
The retina.

distributed throughout the retina to increase light absorption in low-light levels.

Only cones can detect colour. In normal – trichromatic – colour vision, three types of cone are used: red-, green- and blue-sensitive. Deficits cause colour blindness, a genetic, X-linked trait affecting 8% of men and 0.5% of women.

Vascular supply and sensory afferents converge at the optic disc. This part of the retina contains no rods or cones, so it is the 'blind spot'. The blind spot lies medial to the macula, on the nasal portion of the retina.

Refraction

Light entering the eye is refracted (bent) by the curvature of the sclera and cornea, the aqueous humour, the lens and the vitreous humour, so that the image reaching the retina is inverted. Refractive errors cause blurred vision and are caused by changes in the curvature of the cornea or lens, or the composition of the humours, which distort the image before it reaches the retina.

Accommodation

For an object to be seen clearly, light must be focused on to the macula and fovea of the retina, where the cones are most concentrated. This is achieved by accommodation, the adjustment of lens strength by changes in ciliary muscle tension.

- Relaxation of the ciliary muscles increases the tension of zonula fibres, stretching the lens and enabling distance vision
- Contraction decreases tension in the zonula fibres, giving a rounder, fatter lens for near vision

Deficits in lens strength and elasticity underlie most common visual disorders (**Table 1.37**).

The visual pathways

The visual pathways carry sensory information from the retina to the visual cortex (**Figure 1.67**).

Afferents exiting the optic disc form the optic nerve, i.e. cranial nerve II, which travels to the optic chiasm (Greek, 'mark with an X'). Here, the nerves converge and fibres from the nasal retina decussate. At this point information about the right visual field converges on the left and forms the optic tract, and vice-versa.

The optic tracts project from the chiasm to the lateral geniculate nucleus in the thalamus, and the optic radiation from the thalamus to the visual cortices. The radiation is formed of two bundles of fibres, one passing through the temporal lobe, carrying information about the

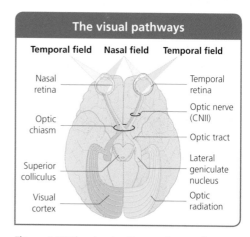

Figure 1.67 The visual pathways. See text for further explanation.

Visual defect	Common name	Deficit	Focus	Corrective lens
Myopia	Short sightedness	Strong lens	In front of retina	Concave
Hypermetropia	Long-sightedness	Weak lens	Behind retina	Convex
Astigmatism		Asymmetry	Imbalanced	Toric
Presbyopia		Reduced elasticity	Increased near point	Magnifying (reading glasses)

Table 1.37 Common deficits in accommodation (the closest point at which an object can be brought into focus)

upper half of the visual field, the other through the parietal cortex carrying information about the lower half of the visual field.

Additional projections from the optic chiasm to the suprachiasmatic nuclei, located in the hypothalamus, which control circadian rhythm. Projections to an area of the brainstem called the pretectum control pupillary and accommodation reflexes, and those to the superior colliculi control movement towards visual stimuli.

When a patient presents with a visual field defect, the nature of the defect usually identifies the location of the lesion within the optic pathways (**Table 1.38**).

Visual pathway lesions and visual field defects		
Lesion location	Lesion location and visual field defect	Name
None		Normal vision
Optic nerve		Unilateral visual loss
Optic chiasm		Bitemporal hemianopia
Optic tract		Homonymous hemianopia
Optic radiation (temporal pathways)		Quadrantanopia
Optic radiation (calcarine)		Quadrantanopia (macular-sparing)

Table 1.38 Correlation between visual field defects and locations of lesions in the visual pathway

Smell

The sense of smell (olfaction) provides information about the external environment through the detection of chemicals carried in the air. Smell alerts people to the presence of danger or food, and helps in the recognition of others. It combines many primary modalities, including floral, fruity and musk, and is linked to memory, emotion and basic sensation.

> **Noxious odours**, such as ammonia, trigger pain receptors and are carried by cranial nerve V rather than the olfactory system.

Air enters the nose and is channelled to the olfactory mucosa by folds of tissue called turbinates (nasal concha). The mucosa contains chemosensory olfactory cells (olfactory receptor neurones) (**Figure 1.68**). Odorants dissolve in the mucus before binding to chemoreceptors on the olfactory cells. Cells generally respond to several odours as they have receptors responsive to many modalities, but optimally to one.

> **Olfactory cells lose their responsiveness (desensitise) very rapidly.** Over the course of a day, a person becomes unaware of the perfume applied in the morning, even though the notes remain for others to smell.

Sensory afferents cross the cribriform plate to the olfactory bulb, continuing along the olfactory tract (cranial nerve I) to the primary olfactory area in the uncus. Projections travel via the thalamus to the primary olfactory cortex and to limbic, frontal and hypothalamic regions for higher processing (**Figure 1.68**).

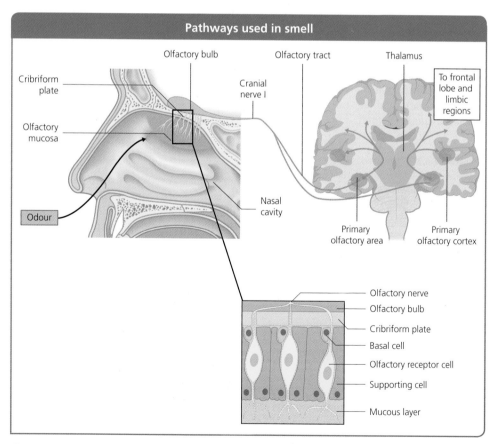

Pathways used in smell

Cribriform plate

Olfactory mucosa

Odour

Olfactory bulb

Cranial nerve I

Nasal cavity

Olfactory tract

Thalamus

To frontal lobe and limbic regions

Primary olfactory area

Primary olfactory cortex

Olfactory nerve
Olfactory bulb
Cribriform plate
Basal cell
Olfactory receptor cell
Supporting cell
Mucous layer

Figure 1.68 Pathways used in smell. See text for futher explanation.

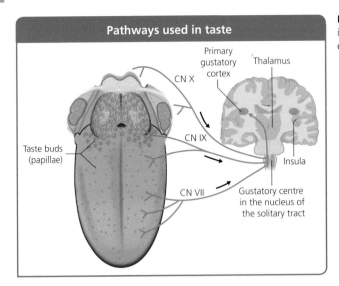

Pathways used in taste

Primary gustatory cortex

Thalamus

CN X

CN IX

Taste buds (papillae)

Insula

CN VII

Gustatory centre in the nucleus of the solitary tract

Figure 1.69 Pathways used in taste. See text for further explanation.

Taste

Taste, like smell, is a chemical sense. It combines five primary modalities: sweet, salt, sour, bitter and umami (meaty). Taste is also associated with somatic sensations, including temperature and consistency (e.g. fatty and liquid), carried by cranial nerve V. Together with the sense of smell, taste provides information about the flavour and nutritional quality of food.

> Taste receptors for all modalities are present on all areas of the tongue. Previously, they were thought to be localised to specific regions.

Taste is detected by sensory cells in the tongue and information is then carried by three cranial nerves (**Figure 1.69**):

■ cranial nerve VII – from the anterior two thirds of the tongue
■ cranial nerve IX – from the posterior third of the tongue
■ cranial nerve X – from the epiglottis and pharynx

These nerves carry the information to the gustatory centres, which are in the nucleus of the solitary tract in the brainstem. The information then passes through the thalamus to the primary gustatory cortex (**Figure 1.69**). Projections to limbic regions allow taste information to be linked to memory and emotional state. Projections to the hypothalamus and brainstem salivatory nuclei (see page 102) control autonomic responses to food intake.

Hearing

Hearing is our quickest sense, enabling us to detect and respond to sound waves 1000 times quicker than to visual information. Sound waves are patterns of vibrations that act on specialised organs situated in the ear. Perception of sound enables sounds to be identified, located and interpreted, and is vital for speech and spoken language.

Anatomy of the ear

The ear is divided into three sections (**Figure 1.70**).

■ The **outer section** (the external ear) comprises the pinna and ear canal, which channel sound into the ear
■ The **middle ear** contains the ossicular chain and Eustachian canal (pharyngotympanic tube), which connects the middle ear to the pharynx to facilitate pressure equalisation between the middle ear and the external environment

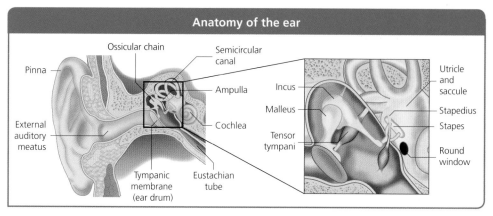

Anatomy of the ear

Ossicular chain

Semicircular canal

Pinna

Ampulla

Incus

Utricle and saccule

Malleus

Stapedius

External auditory meatus

Cochlea

Tensor tympani

Stapes

Round window

Tympanic membrane (ear drum)

Eustachian tube

Figure 1.70 Anatomy of the ear.

■ The **inner ear**, the labyrinth, contains the cochlea and vestibular organs, which have roles in hearing and balance, respectively

The labyrinth has a bony exterior, as shown in **Figure 1.70**, with a smaller but similarly shaped membranous labyrinth within it. Perilymph, a fluid consisting of cerebrospinal fluid and plasma, fills the space between the bony and membranous labyrinth, supporting the latter and maintaining its environment. The membranous labyrinth itself is filled with endolymph, a fluid similar to perilymph but with a high potassium concentration to enable ion flow on activation of the sensory cells (see below).

The spiral part of the labyrinth, the cochlea, is the organ of hearing (see below). The other parts – the semicircular canals, utricle and saccule – are the organs of balance (see page 114).

Transmission of sound

Sound waves travel down the ear canal to the tympanic membrane (eardrum). Vibrations are transmitted across the middle ear via the bony ossicular chain (**Figure 1.70**), which comprises:

■ the **malleus** (Latin, 'hammer')
■ the **incus** (Latin, 'anvil')
■ the **stapes** (Latin, 'stirrup')

The tensor tympani and stapedius muscles attenuate movement of the tympanic membrane and stapes, respectively. This protects the bones against noise damage.

The stapes vibrates against the oval window, which sends waveforms along the cochlea. Vibration causes movement of the basilar membrane situated within the endolymph-filled spiral organ (organ of Corti) within the cochlea (**Figure 1.70**).

This movement causes the cilia of sensory inner hair cells within the organ of Corti to bend against a membrane called the tectorial membrane. The bending of their cilia results in depolarisation of hair cells, generating an action potential which is carried along the axons which form the auditory nerve (part of cranial nerve VIII) (**Figure 1.70**).

Outer hair cells can rapidly change length, in response to strong vibrations, altering the amount of bend they produce on vibration of the basilar membrane, and in this way amplifying or attenuating responses to sound.

The pitch of a sound is ascertained from the distance that its vibration waveform travels along the cochlea. Deep sounds travel further than high ones; think whale song versus mouse squeak.

Sensory afferents travelling in cranial nerve VIII project to the cochlear nuclei and olivary nuclei in the brainstem. They then travel via the inferior colliculus and thalamus to the auditory cortex and association areas in the sensory cortex. Comparison of signals from right and left nerves enables the direction of sound to be determined.

Balance

The ability to detect changes in balance allows correct posture to be maintained; it also enables orientation to the environment. Body position changes constantly; the vestibular system is the specialised organ for detecting the position of the head and controlling adjustments these changes. It has a similar role to that of the proprioceptive organs in the body and has three components:

- The **semicircular canals** are three loops of interconnected fluid-filled canals set at 90° to each other (see **Figure 1.70**); they detect movement along the *x*-, *y*- and *z*-axes
- The **utricle** is a pouch-like structure that detects horizontal head movement and position
- The **saccule** detects vertical head position

The semicircular canals comprise the dynamic labyrinth; they contain structures called ampullae, which detect acceleration and angular head changes. Each ampulla contains a crista ampullaris or ampullary crest. This is fluid filled and contains a

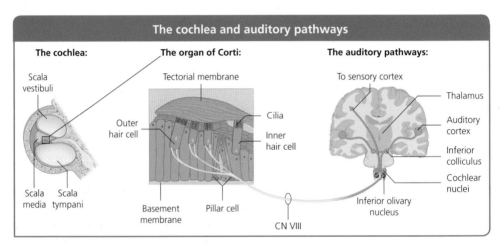

Figure 1.71 The cochlea and auditory pathways. Movement of hair cells against the tectorial membrane in the organ of Corti triggers action potentials which travel along cranial nerve VIII. See text for further explanation

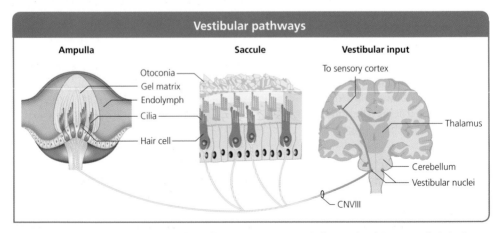

Figure 1.72 The vestibular system supplies information to maintain balance. The christa ampullaris in the ampulla of the semi-circular canals and otoconia in the saccule of the macula detect movement. See text for further details.

gel-like cupula within which lie the cilia of sensory cells (**Figure 1.72**). When the head moves, movement of the fluid bends the cilia and this activates the the hair cells.

The utricle and saccule, which are termed the static labyrinth, monitor head position. They contain macula, specialised epithelium bearing hair cells that protrude into a gel-like substance which has otoconia (ear stones) embedded on its surface (**Figure 1.72**). Gravitational effects on the otoconia move the gel, and this movement activates the hair cells.

> **Vertigo is a spinning sensation when a person is not moving** (not a fear of heights, which is acrophobia). It often presents with balance problems, nausea and vomiting. It is caused by vestibular dysfunction, e.g. due to inflammation and infection the inner ear or vascular changes affecting the brainstem.

Sensory afferents from the dynamic and static labyrinth form the vestibular nerve, which merges with the cochlear nerve to form cranial nerve VIII, and travels to the vestibular nuclei within the brainstem. The vestibulospinal tracts carry information via the thalamus to the parietal cortex and cerebellum for proprioceptive integration.

The vestibulo-ocular reflex

To maintain fixed gaze, vestibular information projects to the abducens (cranial nerve VI, lateral rectus) and oculomotor nuclei (cranial nerve III, medial rectus) to control horizontal eye movement through the vestibulo-ocular reflex.

Nystagmus is the alternating slow and fast eye movements induced by excessive head rotation. The condition is caused by the vestibulo-ocular reflex rapidly adjusting the focus point to compensate for head movement. Nystagmus in the absence of rotation is abnormal.

Answers to starter questions

1. The amount of cerebral folding is a better indicator of intelligence than the ratio of brain to body mass, known as the encephalisation quotient. Folding increases the surface area of the brain, thereby increasing the potential density and connectivity between neurones.

2. The nervous system regulates itself. The brain regulates itself through internal networks, and both the brain and the spinal cord control the activity of the peripheral nervous system. Certain areas, for example the hypothalamus and the insula, maintain set ranges of neural activity, thereby preventing potentially harmful under- or overactivity.

3. The dominant side of the brain is the one responsible for logical and analytical aspects of perception. It is the hemisphere in which the speech centres are located. The left hemisphere is dominant in > 95% of right-handed people and almost 85% of left-handed people, suggesting that the correlation between handedness and speech lateralisation is more complex than initially thought.

4. The firing, on–off pattern of neuronal activation is considered the 'language' of the nervous system. It is similar to the binary code used by computers.

5. Having many types of neurotransmitter enables a high degree of flexibility in cell-to-cell communication, as well as the subtle changes required for the complex behaviour of humans.

Answers *continued*

6. Brain activity and function must be flexible for it to fulfil complex roles, for example in learning and memory formation. This flexibility is conferred by neuronal plasticity, which is the ability to produce new neurones, through neogenesis, and change the structure and function of existing neurones.

7. Many cues, including physical (structural), electrical, cellular and chemical ones, control the development of the brain. Such cues determine its maximum size and the shape and pattern of folding.

8. The adult skull is a rigid, thick, bony box designed to protect the brain from physical insult. In babies, the skull sutures have yet to fuse and are moveable. Between the bone plates of a baby's skull are the fontanelles (soft spots), which are covered with tough membranes to protect the brain without restricting growth.

9. Meninges are vital; they protect and support the brain and spinal cord. They provide stabilising attachments to the skull and vertebral column, reducing the effects of movement. They are also the route of blood drainage and contain cerebrospinal fluid, which nourishes and maintains the integrity of the delicate central nervous system tissue.

10. A body can function at a basic level without a cortex, because control of vital functions such as heart rate, circulation and respiration is a function of the brainstem. Higher neural functions, such as those responsible for decision-making and personality, take place in the cerebral cortex.

11. The idea that a person uses only 10% of their brain is a myth. In truth, 100% of it is used, but areas are active only when they need to be. It would be energetically wasteful to feed the whole brain at times when only certain areas are functioning.

12. In thalamic deep brain stimulation, electrodes attached to pacemakers are implanted in specific areas of the brain. The electrodes produce a regular pattern of signals to stimulate the thalamus. These external signals override the irregular motor or sensory activity underlying the patient's symptoms.

13. The essential bodily functions do not require conscious control from the cortex or fine-tuning by the cerebellum. Sufficient drive to pace and control activity in these circuits is provided by the primitive brainstem, which is highly protected by the dense bone surrounding it.

14. Sleep is controlled by the reticular formation in the brainstem. Deprivation of sleep impairs memory formation, because it prevents the normal 'switch off' of input from the reticular formation to the thalamus and cerebrum. During this period of 'downtime', cortical activity patterns that were produced during daily activities are replayed, making sleep vital for embedding memories.

15. The thin, regular folding of the cerebellum creates a huge surface area, which enables a high density of cells to be closely packed into a small area. This close packing allows rapid processing and integration of neuronal activity to occur and thus rapid adjustments to movements while they are being carried out.

16. Alcohol rapidly alters the cerebellar activity that fine-tunes movement. The effects of alcohol become noticeable within a short time because of the high density and connectivity of cerebellar networks. Even if only a small number of cells are initially affected by the alcohol, they can influence the activity of many others, thereby quickly reducing the ability to control movement precisely. Alcohol also affects the prefrontal cortex, which controls speech, personality and movement, hence the changes to these behaviours.

Answers *continued*

17. The spinal cord used to be considered just a conduit, carrying information from the brain to the peripheral nerves. It is now known to coordinate and fine-tune activity as it enters and leaves the central nervous system.

18. Lower motor neurones originate in the anterior horn of the spinal cord. Projections from the upper motor neurones travel from the cortex and brainstem to connect with the lower motor neurones in the cord. Lower motor neurones are present along the whole length of the cord, so damage to one section affects both upper and lower motor neurones.

19. The ability to feel pain is vital for survival, because it alerts people to physical danger. Patients with congenital insensitivity to pain have no perception of danger, so they often suffer multiple injuries that greatly reduce their life expectancy.

20. Reflex circuits are constantly being activated by sensory input, so the brain dampens their activity to prevent unwanted movement. This concept is called descending inhibition, and its absence explains why damage to this system result in overactivity, seen as increased muscle tone, spasticity and hyper-reflexia.

21. Well-trained athletes use the startle reflex to start moving. This unconscious reflex to a sharp sound, for example that of a starter gun, causes the body to initiate leg movement before the sound is consciously registered and acted on.

22. Reflexes are active circuits that rapidly initiate predictable, unconscious patterns of movement. They are a vital component of survival, because they enable rapid responses to environmental changes.

23. Reflexes can change over time. Babies have 'primitive' reflexes, which allow them to right themselves and suckle, before they develop controlled motor skills. Deep tendon reflexes also change and are often influenced by mental status; a distracted mind increases reflexes by reducing descending inhibition.

24. Hypothalamic activity, which controls activity in the autonomic nervous system, is modified by input from higher centres, such as emotional information from the frontal and temporal lobes. Therefore autonomic activity can be placed under voluntary control; for example, with training it is possible to learn to override the increase in heart rate triggered by fear responses.

25. The enteric nervous system, which controls the gastrointestinal tract, has its own division of the nervous system because it functions independently of the central, peripheral and autonomic nervous systems. However, it can be classed as a subsection of the autonomic nervous system, because it controls unconscious motor behaviours and uses neuronal networks equivalent to the parasympathetic and sympathetic systems.

26. Emotional incontinence, the outbursts of crying or laughing in cases of pseudobulbar palsy, is a consequence of damage to the higher pathways controlling cranial nerve function, for example nerves controlling facial expression and the vocal cords. Emotional incontinence is the emotional equivalent of hyper-reflexia, and is caused by spontaneous activation of reflex emotional circuitry.

27. Compensation for lost sensation does occur. For example, loss of vision is often associated with an increased ability in olfaction or hearing, and loss of hearing is often associated with an increased sense of vibration. This phenomenon probably results from a shift in focus and reduced 'noise in the system', which increases the clarity of the remaining senses.

Answers *continued*

28. Specific anosmias are genetic and caused by selective odorant receptor deficits. For example, 10% of people cannot smell the bitter-almond scent of cyanide, and 2% cannot smell the components of body odour.

Chapter 2
Clinical essentials

Introduction

Just 10 presentations are the subject of 75% of neurological outpatient consultations (**Table 2.1**). All clinicians need to be able to identify, treat or refer the conditions that cause them.

Neurology is predominantly an outpatient-based specialty in which complex patient presentations arising from long-term, often rare conditions are reviewed. Neurosurgery addresses acute and life-threatening surgical emergencies of many types, principally the presentations listed in **Table 2.2**.

Common neurological outpatient complaints	
Presentation	Common causes
Headache and facial pain	Migraine, subarachnoid haemorrhage and tumour
Balance problems	Vertigo and ataxia
Epilepsy and blackouts	Seizures and syncope
Neuropathies	Diabetic neuropathy and inflammatory neuropathy
Movement disorders	Parkinson's disease and tremor
Stroke	Transient ischaemic attack and stroke
Dementia	Alzheimer's disease and vascular dementia
Multiple sclerosis	Optic neuritis and transverse myelitis
Spinal disease	Intervertebral disc protrusions
Functional disorders	Weakness and sensory disturbance

Table 2.1 The 10 presentations that are the subject of 75% of neurological outpatient consultations

Common neurological emergencies	
Emergency	Common causes
Coma	Hypoxia and head injury
Subarachnoid haemorrhage	Aneurysm and arteriovenous malformation
Status epilepticus	Use of certain drugs, hypoglycaemia and tumours
Increased intracranial pressure	Tumours and trauma
Head injury	Subdural haematoma and extradural haematoma
Acute spinal cord syndromes	Trauma and infection
Neurological infection	Meningitis, encephalitis and abscess
Acute neuromuscular weakness	Myasthenia gravis and Guillain-Barré syndrome

Table 2.2 Common neurological emergencies

History taking and examination are diagnostic tools used to differentiate diseases. To be able to detect and understand the major clinical signs and know when to refer a patient to a specialist requires:

- a clear framework of knowledge of basic neuroanatomy and neurophysiology
- an understanding of the main patterns of neuropathology
- knowledge of the common and 'red flag' signs and symptoms and their main causes
- the ability to confidently perform neurological examination of the cranial nerves, upper body and lower body, and to interpret the findings
- a basic understanding of neurophysiological and neuroimaging investigations

Common symptoms and how to take a history

Starter questions

Answers to the following questions are on page 184.

1. What is it like to experience neurological symptoms?
2. Why is the neurological history so important?

Common symptoms

As you listen to the patient give the history, always ask yourself which part of the nervous system could be affected to give the symptoms that they are describing. This approach helps localise the problem.

Consciousness

Loss of consciousness and altered awareness are common; syncope affects about 20% of the population. In contrast, epilepsy affects only 0.75%.

The history taking should attempt to differentiate syncope, seizures and non-epileptic attacks by establishing a detailed picture of the event from start to finish:

- triggers or the situations in which it occurs
- preceding symptoms
- the moment of loss of consciousness
- breathing, colour change, eye movements and whether the eyes are open or closed leading up to, during and after the episode
- responsiveness to verbal or physical stimuli during the episode
- duration
- the nature of any change in muscle tone, posture or movements and their duration during the episode
- the speed of return to normal, and any confusion, disorientation, tearfulness or odd behaviour

The accounts of eyewitnesses are always central to the history. Ask about similar previous episodes, childhood febrile seizures, head trauma and use of prescribed or recreational drugs.

> **A prolonged prodrome** of several minutes of odd symptoms, such as dizziness, light-headedness, nausea and tunnel vision, is far more likely to point to syncope rather than a seizure.

Syncope

This is a sudden transient loss of consciousness with rapid recovery; it is caused by

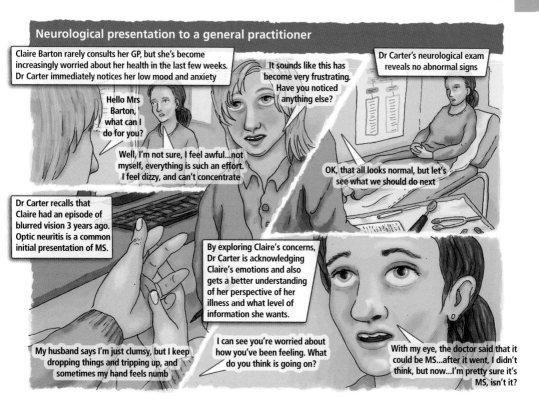

Neurological presentation to a general practitioner

Claire Barton rarely consults her GP, but she's become increasingly worried about her health in the last few weeks. Dr Carter immediately notices her low mood and anxiety

Hello Mrs Barton, what can I do for you?

Well, I'm not sure, I feel awful...not myself, everything is such an effort. I feel dizzy, and can't concentrate

It sounds like this has become very frustrating. Have you noticed anything else?

Dr Carter's neurological exam reveals no abnormal signs

OK, that all looks normal, but let's see what we should do next

Dr Carter recalls that Claire had an episode of blurred vision 3 years ago. Optic neuritis is a common initial presentation of MS.

By exploring Claire's concerns, Dr Carter is acknowledging Claire's emotions and also gets a better understanding of her perspective of her illness and what level of information she wants.

My husband says I'm just clumsy, but I keep dropping things and tripping up, and sometimes my hand feels numb

I can see you're worried about how you've been feeling. What do you think is going on?

With my eye, the doctor said that it could be MS...after it went, I didn't think, but now...I'm pretty sure it's MS, isn't it?

---

global cerebral hypoperfusion. Syncope frequently has cardiovascular causes and is often preceded by light-headedness, closing in of the visual field, tinnitus or autonomic symptoms (e.g. nausea, sweating, pallor and flushing), followed by collapse to the ground. There is frequently urinary incontinence or jerking movements of the limbs. There is then a fairly rapid recovery, over a few minutes, and minimal confusion or disorientation after the event. Specific triggers include standing, coughing, unpleasant sights or procedures (e.g. venepuncture) and prolonged standing.

Seizure

This is a spontaneous, episodic, abnormal discharge of electrical activity in the brain. Seizure results in one or more of:

- abnormal motor, sensory or autonomic features
- altered behaviour and emotion
- altered consciousness

There are many types of seizure. Therefore enquire about specific details and check what the patient means when they use the term 'seizure'.

Usually there is no trigger, but the patient may experience an aura (see page 232), which represents the start of seizure activity in the brain. The nature of the aura, along with the patient's behaviour during a seizure, can help localise the cerebral region of onset (**Figure 2.1**).

> The chief characteristic of seizures is that they are stereotyped recurrent events. This means that each is the same, with no trigger or syncope-like prodrome.

Movement disorder

Problems with motor function are very common and manifest as weakness, slowness, stiffness or with abnormal movements. These each have quite different causes.

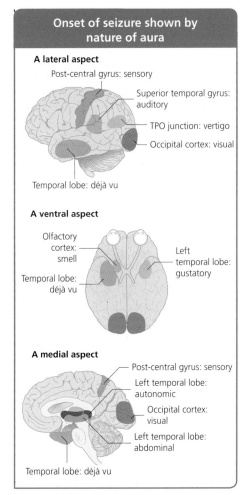

Onset of seizure shown by nature of aura

A lateral aspect

Post-central gyrus: sensory

Superior temporal gyrus: auditory

TPO junction: vertigo

Occipital cortex: visual

Temporal lobe: déjà vu

A ventral aspect

Olfactory cortex: smell

Left temporal lobe: gustatory

Temporal lobe: déjà vu

A medial aspect

Post-central gyrus: sensory

Left temporal lobe: autonomic

Occipital cortex: visual

Left temporal lobe: abdominal

Temporal lobe: déjà vu

Figure 2.1 Localisation of onset of seizure based on nature of aura. TPO, temporal–parietal junction.

Impaired strength of muscular contraction has variable onsets and timings, depending on the cause. The terms -plegia and -paresis describe complete and partial weakness, respectively. Examples are:

■ **hemiplegia,** which is complete paralysis of one side of the body, affecting the face, arm and leg
■ **hemiparesis,** a partial weakness of one side of the body, affecting the face, arm and leg

Fatiguability

This is a progressive worsening of muscle weakness that occurs with repeated muscle use and improves with rest. It is a characteristic feature of myasthenia gravis (see page 438).

Slowness

A general slowing of the movements, or of walking or other specific tasks, is usually a description of bradykinesia. This suggests a parkinsonian syndrome and mandates a check for other features of Parkinson's disease and features associated with Parkinson's plus syndromes (see page 313): symmetrical onset, severe early bladder or bowel symptoms or postural hypotension, cerebellar symptoms, gaze restriction and early falls.

Stiffness

This is a patients' term for increased muscle tone, which may result in difficulty or slowness in moving. It is a core clinical feature of an upper motor neurone lesion.

Abnormal movements

These are common and can be a symptom of systemic illness. It is essential to elicit in the history a careful description of the movements.

The following types of abnormal movements indicate particular causes and are described below:

■ chorea
■ athetosis
■ choreoathetoid movements
■ dystonia
■ tremor
■ myoclonus
■ torticollis
■ restless legs

Chorea

This is the term for brief, irregular (jerking), semipurposeful flowing movements.

Athetosis

The term athetosis describes slower, writhing, non-purposeful, often flowing movements. These movements usually affect the limbs.

Choreoathetoid movements

These movements occur in coexisting chorea and athetosis.

Dystonia

This is intermittent or sustained involuntary muscle contraction resulting in twisting and repetitive movements or abnormal postures. Patients with dystonia describe a limb that does not work, or goes stiff or tight, and the prolonged muscle contraction is often painful. If the condition is intermittent, it may not be evident during assessment. Dystonia is classified according to the body part (or parts) affected and the specific movements or tasks that trigger it (**Table 2.3**).

> **Dystonia** is often misdiagnosed as a functional illness by inexperienced clinicians.

Tremor

This is an involuntary rhythmic movement of a limb or other body part, which the patient often describes as shaking, jerking or twitching. Tremor not associated with disease is classified as essential tremor, which occurs in 10% of people older than 65 years (see page 322).

Myoclonus

This type of movement is a sudden, brief, shock-like contraction or relaxation in muscle tone; it is described by patients as jerking, jumping, seizing or startling. Myoclonus is common in systemic metabolic derangements, such as uraemia in renal failure, or as an adverse effect of medication, for example lithium.

Myoclonus can be isolated ('essential') myoclonus, in which case it is usually benign. Alternatively, it can be a component of epileptic or neurodegenerative disease.

Torticollis

This is neck dystonia causing the head to turn to one side. Torticollis is the commonest adult onset dystonia. The sternocleidomastoid muscle often hypertrophies from sustained contractions. Patients often have a 'sensory trick', whereby touching certain parts of the head stops the dystonia.

Restless legs

This is an irresistible urge to move the legs; it affects 2–15% of the population. The condition usually occurs in bed or at rest and is relieved by movement.

Restless legs can occur as a primary disorder or as part of a neurodegenerative disease. An underlying disease is unlikely if there is a family history of the condition, symptoms improve with dopaminergic therapy or leg movements occur during sleep as well.

> **Tremor and myoclonus do not always signal underlying illness.** However, they often have a serious effect on a patient's confidence and social life.

Sensation

Altered sensation is a common symptom. When non-progressive and in the absence of neurological signs, it is usually benign or part of a functional disorder. However, it can be the predominant or sole symptom of serious diseases, for example multiple sclerosis or Guillain–Barré syndrome, and therefore requires exploration.

Patients seldom report alteration in sensation as a loss from a single sensory modality (pain, temperature, joint position sense or

Classification of dystonia	
By parts affected	By aetiology
■ Focal: one body part affected ■ Segmental: two or more adjacent parts involved ■ Multifocal: two or more non-adjacent parts involved ■ Generalised: widespread muscles involved	■ Primary: dystonia is the only neurological symptom ■ Secondary: nervous system injury or illness (e.g. stroke) is evident ■ Heredodegenerative: symptomatic of a degenerative neurological disease (e.g. Huntington's disease)

Table 2.3 Classification of dystonia

vibration sense; see page 77). They often struggle to describe sensory symptoms. Altered joint position or vibration senses are likely to be reported as balance problems, such as falling, unsteadiness and clumsiness. The history should explore:

- which body part is affected
- how the symptoms have progressed
- how they have fluctuated
- other neurological symptoms

No sensation

Often described as numbness, loss of tactile sensation is a common symptom in functional illness but is also present in cases of central nervous system lesions affecting sensory pathways. For example, a lacunar stroke affecting the internal capsule can cause loss of sensation, with some weakness, on one side of the body.

Paraesthesia

This is the perception of non-painful tactile sensations without an objective cause for them. It is often described as 'pins and needles', prickling, burning, crawling or tingling. If paraesthesia is the sole symptom and is non-progressive, it is unlikely to represent a significant illness. Paraesthesia is common in peripheral nerve diseases, usually bilateral and in a glove-and-stocking distribution (see page 140) or in the distribution of a particular nerve.

> **Stroke** almost always causes a loss of sensation rather than positive abnormal sensations such as paraesthesias.

Saddle anaesthesia

This describes altered sensation over the perineum and is a core clinical feature of cauda equina syndrome (see page 356). Patients may report numbness or dysaesthesia over their anus or genital region, or 'not feeling it when I wipe after using the toilet'.

> **Saddle anaesthesia requires urgent assessment for other features of cauda equina syndrome.** These features include leg or foot weakness, altered bladder or bowel function, and back pain.

Pain

With some causes, such as headache, the description of the pain and associated features is central to diagnosis.

The mnemonic SOCRATES helps explore pain:

- **Site:** where is it, and is it always on the same side?
- **Onset:** how quickly did it reach peak severity from its onset?
- **Character:** is it aching, throbbing, pulsating, dull, sharp or constant?
- **Radiation:** does it move anywhere?
- **Associated features:** are nausea, vomiting, visual disturbance, weakness, other neurological symptoms, systemic symptoms, fever and infective symptoms present?
- **Timing:** is there a temporal pattern? Has the pain changed since it started, and is it continual, episodic, progressing or improving?
- **Exacerbating or relieving factors:** does anything change the pain, such as posture, activity, light and smells?
- **Severity:** how severe is it?

> **The patient's emotional and physical state has a large role in the effect pain has on their life.** Factors such as mood disturbance, social stressors and sleep disturbance should be explored and treated.

Neuropathic pain

This type of pain results from direct damage to the nervous system (see page 462). Neuropathic pain is commonly described as burning, lancinating or electric shock–like sensations.

Muscle cramp and pain

These are common and can occur as part of normal physiological processes, for example with exercise. Prominent or long-standing muscle pains and cramps can be associated with mitochondrial or other muscle diseases.

Headache and facial pain

The history is essential in diagnosing the cause of a headache. Establishing the nature of the headache and associated symptoms (**Table 2.4**), especially the timing of the pain (**Figure 2.2**), is key. It is also necessary to distinguish primary and secondary headaches and to identify those patients who need urgent referral and investigation (see page 209).

Some primary headache disorders are associated with episodes of altered auto-nomic function in the face. Therefore people with headaches should be asked about such episodes.

> **A new headache requires urgent investigation** if the patient presents with any of the following:
> - papilloedema
> - altered consciousness
> - new or progressive confusion or impairment in coordination or cognition
> - new seizures
> - a history of cancer

Migraine aura An aura precedes or coincides with some migraines and indicates focal neurological dysfunction. Common aura symptoms include flashing lights, fortification

Key elements of headache history	
Feature	Key details to cover
Time from onset to peak of headache	Seconds (thunderclap), minutes, hours or days
Location	Unilateral, bilateral, occipital, frontal, diffuse or focal
Nausea	Nausea with or without vomiting: how often?
Associated features	Photophobia, phonophobia, osmophobia, focal weakness or sensory signs or symptoms, visual symptoms, language problems, seizures, reduced consciousness, tearing, conjunctival injection, facial sweating, ptosis, miosis, nasal stuffiness, scalp tenderness or jaw claudication
Preceding symptoms or mood change	Irritability, lethargy, malaise, fever, cognitive decline, progressive or sudden focal neurological deficit, or visual or sensory aura
Character	Throbbing, stabbing, boring, dull, sharp or pressure
Duration	Seconds, minutes or hours
Frequency and regularity	Continuous, intermittent, in bouts, monthly or seasonal
Disability	Non-disabling, interrupts strenuous activity, prevents daily activity, requires rest, makes patient unable to move or disturbs sleep
Precipitating or relieving factors	Coughing, sneezing, straining, exertion, sexual intercourse, pregnancy, menstruation, stress, change in sleep pattern, certain foods, physical stimuli, lying or standing
Number of types of headache experienced	Single stereotyped headaches, two or more distinct experiences, or evolving from one pattern to another
Patient characteristics	Age at onset, gender and smoking history
Medications used	Regular analgesia or analgesia as needed: possibility of medication overuse headache

Table 2.4 Key elements of the headache history

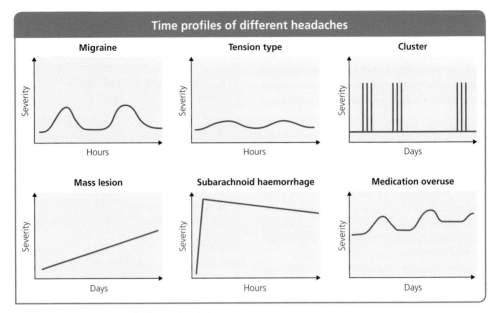

Figure 2.2 Time profiles of different headaches.

spectra (seeing zigzag lines), paraesthesias, motor weakness and dysphasia.

High- or low-pressure headache Headaches can be described as high or low pressure.

- A high-pressure headache is one that worsens on straining, coughing, lying down or sneezing
- A low-pressure headache is a dull or throbbing headache that is exacerbated by standing up and better when lying flat

---

Be alert to the following red flags in the headache history:

- association with neurological signs or symptoms
- high-pressure features (headache exacerbated by straining, coughing or lying down)
- vomiting
- new headache in a patient aged > 50 years.

Thunderclap headache This is any rapidly developing headache that reaches its peak from onset either instantly or within a few seconds. Thunderclap headache requires urgent investigation, because it is frequently a sign of a life-threatening condition such as subarachnoid haemorrhage. There are benign causes, including migraine, but sinister causes must first be urgently ruled out.

Eye pain

Most patients with optic neuritis experience eye pain on eye movement. It is a typical symptom of this condition.

Jaw claudication and scalp tenderness

Pain and tiredness that develop in the muscles involved in chewing during their use and resolves with rest is known as jaw claudication. Scalp tenderness is pain on brushing or stroking the scalp. These are uncommon symptoms and usually indicate temporal arteritis (see page 220). Any patient over 50 years old and presenting with a new headache should be asked about them.

Ear pain (otalgia)

This most often indicates an ear infection. Neurological associations include:

- herpes zoster infection of the ear (Ramsey Hunt syndrome)
- trigeminal neuralgia (see page 220)
- referred pain from a lesion of cranial nerve V, VII, IX or X

Back pain

This is common: 60% of people suffer back pain at any given time. For the vast majority, there is no sinister underlying pathology, so conservative management suffices. Red flags suggesting a sinister cause for back pain are listed on page 342. Back pain is discussed in Chapter 11.

Radicular pain

This is pain that originates in the neck or back and radiates to a specific dermatome. It is common and often caused by a structural lesion affecting nerve roots, for example a herniated intervertebral disc. The affected dermatome identifies the irritated nerve root.

Balance

Problems with balance are a consequence of alteration of proprioceptive input as a result of peripheral nerve, spinal cord, vestibular or cerebellar damage (**Figure 2.3**).

Vertigo

This is the false perception of motion; it is experienced as dizziness, turning or spinning. This common symptom affects about 5% of people.

Table 2.5 summarises common or dangerous causes of vertigo. It can be related to lesions anywhere in the peripheral or central vestibular system. Identifying the cause can be difficult clinically, but the differential diagnosis is narrowed by defining the duration of attacks, triggers, and associated symptoms and neurological signs (see **Table 2.5**).

> Core symptoms and signs of cerebellar dysfunction are VANISHD:
> - Vertigo
> - Ataxia
> - Nystagmus
> - Intention tremor
> - Slurred speech
> - Hypotonia
> - Dysdiadochokinesia

Autonomic function

Isolated autonomic dysfunction is rare. Autonomic dysfunction is usually one of a group of symptoms and signs from a condition such as diabetic neuropathy, the most common cause.

The history should include direct questions about change in bladder, bowel or sexual function (**Table 2.6**). Dysfunction in these areas can be from peripheral or central lesions or secondary to medication use.

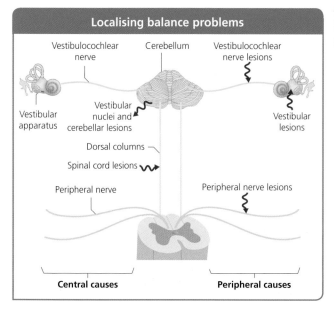

Localising balance problems

Vestibulocochlear nerve

Cerebellum

Vestibulocochlear nerve lesions

Vestibular apparatus

Vestibular nuclei and cerebellar lesions

Vestibular lesions

Dorsal columns

Spinal cord lesions

Peripheral nerve

Peripheral nerve lesions

Central causes

Peripheral causes

Figure 2.3 Peripheral and central lesions contribute to balance problems.

Identification of causes of vertigo		
Condition	Duration of attack	Frequency of attacks
Benign paroxysmal positional vertigo	Initial acute phase hours to days, then 10–15 s	One or two exacerbations per year
Vestibular neuronitis	Several days	One per lifetime
Migraine	Minutes, hours or days	Variable (can be frequent)
Ménière's disease	20 min to 3 h	Recurrent
Brain stem transient ischaemic attack or stroke	Transient ischaemic attack: minutes to hours Stroke: several days	Frequent recurrence of transient ischaemic attacks is rare
Vestibular schwannoma	Weeks	Continuous or recurrent prolonged episodes

Table 2.5 Identification of causes of vertigo

Autonomic function: bladder and bowel history	
Function	Key changes to cover in history
Bladder	Onset: acute, progressing or improving
	Voiding: altered stream
	Initiation: hesitancy
	Termination: dribbling
	Volume passed
	Ability to sense that bladder is full
Bowel	Constipation
	Sensation of need to void
	Urgency
	Ability to hold
Sexual	Libido: normal or reduced
	Erection failure
	Absent ejaculation
	Dyspareunia (pain or discomfort with sexual intercourse)

Table 2.6 Autonomic function: the history should establish any changes in key aspects of bladder and bowel function

Patients often assume that a change in sexual function is not relevant to their other symptoms. They may also be too embarrassed to volunteer information about it. Always ask specifically about sexual function in cases of suspected spinal cord or peripheral nerve diseases.

Special senses

Changes in smell, taste, vision and hearing are the presenting symptoms in many neurological and neurosurgical patients.

Vision

The exact nature, timing, duration and progression of the visual change must be established, because this information narrows the differential diagnosis.

Loss of vision Ascertaining the nature of the loss is essential. For example, transient monocular visual loss has causes ranging from benign, such as migraine, to life-threatening, for example increased intracranial pressure from a tumour (**Table 2.7**).

Blurred vision usually arises from a refractory error of the cornea or lens. However, patients often use the term to report double vision, so clarify the nature of the visual disturbance.

Double vision (diplopia) This is the false visual perception of two of the same object. It is a common neurological symptom with a wide range of causes in a range of locations: brain stem (e.g. as a result of ischaemia), cranial nerves (e.g. because of increased intracranial pressure), orbit (e.g. from orbital cellulitis) and extraocular muscles (e.g. from Graves' ophthalmopathy). It can be monocular (present

Differentiation between types of transient monocular visual loss			
Condition	Type of loss	Duration	Pain
Amaurosis fugax	'Curtain' or 'frosted glass' loss in upper or lower half of visual field of one eye	Seconds to hours	None
Increased intracranial pressure	Brief loss in one or both eyes, varying in region and degree, often with postural changes, coughing or straining	Seconds	Sometimes background headache
Uhthoff's phenomenon	Loss of colour vision or scotoma triggered by heat or exercise	Minutes	None
Migraine aura	Flashing, scintillating, slowly enlarging field defect	Minutes to 1 h; occasionally longer	None or (more usually) typical migraine headache

Table 2.7 Common causes of transient monocular visual loss

with only one eye open) or binocular (present only when both eyes are open). Binocular diplopia is the commonest type.

Photophobia: The dislike or avoidance of light is photophobia. The term is used to describe exacerbation of a headache with exposure to light. Photophobia usually makes patients seek a dark environment. It is a non-specific symptom as well as being a core feature of migraine headaches and the meningism that occurs with subarachnoid haemorrhage or central nervous system infection.

Phonophobia: This is exacerbation of headache by sound. It has the same causes as photophobia.

Spots: Abnormal visual shapes or flashes are common and usually benign, representing the normal ageing of various structures of the eye. But they can be symptoms of significant disease and should be clarified.

- **Floaters** are tiny translucent particles, usually from deposits in the vitreous humour, that can be perceived drifting in the visual field; they are normal, but if they occur in a sudden shower, especially with flashers, they may represent a retinal detachment, which requires urgent ophthalmological review
- **Flashers** are brief flashes of light, often from small areas of retinal detachment
- **Scotomata** are strips or blobs of visual loss in one eye, and usually represent

damage to the retina or optic disc (e.g. in optic neuritis); their presence prompts a thorough neurological review for related symptoms and signs
- **Fortification spectra** are areas of wavy or zigzag lines in the visual field, often as part of a migraine aura; they typically start in one small place, spread over a few minutes to cover a larger area and then resolve, and a typical migraine headache may follow

Hearing

Symptoms of ear disease include the following.

- **Otalgia:** pain in the ear
- **Otorrhoea:** discharge from the ear
- **Aural fullness:** an abnormal sensation of fullness, pressure or discomfort in the ear canal and a key symptom of Ménière disease
- **Tinnitus:** false perception of a tone (often described as ringing, whooshing or pulsing) and a common symptom, affecting 1 in 3 people at some time, most often resulting from noise-induced hearing loss; an association with progressive sensorineural hearing loss suggests an acoustic neuroma or other cranial nerve VIII lesion
- **Hyperacusis:** sensitivity to high-pitched sounds, often resulting in the perception of pain, irritation or discomfort; it is

experienced by 50% of people with tinnitus and associated with cranial nerve VII and VIII dysfunction

■ **Hearing loss (see below):** a common symptom resulting from ageing and excessive exposure to occupational or recreational noise; there are few neurological causes of isolated hearing loss

> **Unilateral adult onset deafness,** with or without vertigo or tinnitus, requires urgent evaluation for underlying structural lesions in the cerebellopontine angle or brain stem.

Loss of hearing Table 2.8 outlines the major types of deafness by cause and their associated clinical features.

Speech, language and swallowing

Speech is the mechanical articulation, and language is the content, fluency and comprehension of speech. Swallowing is a related function, because it employs some of the same muscles and nerves. The first step in evaluating speech or language problems is to clarify exactly what the patient is reporting.

Dysarthria: This is difficulty in articulating words but with normal language content. Causes include motor neurone lesions, cerebellar lesions, neuromuscular junction disorders and muscle disease.

> When a patient reports speech problems, clarify whether the problem is in **thinking or word-finding (dysphasia) or physical articulation (dysarthria).**

Dysphagia: This is difficulty in swallowing; it is common in conditions that cause dysarthria. Isolated dysphagia more often has a non-neurological cause, such as oesophageal tumour, than a neurological one. Pathological processes causing dysphagia and dysarthria often involve the brain stem, lower cranial nerves or the muscles or neuromuscular junctions they innervate; associated symptoms and signs help identify the cause.

Dysphasia: This is language dysfunction and is not caused by articulation problems (**Table 2.9**). The history is often of difficulty finding a word, saying the wrong word or speaking nonsensically. It can be described as:

■ **expressive**, when there is difficulty in producing sensible speech
■ **receptive**, when there is difficulty in understanding language from others
■ **mixed**, when both aspects are seen

Patients tend to present with clinical syndromes of dysphasia (as shown in **Table 2.9**) rather than purely expressive or purely receptive dysphasia.

Dysphasia is seen in any disorder that affects the cerebral cortex or connecting white

Types of deafness		
Type	Structure(s) involved	Causes (associated features)
Conductive (altered conduction of sound waves to the cochlea)	External or middle ear	Ear wax, infection, otosclerosis and Eustachian tube obstruction
Sensorineural (damage to cochlea, central components of hearing or cranial nerve VIII)	Cochlear	Infection, noise (occupational or recreational), toxins (e.g. gentamicin) and age-related presbycusis (high-frequency loss)
	Cochlear nerve	Cerebellopontine angle tumours (tinnitus, facial weakness or numbness), demyelination (other brain stem signs) and tertiary neurosyphilis (vertigo)
Central (lesions in cochlear nuclei and their cortical connections)	Brain stem or cortex	Demyelination and stroke

Table 2.8 The major types of deafness and their associated features

Dysphasia					
Subtype	Speech production	Speech content	Speech reception	Reading	Location
Broca's aphasia	'Broken' (non-fluent)	Some meaningful content	Some understanding	Variable	Frontal operculum
Wernicke's dysphasia	'Watery' (fluent)	Meaningless	Poor understanding	Poor	Posterior superior temporal lobe
Conduction aphasia	Fluent	Some meaningful content	Some understanding	Variable	Inferior parietal lobe

Table 2.9 Subtypes of dysphasia

matter, for example stroke or tumours. If it is of very sudden onset, then stroke is the most likely cause, especially if the clinical picture is a dominant hemisphere stroke (see Chapter 6).

Memory and cognition

Assessment of memory and other cognitive problems is particularly important in patients with neurodegenerative conditions, but many neurological conditions also affect these functions. There are many standardised tools to evaluate memory and cognition. The most commonly used include the mini mental state examination (**Table 2.10**) and the Addenbrooke's cognitive examination. There is much overlap in areas affected by different disease processes, but there are some typical patterns that can point to a particular diagnosis (see page 392).

> **Information from a patient's family or friends is essential when taking a history of cognition.** A patient is often unaware of, downplays or even forgets a problem.

> **Fluctuating orientation and alertness is** the hallmark of delirium. In isolation, it is unusual in dementia.

Systemic symptoms

In patients with new neurological symptoms, it is essential to review systemic symptoms that may indicate a systemic disease, infection

The mini mental state examination	
Cognitive domain	Task
Orientation	Patient asked to name the year, month, day, date, time, country, town, district, hospital and ward
Registration	Examiner names three objects
	Patient repeats until learned
Attention and calculation	Patient subtracts 7 from 100 sequentially or
	Patient spells 'world' backwards
Recall	Patient recalls objects learned earlier
Language	Patient names some common objects
	Patient repeats a simple phrase
	Patient given a three-step command
	Patient given a simple written instruction
	Patient writes a sentence of their making
Visuoperceptual	Patient copies interlocking hexagons

Adapted from Folstein MF, Folstein SE, McHugh PR. 'Mini-mental state'. A practical method for grading the cognitive state of patients for the clinician. J Psychiatr Res 1975; 12:189–198.

Table 2.10 The mini mental state examination

or malignancy. Examples include weight loss and cachexia (wasting syndrome).

Weight loss and cachexia

Patients are often vague or inaccurate about weight loss. Ask if their clothes have become looser or if they have had to tighten belts.

Weight loss is a non-specific symptom of many illnesses but a red flag for cancer, tuberculosis and vasculitis or other systemic autoimmune disease. It often affects patients with significant dysphagia, for example from bulbar motor neurone disease, in which case it does not necessarily imply an underlying tumour.

Fever

Episodic fevers occur in systemic diseases such as vasculitis. Intermittent or continuous fever occurs with infection. Check the duration of fever, how often it has occurred, travel history and infectious exposures.

Neurological history taking

A neurological history follows the format common to other medical assessments: presenting complaint, history of presenting complaint, medical history, drug history, social history, family history and systems review.

History of presenting complaint

There are often multiple significant symptoms, and each one should be covered as a presenting complaint. For each symptom, clearly identify the following.

- Time of onset: be as specific as possible (hour, day, week, month and year)
- Rate of progression: instant or over hours, days, weeks, months or years
- Course of progression: relentless, fluctuating, stepwise or relapsing–remitting
- Exacerbating and relieving factors: for example exercise, rest, noise, heat, lying and standing
- Relation to other symptoms: for example which came first, and how they are related

The details help determine potential causes and rule out categories of illness. **Figure 2.4** illustrates timescales and patterns of symptoms for major aetiological categories.

> 'Listen to your patient; he is telling you his diagnosis,' said William Osler (1849–1919). In some presentations, such as epilepsy, this principle may also extend to the importance of collateral history.

Medical history

This may reveal helpful information because many neurological diseases relapse and remit. Document any relevant childhood illness, such as childhood febrile seizures, which predispose to mesial temporal sclerosis later in life and are a risk factor for epilepsy.

> **Clarify the terms patients use to describe signs or symptoms, particularly medical jargon.** If a specific disease term is mentioned, clarify what the symptoms were and how the presumed diagnosis was reached.

Drug history

Document all current and previous medications. In movement disorders, pay particular attention to the use of drugs that act on the dopaminergic system because, for example, many antipsychotic and antiemetic drugs cause parkinsonism and tardive dyskinesia.

Social history

This reveals the impact of illness on the lives of the patient and their family. Ask patients about:

- employment
- where they live, and with whom
- travel
- usual diet
- stress at home or work
- smoking, alcohol consumption and use of recreational drugs

> **Take elements of the social history at the start of the consultation.** A discussion of employment and who the patient lives with helps establish a rapport and a clearer picture of the patient as a person.

Family history

Use a systematic approach. Start with the patient's children, followed by his or her siblings and their children. Then enquire about the patient's parents, their parents'

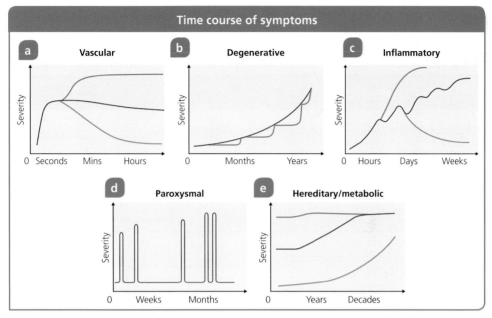

Figure 2.4 The time course of symptoms can indicate the underlying aetiology. (a) Vascular causes typically result in symptoms that have a sudden onset (over seconds) and then stabilise (grey line; e.g. ischaemic stroke) or resolve over minutes to hours (green line). Secondary effects such as cerebral oedema or mass effect can give a staggered pattern (purple line). (b) Degenerative conditions or tumours produce a slow, gradual progression of symptoms that develop over weeks, months or years (grey). Progression can be stepwise as patients become aware of symptoms (purple). (c) Inflammatory and infective causes often result in a subacute and fluctuating onset over days to weeks (grey; e.g. encephalitis): from acute and fulminant (purple; e.g. acute disseminated encephalomyelitis) to a resolving pattern (green; e.g. Guillain–Barré syndrome). (d) Paroxysmal events (e.g. epileptic seizures) produce abrupt episodes. (e) Hereditary conditions can present with a range of patterns, for example a mild problem at birth that progresses over years (grey), severe disability at birth (purple) or late onset (green).

siblings and their children, then the patient's grandparents. Sketch a family tree at the time of asking, because it is easy to forget how the different family members relate to each other.

Occasionally, it is helpful to examine family members of patients with suspected neurological disease, such as Charcot-Marie–Tooth disease, to check for evidence of inheritance.

Neurological systems review

Review any major neurological symptoms that the patient may have overlooked, forgotten or concealed:

- loss of consciousness
- abnormal movements
- headaches

- weakness
- sensory symptoms
- balance problems
- visual disturbance
- seizures
- speech or language problems
- memory or planning problems

General systems review

Review and document major symptoms relating to the cardiac, respiratory, renal, gastrointestinal, respiratory and ophthalmological systems. Ask whether there are other medical problems, and ask about core symptoms in any category that may be relevant from the preceding history.

Common signs and how to examine a patient

Starter questions

Answers to the following questions are on pages 184–185.

3. Do patients always need to be examined during neurological consultations?
4. Has neuroimaging replaced the clinical examination?
5. What is a 'complete' neurological examination?
6. How can neurological examination technique be improved?

Common signs

Lesions at different anatomical sites in the nervous system give characteristic combinations of signs. Localising a lesion to a particular level of the nervous system is the core of clinical assessment. After an assessment of general signs, it is useful to organise signs by functions of the nervous system:

■ consciousness
■ movement
■ motor function
■ sensation
■ pain sensation
■ balance and coordination
■ autonomic functions
■ special senses of vision, hearing, speech and swallowing
■ memory and cognition
■ systemic signs

Consciousness

Epilepsy and syncope are common causes of episodic loss of consciousness but generally do not cause any signs on examination. Altered behaviour, alertness and confusion are common findings in patients with delirium or an encephalopathy.

Encephalopathy

Encephalopathy is a clinical state of decreased attention and consciousness that often fluctuates. It is caused by widespread cortical dysfunction from a huge number of causes, for example infection (i.e. in cases of delirium) or toxins, such as alcohol. Encephalopathy manifests as variable drowsiness, confusion, agitation, and reduced movement and interaction, and it can progress to coma.

Glasgow Coma Scale

Level of consciousness is assessed using the Glasgow Coma Scale (see **Table 2.11**).

Movement

This is assessed throughout the clinical assessment. During the examination, look particularly for the key signs of parkinsonism and for signs of abnormal movements that characterise specific movement disorders.

> **Signs of abnormal movements can be seen at any point of the clinical assessment.** Observe how the patient walks into the consultation room, shakes your hand and moves during history taking.

Tremor

This is an involuntary rhythmic oscillation of a body part. It is helpful to classify tremor as follows:

■ **Rest tremor** is evident when the body part is relaxed

- **A kinetic tremor** occurs during a movement
- **Intention tremor** occurs at the end of a target-directed movement

- **Postural tremor** occurs when adopting a particular position

Common types of tremor are described in Table 2.12.

> Patients with a tremor are often very concerned that they have a serious neurological illness or are dying. Most can be reassured, after sufficient assessment, that their tremor is benign.

Movement signs specific to parkinsonism

Parkinsonism comprises at least two of tremor, rigidity and bradykinesia.

Parkinsonian tremor The characteristic tremor in Parkinson's disease occurs at rest. The tremor is typically a 'pill rolling' movement (in which the thumb and forefinger are rubbed) combined with shaking of the wrists and arms. It is usually a 4–6-Hz tremor.

Rigidity and cogwheeling Continuous involuntary muscle stiffness is known as rigidity. When there is a superimposed tremor and the muscle is passively stretched, the examiner feels a fluctuating, cogwheel-like change in tone. This cogwheeling is common in all causes of parkinsonism.

Bradykinesia This term describes slowed or reduced movements not caused directly by weakness. Bradykinesia often manifests as:

- slowness in walking or turning

Glasgow Coma Scale and Score		
Component	Description	Score
Eyes open (E)	Spontaneously	4
	In response to verbal stimulation	3
		2
	In response to pain	1
	Never	
Best verbal response (V)	Orientated to time, place and person, and converses	5
	Confused conversation (i.e. disorientated but converses)	4
	Inappropriate words	3
	Incomprehensible sounds	2
	No response	1
	Endotracheal tube in place	ET
Best motor response (M)	Obeys commands	6
	Localises pain	5
	Withdraws to pain	4
	Abnormal flexion to pain ('decorticate' posture; see page 164 Figure 2.28)	3
	Abnormal extension to pain ('decerebrate' posture; see page 164 Figure 2.29)	2
	No response	1

Table 2.11 The Glasgow Coma Scale and Score (GCS) ranges from (indicating no response) to 15 (indicating a fully awake state)

Tremor types					
Feature	Physiological	Drug-induced	Essential	Parkinsonian	Cerebellar
Predominant tremor	Postural	Postural or rest	Postural or kinetic	Rest and asymmetrical	Intention
Predominant body part	Upper limbs and bilateral	Upper limbs	Upper limbs and head	Upper and lower limbs	Upper and lower limbs
Head involvement	Uncommon	Uncommon	Common	Very rare	Common
Other features	Worsened by anxiety and caffeine	History of antipsychotic, antiepileptic or antidepressant drug use	Relieved by alcohol consumption; family history in half of cases	Other features of parkinsonism	Other signs of cerebellar disease

Table 2.12 Common types of tremor

- hypomimia (reduced facial expression), which is often a subtle sign, particularly in early disease
- hypophonia (reduced volume of speech), which is evident during the consultation especially during the more advanced stages
- reduced blink rate
- reduced arm swing
- micrographia (progressively shrinking, cramped handwriting)
- progressively smaller movements when opening and closing the finger and thumb

Excess movements

When the history suggests a movement disorder, classification of the patient's movements into the following types is key to identifying potential diagnoses and arranging appropriate investigations:

- chorea
- athetosis
- choreoathetoid movements
- myoclonus
- dystonia
- torticollis

These are described in more detail on page 122.

> **Choreathetosis manifests in many ways.** These include eyebrow lifting, winking, lip movements, cheek puffing, jaw or tongue movements, shoulder or trunk movements, and limb wriggling or jerking.

Motor function

It is the overall combination of signs, rather than a single sign, that helps localise the underlying problem to a lesion affecting either the upper or lower motor neurone. The pattern of signs often allows more precise localisation to muscle, neuromuscular junction, peripheral nerve, root, cord, brain stem or cortex.

> **Always be classifying abnormalities into either upper or lower motor neurone signs during the motor examination.** Further assessment differs considerably for each of these.

Upper motor neurone signs

These indicate dysfunction of the motor system above the α-motor neurone (the lower motor neurone) in the spinal cord, brain stem, cerebellum or cortex. The combination of two or more of these signs in a body part strongly points to an upper motor neurone lesion. In the absence of these signs, it is extremely unlikely that there is such a lesion.

Increased muscle tone (spasticity or hypertonia) Dysfunction of upper motor neurones that send signals to the lower motor neurones in the spinal cord leads to local disinhibition in the cord and a chronically overactive α-motor neurone (see page 85). This effect causes increased tonic contraction of the muscle, resulting in increased resting tone when limbs are moved passively by the examiner (see **Figure 2.20**). Increased muscle tone is a cardinal feature of upper motor neurone lesions. Disorders that affect the lower motor neurone, neuromuscular junction or muscle cannot cause increased tone.

Brisk reflexes These are a consequence of local disinhibition in the spinal cord, which is in turn a result of damage to descending inputs. Tendon reflexes are easily elicited or 'spread' to adjacent muscles, causing them to also contract. Brisk reflexes are a reliable indicator of an upper motor neurone lesion. However, they also frequently occur in healthy or anxious people, so in isolation do not confirm an upper motor neurone lesion. Disorders that affect the lower motor neurone, the neuromuscular junction and muscle do not cause brisk reflexes.

Up-going plantar reflex This is caused by local disinhibition in the spinal cord as a result of damaged descending inputs. The great toe dorsiflexes in response to stroking of the sole of the foot (the normal response is plantar flexion) (see **Figure 2.26**). The direction of the very first toe movement of the toe is taken as the response; patients often find the test unpleasant and quickly withdraw the foot, making it difficult to see the initial movement. Up-going plantar reflex is a sensitive marker of an upper motor neurone lesion, because it is normally absent and is not caused by lower motor neurone lesions.

> Testing the plantar reflex is usually uncomfortable or ticklish for the patient. Try not to repeat it unnecessarily.

Clonus Repetitive or sustained plantar flexion of the ankle occurs when the relaxed ankle is briskly and firmly passively dorsiflexed and held in position by the examiner. A few beats of clonus is normal. Four or more is considered pathological, but this finding does not point to a specific cause.

Pronator drift When the arms are held outwards, with palms upwards and eyes closed, a slow drift of an arm downwards or rotation inwards is known as a pronator drift; it indicates a lesion in the motor cortex (see **Figure 2.14**). Pronator drift results from subtle weakness of the extensor muscles in the arm. It is a common and sensitive sign of a stroke affecting input to the arm but can also be caused by any lesion in the motor cortex.

Forehead sparing In facial weakness caused by a lower motor neurone lesion, the forehead is affected. However, it is spared in upper motor neurone causes because there are bilateral cortical inputs to the portion of the facial nerve nuclei that supplies the forehead muscles.

Lower motor neurone signs

These indicate dysfunction of the motor system at the level of the spinal cord, brain stem, peripheral nerve, neuromuscular junction or muscle.

Reduced muscle tone (flaccidity or hypotonia) The affected muscle is very relaxed and offers little resistance to passive movements. This can arise from any muscle, neuromuscular junction, peripheral nerve or nerve root disorder. It also often occurs in the initial hours of any lesion of the upper motor neurone, before the physiological changes that bring about tonic activation of the lower motor neurone.

Wasting Visible muscle atrophy (loss of muscle mass) is called wasting. Lower motor neurone causes are peripheral nerve or root lesions leading to muscle denervation with consequent loss of the normal trophic factors that usually come from the nerve ending and are essential for maintaining normal muscle tissue. Diseases of the neuromuscular junction do not directly cause wasting, but if very severe and prolonged can result in disuse atrophy.

Fasciculations These are irregular contractions of individual muscle fibres. They are common in healthy people, often precipitated by exercise, caffeine consumption or dehydration. Widespread, persistent or very pronounced fasciculations are more likely to be a pathological sign of denervation and reinnervation of muscles, especially if there are other lower motor neurone signs.

> **Fasciculations in the tongue** are rare and usually caused by lower motor neurone disease.

Reduced reflexes (areflexia) This sign reflects damage to the lower motor neurone, neuromuscular junction or muscle. Such damage results in a weak muscle that is unable to contract when stimulated.

Cortical motor signs

Cortical lesions cause upper motor neurone signs on the contralateral face, arm and leg. However, a small cortical lesion may affect only one or two of the regions.

Flattening of the nasolabial fold Subtle weakness of the facial muscles results in flattening of the crease between the top of the upper lip and the cheek (the nasolabial fold); most commonly present in cases of stroke affecting the face, and in facial nerve palsy.

> **Bell's palsy** often starts with subtle facial weakness and can initially be mistaken for a small stroke. However, it usually becomes obvious within 24 hours.

Brain stem and cranial nerve motor signs

Brain stem lesions usually cause a combination of cranial nerve and limb symptoms attributable to destruction of cranial nerve nuclei and descending and ascending motor and sensory tracts, respectively. Cranial nerves IX–XII are often affected together and are collectively referred to as the lower cranial nerves.

Crossed motor signs This term describes weakness on one side of the face and the opposite side of the body. It occurs when a brain stem lesion affects the ipsilateral facial motor nucleus in the pons and the descending corticospinal tract on the same side, before it decussates in the medulla. This finding is rare and usually caused by an ischaemic stroke or a tumour.

Gaze deviation This is conjugate deviation of both eyes to a particular side. It is common in hemispheric strokes. The eyes deviate away from a hemiparesis in cases of a large cortical lesion, and towards the hemiparesis with a brain stem lesion; therefore gaze deviation is a helpful localising sign.

> The direction of eye deviation relative to signs of paresis helps differentiate cortical and brain stem lesions. In a thalamic or basal ganglia lesion, the eyes deviate towards the paretic side.

Absent corneal reflex The sensory component of the corneal reflex is carried by cranial nerve V and stimulates a bilateral blink mediated by the motor portion of cranial nerve VII. Failure of blinking on one side but not the other implies loss of the motor component on the non-blinking side, i.e. a cranial nerve VII or nuclear lesion on the affected side. The commonest cause is facial palsy, for example Bell's palsy.

> The **functions of cranial nerve VII** can be remembered as 'face, ear, taste, tear': facial weakness, hyperacusis, altered taste and altered eye lacrimation.

Brisk jaw jerk A brisk reflex closing of the jaw indicates an upper motor neurone lesion affecting cranial nerve V, and indicates a pseudobulbar palsy (see Table 13.1).

Deviation of the uvula The uvula normally elevates and remains central when a patient is asked to open their mouth and say 'Ahh'. It deviates towards the normal side in unilateral cranial nerve X lesions and fails to move in bilateral lesions. Deviation occurs in a bulbar or pseudobulbar palsy (see Table 13.1), for example from motor neurone disease.

Spastic (stiff) tongue This is a sign of an upper motor neurone lesion affecting cranial nerve XII. Tongue movement from side to side is slow and stiff. It is common in patients having a stroke, can be present in pseudobulbar palsies and is very rare in isolation.

Altered gag reflex A lack of elevation of the soft palate on stimulation of the pharynx, or an overly pronounced elevation, suggests lower or upper motor neurone involvement, respectively, of cranial nerve X (see **Figure 2.13**). It suggests involvement of cranial nerves IX and X or the medulla as part of a bulbar or pseudobulbar palsy (see Table 13.1).

Dysphonia This is impaired voice production from dysfunction of the vocal cords and usually has a non-neurological cause, such as laryngitis. Rarely, it results from lesions of cranial nerve X or its nuclei as part of a bulbar or pseudobulbar palsy or brain stem stroke.

Speech

Dysarthria (see page 130) most commonly results from a stroke. However, it also has other causes, including other lesions affecting the brain stem or lower cranial nerves.

Swallowing

Dysphagia (difficulty in swallowing) is described on page 130 (see Table 13.1).

Spinal cord motor signs

Spinal cord lesions tend to cause stereo-typed combinations of motor, sensory, and bowel and bladder dysfunction depending on which part of the cord is affected (see page 344). Upper motor neurone signs are present in body parts supplied by motor neurones that originate below the level of the lesion, because of interruption in the spinal cord of descending inhibitor fibres. At the level of the lesion, the lower motor neurone may be affected to give lower motor neurone signs at that level. If the lesion is small and situated in one half of the cord, it causes ipsilateral weakness. In contrast, if the lesion affects both sides of the cord, it causes bilateral weakness.

Nerve root and peripheral nerve motor signs

These cause lower motor neurone signs in the muscles supplied by the affected root or nerve. Few other very specific signs indicate a radiculopathy (nerve root lesion) or neuropathy, but the following are often present in chronic neuropathies.

Inverted champagne bottle Distal leg muscle wasting gives the leg an abnormal appearance; the narrow ankle and wider calf resemble an upside-down champagne bottle. This sign occurs in most chronic motor neuropathies and indicates long-standing motor weakness, which suggests an inherited cause (see page 428).

Pes cavus This is a fixed high arch in the foot; the arch does not flatten when the patient weight bears. About 10% of people have this type of foot, so pes cavus does not always indicate neurological disease. Pes cavus is common in inherited neuropathies (see page 428), along with the inverted champagne bottle appearance; the presence of both strongly suggests an inherited neuropathy.

Neuromuscular junction and muscle motor signs

Patients with muscle and neuromuscular junction disorders often have a characteristic distribution of motor weakness, for example weakness of the eye muscles and bulbar muscles early in myasthenia gravis, and of the proximal arm or leg muscles in muscle disorders. The following signs are also strong pointers to a disorder of muscle or the neuromuscular junction.

Fatiguable muscle weakness (fatiguability) This is muscle contraction that becomes progressively weaker with repetition but improves with brief rest. It is the clinical hallmark of myasthenia gravis and is not present in other conditions. Fatiguable muscle weakness is commonly a ptosis (see page 139) that worsens with sustained up-gaze, diplopia that worsens with sustained gaze, or limb or bulbar weakness that becomes more pronounced with repetitive use of the affected muscles. People who are frail or generally unwell, for example those with sepsis, tire easily, but this should not be mistaken for fatiguability.

Incremental muscle strength This is progressively stronger muscle contraction with repetitive use. It is the clinical hallmark of Lambert–Eaton myasthenic syndrome, often apparent as limb weakness improving with repetitive use. Limb weakness that improves in this way is not a feature of other conditions.

Ophthalmoplegia This is weakness of multiple muscles of eye movements that does not correspond to dysfunction of a single ocular motor nerve. Ophthalmoplegia is uncommon and indicates multiple ocular motor nerve lesions, muscle disease or, most commonly, myasthenia gravis.

Ptosis This is drooping of the upper eyelid. The commonest causes are benign, for example in the case of congenital ptosis resulting from a 'slack' levator muscle. Generally, ptosis caused by a brain stem lesion is bilateral, whereas ptosis caused by lesions affecting cranial nerve III is unilateral. Ptosis caused by muscle and neuromuscular junction problems is also usually bilateral but occurs without the other signs of brain stem lesions.

> **Posterior communicating artery aneurysms often compress cranial nerve III (the oculomotor nerve).** This causes the pupil to dilate and fail to constrict, with varying degrees of ophthalmoplegia (eye muscle weakness) or ptosis, and headache. A unilateral ptosis with a dilated pupil and restricted eye movements is treated as an aneurysm until proven otherwise.

Myotonia This is a muscle contraction that is involuntarily prolonged after voluntary initial contraction. For example, on hand shaking the patient fails to release their grip appropriately, or on direct percussion there is prolonged and sustained muscle contraction. It occurs in myotonic dystrophy before the muscle wasting becomes too advanced, and in other very rare muscle diseases.

Sensory signs

The distribution of sensory loss and the modalities affected are helpful in localising lesions, although there are fewer specific sensory signs to seek than motor signs. The two major sensory pathways are tested:

- the lateral columns, which carry pain and temperature sensation
- the dorsal columns, which carry joint position and vibration sense

Key sensory signs that reliably localise to a particular level of the nervous system are described below.

Hemisensory loss

Cortical lesions involving the somatosensory cortex cause a loss of sensation in multiple modalities on the contralateral part of the body. The face, arm and leg are involved, depending on the extent of the lesion. Thalamic lesions, although rare, can also cause hemisensory loss. The commonest cause is a hemispheric stroke. Another common cause is demyelinating lesions that affect the internal capsule carrying the sensory fibres from the cortex.

Crossed sensory signs This is sensory loss on one side of the face and the contralateral side of the body. It arises when a lesion in the brain stem affects the ipsilateral cranial nerve nucleus, i.e. the spinal trigeminal sensory nucleus, carrying information from the ipsilateral face, and also disrupts the ascending lateral spinothalamic tract. The latter carries information from the contralateral arm and leg, because these fibres cross the midline when they enter the spinal cord.

This is a rare finding but a valuable pointer to a brain stem lesion. In younger patients, demyelination is the commonest cause and in older patients, brain stem stroke syndromes.

Spinal cord sensory level If the trunk has a well-demarcated sensory border below which sensation is abnormal, this is called a sensory level. It is the hallmark of a spinal cord lesion. The border corresponds with the highest level of the spinal cord affected. This is a characteristic and common finding in spinal cord lesions from any cause.

Glove-and-stocking sensory loss This is loss of sensation in the distal limbs in a distribution that corresponds with the areas covered by gloves and stockings. The nature of the loss depends on the size of the nerve fibres affected: pain, temperature and fine discrimination sensation for small fibres, proprioception for large fibres, and all sensory modalities for both sizes.

Facial sensory loss This is common and is often a functional symptom without any underlying pathology. A range of lesions at various points along the trigeminal nerve cause distinct patterns of sensory loss (**Figure 2.5**).

Pain sensation

Abnormal pain perception can manifest as:

- loss of pain perception
- hyperanalgesia (extreme sensitivity to a normally painful stimulus)
- allodynia (the perception of pain in response to a normally non-painful stimulus)

Patients may report marked sensitivity on testing pinprick perception or with the vibration of a tuning fork.

Gait, balance and coordination

Normal gait, balance and coordination depend on intact visual, vestibular, cerebellar and proprioceptive input (see **Figure 2.3**). The following are key signs that indicate disturbance in this system. Gait, balance and coordination also depend on normal motor function; motor signs are considered on pages 136–140.

> **When assessing gait, take care to prevent the patient falling.** If the patient uses a walking aid, let them use it.

General gait, balance and coordination signs

The assessment of gait often helps broadly categorise the cause of balance problems.

Broad-based gait This is an abnormal gait characterised by wide separation of the feet. This type of gait is described as broad- or wide-based, and is commonly present in patients with truncal ataxia. It indicates that the lesion involves the cerebellar vermis.

Narrow-based gait This is characterised by the feet being positioned closer together than normal during walking. Narrow-based gait is usually seen in parkinsonism rather than ataxic syndromes.

High-stepping gait This is characterised by excessively high lifting of the feet from the ground. High-stepping gait is usually caused by the need to lift the affected foot or feet higher than normal during the walking cycle because of the presence of a foot drop on one or both sides, respectively. Bilateral foot drop with a high-stepping gait is most commonly seen in polyneuropathies that affect both legs, such as Guillain–Barré syndrome.

Waddling gait Weakness in the hip girdle muscles results in a tilting pelvic motion on walking: a waddling gait. It is an indication of proximal muscle weakness or hip girdle instability. This type of gait is uncommon; neurological causes include the myopathies, for example dermatomyositis.

Marche à petits pas This uncommon pattern is characterised by very short shuffling steps and upright posture. It is usually caused by diffuse cerebrovascular disease.

Ataxia This is incoordination of movements that is not caused by weakness. It is a non-specific term that includes a wide range of causes.

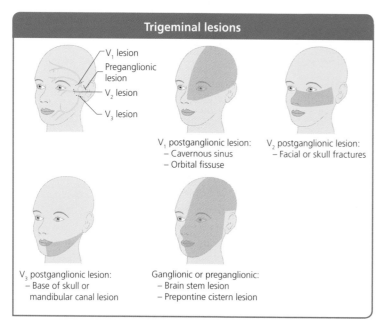

Trigeminal lesions

V₁ lesion
Preganglionic lesion
V₂ lesion
V₃ lesion

V₁ postganglionic lesion:
– Cavernous sinus
– Orbital fissuse

V₂ postganglionic lesion:
– Facial or skull fractures

V₃ postganglionic lesion:
– Base of skull or mandibular canal lesion

Ganglionic or preganglionic:
– Brain stem lesion
– Prepontine cistern lesion

Figure 2.5 Trigeminal nerve lesions. The pattern of facial sensory loss points towards which part of the trigeminal nerve is damaged.

> **Identification of which parts of the body are ataxic helps localise the lesion.** Unilateral ataxia is likely to be caused by a unilateral cerebellar lesion. Bilateral ataxia could be cerebellar or peripheral.

Ataxia is broadly split into cerebellar or sensory ataxia depending on the known or suspected lesion location.

Dysmetria This is impaired coordination resulting in the inability to accurately reach a target, with a tendency to overshoot or undershoot. It is a common sign in cerebellar disease or with significant loss of proprioception from any cause.

Nystagmus The vestibular and visual systems are responsible for normal balance. Vestibular or cerebellar disorders often produce balance problems and may include nystagmus as a sign. Nystagmus is involuntary movement of the eyes, characterised by an initial slower phase in which the eyes drift off a target and a faster corrective saccadic movement back on to the target. It is a common sign in cerebellar disease and in cases of any brain stem lesion affecting the vestibular nuclei.

> **When examining the eyes for nystagmus, remember POCS: P**eripheral lesions cause nystagmus with the fast phase to the **O**pposite side. **C**entral lesions cause nystagmus with the fast phase towards the **S**ame side.

Intention tremor This is a limb tremor in which amplitude increases as the limb reaches its target during a target-oriented movement. Intention tremor is common in cerebellar hemisphere lesions from any cause.

Scanning speech This is a form of dysarthria characterised by broken words and rhythm of speech. It results from poor control over the muscles of speech in significant cerebellar disease, for example multiple sclerosis and stroke.

Dysdiadochokinesia This is impaired ability to perform rapidly alternating hand movements. It is commonly seen in patients with cerebellar hemisphere lesions, as well as those with impaired proprioception from any cause.

Impaired heel–shin coordination Difficulty in lifting the heel of one foot, placing it on the knee of the other, running it down the shin, lifting it off and repeating the movement is a sensitive sign of incoordination of the leg from any cause, for example cerebellar disease and proprioceptive loss.

Peripheral signs of incoordination

Impaired joint position sense as a result of a peripheral neuropathy or spinal cord lesion can result in balance problems, with the following characteristic features on examination.

Pseudoathetosis This rare finding typically occurs only in patients with severe loss of joint position sense from dorsal column lesions, for example in vitamin B12 deficiency, or peripheral neuropathies affecting large diameter fibres. Slow wriggling movements of the fingers are seen when the patient closes their eyes and holds their arms and hands outstretched.

Romberg's sign This describes marked balance impairment brought on when the patient stands with their feet together and closes their eyes. It occurs in any patient who has become dependent on visual feedback to maintain an upright posture.

> **Cerebellar lesions often cause balance and coordination problems.** These problems underlie additional clinical findings that distinguish cerebellar lesions from proprioceptive or vestibular lesions. Patients with cerebellar lesions often also have nystagmus, an intention tremor, slurred speech and dysdiadochokinesia.

Autonomic functions

Routine neurological examination is unlikely to identify any specific autonomic signs. However, when the history raises the suspicion of autonomic involvement, bedside tests of blood pressure and heart rate variation may provide evidence of altered autonomic function. These tests commonly consist of assessments for postural hypotension and heart rate variability during physiological manoeuvres.

Postural hypotension

This is discussed on page 429.

Reduced heart rate variability

The beat-to-beat interval varies depending on the degree of vagus nerve input. Several physiological manoeuvres normally alter the heart rate through the vagus nerve: deep inspiration slows it, and standing from sitting increases it. Loss of these changes suggests autonomic dysfunction from any cause.

Special senses and swallowing

Cranial nerve and nerve nuclei lesions can occur in isolation, but there are often characteristic combinations of findings because anatomically close structures are often affected together. Therefore it is essential to be able to consider the findings together to help localise the lesion. The following are key signs from cranial nerve assessment.

Smell and taste

Changes in smell or taste are rarely the result of neurological disease. Upper airway disease is a far more common cause. Smell and taste changes are formally tested only if they are among the main symptoms reported by the patient.

Anosmia This is loss of the sense of smell and results from dysfunction of cranial nerve I (the olfactory nerve). Anosmia is common after significant head injury, but the patient often has more extensive injuries that dwarf this deficit. Its frequency increases with age for unknown reasons, and it often precedes the major symptoms of parkinsonism by many years.

Altered taste This has many non-neurological causes. However, it is often present in disorders affecting cranial nerve VII (the facial nerve) or

cranial nerve IX (the glossopharyngeal nerve), which carry special gustatory information from the anterior two thirds and posterior third of the tongue, respectively. Altered taste is rare as an isolated symptom but commonly occurs with other symptoms of a seventh nerve palsy or with lower cranial nerve palsies that include those of cranial nerve IX.

Eyes and vision

Disturbances in vision or eye problems are common, and systematic evaluation is required. It is helpful to think of abnormal signs in the following groups:

- general inspection
- acuity
- visual fields
- pupils
- fundi
- eye movements

General inspection

Neurological eye signs that can be found on general inspection, and which should prompt a detailed assessment for potentially very serious conditions, include the following.

- Conjunctival injection: prominent swelling of the conjunctival blood vessels, often with a local ocular cause (e.g. inflammation)
- Proptosis: protrusion of the globe from the orbit, commonly seen in Graves' disease and cases of mass lesions behind the orbit
- Chemosis: oedema of the conjunctiva, most commonly a result of infection or irritation of the cornea

When conjunctival injection, proptosis and chemosis occur together in one eye, the three important neurological conditions to consider are carotid–cavernous fistula, cavernous sinus thrombosis and a trigeminal autonomic cephalgia.

Other neurological eye signs, which are far rarer but important to recognise because they indicate particular diseases, are as follows.

- **Lisch nodules** are an abnormal pigmented hamartoma on the iris in neurofibromatosis type 1 but not neurofibromatosis type 2; these nodules are present in almost all patients with neurofibromatosis type I by late childhood

- **Kayser–Fleischer rings** are rings of copper deposition at the edge of the cornea, apparent as a brownish ring along the edge of each iris; they are found in all patients with Wilson's disease with neurological or psychiatric features, and not in other conditions
- **Raccoon or panda eyes** (periorbital ecchymosis) is bruising around the eyes; this is a sign of a base-of-skull fracture (**Figure 2.6**), especially if it occurs on both eyes after a head injury

Visual acuity

Always document the visual acuity in patients with visual symptoms.

Reduced visual acuity despite correction of refractive errors indicates rapid visual loss. This requires urgent investigation.

Visual fields

Bedside examination of visual fields is not as sensitive as formal automated visual field testing (perimetry). However, it allows identification of areas of field loss, which helps localise the lesion along the visual axis.

The examiner faces the patient head on. Both patient and examiner cover their opposing eyes. The examiner then moves a hat pin into the field of view from the edges, and the patient indicates when they can see it.

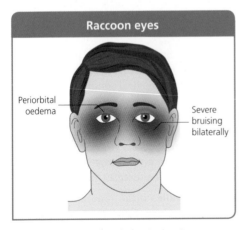

Raccoon eyes

Periorbital oedema

Severe bruising bilaterally

Figure 2.6 Raccoon eyes, which are often seen 2–3 days after a base-of-skull fracture.

Examples of visual field defects include the following.

- **Scotoma** is a discrete blob, band or streak of loss of visual field; it is usually caused by a retinal or optic disc lesion (e.g. optic neuritis, ischaemic optic neuropathy or retinal detachment)
- **Homonymous quadrantanopia or hemianopia** (see Table 1.38) develop when lesions in the occipital cortex or optic radiations cause loss of one quarter or one lateral half of the visual field, respectively; this is common finding, frequently seen in stroke, for example

Pupils

Pupil abnormalities are easily forgotten during a complex clinical assessment. However, they are helpful in localising lesions and identifying a specific cause. They are especially useful in assessment of the drowsy or comatose patient.

Pinpoint pupils The pupils are small and unreactive, most commonly as a result of the use of opiates or other drugs. Pinpoint pupils are also seen in cases of pontine lesions from any cause.

Mid-position pupils Unreactive mid-position pupils suggest a structural, toxic or metabolic lesion affecting the midbrain.

Bilateral dilated and unresponsive pupils These are present in cases of anticholinergic poisoning and in the preterminal stage of brain stem death.

Anisocoria This is the term for pupils of unequal size. Anisocoria is usually normal, especially in the elderly. It may indicate that one pupil is inappropriately large or one is inappropriately small (**Figure 2.7**).

Mydriasis This is an inappropriately large pupil (**Figure 2.7b**). Mydriasis indicates excessive sympathetic input to the pupil or reduced parasympathetic input. If there is normal eye movement and no ptosis, it is often caused by drug use or a relative afferent pupillary defect. If there is normal eye movement and no ptosis but slow accommodation, it is probably a Holmes–Adie pupil. Limited eye movement or ptosis suggests a third nerve palsy.

Miosis The pupil is inappropriately small (see **Figure 2.7c**). This indicates reduced sympathetic input to the pupil.

> Remember 'HAIL ARIS': the Holmes-Adie pupil Is Large at rest and the Argyll Robertson pupil Is Small at rest.

Relative afferent pupillary defect This is pupillary dilation that occurs when a light source is moved from the contralateral eye to the affected eye (see **Figure 2.7d**). It indicates retinal or optic disc disease that limits the pupillary response to direct light on the affected side but does not prevent the consensual response to light in the unaffected eye.

The cause is commonly optic neuritis in the young but more commonly ischaemic optic neuropathy or other unilateral retinal disease in older people.

> **The pupillary fibres of cranial nerve III travel near the outer surface of the nerve fibre,** rendering it vulnerable to external compression or stretching. This may explain why a posterior communicating aneurysm pressing on the outer nerve causes the pupil to dilate.

Light–near dissociation The pupil reacts to either light or accommodation but not both.

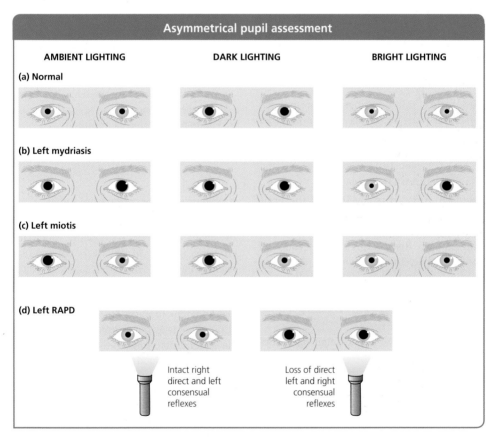

Figure 2.7 Unequal pupils must be assessed in ambient, dark and bright light to determine which is abnormal. (a) Normal pupillary sizes. (b) In left mydriasis, the left pupil is larger in ambient lighting, the right pupil dilates normally in the dark and the left fails to constrict in bright light. (c) In left miosis, the left pupil is smaller in ambient lighting and fails to dilate in the dark, and the right pupil constricts to light normally. (d) In left relative afferent pupillary defect, the left pupil constricts consensually to light in the right eye but not as much through the direct light reflex.

Light–near dissociation is a rare finding and is usually a Holmes–Adie pupil, an Argyll Robertson pupil or a lesion in the dorsal midbrain, as seen in Parinaud's syndrome.

Holmes–Adie pupil This is a mydriatic pupil that does not constrict to light but very slowly constricts to accommodation. It is caused by an idiopathic degeneration of postganglionic nerve fibres. When there is also generalised areflexia, it is called Holmes-Adie syndrome and there is more widespread nerve fibre degeneration.

Argyll Robertson pupil This is a miotic pupil that does not constrict to light but constricts to accommodation. It is associated with tertiary syphilis. Now, with the reduced prevalence of syphilis, this is a rare clinical finding.

Fundi

There are countless fundoscopic signs, but the following are the most common and relevant in neurological disease.

Red reflex This describes the normal red reflection from the retina seen through an ophthalmoscope at a distance. The absence of red reflex in adults is common and suggests a cataract. In children, it is rare and usually signifies a retinoblastoma.

Swollen optic disc Swelling of the optic disc causes venous engorgement, loss of venous pulsation, optic disc haemorrhages, blurred optic disc margins and elevation of the optic disc. This is a common neurological finding, and causes include inflammation, infection and increased intracranial pressure (in which case it is called papilloedema).

Papilloedema This is a swollen optic disc caused by increased intracranial pressure, for example from meningitis or subarachnoid haemorrhage. Papilloedema is usually associated with a headache. Visual loss tends to develop late in the condition, after many weeks or months, and affects peripheral vision first.

Papillitis The optic disc is swollen as a result of inflammation or infection. The commonest cause is optic neuritis, either in isolation or in cases of multiple sclerosis. Papillitis tends to cause pain on eye movement and is associated with early loss of colour vision and visual acuity.

> **Papilloedema** is usually bilateral, causes slowly progressive peripheral field defects and affects acuity only later on. Papillitis, including optic neuritis, affects colour vision and acuity early and usually causes pain on eye movement.

Retinopathy Retinopathy is damage to the retina as a result of inflammation and vascular disease. On fundoscopy, it is visible as changes to retinal vessels and as deposits and haemorrhages.

Hypertensive retinopathy has characteristic findings depending on the stage of retinopathy. These include the following.

- **Silver wiring:** the shiny appearance of sclerotic blood vessels
- **Arteriovenous nipping:** depression of veins where they are crossed by arteries at increased pressure
- **Flame haemorrhages:** ruptured precapillary arterioles and small veins
- **Hard exudates:** yellow flecks on the retina, representing lipid residues from leaking capillaries
- **Soft exudates or cotton wool spots:** whitish or grey fluffy inflammatory lesions

In stage 1 diabetic retinopathy, microaneurysms (bulges in arteries), dot-and-blot haemorrhages (red dots from capillary haemorrhage) and hard exudates (yellow flecks) are present. In stage 2, changes in the macula are also apparent. In stage 3 (proliferative retinopathy), there is also neovascularisation (a tangle of abnormal, fragile vessels) and vitreous haemorrhage (blood in the vitreous humour).

Eye movements

Abnormalities in eye movements indicate a problem in the brainstem, the cranial nerves that control eye movements, the muscles they innervate or the neuromuscular junction. There are numerous types but the following few are those commonly encountered.

Internuclear ophthalmoplegia This is failure to adduct an eye on the affected side on attempted contralateral gaze, along with nystagmus of the contralateral abducting eye. Convergence is normally preserved (**Figure 2.8a**). The commonest causes are stroke and demyelination from multiple sclerosis.

Skew deviation This is vertical misalignment of the eyes in primary gaze. Diplopia is present, with the images separated horizontally. The lesion is usually in the midbrain or posterior fossa; the commonest causes are stroke and demyelination.

> **In diplopia, it may not be immediately clear which eye is misaligned.** To work this out, the false image (from the Paretic eye) is Paler, more Peripheral and more oPaque. The separation of images is maximal in the direction of action of the weak muscle.

Strabismus ('squint') This is horizontal misalignment of the eyes. The commonest form is congenital; because of cortical suppression of one image, the patient does not usually experience diplopia. In acquired causes, commonly lesions of cranial nerve III, IV or VI or the brain stem, there is usually diplopia.

Opsoclonus Opsoclonus is spontaneous, rapid, brief, unpredictable horizontal and vertical eye movements. A very rare sign, the cause is a lesion in the midbrain, for example neuroblastoma in children, or a paraneoplastic phenomenon from small-cell lung tumours in adults.

Eye 'down and out' Dysfunction of the motor component of cranial nerve III causes weakness of all muscles of eye movement except the superior oblique, which is controlled by cranial nerve IV, and the lateral rectus, which is controlled by cranial nerve VI. This dysfunction results in the eye moving down (superior oblique) and out (lateral rectus) at rest (**Figure 2.8b**). There is usually also ptosis on the affected side from weakness of the levator muscle; if the autonomic fibres supplying the pupil are affected, the pupil is dilated and poorly reactive.

Sixth nerve palsy Dysfunction of cranial nerve VI results in difficulty abducting the affected eye (see **Figure 2.8c**), so the patient experiences double vision. The long course of the nerve from the brain stem through the skull means that there are a great many causes of cranial nerve VI dysfunction, including increased intracranial pressure from any cause.

Hearing

Neurological causes of hearing problems also cause dysfunction of the vestibular system if the lesion or injury is in the vestibulocochlear nerve or brain stem nuclei. Isolated hearing loss is more likely to be

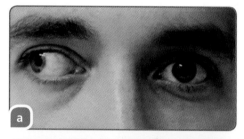

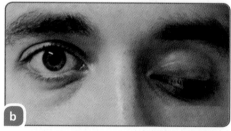

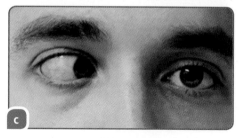

Figure 2.8 Common disorders of eye movements. (a) Internuclear ophthalmoplegia on attempted right lateral gaze. The left eye fails to adduct because of a lesion in the left medial longitudinal fasciculus. (b) Left third nerve palsy. (c) Left sixth nerve palsy.

from cochlear disease. Therefore always assess hearing in conjunction with vestibular function, not in isolation.

Inspection

Check for the obvious redness, swelling and discharge that typify ear infection. Base-of-skull fractures can cause distinct signs in the eyes and ears, and these are sought as part of a thorough assessment of the ears and hearing.

Otorrhoea This is discharge from the ear, most commonly from infections. However, leakage of cerebrospinal fluid from the ear can occur secondary to any traumatic, inflammatory or destructive process affecting the middle cranial fossa.

Haemotympanum This is blood in the external ear canal. It is a common finding in head injuries, in which case it indicates a base-of-skull fracture (**Figure 2.9**).

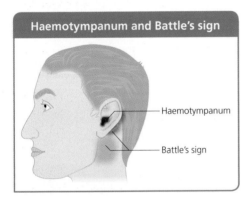

Haemotympanum and Battle's sign

Haemotympanum

Battle's sign

Figure 2.9 Blood in the ear canal (haemotympanum) and around the mastoid process (Battle's sign) are frequently present in base-of-skull fractures.

Battle's sign This is mastoid ecchymosis (bruising around the mastoid process), which is caused by base-of-skull fractures in the middle cranial fossa (**Figure 2.9**).

Hearing loss

Weber's and Rinne's tests are used to help determine which side is affected and whether the hearing loss is conductive or sensorineural (**Figure 2.10**).

Conductive hearing loss This manifests as a negative Rinne's test in the affected ear, and in Weber's test the sound localises to the affected ear. Infection and impacted earwax are the commonest causes.

Sensorineural hearing loss This manifests as a positive Rinne's test, and in Weber's test the tone is heard better in the unaffected ear.

Hyperacusis This does not occur in cases of upper motor neurone causes of facial weakness. Therefore its presence can help distinguish between a lower and an upper motor neurone cause of facial weakness.

Vestibular function

Vestibular disturbances usually result in difficulty in maintaining gaze fixation in response to dynamic head movements. Vestibular function can be tested at the bedside.

Nystagmus This is described on page 142. Nystagmus triggered during Hallpike's test strongly suggests benign paroxysmal positional vertigo or a central vestibular lesion. Hallpike's test involves swiftly tilting a patient's head back over the edge of the bed and to one side whilst looking carefully at their eyes to detect any nystagmus.

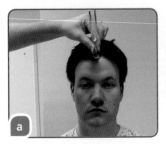 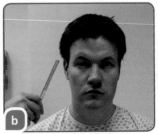 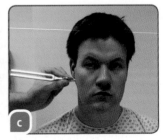

Figure 2.10 Weber's and Rinne's tests. (a) In Weber's test, a vibrating tuning fork is placed on the patient's forehead to test if the sound is heard more strongly on one side. (b) In Rinne's test, the tuning fork is held in front of the ear until it can no longer be heard; it is then placed on the mastoid process (c).

Memory and cognition

Detailed memory and cognitive testing is usually carried out only for patients who report symptoms in these areas or who have conditions that commonly result in cognitive symptoms. The following subsections describe the major signs of cognitive dysfunction.

Language

Assessment and classification of the language disturbance helps localise the lesion and likely cause. Stroke is the commonest cause of the dysphasias and aphasias described below.

Receptive dysphasia This is impaired understanding of speech, with normal speech production. Isolated lesions in the superior temporal gyrus, which is central to language comprehension, cause a predominantly receptive dysphasia.

> Receptive dysphasia varies in degree. Some patients have no understanding of language, some understand simple instructions or words, and others have subtle language problems found only on detailed testing.

Expressive dysphasia Impaired expression of speech, not attributable to dysfunction of the mechanical articulation, is known as expressive dysphasia. It can be subtle, for example mild word-finding difficulties, or extensive, with broken or gibberish speech. Stroke is the most common cause if onset is sudden.

Mixed dysphasia The combination of receptive and expressive dysphasia is the commonest pattern. One form often predominates, but there are usually elements of both on testing. Mixed dysphasia results from disruption of a diffuse network of speech centres mainly in the dominant parietal and temporal lobes.

Broca's aphasia This is a type of expressive dysphasia characterised by some retention of speech comprehension but impaired speech production, with broken, stuttered speech that retains some meaningful content. Lesions involve the dominant posterior inferior frontal gyrus.

Wernicke's aphasia This is characterised by loss of speech comprehension and impaired speech production, with fluid but meaningless speech. Lesions involve the medial temporal lobe.

> Remember the anatomical locations of Broca's and Wernicke's aphasia by remembering that B comes before W in the alphabet Broca's aphasia is caused by damage to the frontal gyrus, which is situated anterior to the medial temporal lobe, which is affected in Wernicke's aphasia.

Neglect

This is inattention to or lack of awareness of one side of the body. Neglect occurs in lesions of the non-dominant parietal cortex from any cause but is most common after a stroke. The inattention can be to tactile stimulation, visual stimulation or both. Sensory extinction is the awareness of sensory stimulation, either tactile or visual, when it is presented to either side independently but not when presented simultaneously to both sides.

Executive function

The frontal lobes are central to many executive functions. Lesions here cause various degrees of 'dysexecutive' behaviour, such as poor memory, inability to plan tasks and disinhibition (e.g. inappropriate sexual behaviour or comments). Frontal release signs are abnormal frontal reflexes and are very common findings in dementia or frontal lobe dysfunction, as listed below. Although non-specific, their presence supports a diagnosis of frontal lobe dysfunction as a cause of the executive dysfunction.

Disinhibition This is wide-ranging loss of normal social graces, appropriateness or inhibitions. Disinhibition is often apparent during the consultation from the patient's unusual, aggressive or sexually forward behaviour. It is common with frontal lobe tumours and other neurodegenerative masses.

Pout reflex This is an abnormal reflex in which the lips are pursed together and pushed forwards when they are pressed by the examiner's finger (**Figure 2.32**).

Palmomental reflex This is an abnormal reflex in which the corner of the mouth of the patient contracts when the ipsilateral palm is stroked (see **Figure 2.31**).

Grasp reflex The grasp reflex is an abnormal reflex in which the patient will grasp on to a finger stroking their open palm without being instructed to do so (**Figure 2.30**).

Apathy Abnormal lack of drive, motivation or action is often seen in frontal lobe disease from any cause. An example is faecal soiling from lack of motivation to go to the bathroom.

Signs of systemic disease

Signs of systemic disease or specific organ dysfunction can help identify:

- a multisystem disorder with a neurological component (e.g. a vasculitis causing a skin rash, renal failure and neuropathy)
- a disease of another organ leading to secondary neurological effects (e.g. pneumonia causing sepsis and encephalopathy)

Therefore a general medical examination is essential in patients presenting with neurological symptoms. Such examinations are beyond the scope of this book, but the key signs of particular relevance to neurological disease are described here.

Skin signs

Skin examination can reveal signs of inherited neurocutaneous syndromes (see page 415), infectious illness (see page 291) or systemic illnesses such as vasculitis (see page 368). However, the skin does not need to be examined in detail unless one of these conditions is suspected.

Purpuric rash These red or purple papules do not fade when pressure is applied, and they can coalesce to form larger areas. The rash represents a small vessel vasculitis in the skin, and is caused by sepsis (e.g. in meningococcal septicaemia; see page 291), idiopathic vasculitis or bleeding disorders (e.g. low level of platelets). In a patient with a new headache and fever, purpuric rash strongly suggests meningococcal septicaemia with systemic sepsis (see page 291).

Gottron's papules

These are scaly erythematous papules, which looks similar to psoriasis, over the dorsum of the knuckles and hands in 80% of patients with dermatomyositis (see page 435), Gottron's papules never occur in other conditions.

Heliotrope rash

This red or purplish rash predominantly over the neck and eyelids is found in 90% of patients with dermatomyositis.

Port wine stain

This is a capillary malformation causing a visible red-purplish 'birthmark', commonly on the face, trunk or arms. It is usually not associated with neurological disease, but in Sturge–Weber syndrome a facial stain with an underlying angioma of the meningeal vessels is associated with seizures, cognitive impairment and glaucoma.

Café au lait spots

These are pale brown lesions that have a range of causes. They are usually seen in neurofibromatosis type 1 (see page 414) and tuberous sclerosis.

Neurofibroma

This is a benign spindle cell tumour of the peripheral nerve sheath, often seen as a violaceous, pedunculated non-tender fleshy skin mass. Neurofibromata are present in almost all adults with neurofibromatosis type 1 (see page 416).

Axillary freckling

Freckles in the armpit or other skin fold creases, is a unique sign of neurofibromatosis type 1 and is present in about 90% of patients by 7 years of age.

Angiofibroma

These small red, brown or skin-coloured papules are seen over the nose and cheeks in > 75% of patients with tuberous sclerosis (see page 417). Angiofibroma most commonly occur over the nasolabial folds.

Ash leaf spots

These are hypopigmented macules seen in 90% of children with tuberous sclerosis, often over the buttocks and trunk.

Shagreen patches

These thick, dimpled areas of skin are seen in 50% of patients with tuberous sclerosis. The presence of shagreen patches is one of the diagnostic criteria for the condition (see page 418).

Observations and vital signs

Measurement of heart rate, blood pressure, temperature, respiratory rate, oxygenation and blood glucose concentration is a standard component of a thorough medical and neurological assessment. It often provides clues to any systemic illness that is a cause or effect of significant neurological disease.

Examination sequences

There is no 'complete' neurological examination. The aim is a targeted assessment of key functions, chosen on the basis of the history and differential diagnosis. For conditions unlikely to produce any clinical signs, for example tension headache, a brief screening examination is appropriate. For other conditions, such as cervical myelopathy, an appropriate routine designed to elicit signs to confirm the suspected diagnosis is required. Therefore examination routines are adapted to the individual patient's history and the clinical context. It is useful to learn the following examination routines in detail and begin to adapt them with practice. The core examination routines are:

- gait and general inspection
- cranial nerves
- upper limbs
- lower limbs
- cerebellum
- higher cortical function

Elements of these routines can be adapted to form more targeted examination routines for specific clinical contexts.

Gait and general inspection

Abnormalities in posture and movement are simple and quick to assess. Problems with posture or movement can result from abnormal sensory input, integration or motor output.

Observe the patient as they walk into the consultation room, or ask them to stand and walk if they are in a chair or bed. Look for any unusual postures of limbs or head and the general pattern, speed and rhythm of movements.

Look for evidence of bradykinesia, such as would be seen in parkinsonism, by asking the patient to repeatedly open and close their hands as wide and as fast as possible. The bradykinetic patient's movements will be progressively slower and smaller.

Look for a tremor by asking the patient to close their eyes with their hands relaxed in their lap. Ask them to count down from 100 in 7s; this will distract them, and any tremor they may have been suppressing will emerge.

Perform Romberg's test to assess proprioception; ask them to put their feet together and close their eyes, but ensure that they do not fall. Patients with loss of joint position sense in the lower limbs, for example from a sensory neuropathy, have marked difficulty in remaining steady in this position with their eyes closed; this result is termed Romberg's positive.

Cranial nerves

The nuclei of cranial nerves III–XII are all within the brain stem, and the cranial nerves pass through various openings in the skull base. Therefore abnormalities in single or multiple cranial nerves point to the brain stem or base of the skull as the site of the problem. The brain stem also contains many limb motor and sensory tracts, which are often also affected when the lesion is in the brain stem (see Figure 1.54).

A quick screen of the cranial nerves is often all that is required, unless the history suggests that an abnormality, such as diplopia, dysphagia, dysarthria, visual problems or facial weakness, is likely to be found. The following summarises key points to assess in the cranial nerves.

Alternating hemiplegia (weakness on one side of the face and in the contralateral limbs) suggests a brain stem lesion above the medulla. The lesion causes ipsilateral cranial nerve signs from damage to ipsilateral nuclei, and contralateral limb weakness resulting from damage to descending corticospinal fibres before they cross in the medulla.

Cranial nerve I

This is rarely assessed. The patient is asked if they can recognise multiple distinct odours, for example orange peel, coffee and chocolate.

Cranial nerves II and III

Assessments of pupillary reflexes, visual acuity and visual fields, as well as fundoscopy, are carried out in most patients. Cranial nerve II carries the afferent limb of the light reflexes, as well as primary visual sensory information. Cranial nerve III carries the efferent limb of the light reflexes and accommodation reflex. The afferent limb of the accommodation reflex comes from cortical centres.

Sequence

The following sequence seems lengthy but, with a little practice, can be performed very rapidly.

Pupils Assessment of the pupils can help determine if there is a lesion in the retina, optic nerve or brain stem.

Note resting size, shape and symmetry in bright and dark light. When the pupils are unequal, this assessment clarifies which pupil is abnormal (see **Figure 2.7**).

Shine a pen torch in each eye to elicit the direct light reflex. This is diminished in any problem with the retina or optic nerve on the affected side.

Note the change in the contralateral pupil; it should also constrict (the consensual reflex). This reflex is reduced on the contralateral side if there is a problem in the contralateral cranial nerve III.

Elicit the accommodation reflex by asking the patient to focus on a finger held a few feet

from their face and moved towards their nose. The reflex can be reduced in cases of lesions in the brain stem nuclei of cranial nerve III.

Test for a relative afferent pupillary defect by shining a pen torch in one eye (eye A) and looking at the consensual reflex in the other eye (eye B). Next move the torch on to eye B and note how the pupil size changes. Do this a few times. Repeat for the other eye (see **Figure 2.7**).

Visual acuity Assessing and documenting acuity is essential in any patient who reports visual symptoms. Test each eye in turn by asking the patient to cover the other eye and read the smallest line they are able to on a Snellen chart.

If the patient is unable to read the largest line on the chart, test if they can count fingers held in front of them, perceive movement of a hand in front of them or perceive light.

Visual fields Formal automated perimetry should be carried out for patients with suspected or confirmed disorders of vision. Bedside testing is done by the examiner sitting at the same level as the patient and using a red hat pin to compare the patient's visual fields with their own.

1. The examiner and patient cover opposite eyes
2. The examiner moves the hat pin into view from outside the field of vision, and the patient indicates when they can see it
3. This is repeated in all four quadrants for each eye in turn

The blind spot is also mapped out in a similar way, asking the patient to indicate when the tip of the pin disappears and reappears.

Scotomata are discrete unilateral sections of visual field loss that arise from retinal or optic nerve disease. Larger quadrants and hemifields of visual loss (quadrantanopia and hemifields, respectively) usually indicate cortical lesions (**Figure 2.11**).

Fundoscopy This allows the retina to be examined and is invaluable in assessing for microvascular disease, for example that caused by diabetes or hypertension, or for optic nerve swelling or atrophy.

1. In a darkened room or with their pupils dilated, ask the patient to focus on a distant object

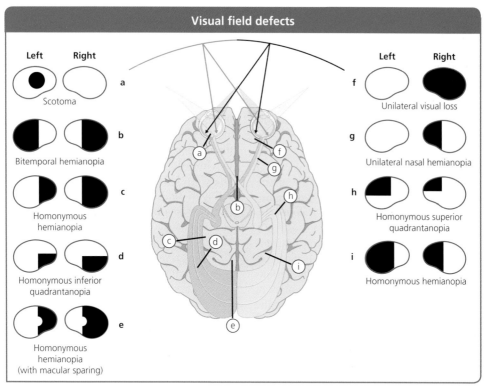

Visual field defects

Left   Right

a   Scotoma

b   Bitemporal hemianopia

c   Homonymous hemianopia

d   Homonymous inferior quadrantanopia

e   Homonymous hemianopia (with macular sparing)

Left   Right

f   Unilateral visual loss

g   Unilateral nasal hemianopia

h   Homonymous superior quadrantanopia

i   Homonymous hemianopia

Figure 2.11 The location of lesions affecting the visual system can be determined by the area of visual loss (black).

2. Look through the ophthalmoscope at each of their eyes in turn from a couple of feet (60 cm) to detect the red reflex; this is commonly lost in cases of cataract
3. Close in and identify an artery or vein and follow it back to the optic disc; inspect the disc and rest of the retina systematically

Fundoscopy is difficult to master, but with practice anyone can become proficient at identifying the common and important signs.

Cranial nerves III, IV and VI

Eye movements are controlled by cranial nerves III, IV and VI, and are assessed together by examining eyelid and eye position and movements (see Figure 1.55). Careful assessment can distinguish between isolated third, fourth or sixth nerve palsies, more complex combinations of these or weakness from muscle or neuromuscular junction disease.

First note any ptosis; bilateral is usually muscle or neuromuscular junction disease, and unilateral is often from a third nerve palsy. Then test how fully the eyes move in each direction of gaze by asking the patient to follow your finger with their eyes. Limited movement in a particular direction shows that a specific muscle is not working. When a particular extraocular nerve is dysfunctional, its innervated muscles will be weak (see Figure 1.55).

Down-and-out eye, oculomotor palsy and third nerve palsy

These are discussed on page 147.

Trochlear nerve palsy and fourth nerve palsy

Fourth nerve palsy presents with impaired depression and intorsion of the affected eye, often with a compensatory head tilt away from the affected side. It most commonly has a congenital cause or is a result of head trauma.

Abducens nerve palsy and sixth nerve palsy

With a sixth nerve palsy, the affected eye is slightly adducted in primary gaze and there is impaired abduction on attempted lateral gaze to the affected side (**Figure 2.8b**). Cranial nerve VI has a long intracranial course and is often affected by any cause of increased intracranial pressure.

Cranial nerves V and VII

Cranial nerve V is largely sensory, and cranial nerve VII is largely motor. Both mainly involve the face and are conveniently assessed together.

Cranial nerve V is tested by gently touching the face with a pin in each division of the nerve and asking whether it is felt normally. Lesions result in sensory loss on testing pinprick or temperature sensation in one or more of the three divisions: ophthalmic, maxillary and mandibular (see Figures 1.56 and 1.57). There can be wasting of the masseter and temporalis muscles along with weakness of jaw opening. The jaw jerk test is performed by gently tapping a finger placed on the patient's chin with their jaw open (**Figure 2.12**). A brisk closing of the mouth is abnormal and indicates an upper motor neurone lesion.

Lesions of cranial nerve VII cause an ipsilateral facial weakness that is seen when the patient is asked to wrinkle their forehead, close their eyes, puff out their cheeks and whistle.

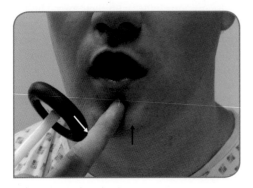

Figure 2.12 The jaw jerk reflex is tested by placing the finger on the loosely open jaw and tapping on the finger gently with a tendon hammer (white arrow). The jaw is observed for brisk reflex closure (black arrow).

Brain stem nuclei or cranial nerve lesions cause the full face to be affected, including the forehead. In contrast, contralateral motor cortex lesions spare the forehead (the ipsilateral motor cortex also innervates the lower motor neurones controlling the forehead muscles, which therefore continue to work) while affecting the mouth and lower facial muscles.

The facial nerve also innervates the stapedius muscle of the ear and carries taste sensation from the anterior two thirds of the tongue. Therefore lower motor neurone lesions also result in sensitivity to high-pitched sounds (hyperacusis) and altered taste.

> Remember: the **functions of the facial nerve** are 'face, ear, taste and tear'.

Cranial nerve V carries sensation from the cornea as part of the corneal reflex, whereas cranial nerve VII controls the muscles involved in the eyelid-blinking part of this reflex.

Cranial nerve VIII

Damage to the auditory and vestibular nerves results in hearing loss (the auditory portion) and nystagmus or balance problems (the vestibular portion).

The auditory portion of the nerve is assessed at the bedside by inspection with an otoscope to look for wax, scars, or discharge or debris in the ear canal and by quietly whispering a number in each ear. Weber's and Rinne's tests can also be performed to determine whether hearing loss is conductive or sensorineural (see **Figure 2.10**).

The vestibular portion of the nerve is assessed by looking carefully for nystagmus. Lesions in the vestibular nerve or its nuclei can also cause abnormal balance and an abnormal, imbalanced gait evident when observing the patient walk.

Cranial nerves IX, X and XII

These three nerves (the lower cranial nerves) are tested together, because they are often affected together. Dysfunction results in dysarthria, hoarseness, weak cough, dysphagia and wasting or spasticity of the tongue.

These symptoms are described as a bulbar palsy if caused by a lower motor neurone lesion, or a pseudobulbar palsy if resulting from an upper motor neurone lesion.

Lower cranial nerve function is tested by:

- tongue inspection for abnormal dryness or fasciculation
- inspection of the uvula (it should rise symmetrically when the patient says 'Ahh')
- listening for any dysarthria or hoarseness

The gag reflex involves sensory fibres from cranial nerve IX and motor fibres from cranial nerve X, and is tested by stimulating the back of the palate and looking for a reflex gag (**Figure 2.13**). Absence of the gag reflex suggests a lower motor neurone or sensory lesion. Exaggeration of the reflex suggests an upper motor neurone lesion.

Cranial nerve XI

This is a purely motor nerve that supplies some of the muscles of the neck. Weakness on shoulder shrugging or head turning, or wasting or fasciculations of the sternocleidomastoid or trapezius muscles, points to a lesion of cranial nerve XI.

Limb examination

Examination of the limbs can identify problems at any level of the nervous system from muscle to cortex, and is usually performed in every patient. It follows a standard sequence: inspection, tone, power, reflexes, coordination and sensation. Bear in mind the following general points.

Inspection

Ensure that the limbs are sufficiently exposed to look carefully at muscle bulk, fasciculations, scars, deformities, etc.

Tone

Ask the patient to relax their limb and passively move it to feel for the resting tone.

> **Patient anxiety may be mistaken for pathological increased tone.** To distinguish the two, try to distract or talk to the patient when assessing tone.

Power

This is a central part of the neurological examination and needs to be mastered. It should be practiced until the sequence of muscles to be tested becomes second nature.

- Attempt to test 'like with like', i.e. provide more force when testing stronger muscles than weaker ones before declaring a muscle normal or weak
- Give clear instructions; show the patient or move their limb into the position you wish to test
- By testing a few different muscles from each peripheral nerve and myotome, it is possible to localise the lesion more precisely
- Grade each muscle tested according to the Medical Research Council power grade (**Table 2.13**)

Reflexes

In the upper limbs, reflexes can be normal, reduced, absent or increased. If absent initially, the reflex must be retested with reinforcement: have the patient clench their teeth tightly just before testing the muscle, or hold their hands together and pull. This increases background tone and may bring out a reduced reflex.

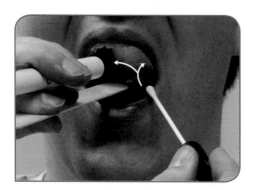

Figure 2.13 The gag reflex is tested by using a tongue depressor and torch to visualise the pharynx and then touching each side in turn with a cotton swab to check if the patient can feel both sides (the afferent limb is through cranial nerve IX), noting contraction of the soft palate (the efferent limb is through cranial nerve X).

UK Medical Research Council muscle power grading scale	
Grade	Description
0	No movement
1	Flicker of muscle contraction
2	Movement only with gravity eliminated
3	Can overcome gravity but no resistance
4	Some resistance but can be overcome by examiner
5	Normal strength

Table 2.13 Grading muscle power: the UK Medical Research Council scale

With the patient as relaxed as possible, place a finger over the tendon of the muscle being tested. The muscle should be slightly stretched but not completely extended.

Swing the tendon hammer firmly on to your finger.

Coordination

Smooth coordination requires integrated proprioceptive, vestibular and visual input along with intact motor function. Dysfunction anywhere in this system can impair coordination. Significant weakness can limit the ability of a patient to coordinate a limb without there being actual poor coordination.

Sensation

It is easy to get lost when assessing sensation but learning an efficient routine allows this stage to be performed accurately and quickly.

- Always start distally and work proximally, starting 'mid limb' leaves you uncertain where to go next
- Give patients clear and simple instructions when asking about what they can feel (e.g. 'Can you feel anything?' and 'Does it feel like a sharp pin?')
- Test at least one modality from each of the dorsal columns and lateral columns rather than multiple modalities from the same sensory pathway
- Test each major peripheral nerve
- Test each dermatome if the history suggests a radiculopathy or myelopathy

If the patient reports altered sensation, compare it with the other side, asking them 'Does it feel the same on both sides?'

- If there are any areas of abnormal sensation, move in a proximal direction until normal sensation is felt; map out any abnormal areas in this way
- The hallmark of peripheral nerve root lesions (e.g. from a herniated intervertebral disc) is pain radiating from the back or neck into the area supplied by the affected nerve root, along with variable sensory loss and motor weakness (**Table 2.14**); this area of skin is often very sensitive to touch, so be gentle when examining someone with a suspected nerve root entrapment

Upper limbs

After the arms are inspected for muscle wasting, abnormal posturing or movements, and for fasciculations, the patient then holds their arms up in front of them with their palms face up and closes their eyes (**Figure 2.14**). Any downward drift (pronator drift) of an arm indicates an upper motor neurone lesion in the corticospinal tract.

Tone

This is assessed by passively moving each arm in turn.

Power

This is tested by examining particular muscles in sequence. **Table 2.15** and **Figures 2.15–2.18** show the instructions to give and which muscles, nerves and roots are being tested.

Reflexes

The biceps (C5–C6), triceps (C6–C7) and supinator (C5–C6) reflexes are tested as shown in **Figure 2.19**.

Coordination

This is assessed by asking the patient to touch their nose with their finger and then reach forwards and touch the examiner's upheld finger. Secondly, ask them to clap one hand on the other, flipping the hand each time.

Disc herniation				
Affected disc	Affected spinal root	Sensory changes	Motor deficit	Reflex lost
C4–C5	C5	Shoulder and lateral upper arm	Deltoid, supraspinatus and infraspinatus	Supinator
C5–C6	C6	Lateral aspect of forearm, thumb and forefinger	Biceps and brachioradialis	Biceps
C6–C7	C7	Dorsal aspect of forearm, and middle finger	Triceps and extensor muscles of wrist and fingers	Triceps
C7–T1	C8	4th and 5th digits and medial aspect of palm	Intrinsic muscles of the hand, and thumb flexor	–
L1–L2	L2	Anterior upper thigh	Hip flexion	–
L2–L3	L3	Anterior thigh and knee	Knee extension	–
L3–L4	L4	Medial calf	Knee extension	Patellar
L4–L5	L5	Lateral calf, and big toe	Ankle and big toe dorsiflexion	–
L5–S1	S1	Posterior calf, sole of foot and lateral little toe	Ankle plantar flexion	Achilles
–	S2–S4	Groin, perineal and perianal regions	External anal and bladder sphincters	Anal

Table 2.14 Typical findings in intervertebral disc herniations

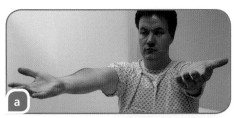
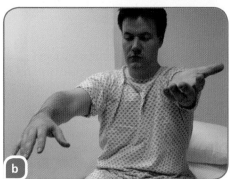

Figure 2.14 Checking for pronator drift. (a) The patient holds their arms up, palms up and wide apart. (b) On closing their eyes, the arm pronates and flexes slightly at the elbow.

Difficulty in smoothly alternating the clapping hands in this manner is called dysdiadochokinesia and is often seen in cases of cerebellar lesions.

Sensation

This is tested by asking if the patient can feel a sharp pinprick in areas of each of the major peripheral nerves and dermatomes; this tests the anterolateral system. Sensation is also tested by checking joint position or vibration sense in the same areas; this tests the dorsal column system.

Lower limbs

As in the upper limb examination, the patient is exposed and inspected for signs of muscle wasting, fasciculations, posturing, abnormal movements and deformity.

Tone

This is assessed by rolling each leg in turn, looking to see how loosely the ankle joint moves, and then swiftly pulling up the thigh to see if the foot is lifted off the couch (this indicates increased tone) or slides up the couch (the normal response) (**Figure 2.20**).

Power

This is assessed by systematically testing the strength in a series of muscles. **Table 2.16** and **Figures 2.21–2.24** show the instructions

Muscle testing sequence in upper limb examination

Instruction	Muscle	Muscle action	Nerve	Root
Lift your elbows up and out	Deltoid	Shoulder abduction	Axillary	C5–C6
Make your arms like a boxer's	Biceps brachii	Elbow flexion	Musculoskeletal	C5–C6
Make your arms like a boxer's	Triceps	Elbow extension	Radial	C7
Make fists and cock your wrists back	Extensor carpi radialis longus	Wrist extension and abduction	Radial	C6
Make fists and cock your wrists back	Extensor carpi ulnaris	Wrist extension and adduction	Radial	C7
Keep your fingers out straight	Extensor digitorum	Finger extension	Radial	C7
Stick your thumbs out to the side	Extensor pollicis brevis	Thumb abduction	Radial	C7
Shake my hand: don't let me turn it	Pronator teres	Forearm pronation	Median	C7
Grip my finger tips	Flexor digitorum profundus I and II	Flexion of distal phalanx	Median	C8
Bend your thumbs	Flexor pollicis longus	Flexion of thumb	Median	C8
Touch you thumbs to the base of you little finger	Opponens pollicis	Thumb opposition	Median	T1
Spread your fingers wide	Flexor carpi ulnaris	Finger abduction	Ulnar	C8
Spread your fingers wide	1st dorsal interosseous	Finger abduction	Ulnar	T1
Keep your fingers together	2nd palmar interosseous	Finger adduction	Ulnar	T1
Keep your thumb on your palm	Adductor pollicis	Thumb adduction	Ulnar	T1

Table 2.15 Muscle testing sequence in upper limb examination

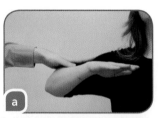

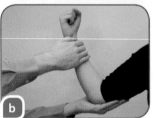

Figure 2.15 Assessment of power of the muscles supplied by the axillary and musculoskeletal nerves. Muscles, spinal roots and nerves are, respectively: (a) deltoid, C5–C6, axillary; (b) biceps, C5–C6, musculoskeletal.

to give and muscles to test along with their innervating peripheral nerves and roots.

Reflexes

The patellar (L2-L4), Achilles (S1) and plantar reflexes (L5–S1; also called Babinski's reflexes) are tested as shown in **Figures 2.25** and **2.26**. The normal plantar reflex is for the great toe to initially flex and curl up (a 'down-going' or 'flexor' plantar response; see **Figure 2.26b**). In upper motor neurone lesions, the initial movement of the toe is upwards (the 'up-going' or 'extensor' plantar response; see **Figure 2.26c**). Clonus is an abnormally prolonged and repetitive contraction of gastrocnemius when the ankle is

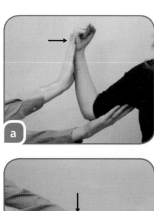
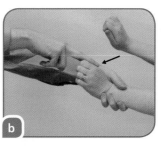
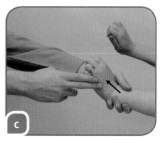

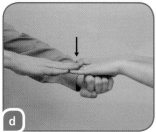
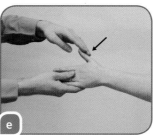

Figure 2.16 Assessment of power of the muscles supplied by the radial nerve. Arrow indicates direction of force exerted by examiner. Muscles, spinal roots and nerves are, respectively: (a) triceps, C7, radial; (b) extensor carpi radialis longus, C6, radial; (c) extensor carpi ulnaris, C7, radial; (d) extensor digitorum, C7, radial; (e) extensor pollicis brevis, C7, radial.

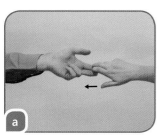
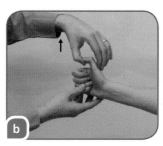
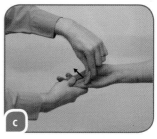

Figure 2.17 Assessment of power of the muscles supplied by the median nerve. The arrow indicates the direction of force exerted by the examiner. Muscles, spinal roots and nerves are, respectively: (a) flexor digitorum profundus I and II, C8, median; (b) flexor pollicis longus, C8, median; (c) opponens pollicis, T1, median.

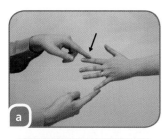
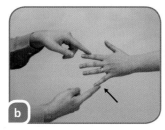
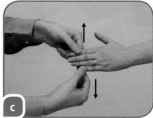

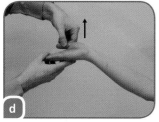

Figure 2.18 Assessment of power of the muscles supplied by the ulnar nerve. The arrow indicates the direction of force exerted by the examiner. Muscles, spinal roots and nerves are, respectively: (a) first dorsal interosseous, T1, ulnar; (b) flexor carpi ulnaris, C8, ulnar; (c) second palmar interosseous, T1, ulnar; (d) adductor pollicis, T1, ulnar.

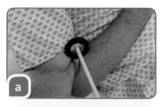
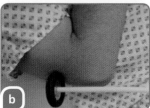
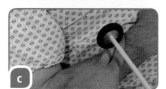
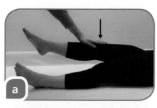

Figure 2.19 Reflexes of the upper limb reflexes. Position in which to test the stretch reflex of (a) biceps, (b) triceps and (c) supinator.

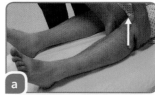
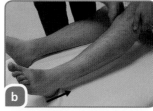
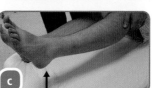

Figure 2.20 Assessment of tone in the legs. (a) The examiner briskly lifts up the knee (white arrow). (b) With normal tone, the heel drags up the bed. (c) With increased tone, the heel lifts off the bed.

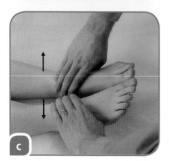

Figure 2.21 Assessment of power around the hip. The arrow indicates the direction of force exerted by the examiner. Muscles, spinal roots and nerves are, respectively: (a) iliacus, L1-L2, femoral; (b) gluteus maximus, L5–S1, inferior gluteal; (c) adductors, L2-L3, obturator.

Coordination

In the legs, coordination is assessed by asking the patient to lift their heel, place it on the opposite knee and run it up and down their shin, or by asking them to tap out a rhythm with their foot.

Sensation

This is assessed using pinprick testing (of the anterolateral system) and vibration and joint position testing in the same manner as in the upper limbs.

Localising lesions from limb signs

Patterns of abnormalities in the limb examination are very helpful in identifying which part of the nervous system is affected. **Table 2.17** shows the typical patterns of abnormalities found on limb examination depending on the location of the lesion.

Spinal cord lesions produce distinct patterns of sensory and motor dysfunction depending on precisely where the lesion is (**Figure 2.27**).

passively dorsiflexed by the examiner and held in position. This abnormal reflex is an upper motor neurone sign.

Muscle testing sequence in lower limb examination				
Instruction	Muscle	Muscle action	Nerve	Root
Push your leg into the couch	Gluteus maximus	Hip	Inferior gluteal	L5–S1
Don't let me separate your legs	Adductors	Adduction at hip	Obturator	L2–L3
Lift your leg up	Iliacus and psoas major	Hip flexion	Femoral	L1–L2
Bend your knee, and don't let me bend it more	Quadriceps	Extension at knee	Femoral	L3–L4
Bend your knee, and don't let me turn your leg out	Gluteus medius and minimus	Internal rotation of thigh	Superior gluteal	L4–L5
Bend your knee, and don't let me straighten it	Hamstrings	Flexion at knee	Sciatic	S1
Push your foot down	Gastrocnemius	Plantar flexion at ankle	Tibial	S1–S2
Turn your foot in	Tibialis posterior	Inversion of foot	Tibial	L4–L5
Curl your toes	Small muscles of the foot	Cupping of foot	Tibial	S1–S2
Point your foot towards your head	Tibialis anterior	Dorsiflexion at ankle	Deep peroneal	L4
Point your big toe towards your head	Extensor hallucis longus	Extension of the toe	Deep peroneal	L5
Turn your foot out	Peroneus longus and brevis	Eversion of foot	Superficial peroneal	L5–S1

Table 2.16 Muscle testing sequence in lower limb examination

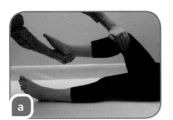
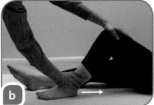
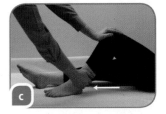

Figure 2.22 Assessment of power around the knee. The arrow indicates the direction of force exerted by the examiner. (a) Gluteus medius and minimus, L4–L5, superior gluteal. (b) Quadriceps, L3–L4, femoral. (c) Hamstring, S1, sciatic.

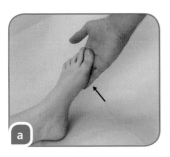
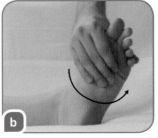
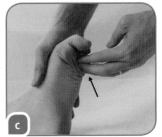

Figure 2.23 Assessment of power of the muscles of the tibial nerve. The arrow indicates the direction of force exerted by the examiner. Muscles, spinal roots and nerves are, respectively: (a) gastrocnemius, S1–S2, tibial; (b) tibialis posterior, L4–L5, tibial; (c) small muscles of the foot, S1–S2, tibial.

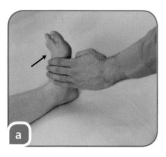
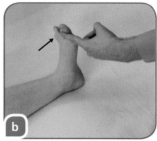
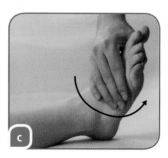

Figure 2.24 Assessment of power of the muscles supplied by the peroneal nerve. The arrow indicates the direction of force exerted by the examiner. Muscles, spinal roots and nerves are, respectively: (a) tibialis anterior, L4, deep peroneal; (b) extensor hallucis longus, L5, deep peroneal; (c) peroneus longus and brevis, L5–S1, superficial peroneal.

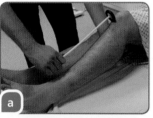

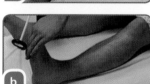

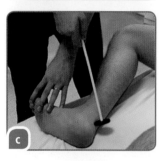

Figure 2.25 Reflexes of the lower limb. Examples of how to test the (a) knee jerk and (b) and (c) ankle jerk.

Many drugs, for example statins, and metabolic diseases, such as hypothyroidism, can cause a **myopathy with classic proximal limb weakness.**

Peripheral nerve or nerve root lesions tend to cause loss of power and sensation in the muscles and skin innervated by the affected neurones. In polyneuropathies, this tends to cause a glove-and-stocking distribution of sensory loss and distal more than proximal weakness. In focal nerve or nerve root entrapment, the weakness and sensory loss occurs in a more discrete, focal distribution.

Pyramidal weakness

Motor cortex lesions produce weakness that affects the extensors more than the flexors in the upper limb, and affects the flexors more than the extensors in the lower limb. This causes a characteristic flexion of the elbow and wrist and extension of the hip, knee and foot on the affected side; this is known as pyramidal weakness.

Decorticate posture

This is the combination of a contralateral flexed elbow, wrist, and extended ankle and knee, along with eyes deviated away from the flexed arm. The term is used when this occurs with decreased consciousness or coma, in which case it is usually bilateral, with the eyes looking straight ahead (**Figure 2.28**).

Decerebrate posture

This is the combination of a contralateral extended and pronated elbow, wrist, knee and ankle with neck extension. The term is used when the posture occurs with decreased consciousness or coma, in which case it is usually bilateral (**Figure 2.29**). It differs from the decorticate posture in that the arm is extended, not flexed, and the head is extended.

Like the decorticate posture, decerebrate posture indicates severe brain injury from

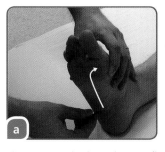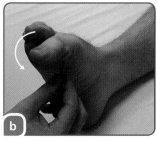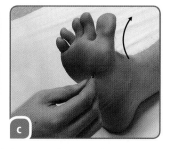

Figure 2.26 Checking plantar reflexes. (a) Stroking the sole of the foot (white arrow) elicits either (b) normal plantar flexion of the great toe or (c) abnormal dorsiflexion of the great toe and fanning of the toes.

Limb examination abnormalities and lesion location						
Lesion location	Limb examination findings					
	Tone	Power		Reflexes	Coordination	Sensation
Lower motor neurone lesions						
Muscle	+/–	Proximal		+/–	+	+
Neuromuscular junction	+/–	Fatiguable		+/–	+	+
Peripheral nerve		Distal or focal			+/–	+/– focal loss
Spinal root		Focal			+	Painful
Upper motor neurone lesions						
Spinal cord	++	Paraplegia or tetraplegia		++	–	–
Brain stem	++	Ipsilateral face and contralateral limb		++	–	–
Cortex	++	Contralateral face and limb		++	+/–	+/–

+, normal; -, reduced; +/-, normal or reduced; ++, increased.

Table 2.17 Use of patterns of limb examination abnormalities to localise lesions

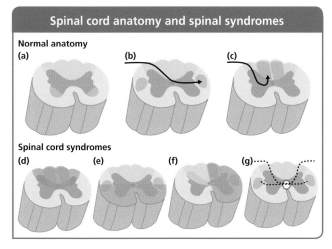

Spinal cord anatomy and spinal syndromes

Normal anatomy
(a)   (b)   (c)

Spinal cord syndromes
(d)   (e)   (f)   (g)

Figure 2.27 Spinal cord anatomy and spinal cord syndromes. (a) Ventral horn: cell bodies of lower motor neurones (blue). (b) Lateral columns (blue) receive pinprick and temperature sensation input from the contralateral body through fibres crossing the midline through the anterior commissure. (c) Dorsal columns (blue) receive joint position sense and vibration sense from the ipsilateral body through fibres that cross at the medulla. (d) Posterior cord syndrome: loss of joint position and vibration senses below the lesion. (e) Anterior cord syndrome: loss of pinprick and temperature sensation and weakness below the lesion. (f) Lateral cord syndrome: loss of ipsilateral joint position and vibration, and contralateral pinprick and temperature sensation and weakness below the lesion. (g) Central cord lesion: disruption of the crossing pinprick and temperature fibres supplying the lateral columns.

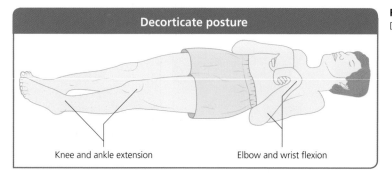

Figure 2.28
Decorticate posture.

Decorticate posture

Knee and ankle extension

Elbow and wrist flexion

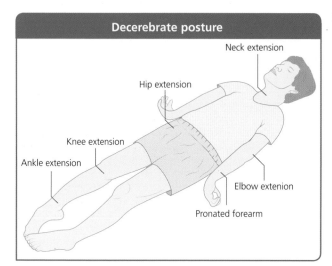

Figure 2.29 Decerebrate posture.

Decerebrate posture

Neck extension

Hip extension

Knee extension

Ankle extension

Elbow extenion

Pronated forearm

structural or traumatic injuries. Both postures can also be present in diffuse metabolic injury to the brain caused by toxins or hypoxia.

Cerebellum

Many aspects of the function of the cerebellum are covered by the history and examination of the gait, cranial nerves and limbs. If the history suggests cerebellar disease, or if this is the initial impression on examination, it is worth using the following routine to more fully elicit cerebellar signs. These steps can be remembered with the mnemonic VANISHD: Vertigo, Ataxia, Nystagmus, Intention tremor, Slurred speech, Hypotonia, Dysdiadochokinesia.

Vertigo

If not specifically covered in the history, ask whether the patient experiences any vertigo. If so, when does it occur, how long does it last, and what are its triggers, relieving factors and associated symptoms?

Ataxia

Look for ataxia by assessing gait and upper and lower limb coordination.

Nystagmus

Look again at the eyes for any nystagmus.

Intention tremor

This may have been identified as part of the upper or lower limb examination. If not, look for it by assessing limb coordination and noting whether the limb wavers as it approaches the target.

Speech

Cerebellar disease often causes dysarthria, heard as slow, slurring or stuttering speech. If not evident in the history, ask the patient to repeat phrases including:

- 'baby hippopotamus'
- 'yellow lorry, red lorry'
- 'British constitution'

Hypotonia

Assess tone in the arms and legs. Cerebellar lesions often initially cause reduced tone, which then develops into increased tone over days to weeks.

Dysdiadochokinesia

Ask the patient to clap one hand on the other as described in the upper limb examination.

Higher cortical function

Assessment of higher cortical function allows objective measurements of response to treatments. It can also help determine a patient's ability to consent to investigations and treatments.

Formalised cognitive assessments include the revised Addenbrooke's cognitive assessment, the Montreal cognitive assessment and the mini mental state examination (see **Table 2.10**).

Any pathology that causes cortical dysfunction, for example hemispheric stroke, Alzheimer's disease and primary brain tumour, can result in cognitive changes. Recognition of these changes can help localise a disease process in the cortex.

Cortical release signs

These are physical signs that often accompany neurodegenerative disease.

Grasp reflex

Stroke the patient's open hand with your finger or the end of a tendon hammer. Observe for a reflex clasping of the hand (**Figure 2.30**).

Palmomental reflex

Stroke the thenar eminence with the end of a tendon hammer, observing the ipsilateral chin for any small reflex contraction (**Figure 2.31**).

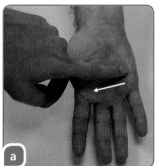
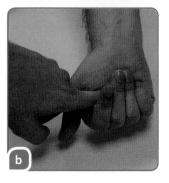

Figure 2.30 Grasp reflex: involuntary grasping of objects passing through the hand.

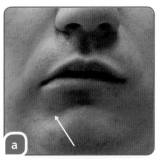
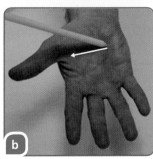

Figure 2.31 Palmomental reflex: a small ipsilateral contraction of the chin on stroking the palm.

Pout reflex

Press firmly on the patient's closed lips and note any reflex pouting (**Figure 2.32**).

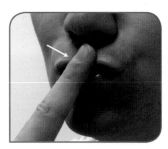

Figure 2.32
Pout reflex. On pressing the lips, the patient involuntarily forms a pout.

Investigations

Starter questions

Answers to the following questions are on page 185.

7. What effects do neurological tests have on patients?
8. Why might investigations not be in the best interests of a patient?

Specialised investigations help localise a lesion and determine its cause.

Neuroradiology

Clinical neuroradiology is used in both the diagnosis and treatment of disease. Interventional radiology is a subspecialty within radiology in which minimally invasive procedures are carried out under imaging guidance. This allows instruments such as needles or catheters to be guided to the target without open surgery, thereby reducing infection rates and enhancing recovery times.

Ionising radiation

X-rays are high-energy photons. As they pass through tissue, their energy is sufficient to ionise atoms by displacing electrons and disrupting molecular bonds, therefore they are potentially harmful to tissues. The effects of radiation are divided into:

■ stochastic effects, which occur by chance and include genetic damage and cancer

■ deterministic effects, which have a clear relationship with X-ray dose (**Table 2.18**) and include skin erythema and burns, cataracts, radiation sickness and death at high doses

Stochastic effects have no threshold: any dose can cause genetic damage. This is why it is vital to use as low a dose as reasonably practicable, especially in children.

Plain radiography

X-rays are differentially absorbed (attenuated) according to tissue density: metal and bone have greatest absorption (attenuation), soft tissue has much lower absorption, and air has the lowest. This generates the contrasts seen when X-rays have passed through the patient and strike the X-ray film or digital detector. Plain radiographs do not show soft tissues well, so they have a limited direct role in neuroradiology. Examples of their use include assessment of ventriculoperitoneal shunts, fractures and skeletal abnormalities.

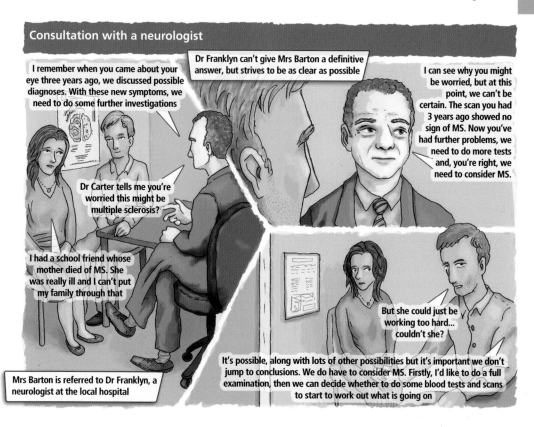

Consultation with a neurologist

Mrs Barton is referred to Dr Franklyn, a neurologist at the local hospital

Dr Franklyn can't give Mrs Barton a definitive answer, but strives to be as clear as possible

I remember when you came about your eye three years ago, we discussed possible diagnoses. With these new symptoms, we need to do some further investigations

Dr Carter tells me you're worried this might be multiple sclerosis?

I had a school friend whose mother died of MS. She was really ill and I can't put my family through that

I can see why you might be worried, but at this point, we can't be certain. The scan you had 3 years ago showed no sign of MS. Now you've had further problems, we need to do more tests and, you're right, we need to consider MS.

But she could just be working too hard... couldn't she?

It's possible, along with lots of other possibilities but it's important we don't jump to conclusions. We do have to consider MS. Firstly, I'd like to do a full examination, then we can decide whether to do some blood tests and scans to start to work out what is going on

Radiation dosage	
Source of exposure	Dose
Sleeping next to someone	0.05 µSv
Dental X-ray	0.005 mSv
Chest X-ray	0.02 mSv
Transatlantic flight	0.07 mSv
CT scan of the head	1.4 mSv
UK average annual radiation dose	2.7 mSv
Whole body CT scan	10 mSv
Level at which changes in blood cells can be readily observed	100 mSv
Severe radiation poisoning	2 Sv

CT, computerised tomography.

Table 2.18 Radiation dosage exposures

Fluoroscopy and cerebral angiography

Fluoroscopy is an adaptation of plain radiography that uses an image intensifier and real-time display instead of an X-ray film to produce dynamic images. Structures may be enhanced and anatomy shown by administering contrast agents. Iodinated contrast is nephrotoxic, and there is a risk of anaphylaxis.

Neuroradiological applications include image-guided lumbar puncture and biopsy, but the main use is cerebral angiography. This technique visualises the intracranial vessels by the use of iodine-based contrast injected into the arteries, typically through a catheter placed in the common femoral artery in the groin.

Digital subtraction angiography

This technique improves visualisation of intracranial vasculature. An initial 'mask' image is obtained and imaging is repeated after injection of contrast. By digitally subtracting the pre-contrast image from the post-contrast one, structures such as bone and soft tissue, which would otherwise obscure the image, are removed. Digital subtraction angiography is used to visualise vascular pathologies. It produces much higher resolution images than those obtained by computerised tomography (CT) angiography.

The catheter used for digital subtraction angiography may also be used to deploy stents or coils into vascular abnormalities, including aneurysms. This forms the basis of interventional neuroradiology.

Computerised tomography

In CT, as in plain radiography, X-rays are used to penetrate tissue. In CT, the X-ray detectors rotate around the patient to acquire multiple images from different projections. These images are assembled by computer into cross-sectional images in the axial plane (tomograms). Data can also be manipulated in additional planes (multiplanar reformatting) to produce coronal and sagittal reformats as well as three-dimensional images. Early CT scanners took 5 min to scan the head, and hours to process the data. Now, a scan takes about a second.

Sir Godfrey Hounsfield developed the first human CT scan in 1971. The scan showed a cystic tumour in the frontal lobe, which previously could have been seen only during surgery. This achievement won him a Nobel Prize in 1979.

Computerised tomography has several advantages over conventional radiography. The superimposition of structures is avoided, and the greater contrast facilitates differentiation between tissue types. CT images may be digitally manipulated to enhance contrast between tissues (**Figure 2.33**).

The main neuroradiological application of CT is the identification of haemorrhage, infarction, hydrocephalus and tumours. Images of tumours can be enhanced by administering intravenous iodinated contrast, which is able to cross the blood–brain barrier because of the tumour's excessive vascular permeability.

CT angiography

This has been made possible by the speed of

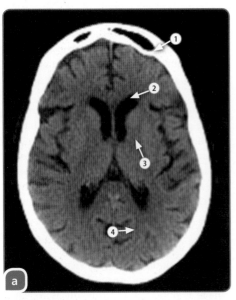
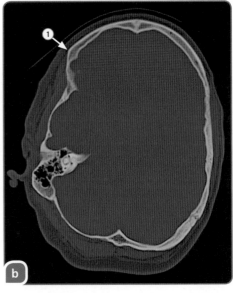

Figure 2.33 Axial computerised tomography scan of the brain, showing the effects of changing window width and level to highlight (a) brain parenchyma and (b) bone. ①, bone; ②, cerebrospinal fluid; ③, white matter; ④, grey matter.

modern CT scanners, which allows images to be acquired while the contrast is still in the vessels. CT angiography is used to identify aneurysms, stenosis and vascular malformations. It lacks the high spatial resolution of conventional catheter angiography using X-rays but is less risky, less invasive, quicker and more cost-effective. CT angiography shows vascular anatomy more clearly than magnetic resonance imaging (MRI) or ultrasound.

Disadvantages of CT

Computerised tomography is a high-dose technique, delivering 1.4 mSv per head scan; for comparison, the risk of developing a fatal cancer is 1:1000 to 1:2000 per 10 mSv. This risk must be balanced against the likely benefits. Iodinated contrast is nephrotoxic, so caution is required for its use in patients with impaired renal function. Anaphylaxis is also a risk.

Magnetic resonance imaging

This technique uses strong magnetic fields, i.e. non-ionising radiation, to discriminate between different tissues on the basis of the behaviour of the constituent hydrogen atoms.

The strength of a magnetic field is measured in tesla (T): 1 T is 30,000 times the strength of the Earth's magnetic field. The typical magnetic strength of MRI scanners are in the order of 1.5–3 T. Consequently, MRI is contraindicated in patients with pacemakers, cochlear implants, intraocular foreign bodies, intracranial aneurysm clips (but not coils) and certain metallic prostheses, because these would move in the magnetic field. All ferromagnetic items, for example credit cards, and electronic devices are removed before entering the MRI room.

Basic principles of MRI

Hydrogen nuclei (protons) are positively charged and behave like magnets. In the MRI scanner, the magnetic moments of the body's hydrogen nuclei align parallel to the magnetic field, i.e. they become longitudinally magne-

tised, spinning like a top (precessing) (**Figure 2.34a**). A second electromagnetic pulse (a radiofrequency) at an angle to the main magnetic field, and at the same frequency as hydrogen nuclei, causes them to resonate. The hydrogen nuclei do not move, but their magnetic moment realigns in a transverse direction (transverse magnetisation) and they are said to be 'in phase' (**Figure 2.34b**).

When the transverse radiofrequency pulse is switched off, the hydrogen nuclei repel each other. This repulsion causes them to lose their transverse magnetisation and become 'dephased', a process called T2 relaxation. They simultaneously regain longitudinal magnetisation (**Figure 2.34c**); this is called T1 relaxation. The hydrogen nuclei in different tissues undergo these changes ('relax') at different rates; as they do so, their magnetic moments move in the MRI receiver coil, and this movement induces an electrical current that generates the images.

Types of MRI

The T1 and T2 relaxation processes are exploited for the basic MRI sequences: T1- and T2-weighted imaging (**Figure 2.35**). Many other MRI sequences are derived from these two basic sequences. For example, because different tissues have characteristic T1 and T2 times, the signal from specific tissues may be suppressed.

- **FLAIR** (fluid-attenuated inversion recovery) suppresses water and cerebrospinal fluid and is useful in identifying periventricular abnormalities such as multiple sclerosis plaques (**Figure 2.36**)
- **STIR** (short tau inversion recovery) suppresses fat, and is used in spinal imaging to suppress the fat signal in bone marrow (**Figure 2.37**), thereby highlighting bone lesions
- **Diffusion weighted imaging** (often called the 'stroke sequence') is used to help diagnose stroke; newly infarcted cells swell and absorb extracellular water, resulting in restricted diffusion and a characteristic bright signal on diffusion-weighted imaging sequences

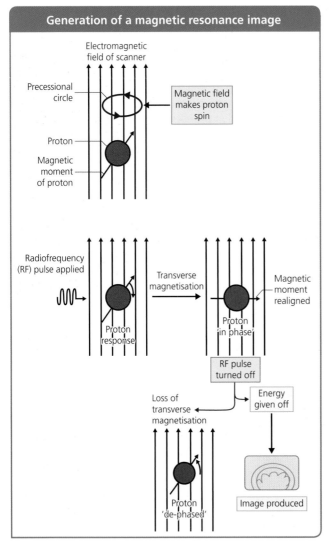

Generation of a magnetic resonance image

Electromagnetic field of scanner

Precessional circle

Magnetic field makes proton spin

Proton

Magnetic moment of proton

Radiofrequency (RF) pulse applied

Proton response

Transverse magnetisation

Proton in phase

Magnetic moment realigned

RF pulse turned off

Loss of transverse magnetisation

Energy given off

Proton 'de-phased'

Image produced

Figure 2.34 Generation of a magnetic resonance image. Protons precess (spin) when placed in a magnetic field. A radiofrequency pulse delivered at a specific frequency tips these protons. The rate at which the protons return to their starting position, and the characteristic energy emitted as they recover, varies between tissues.

Functional MRI

This type of MRI is used to measure changes in brain activity by detecting corresponding changes in cerebral blood flow. One functional MRI sequence is BOLD (blood oxygenation level–dependent). This exploits the facts that deoxyhaemoglobin and oxyhaemoglobin have different magnetic properties, and their proportions in brain tissue are different during activity and at rest. These phenomena allow identification of areas responsible for certain tasks; for example, visual stimulation activates the visual cortex in the occipital lobe.

Functional MRI is experimental, and there is controversy regarding its reliability and what it exactly measures.

Positron emission tomography

Positron emission tomography (PET) is a nuclear imaging method used primarily in the detection of cancer and its metastases. Rather than showing anatomy, it shows function by visualising metabolic activity in the body.

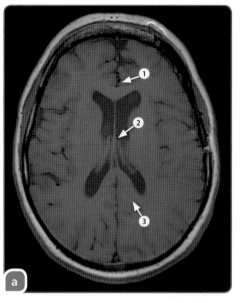
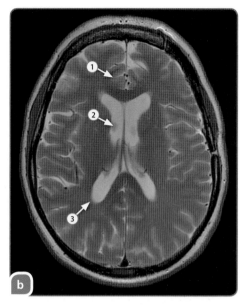

Figure 2.35 T1- and T2-weighted axial magnetic resonance images of the brain. (a) On T1-weighted images, cerebrospinal fluid is dark, and white matter has a higher signal than grey matter because of differences in fat content within myelin. (b) On T2-weighted images, the cerebrospinal fluid and oedema are bright, and white matter is darker than grey. ①, grey matter; ②, cerebrospinal fluid; ③, white matter.

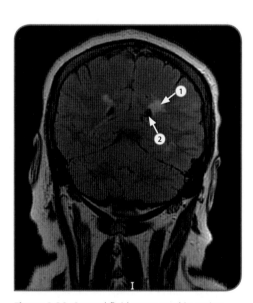

Figure 2.36 Coronal fluid-attenuated inversion recovery (FLAIR) sequence of the brain, showing suppression of the signal from cerebrospinal fluid ②, thereby highlighting oedema ①.

Basic principles of PET

A glucose analogue, fluorodeoxyglucose, labelled with a radioactive isotope (typically fluorine-18, ^{18}F), is injected intravenously and accumulates in metabolically active tissues.

^{18}F undergoes radioactive decay by emitting a positron (an antimatter electron). Its subsequent collision with an electron annihilates both particles and emits two high-energy gamma photons (511 keV) in opposite directions. The photons are detected by a bank of scintillation crystals, which create a flash of light when a gamma photon reaches them; this light is then converted into an electrical signal. The simultaneous detection of two gamma photons in opposite detectors allows accurate localisation of their origin.

Positron emission tomography scans are often done alongside a CT scan to permit more accurate anatomical localisation of abnormalities.

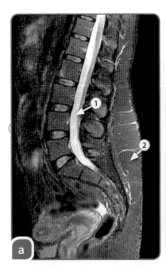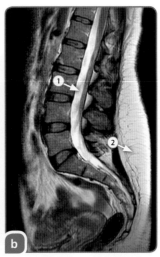

a

b

Figure 2.37 Sagittal T2W short tau inversion recovery (STIR) sequence of the lumbar spine (a) compared with normal T2W image (b), showing suppression of fat signal in the STIR sequence with resulting dark signal (a) compared with the normal T2W sequence where the fat signal is not suppressed and appears bright (b). ①, cerebrospinal fluid; ②, fat.

Clinical applications of PET

Before the advent of functional MRI, PET was used to localise the source of seizures; the seizure focus shows reduced metabolic uptake after a seizure. Novel PET agents have also been used to identify amyloid plaques in the brains of patients with Alzheimer's disease.

The main limitations of PET are its high radiation dose (as high as 20 mSv) and low spatial resolution.

Ultrasound

In ultrasonography, high-frequency sound waves (2–18 MHz) are used to provide real-time images of soft tissue. Sound waves are reflected or absorbed according to tissue type. Reflected sound waves are transformed into an image. No ionising radiation is used, but the technique is limited by considerable interobserver variability and patients' body habitus.

In neuroradiology, the use of ultrasound is limited and largely restricted to the assessment of blood flow in the carotid and vertebral arteries (**Figure 2.38**). Intracranial arteries are largely inaccessible, because sound waves cannot penetrate the adult skull. However, ultrasound does have a role in paediatric neuroimaging, because the sound waves can pass through the soft fontanelles in infants.

Neurophysiology

Clinical neurophysiological studies are based on the ability to measure electrical activity in the brain, nerve and muscles to detect and characterise patterns of nervous system dysfunction. Unlike radiology, which largely identifies structural abnormalities, neurophysiology identifies abnormalities in the function of the nervous system.

Electroencephalography

This is non-invasive recording of the activity of cortical neurones through 21 electrodes placed on the scalp. The recordings are displayed in various standardised ways called montages. Simultaneous video recording is often used for evidence of clinical correlates.

Electroencephalography (EEG) is used in investigation of disorders such as suspected epilepsy (to identify the syndrome), coma, parasomnias and encephalopathies. Prolonged recordings are possible with the use of an ambulatory EEG monitor, which the patient wears and activates during an event. EEG recordings can also be made over multiple days in an in-patient unit with 24-h EEG and video recording. Prolonged recording is often helpful for investigating the nature of seizures when diagnosis is uncertain. Before epilepsy

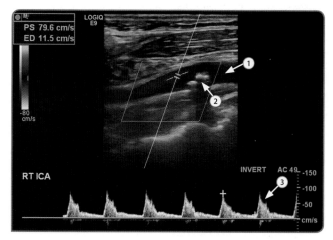

Figure 2.38 Doppler sonography excels in showing vascular narrowing (stenosis) of the carotid arteries. This image shows a calcified atheromatous plaque in the internal carotid artery. ①, internal carotid artery; ②, atheroma; ③, vascular waveform.

surgery, EEG is essential for definitive identi-fication of the site of seizure onset.

Invasive intracranial electrode placement is carried out in selected surgical cases to further clarify the precise location of seizure onset.

Nerve conduction studies and electromyography

The electrical activity of the nerves and mus-cles is measured in nerve conduction studies (NCS) and electromyography (EMG), respec-tively. A recording probe is placed on the skin over a muscle or section of nerve while another probe is placed elsewhere on the skin over the same muscle or nerve to stimu-late it.

Nerve conduction studies are used to iden-tify which nerves are dysfunctional, whether there is sensory or motor involvement and whether there is demyelination, axonal dam-age or both. This information can significantly inform diagnosis and can be used for monitor-ing clinical course.

Electromyography is used to identify pri-mary muscle disease or secondary effects from nerve dysfunction. It also identifies key features of neuromuscular junction disorders such as myasthenia gravis.

Some patients find NCS and EMG uncom-fortable, and some particular applications of it are more painful than others. However they are generally very well tolerated.

> **Demyelinating neuropathies slow nerve conduction and prolong the action potential.** Severe demyelination can cause conduction block (a loss of signal distal to the point of demyelination).

Evoked potentials

Evoked potential studies measure the cor-tical electrical activity evoked by stimu-lating particular sensory modalities. In visual evoked potential studies, the retina is stimulated by flashing images and the time delay and amplitude of the visual cortical response is recorded. The results are help-ful for identifying a subclinical optic neuri-tis and can aid in the diagnosis of multiple sclerosis.

Less common are auditory and somato-sensory evoked potential studies, in which are measured the cortical response to hear-ing and tactile sensation, respectively. The results of such studies can help clarify whether there is abnormal electrical func-tion in the nervous system in cases of doubt, for example in patients with functional sen-sory loss.

Cerebrospinal fluid analysis

Abnormalities in the total volume, flow and constituents of cerebrospinal fluid occur in a range of neurological disorders.

Lumbar puncture

Cerebrospinal fluid is obtained through lumbar puncture. The patient lies on one side in the fetal position. The L4 and L5 spinous processes are identified, and under sterile technique and local anaesthetic a fine needle is inserted between the vertebrae and advanced beyond the dura to collect the fluid.

Post-dural puncture headache occurs in 10% of patients and can be severe and prolonged. It is treated with strict bed rest, caffeine, and in resistant cases a blood patch. Far rarer are epidural haematomas and infection.

Cerebrospinal fluid tests

The basic variables measured are opening pressure of the cerebrospinal fluid, cell count, culture results, and protein and glucose concentration. Cerebrospinal fluid pressure is increased in many conditions, and very high levels may necessitate surgical treatment (see page 187).

Cerebrospinal fluid normally contains no white or red blood cells, and no organisms. Very high white cell counts are found in bacterial infections, less so in viral infections. Most inflammatory processes increase cerebrospinal fluid protein concentration, and bacterial infections of the central nervous system result in a low cerebrospinal fluid glucose concentration.

Viral polymerase chain reaction studies are required in cases of suspected infection of the central nervous system to check for a range of viruses, including herpes simplex virus and varicella-zoster virus.

The following additional tests are helpful in specific circumstances.

Oligoclonal bands

Many autoimmune diseases affecting the central nervous system, including multiple sclerosis, are associated with the presence of 'bands' in the cerebrospinal fluid when the samples are analysed by electrophoresis, a technique for separating proteins by size. These oligoclonal bands represent increased levels of immunoglobulin produced by abnormal B cells and the particular pattern may suggest a specific autoimmune disease.

Spectrophotometry analysis

A yellowish discoloration results from the presence of a breakdown product of red blood cells: xanthochromia. The presence of xanthochromia in the cerebrospinal fluid is a sensitive indicator of intracranial haemorrhage. In cases of subarachnoid haemorrhage, the test result will become positive after about 12 h from its onset.

Other laboratory tests

Almost any systemic illness can cause neurological dysfunction. Consequently, basic haematological and biochemical tests are routinely carried out in patients presenting with neurological illness.

Encephalopathies often present with abnormalities of urea and electrolytes, liver function tests and thyroid function tests that indicate the underlying cause. A full blood count is essential to seek evidence of infection, i.e. an increased white cell count, or occult malignancy, i.e. low haemoglobin, that may be causing the neurological symptoms.

More specialised tests include genetic tests, for example for Huntington's disease and myotonic dystrophy, and tests for rare biochemical abnormalities found in genetic metabolic diseases, for example high phenylalanine levels in phenylalanine hydroxylase deficiency.

Antibody tests

Blood tests for antibodies implicated in neurological and systemic disease are frequently done, because there are many known associations. In some instances, the results guide immunosuppressive treatment. Some tests are for autoantibodies that directly damage the nervous system, for example anti-acetylcholine receptor antibodies in myasthenia gravis, and others for antibodies that do not directly cause neuronal damage, for example anti-thyroid peroxidase antibodies in Hashimoto's encephalopathy.

Biopsy

Biopsy of brain, nerve, muscle, skin and other organs is rarely carried out but can be essential in establishing an exact diagnosis and determining appropriate treatment in diagnostically challenging cases.

Brain biopsy

This is usually done through stereotactic surgery (see page 184) when a specific tissue diagnosis is likely to significantly affect treatment, such as chemotherapy targeted at a specific tumour or antibiotic therapy for a specific bacterial infection.

Nerve biopsy

This type of biopsy is rarely required to diagnose a neuropathy. It is usually reserved for confirming a suspected diagnosis of a vasculitic neuropathy.

Muscle biopsy

Biopsies of muscle are common. They are carried out in most cases of chronic myopathies when there is no clear cause or clinical diagnosis. Muscle biopsy can be done under local anaesthetic.

Skin biopsy

Skin biopsies are less invasive than the above and can sometimes give the pathological clue to a systemic illness such as vasculitis or lymphoma.

Management options

Starter questions

Answers to the following questions are on page 185.

9. Are neurological diseases incurable?

10. Why is neuroregeneration seen as the 'Holy Grail' of treatment?

For many neurological conditions, treatment is supportive rather than curative. For others, disease-modifying or curative non-surgical therapies are available. Identifying which patients would benefit from one of these treatments is central to clinical neurology practice.

Neurosurgery is often high risk and restricted to:

- life-saving treatment of critically ill patients, for example extraventricular drainage through a burr hole in cases of acute hydrocephalus
- use of lower risk techniques when there is a potentially life-transforming benefit that clearly outweighs risk, for example lumbar discectomy for an acute disc prolapse

Neurorehabilitation

Neurorehabilitation is a mix of supports and therapies that maximise a patient's quality of life and capability after a serious neurological injury or diagnosis. Specialist inpatient and outpatient services are essential for long-term recovery from neurological illness. Neurorehabilitation consultants coordinate a team of specialist physiotherapists, occupational therapists, speech and language therapists and psychologists. Intensive inpatient therapy and regular outpatient sessions help establish and maintain patients at their best level of function. It is an essential part of the management of cerebral palsy, stroke, Parkinson's disease, multiple sclerosis and brain injury.

An acute neurological disability or a diagnosis of a chronic neurodegenerative disease is life-shattering for most people who experience it. Often support from other people with the condition, or from understanding specialist nurses, goes a long way to help people face their own challenges.

Disease-modifying treatments

This section describes the more commonly used treatments for changing the short-, medium- and long-term outcome of disease.

Fibrinolytic drugs

Tissue plasminogen activator is the only fibrinolytic drug licensed for use in ischaemic stroke.

Tissue plasminogen activator

Thrombolysis is used within 4.5 h of acute ischaemic stroke to reduce disability in survivors (see page 252). In cases of large carotid or basilar artery occlusions, tissue plasminogen activator can be given by intra-arterial administration and occasionally through a catheter to physically remove the clot if the intravenous therapy does not clear the blockage.

Mode of action Tissue plasminogen activator cleaves zymogen plasminogen to yield the protease plasmin. Plasmin degrades fibrin, a major component of arterial blood clots, into inactive proteins; this process is called fibrinolysis.

Indications Tissue plasminogen activator is administered to patients with acute ischaemic stroke, confirmed by CT, within 4.5 h of symptom onset.

Adverse effects The most significant complication is intracerebral or gastro-intestinal bleeding. One in 10 patients has minor intracerebral bleeding with minimal clinical consequences. One in 100 has major intracerebral haemorrhage.

Interactions Bleeding risk is increased with the use of antiplatelet or anticoagulant agents.

Immunosuppressive therapies

Immunosuppressant agents are a diverse group of drugs that have the effect of impairing normal or pathological aspects of the immune response. The usual aim is to control disease as far as possible while minimising adverse effects. For many diseases, high-quality evidence for the use of specific immunosuppressants is limited. The major indications, adverse effects and interactions of commonly used immunosuppressive therapies are shown in **Table 2.19**.

Immunosuppressive therapies for neurological conditions			
Drug(s)	Common indications	Adverse effects	Interactions
Corticosteroids	Multiple sclerosis relapse Chronic inflammatory demyelinating polyneuropathy Myasthenia gravis	Weight gain Osteoporosis Diabetes Gastric ulceration	Many minor interactions
Intravenous immunoglobulin	Guillain–Barré syndrome Myasthenia gravis	Flu-like symptoms Thrombosis	Limits vaccinations
Plasma exchange	Refractory inflammatory diseases	Electrolyte disturbance Coagulopathy	Removes drugs present in plasma
Methotrexate	Myasthenia gravis Dermatomyositis	Bone marrow suppression Liver toxicity Lung fibrosis Spina bifida (in fetus)	Trimethoprim increases toxicity Non-steroidal anti-inflammatory drugs
Cyclophosphamide	Vasculitis Refractory inflammatory diseases	Haemorrhagic cystitis Bone marrow suppression	Clozapine increases toxicity

Table 2.19 Commonly used immunosuppressive therapies in neurological conditions

Multiple sclerosis therapies

There are a range of established and emerging immunomodulating therapies. These include older medications such as the interferons (e.g. interferon-β) and glatiramer acetate in relapsing–remitting multiple sclerosis. Newer medications for multiple sclerosis include intravenous monoclonal antibodies such as natalizumab and alemtuzumab.

Interferon-β

This is given by subcutaneous injection, the frequency depending on the formulation. Interferon-β reduces relapses by about one third.

Mode of action Interferon-β changes many aspects of the immune system. Its effects include broadly altering receptor signalling and T-cell activity.

Indications Interferon-β is given to patients with relapsing–remitting multiple sclerosis who have had at least two relapses over 3 years.

Adverse effects Flu-like adverse effects and irritation at the injection site are common. About 10% of patients develop depression.

Interactions Interferon-β decreases renal clearance of zidovudine and can cause severe immunosuppression.

Natalizumab

This is given as a monthly injection. Natalizumab reduces relapse rate by 70–90%.

Mode of action Natalizumab is a humanised monoclonal antibody directed against very late antigen 4 (VLA-4), an adhesion molecule central to the migration of activated lymphocytes across the blood–brain barrier. Natalizumab prevents movement of lymphocytes into the central nervous system, and thereby prevents relapsing inflammation.

Indications Natalizumab is given to patients with relapsing–remitting multiple sclerosis who have had two or more disabling relapses in 1 year.

Adverse effects With natalizumab, adverse effects are rare. In patients with latent, asymptomatic central nervous system infection with the JC virus, prolonged use of natalizumab (> 2 years) increases the risk of progressive multifocal leucoencephalopathy.

Interactions Inhaled beclometasone increases the risk of natalizumab toxicity.

Fingolimod

This is one of a number of new oral disease-modifying drugs for the treatment of multiple sclerosis. Fingolimod is taken as an oral tablet four times daily and reduces relapses by about 60%.

Mode of action Fingolimod is a sphingosine 1-phosphate receptor modulator that stops lymphocytes leaving lymph nodes, thereby reducing lymphocyte migration into the central nervous system.

Indications Fingolimod is given to patients who have had two or more relapses in 2 years.

Adverse effects These include headache, herpes infections, depression, bradycardia and leucopenia.

Interactions There is a risk of heart block with fingolimod and amiodarone, disopyramide and beta-blockers.

Supportive treatments

For many neurological and neurosurgical conditions, long-term symptoms are not cured but rather managed through the use of a range of medications.

Neuropathic pain agents

Table 18.2 details common treatments for neuropathic pain and the order in which they are used.

Antispasticity agents

Spasticity is a common symptom in any condition causing long-term motor weakness and immobility. Physiotherapy and splinting of limbs can help maintain good tone and posture, but when spasticity is severe, medication may be useful.

Baclofen

This is a widely used antispasmodic agent.

Mode of action Baclofen activates central nervous system $GABA_B$ receptors, and thereby inhibits spinal cord reflex arcs and tonic muscle activation.

Indications Baclofen is used as first-line treatment for neuromuscular spasticity.

Adverse effects Drowsiness is common, affecting up to 60% of patients, but lessens over time. Nausea and confusion are experienced by up to 10%.

Interactions Concurrent use of other GABA receptor agonists brings a risk of over-sedation.

Drugs used to treat Parkinson's disease

Most of these act to improve motor symptoms by increasing dopaminergic activity in the brain. They are described on pages 317 in Chapter 9.

Neuromuscular junction transmission enhancers

Symptomatic therapy for neuromuscular junction weakness uses pyridostigmine. This acetylcholinesterase inhibitor prolongs the action of acetylcholine at the neuromuscular junction.

Pyridostigmine

This is the acetylcholinesterase inhibitor of choice for the treatment of myasthenia gravis. Neostigmine, a subcutaneous acetylcholinesterase inhibitor, is rarely used because of its high potency and potential for causing significant bradycardia.

Mode of action Pyridostigmine inhibits the action of acetylcholinesterase at synapses. In this way, it prolongs the action of released acetylcholine and therefore muscle contraction.

Indications Pyridostigmine is used in myasthenia gravis as a standard symptomatic therapy.

Adverse effects The signal boost also occurs at non-motor synapses. Therefore pyridostigmine causes predictable, dose-dependent adverse effects at autonomic nerve terminals. These effects include nausea, abdominal pain, diarrhoea, salivation, urinary frequency and bradycardia.

Interactions Pyridostigmine has few direct clinically significant interactions. However, patients with myasthenia gravis are sensitive to the effects of many drugs on the neuromuscular junction, so great care needs to be taken when starting them on any new medication.

Drugs used to treat neurodegenerative dementia

Centrally acting acetylcholinesterase inhibitors and the glutamate receptor antagonist memantine can slow progression at different stages of Alzheimer's disease. In the past, there was a history of prescribing atypical antipsychotic drugs for behavioural problems in patients with dementia. However, this practice is associated with a high incidence of severe adverse effects in older people, including stroke and death. Therefore, in the UK, only risperidone is licensed for use in patients with Alzheimer's disease, and this is restricted to short-term treatment in specific circumstances.

Acetylcholinesterase inhibitors

Loss of widely projecting cholinergic neurons is central to the early pathology of Alzheimer's disease. Drugs which stop the breakdown of acetylcholine by inhibiting the enzyme which degrades it, acetylcholinesterase, have been shown to slow the progression of some aspects of Alzheimer's disease.

Mode of action Donepezil, galantamine and rivastigmine are reversible inhibitors of acetylcholinesterase that are active in the central nervous system. They enhance the disrupted cholinergic transmission which is a core part of the neurodegenerative pathogenesis in Alzheimer's disease.

Indications Donepezil, galantamine and rivastigmine are used to treat mild to moderate Alzheimer's disease. Rivastigmine is also used in mild to moderate dementia associated with Parkinson's disease.

> Patients on **acetylcholinesterase inhibitors for dementia** require regular cognitive assessments to help judge whether they are benefitting from these drugs.

Adverse effects Gastrointestinal disturbances are the most common adverse effects of acetylcholinesterase inhibitors.

Interactions Galantamine plasma concentration is increased by various antibiotics, including erythromycin.

Memantine

Memantine inhibits glutamate signaling at NMDA receptors. Its use in dementia is controversial due to a lack of very clear benefit in clinical trials. Nonetheless there is some evidence that it is beneficial in some stages of Alzheimer's disease.

Mode of action Memantine is a noncompetitive glutamate receptor antagonist that decreases N-methyl-D-aspartic acid (NMDA) receptor–related calcium influx, and thereby reduces neuronal toxicity from calcium accumulation.

Indications Memantine is indicated in cases of moderate to severe Alzheimer's disease in which acetylcholinesterase inhibitors are contraindicated or not tolerated.

Adverse effects Confusion, dizziness, drowsiness and hallucinations occur in a small minority of patients (< 5%).

Interactions Memantine should not be used with ketamine (which is occasionally used for anaesthesia), because of the risk of central nervous system toxicity.

Antiepileptic medications

The aim of drug therapy is to render patients seizure-free without any adverse effects.

This often cannot be fully achieved, but what is attained is minimal seizures with minimal adverse effects. A range of antiepileptic drugs are available, but information on their relative efficacy is limited.

Levetiracetam

Levetiracetam is a relatively new anti-epileptic drug that has jumped to the forefront of epilepsy drug treatment. It has many of the characteristics of the ideal anti-epileptic drug: rapid onset of action; minimal drug interactions; minimal teratogenicity; minimal side effects and efficacy in a range of seizure types.

Mode of action Levetiracetam binds to presynaptic calcium channels to inhibit neurotransmitter release at central nervous system synapses.

Indications Levetiracetam is used as monotherapy or add-on therapy in all types of partial onset seizures.

Adverse effects Confusion and sedation are the commonest adverse effects and tend to be minor. Rarely, levetiracetam worsens severe depression.

Interactions No significant drug interactions are known.

> **Levetiracetam is commonly used to treat seizures in very ill hospital patients.** This is because it has no drug interactions, can be given intravenously and is rapidly effective.

Sodium valproate

Sodium valproate is very effective in controlling many types of seizures. Unfortunately the relatively high risk of teratogenicity limits its use in women of childbearing age. It also has dangerous interactions with other commonly used drugs.

Mode of action The main action of sodium valproate is inhibition of sodium channels.

Indications It is used to treat partial onset or primary generalised seizures.

Adverse effects Teratogenicity is commoner with sodium valproate than with most other antiepileptic drugs; it is associated with a risk of birth defects of up to 10%. Therefore sodium valproate is usually avoided in women of childbearing age. Nausea is common, and the drug can rarely cause liver dysfunction.

> **Young women starting sodium valproate** must be informed of the risks of it causing birth defects.

Interactions Carbapenems significantly reduce the level of valproate, so they should be avoided. Carbamazepine, another antiepileptic drug, also reduces the level of valproate. Valproate increases the levels of carbamazepine active metabolites.

Phenytoin

Phenytoin is now rarely used as a long-term anti-epileptic drug in developed countries because of the need for drug level monitoring, the high incidence of side effects and the availability of newer drugs. Nevertheless it is still frequently used for short periods in status epilepticus where it is very effective.

Mode of action Phenytoin is a sodium channel blocker.

Indications Phenytoin is not commonly used for long-term treatment, because of its adverse effect profile. It is effective in cases of partial onset and primary generalised seizures other than absence seizures. Phenytoin is used in the treatment of status epilepticus. It can be used in pregnancy, if essential, but carries a risk of fetal developmental problems.

> **Phenytoin is used as part of the acute treatment of status epilepticus, despite having a number of adverse effects when used long term.** It can be given intravenously and has rapid onset of action.

Adverse effects Bradycardia can rarely occur during intravenous infusion. Leucopenia can also occur with long-term use. Drowsiness is common, and there is a narrow therapeutic index that requires blood monitoring. Long-term use can cause coarsening of facial features, gingival hypertrophy, acne and hirsutism.

Interactions Phenytoin interacts with many antibiotics, including clarithromycin, ciprofloxacin and trimethoprim, as well as many other drugs.

Drugs used to treat headache

Headache is discussed in detail in Chapter 4, and Table 4.4 summarises commonly used migraine therapies. The common first-line therapies for acute migraine attacks and for prophylactic treatment include the following.

Simple analgesics: aspirin, paracetamol (acetaminophen) and non-steroidal anti-inflammatory drugs

Simple analgesics are often effective treatments for migraine, especially in their dispersible form. They have relatively few side effects or drug interactions.

Mode of action Aspirin, paracetamol (acetaminophen) and other non-steroidal anti-inflammatory drugs (NSAIDs) probably all act through inhibition of vasoactive substances such as prostaglandin.

Indications Simple analgesics are used as first-line therapy for any migraine.

Adverse effects Aspirin and NSAIDs can cause gastrointestinal disturbance, such as dyspepsia or ulceration. Asthma can be exacerbated by NSAIDs.

> **Aspirin is frequently used to treat migraine in pregnant women.**
> However, it should be avoided closer to labour, because it increases the risk of significant bleeding.

Interactions Aspirin and NSAIDs increase the risk of gastrointestinal bleeding when used with other antiplatelet or anticoagulant agents.

Triptans

This class of drug is used as a second line treatment for migraine or in cluster headache.

Mode of action Triptans act as agonists at 5-HT$_1$ receptors and modulate central pain pathways activated in migraine.

Indications Triptans are used to treat acute migraine attacks that do not respond to simple analgesics. They are also effective in cluster headache.

Adverse effects Triptans cause a degree of vasospasm and should be avoided in patients with coronary artery disease or uncontrolled hypertension.

> **Patients often respond to an alternative triptan if the first one tried does not work.** Triptans can be very effective, so a few types are usually tried.

Interactions Monoamine oxidase inhibitors reduce the breakdown of triptans and should be avoided.

Beta-blockers (e.g. propranolol)

Beta-blockers are a commonly used and effective drug for preventing migraine.

Mode of action Beta-blockers modulate the adrenergic nervous system and cranial and extracranial blood flow.

Indications They are a preventive treatment for frequent, disabling migraine attacks.

Adverse effects Hypotension, bradycardia, vivid dreams and lethargy are common adverse effects. They can limit the dose used or necessitate switching to an alternative preventive therapy.

> With all **preventive therapies**, it is crucial to start at low doses and increase slowly to minimise adverse effects.

Interactions Other antihypertensive agents exacerbate the hypotensive effect of beta-blockers.

Amitriptyline

Amitriptyline is widely known for its use as an anti-depressant but it is also widely used for neuropathic pain and migraine.

Mode of action Amitriptyline inhibits abnormal cortical activity and other central pathways activated in migraine.

Indications It is used as preventive treatment for frequent, disabling migraine attacks.

Adverse effects
Sedation, dry mouth and weight gain are common adverse effects.

> **Preventive therapies for migraine** may take 3–6 months to reduce headache frequency or severity.

Interactions Combining amitriptyline with serotoninergic drugs increases the risk of serotonin syndrome (a very rare and life-threatening metabolic disturbance triggered by certain combinations of drugs).

Antiepileptic drugs (e.g. topiramate and valproate)

Several anti-epileptic drugs have been shown in clinical trials to reduce the frequency and severity of migraines. The precise mechanisms are not clearly understood but altering central pain pathways in the trigeminal system are likely to be involved.

Mode of action Antiepileptic drugs modulate central glutamate and GABA neurotransmitter pathways whose abnormal activation is central to the pathogenesis of migraine.

Indications These drugs are used as preventive treatment for frequent, disabling migraine attacks.

Adverse effects Sedation, poor concentration and tremor are common adverse effects for several antiepileptic drugs. Topiramate reduces appetite and predisposes to renal calculi, whereas valproate promotes weight gain.

Interactions Antiepileptic drugs have a wide range of interactions. These are reviewed before any individual patient starts such therapy.

Verapamil

Verapamil is used in patients with cluster headache who do not respond to triptans. The exact mechanisms of action in cluster headache are not understood.

Mode of action Verapamil blocks voltage-gated calcium channels and alters cerebral vascular tone.

Indications It is used as preventive treatment for frequent cluster headache.

Adverse effects Flushing, dizziness and fatigue are common.

Interactions Combining beta-blockers and verapamil can lead to severe bradycardia. Erythromycin levels are increased by verapamil.

Neurosurgery

Many risks are associated with neurosurgical procedures, including intracranial infection, haemorrhage and direct neurological injury from damage to nervous tissue. Recovery of neurological function after a major procedure such as a craniectomy is a prolonged process and never guaranteed.

Generally, the older the patients and the greater their medical co-morbidities, the less likely they are to survive a neurosurgical procedure. There comes a point at which there is no reasonable possibility of surviving such a procedure and it should not be attempted, even if the patient is dying.

Patients on blood-thinning medications, for example warfarin, aspirin and clopidogrel, need their coagulation function normalised before surgery to reduce the risk of bleeding. This can be achieved by waiting for the drugs to clear from the system or, particularly in emergency surgery, by infusion of blood products.

Common neurosurgical techniques

The following techniques are commonly used on their own or as part of more complex surgeries.

Burr holes

These are small holes drilled through the skull. They are used:

- as a therapeutic procedure (e.g. to allow direct drainage of a localised extradural haematoma)
- as part of other procedures (e.g. to insert an extraventricular drain)
- as a way to remove a section of skull by connecting a series of burr holes to allow further work

Drilling a burr hole is a relatively minor neurosurgical procedure. However, it is not undertaken lightly, because of potentially fatal complications such as haemorrhage or infection.

Craniotomy and craniectomy

In a craniotomy, a portion of the skull is removed to allow access for a procedure, such as evacuation of a haematoma or removal of a tumour. The portion is then replaced.

In craniectomy, part of the skull is removed and the skin subsequently closed without replacing the skull at that time; it is performed with the aim of decompressing the brain in situations of intractable intracranial pressure (ICP) elevation when other medical measures of ICP control have been exceeded (e.g. severe traumatic brain injury, malignant cerebral oedema following a large stroke). Craniectomy is generally a more invasive and traumatic procedure than craniotomy, requiring a more protracted recovery with potentially more complications. It can be a primary therapeutic procedure in itself, as in the decompression example, or a prelude to gaining access to the brain parenchyma for other procedures, such as open biopsy, open mass lesion resection and lobectomy (**Figure 2.39**).

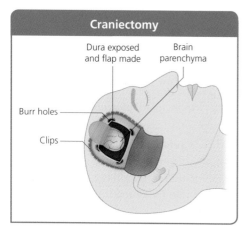

Craniectomy

Dura exposed and flap made

Brain parenchyma

Burr holes

Clips

Figure 2.39 Craniectomy. A scalp flap followed by burr holes in the skull. A portion of skull is removed and the underlying dura opened. Subdural haematomas can be removed or the underlying brain parenchyma accessed for tumour removal, vascular surgery or any other procedure.

Intracranial pressure monitoring and treatment

There are numerous clinical scenarios that may require intermittent or continuous measurement of intracranial pressure, e.g. traumatic brain injury. There are a range of techniques available to do this which vary in their invasiveness and accuracy.

Pressure monitoring

The most commonly used devices are a small 'bolt' placed under the skull through a small hole, and a small pressure transducer placed directly into the brain parenchyma. These allow continuous measurement of fluctuations in intracranial pressure to guide surgical or medical management of increased pressure.

Controlling intracranial pressure

In conditions in which the balance between cerebrospinal fluid production and removal is disrupted and leads to increased intracranial pressure, controlled removal of the fluid may be needed.

Extraventricular drains These are used in an emergency setting when a temporary method for draining cerebrospinal fluid is required to control and prevent ICP elevation, for example cases of acute hydrocephalus from an obstructed 4th ventricle, subarachnoid haemorrhage, traumatic brain injury and meningitis. A burr hole is made and a catheter inserted into part of the lateral ventricle thereby allowing external drainage of ventricular CSF.

Ventricular–peritoneal, ventricular–atrial and ventriculo-pleural shunts These are used for longer term regulation of cerebrospinal fluid drainage in hydrocephalus. A shunt tube is inserted, with one end (the 'proximal' end) in an extraventricular drain, into the ventricle and the other end (the 'distal' end) placed in the peritoneal cavity (for a ventricular–peritoneal shunt), and the rate of flow is valve-controlled. Alternatively, this end is placed in the right atrium (for a ventricular–atrial shunt) or the lung pleural cavity (for a ventricular-pleural shunt).

Stereotactic surgery

In this type of surgery, an external frame is attached to the patient and used to selectively target a particular brain region of interest, for example during biopsy of a tumour, or during targeting and insertion of electrodes for deep brain stimulation (e.g. Parkinson's disease). Advanced MRI and CT techniques are used to localise and plan the surgery.

Radiotherapy can also be targeted to specific brain regions; this is stereotactic radiotherapy. For example, in gamma knife surgery, hundreds of separate beams of low-dose gamma radiation are focused from different directions on to the target area. This minimises the radiation exposure of non-target areas.

Specific neurosurgical procedures

Two common neurosurgical procedures are described here; others are described in the appropriate chapters (e.g. for carotid endarterectomy in ischaemic stroke, and neurosurgical clipping and endovascular coiling for intracranial arterial aneurysms, see Chapter 6).

Tumour and abscess removal

Neuroimaging provides a high degree of certainty in identifying the nature of mass lesions in the central nervous system, but biopsy is usually required to differentiate tumours from abscesses. A small burr hole is made under stereotaxic guidance. The mass is usually debulked, i.e. as much of the lesion is removed as possible during the procedure. Histological analysis then confirms the nature of the lesion and guides further therapy.

Spinal decompression surgery

Neurosurgical decompression of a herniated disc, osteophyte bars or other localised structural lesions that compress the spinal cord and/or nerve roots is a common procedure. Decompression is often effective at improving pain and motor weakness, and hence mobility and quality of life, but less effective at restoring sensory loss. Patients without structural lesions on neuroimaging are unlikely to benefit from disc surgery for back or neck pain. Other procedures performed in the spine include removal of tumours, drainage of infections and fixation of fractures or spinal instability with screw fixation and implantation of metal work.

Functional neurosurgery

Deep brain stimulation is an emerging technique that uses stimulators inserted into specific brain regions to interrupt normal or pathological transmission. The technique has been most extensively and successfully used in treating the tremor of Parkinson's disease in selected patients, but it has also been used to treat neuropathic pain, dystonia, other tremor and even depression.

The patient is awake during surgery to aid in placement of the stimulator through a small burr hole, using stereotaxic and combined CT and MRI guidance.

Answers to starter questions

1. Most people find neurological symptoms such as numbness, tingling, visual loss, fortification spectra and weakness terrifying. Even transient symptoms can cause a great deal of anxiety, because people often worry that they have a serious and possibly life-threatening illness.

2. With enough time, a condition will declare itself by the pattern of fluctuation, progression and symptoms. The history is a retrospective analysis of how the disease has behaved, and it gives the most clues to the underlying problem.

3. In many neurological consultations, an examination will not help establish a diagnosis. For example, an examination will add no useful information in the case of new onset epilepsy with no serious underlying cause. A differential diagnosis is often reached from the history alone, with little possibility of the examination altering it. However, an examination is always carried out in order to be thorough and to reassure the patient that they have received a complete assessment.

4. As access to neuroimaging has improved and the techniques have become more refined, the need to correlate subtle abnormalities detected on scans with any examination findings has become more important, not less, because not every abnormality on a scan is relevant. Imaging is always used as a supportive tool rather than an exclusively diagnostic one.

Answers *continued*

5. There is no such thing as a complete neurological examination. For each individual patient, the extent of the examination is determined by the history and differential diagnosis, as well as by the clinician's knowledge of what is likely to be found, and what is useful to find, on examination. Knowing what to examine and what to leave out is a key clinical skill that comes only with experience.

6. Practice, practice, practice! Performing the neurological examination routine over and over until it is second nature allows the clinician to focus not on 'what to do next' but on 'what do these signs mean?' Stroke wards and general medical wards are good places to review patients with neurological signs.

7. For some patients, having neurological investigations reassures them that they are being taken seriously and assessed thoroughly. For others, it provokes fear and anxiety because they interpret the need for investigation as a sign that they have a significant illness. Always let the patient know why you are carrying out particular tests.

8. Most neurological tests are not 100% sensitive or specific. This can cause more confusion than clarity if a test is requested unnecessarily, or commit a patient to more invasive investigations if unexpected results are found. If a particular test is to help in management, its results should answer a clear and specific question.

9. Some neurological conditions are ultimately fatal, and for many patients treatment is supportive rather than curative. However, many conditions are curable, and specific therapeutic options are available. Examples are monoclonal antibody therapy for multiple sclerosis, and deep brain stimulation for Parkinson's disease.

10. Neurones in the central nervous system have limited ability to regenerate. If treatments could enable major regeneration of brain tissue, then recovery from many conditions would be radically transformed. Fixed brain injuries such as trauma and stroke would benefit from having new neuronal tissue to use for recovery, and neurodegenerative processes such as those in Parkinson's disease and motor neurone disease could be halted or reversed.

Chapter 3
Increased intracranial pressure and traumatic brain injury

Starter questions

Answers to the following questions are on page 207.

1. Can the body prevent increased intracranial pressure (ICP)?
2. Why can infants and the elderly tolerate potentially high ICP for longer?
3. Can steroids be used to control ICP after brain trauma?

Introduction

Intracranial pressure (ICP) is the pressure inside the skull, i.e. the pressure of the brain, cerebral blood and cerebrospinal fluid. It is measured in millimetres of mercury (mmHg). Clinical features of raised ICP are significant in many neurological and neurosurgical presentations.

Traumatic brain injury is a leading cause of death and disability. If the injury is severe, only 30% of patients make a 'good recovery', i.e. they have minor neurological deficits but can resume a normal life. Most of the other 70% never return to their previous lifestyle or occupation. Primary prevention of traumatic brain injury focuses on enforcement of road traffic safety legislation, such as that related to speed limits and the use of seatbelts and motorcycle helmets.

Case 1 Headache and vomiting

Presentation

Bill Jameson, aged 74 years, presents to the emergency department. His son states that 'he hasn't been right' since falling down the steps and hitting his head 4 weeks ago.

Initial interpretation

The history suggests a head injury. The cause needs to be ascertained, and Mr Jameson assessed for complications of a head injury (**Table 3.1**).

History

Mr Jameson has difficulty expressing his thoughts (expressive dysphasia), but he understands commands. His son clarifies his statements. Mr Jameson slipped on his socks while dressing. Immediately after the fall, he felt well; he neither lost consciousness nor vomited. He did not have any seizures, weakness or neurological deficit. He had no leakage of fluid from his nose or ear, and no external signs of injury.

About 3 weeks after the fall, Mr Jameson started to complain of headaches. These were worse in the morning; on waking, he felt nauseous and vomited occasionally. He also started stumbling in the past week.

In the past 3 days, his right arm and leg have not moved, and his ability to communicate through speech has decreased. Initially, he was just slow to find the right word, but in the past 24 h he has had real difficulty speaking.

Interpretation of history

The initial history suggests that the fall was mechanical and unrelated to an underlying pathology. Mr Jameson's immediate neurological status was good, with no features to suggest an immediate intracranial bleed.

Headache associated with nausea and vomiting strongly suggests increased ICP. Speech difficulties and weakness on the

Taking a history of head injury	
Category	History sought
Mechanism of injury	Does the mechanism (e.g. simple fall, assault and road traffic accident) suggest severity of trauma and likelihood of major traumatic brain injury?
Neurological status at scene of injury	Does patient have an altered level of consciousness (e.g. determined by Glasgow coma scale score)?
	Immediate neurological deficits?
	Signs of an 'open' skull fracture?
Presence of neurological complications	Nausea and vomiting (a feature of increased intracranial pressure)?
	Seizures or signs of basal skull fracture?
	Symptoms of memory loss?
Management to date	Was patient taken to hospital?
	Was brain imaging done?
	What management was instituted?
Current status	What are the neurological complications or deficits?
Drug and social history	Does patient drink alcohol or take blood-thinning medications? (These increase risk of an intracranial bleed)

Table 3.1 Key aspects of the history after a traumatic head injury

Case 1 *continued*

right side over the past week, i.e. nearly 3 weeks after falling, also suggest an intracranial lesion (see page 43).

Symptoms evolving over days to weeks suggest a chronic cause for the focal neurological deficits. No obvious features of infection are present, and although tumour is possible, the main differential diagnosis to exclude is an old intracranial haemorrhage, a chronic subdural haematoma, especially given Mr Jameson's age and traumatic head injury 4 weeks ago.

Further history

Mr Jameson takes aspirin and drinks half a bottle of wine every day. Aspirin increases the risk of intracranial haemorrhage after trauma. Regular alcohol use also increases the likelihood of intracranial haemorrhage, because the resultant brain atrophy stretches subdural veins, thereby increasing their propensity to rupture.

> **Intracranial haemorrhage must be suspected in any patient who has sustained a traumatic head injury and who takes blood-thinning medication**, such as aspirin, clopidogrel and especially warfarin. These drugs are commonly prescribed for the elderly but significantly increase the risk of intracranial haemorrhage.

Examination

Mr Jameson's eyes are open spontaneously. He obeys commands but makes only sounds, not words; he is unable to verbalise. He has severe right-sided weakness, along with brisk reflexes in his arms and legs. Fundoscopy reveals mild papilloedema (**Figure 3.1**).

Interpretation of findings

Mr Jameson's Glasgow coma scale score is E4 (eyes open spontaneously) V2

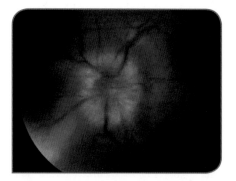

Figure 3.1 Papilloedema, a swollen optic disc, seen on fundoscopy. The disc margins are blurred and the vessels distorted.

(verbal response: incomprehensible sounds) M6 (motor response: obeys commands), giving a total of 12/15) (see page 453). He has expressive dysphasia and right-sided motor symptoms, which suggest an intracranial lesion affecting the left side of his brain. Headache, nausea and/or vomiting and papilloedema are the three cardinal features of increased ICP.

Mr Jameson requires an urgent computerised tomography (CT) scan of his head. His coagulation variables and liver function need to be checked, and his platelets cross-matched in case surgery is required.

Investigations

The CT scan shows a large left-sided collection that is darker (hypodense) than the surrounding brain (**Figure 3.2**). The fluid collection is pushing the brain from left to right. The left lateral ventricle appears smaller than the right and is pushed more towards the midline. The radiologist reports a left-sided chronic subdural haemorrhage.

Diagnosis

The neurosurgical team is consulted and decides that urgent surgical evacuation of the bleed is required. Platelets are

Case 1 *continued*

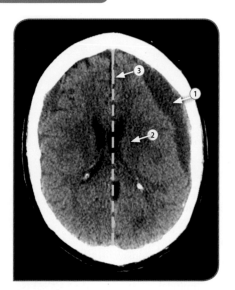

infused immediately to reverse the effects of aspirin, and burr hole evacuation of the chronic subdural haematoma is carried out: two 2 cm holes are made in the skull, the dura is opened and the blood washed out. The fluid was under high pressure and came out spontaneously. Saline was then flushed into the burr holes until clear fluid came out. The emergence of clear fluid confirms removal of all blood breakdown products.

Mr Jameson recovers rapidly; he can walk after 3 days and is discharged. At his 8-week review, he is well, with no headaches.

Figure 3.2 Axial computerised tomography scan showing left-sided chronic subdural haematoma ① with crescent-shaped hypodense appearance. The posterior aspect of the left lateral ventricle is compressed and starting to become effaced ② and midline shift from left to right ③ indicate increased intracranial pressure and mass effect.

Increased intracranial pressure

Intracranial pressure is the pressure in the skull cavity (see page 39). Cerebral perfusion pressure is the pressure gradient driving cerebral blood flow, which provides oxygen and nutrients to the brain and removes waste products from it.

At a fixed blood pressure, a rise in ICP will decrease cerebral perfusion pressure. Therefore an uncontrolled increase in ICP must be prevented to preserve the brain's blood supply, driven by cerebral perfusion pressure, and thus brain function.

Aetiology

Increased ICP is caused by an uncompensated increase in volume of any of the three components of volume in the intracranial cavity:

- the brain (V_{brain})
- cerebral blood (V_{blood})
- cerebrospinal fluid (V_{CSF})

Causes of increased ICP are listed in **Table 3.2.**

Brain compliance is the ability of the brain to tolerate additional intracranial volumes without significant increase in ICP. ICP increases once compliance has been exhausted.

Cerebrospinal fluid is the key component in the mechanism to compensate for additional intracranial volume to prevent raised ICP. Intracranial cerebrospinal fluid is squeezed out into the lumbar cistern to reduce V_{CSF} Once the maximum volume of cerebrospinal fluid that can be expelled has been removed, ICP starts to increase exponentially (**Figure 3.3**).

Causes of increased intracranial pressure	
Aetiology	Examples
Increase in brain volume (V_{brain})	Tumours (e.g. metastases and primary brain tumours)
	Infection (e.g. cerebral abscess)
	Cerebral oedema (e.g. after stroke or ischaemic injury, trauma, infection, hydrocephalus and status epilepticus)
Increase in cerebral blood volume (V_{blood})	Intracranial haemorrhage (e.g. acute or chronic subdural haematoma, extradural haematoma, intracerebral haemorrhage, subarachnoid haemorrhage and intraventricular haemorrhage)
	Obstruction to venous outflow (e.g. cerebral venous thrombosis, including sinus thrombosis)
Increase in cerebrospinal fluid (V_{CSF})s	Hydrocephalus (e.g. communicating or non-communicating obstructive hydrocephalus)
	Increased CSF production (e.g. tumours of ventricular choroid plexus; these are very rare!)
	Impaired CSF drainage as a result of obstruction of arachnoid granulations (e.g. after meningitis or subarachnoid haemorrhage)
	Idiopathic intracranial hypertension

CSF, cerebrospinal fluid.

Table 3.2 Causes of increased intracranial pressure

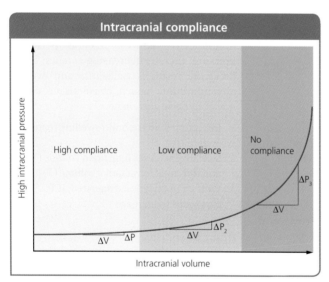

Figure 3.3 The intracranial pressure (ICP)–volume curve shows compliance and compensation in the brain. The change in volume (ΔV) initially causes very little, if any, change in pressure (ΔP). As compliance decreases, ΔP_2 per ΔV steadily increases. When no further compliance (i.e. buffering capacity) is available, for the same ΔV, the ΔP_3 is significantly higher and starts to increase exponentially.

Normal ICP is suggested on imaging **(Figure 3.4)** by the absence of midline shift, normal cerebrospinal fluid spaces (sulci and open basal cisterns) and normal differentiation between grey and white matter.

Age

Buffering capacity varies greatly between patients and by age. During ageing, the brain shrinks (cortical atrophy), so V_{brain} decreases and more space, filled with cerebrospinal fluid, becomes available inside the skull. Therefore elderly patients can tolerate larger

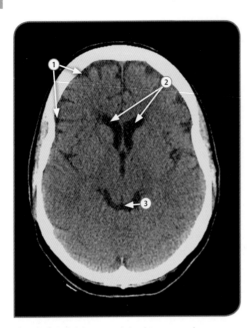

Figure 3.4 Axial computerised tomography scan of a brain at the level of the lateral ventricles. (1) The cerebrospinal fluid spaces surrounding the sulci and gyri are clearly visible and the sulci and gyri, as a result, also appear visible. (2) Lateral ventricles visible and not compressed. (3) Basal cisterns are open with cerebrospinal fluid visible.

pathological lesions, such as traumatic haemorrhage, than young patients can.

Cerebral blood flow

Maintenance of constant cerebral perfusion (see page 38) is critical for normal brain function. Normal cerebral blood flow is 50 mL/100 g of brain tissue/min; cerebral blood flow <23 mL/100 g causes reversible neurological deficits, and irreversible brain tissue death occurs if it decreases to <8 mL/100 g. Cerebral blood flow depends on cerebral perfusion pressure, which in turn depends on mean arterial pressure and ICP.

The mean arterial pressure (MAP) is the average arterial blood pressure in a single cardiac cycle. It is calculated from the systolic and diastolic blood pressures (SBP and DBP):

$$MAP = DBP + \tfrac{1}{3}\,(SBP - DBP)$$

Mean arterial pressure is used to calculate cerebral perfusion pressure (CPP):

$$CPP = MAP - ICP$$

Normal ranges of these values are as follows.

- Systolic blood pressure/diastolic blood pressure = 120/80 mmHg
- Mean arterial pressure: ~93 mmHg
- ICP = 8–12 mmHg
- Cerebral perfusion pressure = 80–85 mmHg

Clinical features

The symptoms and signs of increased ICP depend on the amount of compensation available, i.e. the degree of brain compliance, and how quickly ICP increases.
The classic features of increased ICP are:

- headache
- nausea and/or vomiting
- altered level of consciousness
- papilloedema

Acutely increased ICP may present as one of the brain herniation syndromes (**Table 3.3**).

Complications of intractable increases in ICP

Excessive ICP that continues to increase dramatically reduces cerebral perfusion pressure, thereby decreasing cerebral blood flow. The result is ischaemia and eventually infarction, which cause tissue death. A vicious cycle can ensue.

1. Infarction leads to brain swelling (cerebral oedema)
2. Swelling increases total brain volume (V_{brain}) and thus total intracranial volume (V_{total})
3. With compensation exhausted, ICP continues to increase

Brain herniation

The intracranial space is divided into compartments by folds of the dural layer of the meninges (see page 27). The skull is a closed box, so intractable increases in ICP cause parts of brain to shift between compartments (i.e. herniation; **Figure 3.5**). Vital structures can become compressed against the bone or tough dura mater, leading to life-threatening neurological deficits (**Table 3.3**).

Brain herniation syndromes

Description of herniation	Critical brain structures compressed	Complications and features
Cingulate: medial part of frontal lobe (cingulate gyrus) passes under falx cerebri to opposite side	Anterior cerebral artery	Hemiparesis
	Frontal horn of lateral ventricle	
Tentorial (uncal): medial part of temporal lobe (uncus) passes through tentorial incisura	Midbrain structures	Depends on compression
	Ipsilateral cranial nerve III	Ipsilateral fixed, dilated pupil
	Ipsilateral cerebral peduncle	Contralateral hemiparesis
	Reticular activating formation	Reduced level of consciousness
	Ipsilateral posterior cerebral artery	Blindness caused by occipital lobe infarction
Central: diencephalic structures (e.g. thalamus) through tentorial incisura	Midbrain vertical gaze centre	Loss of vertical up-gaze
	Hypothalamic sympathetic pathways	Bilateral fixed and small pupils
	Cardiorespiratory centres	Abnormal respiratory patterns, Cushing's reflex and cardiac arrest
Tonsillar: cerebellar tonsils pass through foramen magnum and compress lower brain stem	Medulla	Depends on structures
	Cardiorespiratory centres	Abnormal respiratory patterns, Cushing's reflex and cardiac arrest

Table 3.3 Features of the major brain herniation syndromes

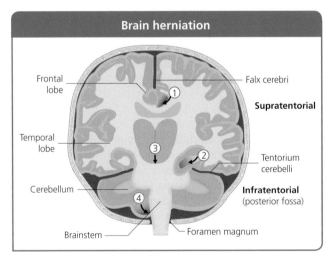

Brain herniation

Frontal lobe — Falx cerebri

Supratentorial

Temporal lobe

Tentorium cerebelli

Cerebellum — **Infratentorial** (posterior fossa)

Brainstem — Foramen magnum

Figure 3.5 Sites of brain herniation. In cingulate (or sub-falcine) herniation ①, the right or left side of the brain moves under the falx to the opposite side. In tentorial (uncal) herniation ②, the uncus (the most medial aspect of the temporal lobe) moves through the tentorial incisura (the hole in the tentorium) to the infratentorial compartment. In central herniation ③, parts of the diencephalon (e.g. thalamus) move down through the tentorial incisura from supra- to infratentorial. Tonsillar herniation (true coning) ④ occurs when the cerebellar tonsils pass through the foramen magnum and crush the lower brain stem and its cardiac and respiratory centres.

Diagnostic approach

Any patient with features of increased ICP requires an urgent brain CT. MRI may also be required. A check for papilloedema and evaluation of visual acuity are essential.

Investigations

Investigation is designed to evaluate the severity of increased intracranial pressure and elucidate the cause. The safest first investigation is a CT scan to rule out a space occupying lesion.

> **Cushing's reflex results from compression of the cardiorespiratory centres in the medulla (see page 60). This effect causes Cushing's triad:**
>
> - hypertension
> - bradycardia
> - abnormal respirations
>
> Cushing's triad indicates severely increased ICP, tonsillar herniation and an imminent risk of cardiorespiratory arrest. Patients require urgent resuscitation, stabilisation of their condition and immediate imaging to find the cause.

Imaging

Imaging features of increased ICP include the following (**Figure 3.6**):

- midline shift
- loss of normal cerebrospinal fluid spaces (e.g. closed basal cisterns)

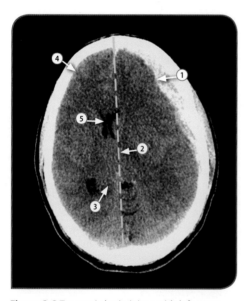

Figure 3.6 Traumatic brain injury with left acute subdural haematoma ①. The clot is hyperdense (i.e. white) and crescent-shaped, and extends over the cerebral hemisphere because the suture lines of the inner surface of the skull do not limit it. Features of increased intracranial pressure include midline shift ②, obliteration of basal cisterns ③, lack of cortical sulci ④ and effaced and partially compressed ventricles ⑤.

- change in ventricle size (e.g. either enlarged from hydrocephalus or collapsed or effaced because of brain swelling)
- loss of normal differentiation between grey and white matter

> **Lumbar puncture** is contraindicated in any patient with features of increased ICP until imaging has excluded a space-occupying lesion. This is because of the risk of cerebral herniation in the presence of a mass lesion.

Management

The management of increased ICP depends on aetiology. Definitive intervention is treatment of the cause, such as removal of a tumour. Initial management can include artificial ventilation and medications to temporarily limit ICP increases.

Artificial ventilation

Both carbon dioxide (CO_2) and oxygen (O_2) affect cerebral blood flow and volume by changing blood vessel diameter. Increased CO_2 and decreased O_2 cause cerebral dilation, and therefore increase both cerebral blood flow and cerebral blood volume. This increases O_2 supply and CO_2 removal. However, it also increases V_{blood} and thus V_{total} and, importantly, ICP. This can lead to a vicious circle if ICP is already high.

Patients with increased ICP resulting from acute brain injury are not allowed to reduce their respiration, i.e. to hypoventilate, because the resulting decrease in O_2 and increase in CO_2 would further increase ICP.

In life-threatening increased ICP with signs of brain herniation (see page 193), the patient is placed on an artificial ventilator with a short period of excessive ventilation (hyperventilation) to decrease CO_2 level, i.e. to 'blow off' CO_2. This treatment causes cerebral blood vessels to constrict, thereby reducing cerebral blood flow, cerebral blood volume, V_{blood} and V_{total}, and therefore ICP. This is a temporary treatment, because it can eventually cause ischaemia and infarction if prolonged.

Medication

Corticosteroids reduce cerebral oedema associated with tumours. Mannitol, an osmotic diuretic, causes the absorption of fluid from the central nervous system; the fluid is then excreted by the kidneys.

No medication should be started without discussion with a neurosurgeon, neurological intensive care physician or neurologist, because of possible contraindications. For example, corticosteroids are contraindicated in traumatic brain injury, because they increase mortality and worsen outcome.

Surgery

The aim of surgical treatment is to decrease ICP by removing the additional volume from the underlying pathology, and thus reduce intracranial volume. For example, removal of a tumour reduces additional V_{brain}, and removal of a haematoma reduces additional V_{blood}.

A decompressive craniectomy is surgery in which a piece of skull is removed to create space (Figure 3.7). The operation is associated with considerable morbidity and is used only in life-threatening circumstances.

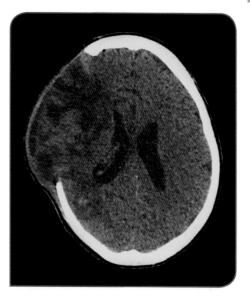

Figure 3.7 Axial computerised tomography scan showing a decompressive craniectomy, a treatment for intractable increases in intracranial pressure. A bone of the skull has been removed to increase the available intracranial volume and convert the closed box to an open one.

Traumatic brain injury

Traumatic brain injury is classified by mechanism, site and severity of injury (**Table 3.4**). Additional injuries to the spine, spinal cord and other systems are investigated and managed appropriately.

Concussion is an alteration of consciousness without any structural damage to the brain after a blunt traumatic brain injury. The condition may include amnesia, confusion and loss of consciousness. Over 75% of cases of traumatic brain injury presenting to emergency departments are concussions or other forms of mild traumatic brain injury.

Epidemiology

In the UK, 1500 per 100,000 people attend emergency departments annually with head injuries. Of these, 300 require hospital admission and 15 require admission to specialist neurosurgical units.

Aetiology

Road traffic accidents are the leading cause of traumatic brain injury, followed by falls and assaults.

Pathogenesis

Traumatic brain injuries can be classed as:

Traumatic brain injury: classification		
Major category	Subcategory	Example(s)
Mechanism of injury	Blunt	Impact of moving head against static surface (e.g. ground) or static head struck by moving object (e.g. hammer)
	Penetrating	Gunshot wound
	Acceleration–deceleration	Diffuse brain injury after road traffic accident
Site of injury	Skull	Base-of-skull fracture (e.g. anterior, middle or posterior fossa)
	Brain	Extra-axial lesion: extradural, acute or chronic subdural haemorrhage
		Intra-axial lesions: contusion, intracerebral haemorrhage, diffuse axonal injury and cerebral oedema
Severity of injury, based on Glasgow coma scale score at presentation	Mild	Score of 14–15
	Moderate	Score of 9–13
	Severe	Score of 3–8

Table 3.4 Classification schemes for traumatic brain injury

- primary injuries occurring at the time of trauma
- secondary injuries that evolve after the initial trauma (**Figure 3.8**)

Primary brain injury

This type of injury includes:

- injury to the scalp, skull and blood vessels inside or outside the dura, with subsequent extra-axial (i.e. extradural or subdural) haemorrhage
- injury to the brain, with intra-axial haemorrhage and complications (e.g. contusion, intracerebral haemorrhage and intraventricular haemorrhage with hydrocephalus)
- brain deformation and shearing caused by rotational acceleration–deceleration forces, leading to diffuse axonal injury

Secondary brain injury

This develops after the initial injury. It includes cerebral oedema, impaired cerebral blood flow and cell damage. Risk factors that should be identified to prevent or limit secondary brain injury include:

- increased ICP
- hypoxia (reduced oxygenation)
- hypovolaemia (reduced blood volume and blood pressure)
- hypercapnia (increased CO_2)
- seizures
- hydrocephalus
- metabolic abnormalities (e.g. of glucose and sodium)
- pyrexia (high temperature)

Clinical features

Patients with a traumatic brain injury often have an altered level of consciousness. This is assessed using the Glasgow coma scale; the score is used to categorise injury severity. Patients may also have focal neurological deficits or present with seizures. Meticulous assessment is essential (**Table 3.5**), and includes checking for skull base factures (**Table 3.6**). Signs of a skull base fracture include 'raccoon eyes' (see Figure 2.6) and Battle's sign (see Figure 2.9). Raccoon eyes occur as meningeal tearing (usually due to an anterior cranial fossa fracture) allows venous sinus bleeding (ecchymosis) into cranial sinuses and periorbital soft tissue. Battle's sign is ecchymosis visible as mastoidal bruising, due to fracture of the middle cranial fossa.

Diagnostic approach

All patients who have experienced major trauma, including isolated traumatic brain injury, are initially assessed, resuscitated and

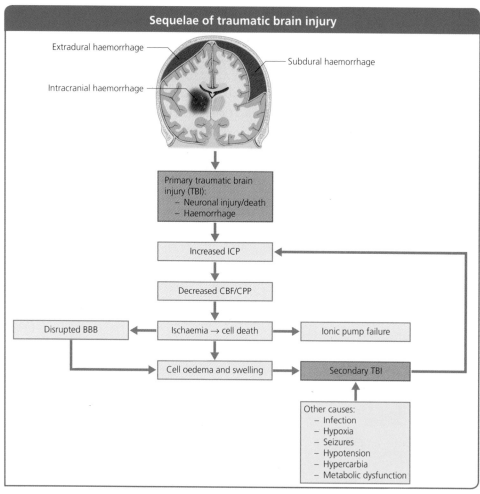

Figure 3.8 Sequelae of traumatic brain injury. BBB, blood-brain barrier; CBF, cerebral blood flow; CPP, cerebral perfusion pressure; ICP, intracranial pressure.

Examination of a patient with traumatic brain injury	
Site	Examination
Scalp	Look for lacerations, foreign bodies and evidence of depression of underlying skull bones
	Cover any open wounds with antiseptic-soaked dressing
	Identify any bleeding from the scalp, and control it with pressure
Skull	Assess for features of skull base fracture (see Table 3.6)
Brain	Determine level of consciousness (the patient's Glasgow coma scale score)
	Examine pupils for size and reactivity to light
	Cranial nerve assessment
	Assess peripheral neurological status (tone, power, reflexes, coordination and sensation, if possible)
Spine	Assess the whole spine (with maintenance of spinal precautions) to identify any tenderness suggesting fracture
	Do a digital rectal examination to assess for sphincter dysfunction and spinal cord injury

*In a patient with severe depression of consciousness level, it may not be possible to carry out a complete assessment; aim to be as complete as possible.

Table 3.5 Neurological examination in a patient with traumatic brain injury*

stabilised following Advanced Trauma Life Support protocols (**Table 3.7**). In the initial primary survey, this means identifying and treating life-threatening injuries affecting:

■ the airway (e.g. airway obstruction)
■ breathing (e.g. tension pneumothorax)
■ the circulatory system (e.g. cardiac tamponade)

The spine must also be stabilised, for example with a cervical collar or bilateral supporting foam blocks, to prevent aggravating any spinal injury that may be present.

Investigations

Computerised tomography imaging is the definitive way to evaluate brain and skull

Clinical features of skull base fracture	
Skull base region	Fracture feature(s)
Anterior (fossa) skull base	Subconjunctival haemorrhage
	Bilateral periorbital bruising ('panda bear eyes' or 'racoon eyes')
	Cerebrospinal fluid rhinorrhoea (leakage of cerebrospinal fluid through the nose)
	Palsy of cranial nerve I (the olfactory nerve)
Middle (fossa) skull base	Palsies of cranial nerve VII (the facial nerve) and cranial nerve VIII (the vestibulocochlear nerve)
	Bruising behind the ear (Battle's sign)
	Blood in the middle ear (haemotympanum)
	Cerebrospinal fluid otorrhoea (leakage of cerebrospinal fluid through the ear)
Posterior (fossa) skull base	Palsies of the lower cranial nerves

Table 3.6 Clinical features suggesting a skull base fracture

ATLS principles	
ATLS sequence	Description
Primary survey and primary resuscitation	ABCDE approach to resuscitate the patient and to identify and stabilise life-threatening injuries: Airway, Breathing, Circulation, Disability, Exposure*
AMPLE history	History of events surrounding the trauma and current management instituted:
	Allergies
	Medications
	Past medical history
	Last meal
	Events surrounding injury (mechanism, management, etc.)
Initial investigations	Trauma scan (CT of head, cervical spine, chest, abdomen and pelvis)
	Blood tests (full blood count, urea and electrolytes, liver function tests, arterial blood gases (to assess oxygen and carbon dioxide levels), grouping and saving of blood (to obtain blood products from the blood bank for potential use) and cross-match of blood products
Secondary survey and secondary resuscitation	Full head-to-toe assessment to identify any other systemic injuries
	Other imaging studies, if indicated (e.g. X-rays of bones)
Definitive management	Transfer to definitive management, depending on the pathology

CT, computerised tomography.

*The initial tenets of assessment in any emergency.

Table 3.7 Principles of Advanced Trauma Life Support for evaluating patients with major trauma

injuries. The results indicate urgency of treatment.

Management

Management of traumatic brain injury requires an understanding of intracranial physiology and ICP. The critical aims are to:

- rapidly resuscitate, investigate and treat after discussion with a neurosurgeon
- arrange prompt transfer to a neurosurgical unit, if indicated
- investigate and appropriately manage any associated spine and spinal cord injuries (for which there is a high risk)
- maintain cerebral perfusion pressure (a target of ≥ 65 mmHg is used in traumatic brain injury)
- control ICP (target < 20 mmHg) to prevent secondary brain injury (**Table 3.8**)
- maximise long-term recovery with neurorehabilitation

Once the patient has recovered from the initial injury, neurorehabilitation is provided by neurorehabilitation physicians, physiotherapists and occupational therapists.

Medication

Table 3.8 summarises medical options for controlling increased ICP. Corticosteroids are contraindicated in acute traumatic brain injury, because they increase mortality and worsen outcome. The role of prophylactic antibiotics to prevent infection is controversial, but they are usually used in:

- compound ('open') skull fractures
- penetrating brain injury
- breech of the dura
- gross contamination

Surgery

The surgical options for traumatic brain injury depend on the pathology, and for most patients include one or more of the following:

- elevation of depressed skull fractures
- burr hole drainage of chronic subdural haematoma

Management of ICP in traumatic brain injury		
Principle	Techniques	Mechanism
Conservative	Elevate the head end of the patient's bed to above 30°	Promotes drainage of venous blood from the brain, thereby reducing ICP
	Treat other systemic complications (e.g. infection and electrolyte disturbances)	Any systemic insult can cause secondary brain injury
Medical	Control temperature, prevent seizures and provide sedation	Decrease cerebral metabolic activity
	Keep carbon dioxide at the lower end of the normal range	Prevents increase in cerebral blood flow by vasoconstriction, thereby reducing ICP
	Infuse bolus dose of mannitol (0.5 g/kg)	Osmotic diuretic to absorb fluid from the brain, thereby decreasing intracranial volume and ICP
	Barbiturates to induce coma	Decrease cerebral metabolic activity
	Hypothermia	Decrease cerebral metabolic activity
Surgical	Evacuation of mass lesion (e.g. acute subdural haematoma)	Relieve mass effect and cause for oedema
	CSF diversion (e.g. external ventricular drain)	Removes CSF, thereby reducing ICP and increasing compliance
	Decompressive craniectomy (removal of part of the skull)	Creates space to accommodate brain oedema

CSF, cerebrospinal fluid.

Table 3.8 Approaches to management of increased intracranial pressure (ICP) in the setting of traumatic head injury

- craniotomy and evacuation of acute intracranial haemorrhage (see page 182)
- decompressive craniectomy
- repair of cerebrospinal fluid leak

Prognosis

Secondary and iatrogenic complications are common (**Table 3.9**). Acute stage management is only a small step. It is often followed by a long and challenging phase of neurological rehabilitation to enable the patient to recover as much neurological function as possible.

The decision whether or not to operate on a patient who has had a traumatic brain injury can be difficult. In cases of devastating neurological injury indicating poor outcome, for example with a poor Glasgow coma scale score and a likely Glasgow outcome score (GOS) of 2 or 3, is it better to not offer any treatment and let the patient die peacefully?

Traumatic brain injury complications	
Complication	Description
Epilepsy	Traumatic brain injury increases seizure risk, especially in severe cases and cases of depressed skull fracture and traumatic intracranial haemorrhage
Hypopituitarism	Chronic impairment of pituitary function in 20% of patients
Cognitive dysfunction	Impairment of memory, concentration and attention
Neurological deficits	Cranial nerve and motor deficits (e.g. hemiparesis)
Neuropsychiatric	Depression and mood disturbance

Table 3.9 Complications after traumatic brain injury

Extradural haematoma

An extradural haematoma is a bleed in the extradural space (outside the dura) between the dura and the inner table of the skull. It is also known as epidural haematoma.

Epidemiology

Extradural haematoma accounts for 1% of emergency head trauma admissions in the USA. Men are more likely to be affected than women, at a ratio of 4:1. The condition usually occurs in young adults.

Aetiology

The commonest cause for extradural haematoma is a skull fracture at the pterion, which can lacerate the middle meningeal artery running beneath it. This damage causes acute haemorrhage, and the blood collects in the extradural space. Other causes include dural venous sinus injury and bleeding from diploic veins in the skull after a fracture.

Clinical features

The features of evolving extradural haematoma are as follows.

1. Initial transient loss in consciousness and then recovery; this is the start of the lucid interval in most cases
2. Continued bleeding overcomes the body's ability to compensate; ICP increases, thereby worsening headache, nausea and vomiting
3. Consciousness level starts to deteriorate, with increasing drowsiness and decrease in Glasgow coma scale score; this is the end of the lucid interval
4. Eventually, features of brain herniation develop; these are most commonly tentorial (see **Table 3.3**), with ipsilateral fixed dilated pupil and contralateral hemiparesis

If untreated, extradural haematoma leads to coma, tonsillar herniation and cardiorespiratory arrest.

Diagnostic approach

A suspected extradural haematoma is a neurosurgical emergency; it indicates urgent CT of the head (**Figure 3.9**). The haemorrhage is classically:

- hyperdense (i.e. white)
- biconvex (lenticular) in shape
- limited to the suture lines of the inner surface of the skull, as a result of the attachments of the dura

Management

Extradural haematomas are evacuated immediately. Delay results in death or severe disability. If the patient is in a coma and has signs of brain herniation, urgent ICP control measures (e.g. mannitol infusion and hyperventilation) are required while they await surgery.

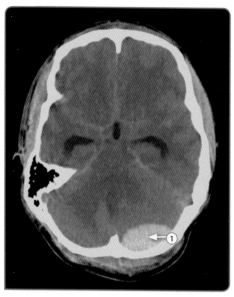

Figure 3.9 Axial computerised tomography scan of brain, showing a left-sided acute extradural haematoma overlying the left cerebellum. The clot ① is usually hyperdense (i.e. white), biconvex and lens-like in appearance. It is limited by and does not cross the suture lines of the inner surface of the skull. The commonest location of an extradural haemorrhage following trauma is usually overlying the frontotemporal region and is usually due to fracture of the pterional region of the skull with rupture of the middle meningeal artery underneath.

Acute subdural haematoma

Subdural haematomas are bleeds in the subdural space, between the dura and arachnoid (see page 27). They are classified by how long it takes before clinical signs appear after the injury, and by their appearance on CT (**Table 3.10**).

Acute subdural haematoma commonly occurs in young patients after a road traffic accident, and in elderly patients after a fall.

Aetiology

Compared with extradural haematoma, acute subdural haematoma represents more severe trauma and damage to the brain. It is most often caused by acceleration–deceleration forces during trauma; these forces cause haemorrhage by tearing bridging veins that traverse the subdural space.

Classification of subdural haematoma			
Features	Acute	Subacute	Chronic
Time from injury (days)	0–5	6–20	> 21
Appearance on CT scan	Hyperdense (i.e. white)	Isodense ('brain grey', becoming progressively darker)	Hypodense (i.e. dark black)

Table 3.10 Classification of subdural haematoma based on time from initial injury and appearance on computerised tomography (CT)

Clinical features

Most patients presenting with acute subdural haematoma are in coma. The lucid interval is less common with acute subdural haematoma than with extradural haematoma.

The following are CT features of acute subdural haematoma (see **Figure 3.6**):

■ hyperdense (i.e. white) appearance
■ crescent-shaped mass overlying the cerebral hemisphere
■ not limited by suture lines of the skull
■ may have other signs of intracranial injury (e.g. contusions and diffuse axonal injury)

Management

Evacuation of all acute subdural haematomas that are >10 mm in maximal diameter or causing >5 mm of midline shift is recommended, regardless of level of consciousness.

Post-operative ICP monitoring and control in neurointensive care is often required.

If brain oedema is anticipated, decompressive craniectomy may be carried out during the initial operation to reduce the risk of increased ICP and secondary brain injury.

Prognosis

Patients with an acute subdural haematoma that requires surgery have a 40–60% chance of survival. This compares to 90% for patients with extradural haematoma.

> **Acute subdural haematoma may occur in patients on warfarin with a history of only minor head trauma.** Anticoagulant therapy increases the risk of acute subdural haematoma 7-fold in men and 26-fold in women.

Chronic subdural haematoma

Chronic subdural haematoma is a subdural bleed that has liquefied (over weeks). It presents mainly in elderly patients. Risk factors other than older age include:

■ alcohol abuse
■ use of an anticoagulant (e.g. warfarin)
■ abnormal coagulation function
■ risk of frequent falls

Acute subdural blood is eventually broken down by an inflammatory response to produce a chronic subdural haematoma: a dark 'motor oil–like' fluid collection that does not clot. The blood breakdown products exert osmotic pressure. This attracts water, which leads to enlargement of the collection.

> **The cerebral atrophy that occurs with age stretches the delicate bridging veins that run across the subdural space from arachnoid to dura.** In an elderly person, even a minor trauma or fall can tear these veins, leading to subdural haemorrhage. However, the same atrophy means that volume increases are better tolerated.

Clinical features

Patients present with features of increased ICP with or without focal neurological deficits.

The CT appearance of chronic subdural haematoma reflects the breakdown of blood over time (see **Figure 3.2**).

■ The haematoma is hypodense (i.e. dark) compared with surrounding brain
■ It is a crescent-shaped mass overlying the cerebral hemisphere
■ Significant mass effect and midline shift may be visible

Management

Treatment is indicated if there are symptoms such as severe headache or focal neurological deficits. Correction of underlying coagulopathy, if present, is followed by surgical evacuation.

Traumatic intraparenchymal haemorrhage

Traumatic intraparenchymal haemorrhages occur in brain tissue itself (**Table 3.11**). They include haemorrhagic contusions, intracerebral haemorrhages and 'burst lobe'. They irritate brain tissue and appear as discrete areas of hyperdense (i.e. white) lesions on CT.

Clinical features

In the first couple of days, an intraparenchymal contusional haemorrhage often causes less mass effect. Later, they frequently 'blossom' and enlarge to cause a marked increase in ICP that can be fatal (**Figure 3.10**). Clinical progress correlates with this: the patient initially appears well; however, after hours or days they may suffer life-threatening neurological deterioration, such as a brain herniation syndrome.

Intraparenchymal lesions associated with traumatic brain injury	
Lesion	Description
Haemorrhagic contusion	Discrete area (1–20 mm) of bleeding
	Small ruptured parenchymal vessel surrounded by necrotic brain
	Inferior surfaces of frontal and temporal lobes, where sudden deceleration has caused brain to impact bony prominences
Intracerebral haemorrhage	Area of haemorrhage > 20 mm
	Usually frontal and temporal lobes
Burst lobe	Combination of severe haemorrhagic contusion and/or intracerebral haemorrhage, with an adjacent acute subdural haematoma

Table 3.11 Intraparenchymal lesions associated with traumatic brain injury

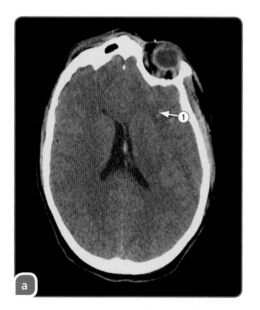

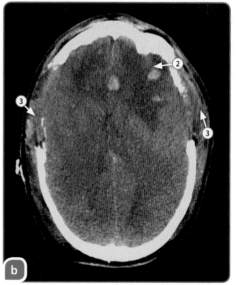

Figure 3.10 'Blossoming' of a traumatic intraparenchymal haemorrhage with oedema. (a) Initial computerised tomography (CT) scan showing only minor left frontotemporal lobe contusions ①. (b) A subsequent axial CT scan showing evolving and worsening frontotemporal contusions with oedema ② and mass effect that required bilateral decompressive craniectomies ③ to relieve severe increased ICP.

Management

Initial management is close neurological observation and monitoring for increased ICP.

Surgical evacuation of contusions is difficult; they are often multiple, so it is difficult to resect between contusion and normal brain. Larger intraparenchymal haemorrhages, for example intracerebral haemorrhages, are easier to remove.

If deterioration occurs, ICP management measures are implemented. These include decompressive craniectomy, if indicated.

Surgery

This is sometimes carried out in cases of:

- a large haemorrhagic volume (>50 mL)
- progressive neurological deterioration referable to the lesion, and either signs of mass effect on CT or medically refractory increased ICP

Diffuse axonal injury

Diffuse axonal injury occurs when the brain has been subjected to rapid acceleration–deceleration forces, most often in a road traffic accident. These shearing forces cause widespread stretching and tearing of axons and their myelin sheaths.

Clinical features

Diffuse axonal injury can be devastating. Patients are usually severely obtunded and may remain in a vegetative state, with little chance of recovery.

Computerised tomography sometimes shows diffuse multiple petechial (dot) haemorrhages in characteristic locations, including the:

- cerebral hemispheres
- corpus callosum
- dorsolateral brain stem

Management

Management is supportive. The neurological prognosis of diffuse axonal injury is usually very poor.

Hydrocephalus

Hydrocephalus (Greek: hydro, 'water'; kefale, 'head') results from impaired flow or absorption of cerebrospinal fluid, or rarely its overproduction (see page 31). It leads to intracranial accumulation of cerebrospinal fluid, which increases ventricular size and ICP (see page 190).

This common neurosurgical condition can develop at any age from the fetal period to adulthood.

Aetiology

Hydrocephalus can be congenital or acquired. Its causes are shown in **Table 3.12**. The accumulation of cerebrospinal fluid can be the consequence of:

- blockage of flow
- inadequate reabsorption
- excess production (very rarely)

Obstructive non-communicating hydrocephalus

Cerebrospinal fluid flow is obstructed by a blockage in the ventricular system or outflow from the ventricular system. The cerebrospinal fluid in the ventricles does not communicate with the subarachnoid space.

Communicating hydrocephalus

Hydrocephalus is communicating when there is no blockage of cerebrospinal fluid

Aetiology of hydrocephalus		
Category	Non-communicating	Communicating
Vascular	Intracranial haemorrhage (e.g. intraventricular haemorrhage and intracerebral haemorrhage)	Subarachnoid haemorrhage
Infection	Infective space-occupying lesion (e.g. cerebral abscess and cyst)	Infectious meningitis (e.g. fungal or bacterial, for example in tuberculous meningitis)
Tumours	Any tumour in (e.g. colloid cyst and meningioma) or outside (e.g. glioma and metastasis) the ventricular system	Carcinomatous infiltration of the meninges (e.g. in cases of severe metastatic disease)
Congenital	Stenosis of the ventricular system (e.g. aqueduct of Sylvius and foramina of Magendie and Luschka)	

Table 3.12 Causes of hydrocephalus depending on whether it is communicating or non-communicating

flow between the ventricles and the subarachnoid space, but rather the problem is impaired cerebrospinal fluid absorption by arachnoid granulations. Therefore the cerebrospinal fluid in the ventricles communicates with that in the subarachnoid space.

Clinical features

These depend on the age of the patient and how quickly symptoms develop.

Acute hydrocephalus

This type of hydrocephalus presents with features of increased ICP (see page 192). Patients develop acute headache associated with nausea, vomiting or both, as well as a deterioration in consciousness level. There may also be:

- features of brain herniation syndromes (see page 193)
- irritability in infants and young children
- 'sunsetting' eyes (impairment of upward gaze causes the eyes to spontaneously look down; this sign is caused by pressure on midbrain vertical gaze centres)

Children younger than 18 months have skull bones that are still unfused. Increased ICP causes an increase in head circumference, a common reason for physicians to refer infants to neurosurgeons for likely hydrocephalus.

Chronic hydrocephalus

In infants and young children, chronic hydrocephalus generally presents with progressive deterioration in higher neurological functions (e.g. failure to thrive, developmental delay and worsening performance in school) and persistent pressure headaches. Acute-on-chronic deterioration may occur, with acute features. Adults also present with similar symptoms.

Diagnostic approach

The aims are to:

- confirm the presence of acute hydrocephalus
- define the condition as communicating or non-communicating
- establish the cause

Investigations

Computerised tomography is the first-line investigation (**Figure 3.11**).

- In non-communicating hydrocephalus, ventricular enlargement occurs proximal to the site of obstruction; the cause of the obstruction (e.g. tumour, aqueduct stenosis and haemorrhage) should be ascertained
- In communicating hydrocephalus, there is usually generalised dilatation of all ventricles, with no obvious obstructing lesion

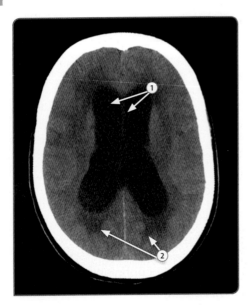

Figure 3.11 Axial computerised tomography scan of hydrocephalus, showing ① dilated lateral ventricles and ② periventricular oedema surrounding the frontal and occipital horns of lateral ventricles.

■ Further imaging with MRI may be required; neonates and infants with an open anterior fontanelle have ultrasound scanning through this area to assess and monitor ventricular size

Management

Surgery is the mainstay of treatment for hydrocephalus. Techniques depend on the underlying cause, and whether hydrocephalus is communicating or non-communicating.

Surgery

The commonest technique is cerebrospinal fluid diversion with a ventriculoperitoneal shunt or endoscopic third ventriculostomy.

Ventriculoperitoneal shunt

A catheter is inserted into the ventricle to drain excess cerebrospinal fluid to the peritoneum. Risks include infection, bleeding, blockage, fracture and breakage, and shunt failure.

> **Patients with a ventriculoperitoneal shunt can present with features of acute hydrocephalus.** These indicate shunt failure as a result of blockage, obstruction, fracture and breakage, or shunt infection. Imaging is used to seek mechanical breaks in the shunt and extrusion from the ventricle or peritoneal spaces. Cerebrospinal fluid may be sampled to test for infection.

Endoscopic third ventriculostomy

In this minimally invasive technique, a hole is made in the floor of the 3rd ventricle. This creates an alternative channel for cerebrospinal fluid to enter the subarachnoid spaces and be reabsorbed by arachnoid granulations.

A successful endoscopic third ventriculostomy can prevent the need for permanent shunting. It is useful when there is an obstruction distal to the 3rd ventricle, for example in aqueduct stenosis, but not in cases in which cerebrospinal fluid reabsorption problems predominate, such as communicating hydrocephalus after meningitis or subarachnoid haemorrhage.

Answers to starter questions

1. When a pathological process increases intracranial volume, the body initially prevents ICP rise by removing cerebrospinal fluid. However, if the intracranial volume continues to increase, a point is reached at which this compensatory mechanism becomes exhausted and the pressure starts to increase exponentially. The body's ability to maintain a constant intracranial volume depends on the patient's age and the pathological process.

2. Infants younger than 18 months have skulls that are incompletely fused. Their 'open skull' confers greater compliance to increases in intracranial volume, which manifest as increased head circumference. Older people are also better able to tolerate increases in intracranial volume. This increased compliance is a consequence of the brain atrophying with age, which decreases brain volume in proportion to total intracranial volume.

3. Steroids are useful for reducing ICP in cases of cerebral oedema caused by tumour. However, they are contraindicated in acute traumatic brain injury, because they are associated with poorer outcomes after 6 months.

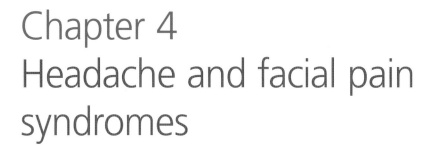

Chapter 4
Headache and facial pain syndromes

Starter questions

Answers to the following questions are on page 224.

1. Why do people get migraines?
2. Why do some people experience autonomic symptoms with migraine?
3. Can headaches be considered disabling conditions?

Introduction

Nearly everyone has a headache at some point in their life. A quarter of the population have frequent disabling headaches, making recurrent headache one of the most prevalent chronic neurological conditions. It is associated with depression, stress and anxiety, as well as time off work and loss of employment.

Headaches are either primary or secondary:

- **Primary headache** occurs in the absence of significant pathology

- **Secondary headache** is a symptom of underlying disease, including infections, tumours and increased intracranial pressure

The approach to headache is to exclude a secondary cause, identify the type of headache and assess the effect on the patient. Therapy is then directed accordingly.

Case 2 Headache

Presentation

Aileen Hastings, aged 21 years, presents to the emergency department complaining of severe generalised headache and nausea.

Initial interpretation

Presentation of a new headache requires careful assessment to differentiate a primary headache syndrome, such as migraine, from secondary headache arising from a cause such as subarachnoid haemorrhage. Questions need to cover speed of onset, the nature of the pain, associated features, exacerbating and relieving factors and a general medical history to narrow the differential diagnoses.

History

Aileen has a 3-month history of generalised headache, which developed over several weeks. The headache is dull, all over her head but worse frontally, and associated with occasional nausea but no vomiting. It is worse when lying down, coughing or straining. There is no eye watering, nasal discharge or photo- or phonophobia, and she has no positive visual or other neurological symptoms.

Interpretation of history

This is a gradual onset headache rather than a more worrying acute event. The latter would suggest a cerebrovascular event, which would cause a thunderclap headache (a sudden and severe headache).

The effect of posture changes and nausea could suggest a high-pressure headache. However, Aileen has no symptoms of neurological deficits suggesting an intracranial mass lesion. There are no features of migraine or cluster headache. Migraine would present with a pulsatile severe headache with nausea and photophobia. Cluster headache would present with episodic very severe one-sided retro-orbital stabbing pains with eye watering, ptosis and facial sweating.

Further history

Aileen has a history of acne, for which she takes oral tetracycline regularly. She has gained 8 kg in weight in the past year and is obese.

Examination

On general inspection, Aileen is noted to be obese. Systemic examination is normal. Pupils are reactive and eye movements normal. Visual acuity is normal. However, she has enlarged blind spots bilaterally, and a field defect is detected during bedside assessment (**Figure 4.1**). Fundoscopy reveals bilateral swollen optic discs, which suggests papilloedema. The remainder of the neurological examination is normal.

Interpretation of findings

The enlarged blind spot, field defect and swollen optic discs in the context of a potential high-pressure headache strongly suggest increased intracranial pressure. Patients are very frequently unaware of field defects, because they develop gradually. The lack of other neurological findings is somewhat reassuring but does not exclude serious underlying pathology.

High body mass index and recent weight gain, along with the use of tetracycline, increase the possibility of idiopathic intracranial hypertension (**Table 4.1**). A cerebral venous sinus thrombosis can present with the same history and examination. Other serious causes of increased

Case 2 *continued*

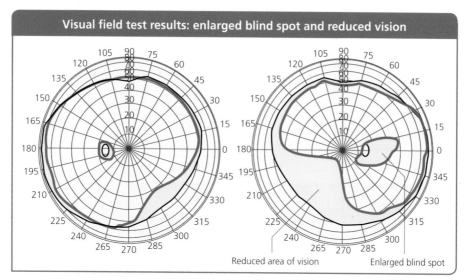

Visual field test results: enlarged blind spot and reduced vision

Reduced area of vision   Enlarged blind spot

Figure 4.1 Visual field test results. Normal visual fields and blind spots are in black, and the results in blue. There is an enlarged blind spot on the left and an area of reduced vision caused by pressure on the inferior nasal fibre.

Medications causing intracranial hypertension	
Medication	Common indication(s)
Isotretinoin	Acne vulgaris
Tetracycline	Acne vulgaris
Prednisolone	Many
Tamoxifen	Breast cancer
Beclomethasone	Asthma
Minocycline	Acne vulgaris

Table 4.1 Medications associated with idiopathic intracranial hypertension

intracranial pressure, such as a tumour, also need to be excluded.

Investigations

A computerised tomography (CT) scan of the brain with contrast excludes a mass lesion. A CT venogram to visualise the cerebral veins is normal, thereby excluding cerebral venous sinus thrombosis.

Lumbar puncture is carried out. The intracranial pressure on insertion of the needle (the opening pressure) is very high, at 52 cm H_2O. Once 20 mL of cerebrospinal fluid is removed, the pressure on withdrawing the needle (the closing pressure) is 16 cm H_2O. After the procedure, both the headache and the results of formal visual field testing have improved.

The results of cerebrospinal fluid analysis show glucose concentration and cell count are normal.

Diagnosis

A diagnosis of idiopathic intracranial hypertension is made on the basis of the nature of the headache and the increased intracranial pressure in the absence of a cause other than obesity and tetracycline use. Aileen is reassured that her condition is not life-threatening, but she is told that her vision is under threat if the pressure is not controlled in the long term.

Aileen is advised to lose weight, and the tetracycline is stopped. As an interim measure, she is started on acetazolamide, a

Case 2 *continued*

carbonic anhydrase inhibitor that reduces production of cerebrospinal fluid. A few weeks later, repeat visual field assessment shows improvement.

> **Obesity probably increases intracranial pressure by increasing the peripheral conversion of androgens to oestrogens in body fat.** Higher levels of oestrogens are known to increase the level of spinal fluid production.

Case 3 Throbbing headache and reduced vision

Presentation

Stephanie Peterson, a 41-year-old police officer, attends the emergency department with a severe headache, change in vision, nausea and photophobia.

Initial interpretation

The differential diagnosis for this presentation is broad; it includes both primary headache syndromes and secondary headaches arising from serious pathology. A full and detailed headache history is essential to establish the cause of the headache.

History

The headache started 3 days ago and progressed to its peak intensity over 4 h. The pain is over the left frontal region. It is pulsatile, and she rates its severity as 8 out of 10 at its worst. The pain has waxed and waned since the headache's onset but has stayed at least 5 out of 10 in severity.

Stephanie has missed work and spent most of the time in bed, because normal activities and light aggravate her symptoms. Throughout, she has felt very nauseated and has vomited five times.

Shortly before the pain started, she noticed a 'blind spot' in her vision.

She says that the right upper portion of her vision is blurred and she cannot see things there properly. This symptom developed slowly and spread from the centre outwards. She has no other neurological symptoms.

Interpretation of history

Stephanie has described a severe pulsatile unilateral headache associated with nausea and vomiting and photophobia, and aggravated by physical activity. The onset was gradual. These features seem typical for a migraine headache.

Her description of the visual field disturbance is also typical of a migraine aura, except for its duration, which is a little prolonged. This raises the possibility of a secondary headache caused by an ischaemic or haemorrhagic stroke, structural lesion or central nervous system infection.

The key to determining the cause is to ascertain:

- if she has had similar headaches before
- if she has had a migraine aura, how long it normally lasts
- family history
- risk factors for stroke
- any other symptoms suggesting a focal neurological lesion

Case 3 *continued*

Further history

Many years ago, Stephanie's general practitioner diagnosed migraine, and she suffers similar headaches roughly once every 2 months. She takes prophylactic propranolol, because the weekly migraines she used to have were interfering with her work. However, her migraine headaches are not normally as severe or prolonged as this presentation, and they usually respond to aspirin. This time, she started taking regular dihydrocodeine on the 2nd day.

She has no risk factors for stroke; she is a non-smoker with normal blood pressure and no family history of stroke. She has no family history of migraine, and no infective symptoms.

Examination

Stephanie is in clear discomfort, and is mildly photo- and phonophobic. She has no neck stiffness. There is no redness, swelling or watering of her eyes. General neurological examination reveals only a right upper quadrantanopia (loss of an quarter of the visual field) on visual field testing (**Figure 4.2**). Systemic examination is normal.

Interpretation of findings

The presentation is very probably a migraine, based on the absence of additional neurological findings and signs or symptoms of systemic infection. Nonetheless, it is more prolonged than Stephanie's usual migraines, and there is a persistent visual field defect. These features warrant an urgent magnetic resonance imaging (MRI) to exclude a stroke or other secondary cause.

Investigation

Stephanie is admitted for pain management and neuroimaging. An MRI scan of her brain is normal. Her opioid medications are stopped, because they are usually ineffective for migraine headaches. She is given sumatriptan, and her headache and visual field defect resolve over 24 h.

Diagnosis

With the more serious differential diagnoses excluded, migraine is diagnosed. Stephanie is educated on the use of triptans.

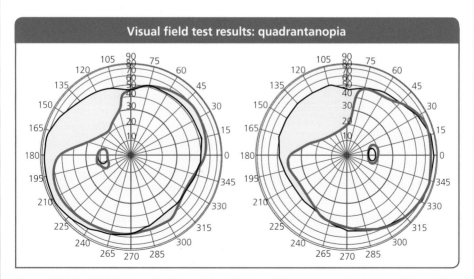

Figure 4.2 Visual field test results. Normal visual fields and blind spots are in black, and the results in blue. There is a superior homonymous quadrantanopia.

Migraine

Migraines are recurrent episodes of head and facial pain, nausea and vomiting, with varying degrees of autonomic features and transient neurological symptoms. These episodes are associated with altered neuronal and neurovascular activity. Migraine is the commonest cause of headaches leading to disability and the disruption of daily activity.

Migraine mimics and chameleons can make diagnosis difficult (**Table 4.2**).

■ Migraine mimics are conditions that mimic migraines
■ Migraine chameleons are migraines that mimic other conditions

Some migraines are preceded or accompanied by an aura.

Migraine mimics and chameleons	
Type	Feature(s)
Mimics	Distinguishing clinical feature(s)
Trigeminal autonomic cephalgias	Agitation, including the desire to move around
Acute glaucoma	Painful, tender, firm eye with visual loss and haloes
Carotid artery dissection	Neck pain and Horner's syndrome
Structural lesions	Early morning headaches, vomiting without nausea and visual obscurations
Meningitis	Systemic signs and symptoms
Giant cell arteritis	Age > 50 years, scalp tenderness, jaw claudication and systemic symptoms
Chameleons	Feature(s) of the migraine that cause confusion
Transient ischaemic attacks	Transient visual loss
Stroke	Visual loss, motor weakness and dysphasia
Epilepsy	Visual, olfactory or gustatory aura
Vestibular disorders	Vertigo
Multiple sclerosis	Intermittent sensory disturbance

Table 4.2 Migraine mimics (headache-causing disorders that can be mistaken for migraines) and migraine chameleons (unusual migraines that present with features suggesting an alternative disorder)

Epidemiology

Migraine affects 15-20% of women and about 5% of men.

Aetiology

There is a strong familial tendency to have migraines. Many genes probably underlie this predisposition.

Many patients identify specific triggers for their attacks, such as chocolate, cheese and wine. However, it is unclear if these are true triggers or a craving associated with the prodrome of the migraine.

Pathogenesis

Migraines result from a complex interaction between genetic predisposition, abnormal cortical and subcortical electrical activity, and altered processing in peripheral structures (e.g. the cervical, occipital and trigeminal nerves and their central connections).

The aura

The migraine aura is caused by a wave of cortical spreading depression. This is a slowly moving wave of decreased neuronal function that sweeps over the cortex and probably corresponds with the aura. The association between the cortical spreading depression and headache symptoms is less clear.

The headache

Migraine pain arises from abnormal activity of the cervical, occipital and trigeminal nerves and abnormal central processing in their brain stem nuclei. These phenomena are probably triggered by the cortical spreading depression.

Some neurones in the trigeminal ganglion innervate dura and dural vasculature along with the area around the eye. Also, central trigeminal nuclei receive input from occipital nerve fibres and cervical nerve fibres. Therefore activation in this system accounts for the perception of pain around the eye and head.

Figure 4.3 shows some of the structures central to pain perception in migraine.

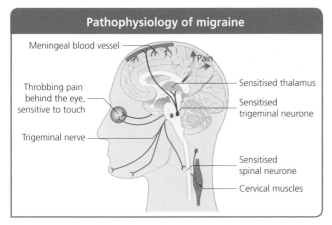

Figure 4.3 Migraine is a consequence of abnormal peripheral sensitisation of trigeminal, cervical and occipital fibres, central brain stem and spinal cord nuclei, and other brain regions including the thalamus. Abnormal activation of the trigeminal and facial nerves and their nuclei results in hypersensitivity in the structures they innervate along with the autonomic features of migraine.

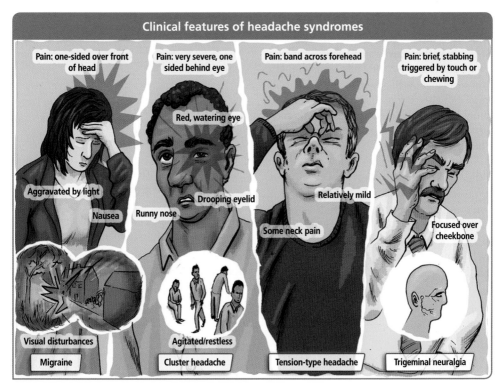

Figure 4.4 Typical features of migraine, cluster headache, tension-type headache and trigeminal neuralgia.

Clinical features

Migraines are highly variable. They usually consist of a throbbing or pulsatile headache that gradually develops over 30 min to a few hours. The headache is usually accompanied by varying degrees of photophobia, phonophobia, nausea and vomiting.

Aggravation of pain by movement is the most characteristic feature of migraine. Patients experiencing a migraine prefer to lie down and seek a dark, quiet place (**Figure 4.4**).

> Adults with **recurrent headaches that began in childhood** almost always have migraine.

Many patients have a migraine prodrome. This phase, which can last several days, leads up to

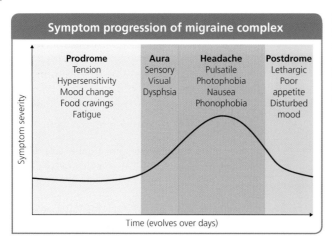

Figure 4.5 The migraine complex comprises a prodrome of mood and appetite changes, an aura or altered sensory perception; a headache phase; and a postdrome of further fatigue and mood changes.

the headache and may include aura symptoms (e.g. visual disturbance), altered mood, sleepiness, food cravings, irritability or fatigue. After the headache itself, there is often a similar period of altered mood, appetite changes and fatigue; this is the postdrome. The combined symptoms from prodrome to postdrome are the migraine complex (**Figure 4.5**).

Migraine without aura

Over 80% of patients with migraine experience no aura. The International Classification of Headache Disorders (ICHD), used widely in clinical trials, defines migraine according to the following criteria:

- episodic attacks
- duration of 4–72 h
- two or more of:
  - pulsating
  - unilateral
  - moderate
  - severe intensity
  - aggravated by movement
- at least one of nausea and/or vomiting, and photophobia with phonophobia

However, in clinical practice there is a spectrum; migraines can be bilateral, mild, non-pulsatile, continuous and last < 4 h or > 72 h.

Migraine with aura

There are many types of aura. They are often mistaken for symptoms of other neurological conditions, including stroke and multiple sclerosis (see **Table 4.2**).

Auras are usually stereotypical (repeated in the same pattern) for each patient. Symptoms can be:

- positive (e.g. zigzag lines in vision, and pins and needles in hands or feet)
- negative (e.g. blind spots, and numb hands or feet)

They may develop over several minutes and last less than an hour. The headache then usually follows within an hour, but it may be absent.

Some subtypes of migraine have distinct symptoms and signs (**Table 4.3**).

Diagnostic approach

Diagnosis is usually possible from the history. Three or more of the following symptoms strongly suggest migraine:

Migraine subtypes	
Subtype	Symptoms and signs
Acephalic	Migraine aura without subsequent headache
Basilar	Brain stem signs, and reduced level of consciousness
Chronic	Migraine on ≥ 15 days/month for 3 months
Hemiplegic	Hemiplegic aura
Status migrainosus	Severe attack lasting > 3 days

Table 4.3 Migraine subtypes

- pulsatile headache
- duration of 4–72 h
- unilateral pain
- nausea and/or vomiting
- disabling intensity
- family history of migraine

Cases of recurrent typical migraine attacks with stereotypical features and a normal neurological examination may not need further investigation.

Investigations

An MRI of the brain and a lumbar puncture are indicated for patients with:

- new headache (if they are > 50 years old)
- fever
- thunderclap headache (maximum intensity reached in < 5 min)
- neurological deficit
- new cognitive dysfunction
- drowsiness
- significant change from previous headaches
- a compromised immune system

Time is often the best tool for identifying a particular headache syndrome. Assuming that no worrying features are present, observation of the pattern and development of symptoms over time often clarifies the nature of the headache syndrome.

Management

Headache diaries can be used to clarify the frequency, severity, nature and associated symptoms of migraine, for example by showing the headache to be more or less frequent than initially thought. In women, headache diaries can reveal patterns related to the menstrual cycle.

Therapies are used for either acute attacks or as preventive measures (**Table 4.4**). First-line medications taken at the onset of headache include simple analgesic and antiemetic drugs. Second-line drugs include triptans, for example sumatriptan. Opioids are generally ineffective and often lead to medication overuse headache (see page 223).

Preventive therapies

These include:

- beta-blockers such as propranolol
- antidepressant drugs such as amitriptyline
- antiepileptic drugs such as topiramate

If these therapies are ineffective, patients may benefit from greater occipital nerve block injections or botulinum toxin type A injections around the neck, scalp and face.

Physical scalp and occipital nerve stimulators are an active area in migraine therapy research. The rationale is that stimulation of peripheral occipital nerve branches down-regulates central sensitisation pathways, thereby relieving migraine symptoms.

Migraine therapies		
Therapy	Indication	Dose or route
Paracetamol (acetaminophen)	Acute attack	1 g as needed
Aspirin	Acute attack	300–900 mg as needed
Domperidone	Acute attack (nausea)	10 mg as needed
Metoclopramide	Acute attack (nausea)	10 mg as needed
Triptans	Acute attack	Various doses and routes (e.g. sumatriptan 25 mg)
Beta-blockers	Preventive	Various (e.g. propranolol 40 mg twice daily)
Antidepressant drugs	Preventive	Various (e.g. amitriptyline 10 mg at night)
Antiepileptic drugs	Preventive	Various (e.g. topiramate 25 mg at night)
Greater occipital nerve block	Preventive	Injections of local anaesthetic and steroid
Botulinum toxin type A	Preventive	Injections on scalp, neck and face

Table 4.4 Common migraine therapies

Tension-type headache

Most headaches are tension-type headaches. These are characterised by a band of pain or pressure around the forehead, with no other neurological features.

Epidemiology

Tension-type headaches are experienced by up to 80% of the population. They are rarely severe, and most people can self-manage them at home. This type of headache affects women and the young more than men and older patients.

Aetiology

The cause of tension-type headache is poorly understood, but aetiological factors include:

- contracted cranial muscles
- stress
- inappropriate prescription lenses
- increased pericranial myofascial tissue sensitivity
- sensitisation of sensory inputs

The variability of this type of headache both within and between individual patients may result from increased sensitivity to nociceptive inputs in central pain centres.

Clinical features

Patients typically have pain around the forehead but no nausea, vomiting or autonomic symptoms. ICHD criteria include:

- 10 episodes occurring on average on < 1 day/month

- duration of 30 min to 1 week
- only one of photophobia or phonophobia
- two or more of:
    - mild to moderate
    - non-pulsating (band, tightness or pressure)
    - bilateral
    - not aggravated by activity
    - no nausea or vomiting

Diagnostic approach

Patients with persistent tension-type headaches are screened for depression and anxiety, which can perpetuate symptoms. Serious secondary causes, including tumours, are considered but there is usually no need for investigations.

> Patients with a new chronic tension-type headache are often anxious about the possibility of an underlying life-threatening cause. Reassurance requires a clear explanation that there are no features to suggest a sinister cause, and that the symptoms are common and overwhelmingly usually benign.

Management

Most patients self-manage their headache with simple analgesia. Opioids and frequent use of analgesic drugs are avoided to prevent medication overuse headache (see page 223).

Patients with severe forms of headache that fail to respond to simple analgesia may actually have migraine (see page 214).

Cluster headache

Cluster headaches are recurrent attacks of severe orbital pain associated with cranial autonomic disturbances on the same side of the head as the pain. They are a type of trigeminal autonomic cephalgia (**Table 4.5**).

The trigeminal autonomic cephalgias are a group of clinically overlapping syndromes of recurrent bouts of severe headache with associated facial autonomic features. The different types overlap in their features but can usually be distinguished clinically and by their response to treatments.

Features of trigeminal autonomic cephalgias			
Feature	Cluster headache	Paroxysmal hemicrania	SUNCT
Frequency (per day)	1–3	5–8	> 10 (may be hundreds)
Duration	Hours	Minutes	Seconds
First-line treatment	Verapamil	Indometacin	Lamotrigine
Indometacin responsiveness	Occasional (rare)	Dramatic: complete resolution	Rare

SUNCT, short-lasting, unilateral, neuralgiform headache attacks with conjunctival injection and tearing.

Table 4.5 Features of the trigeminal autonomic cephalgias

Epidemiology

Cluster headache has a prevalence of 15 per 100,000 people, with a male predominance (4:1). Increased prevalence in close family members suggests an inherited component.

Aetiology

The cause of cluster headache is unknown.

The facial pain of cluster headache is a consequence of activation of the ophthalmic branch of the trigeminal nerve. The autonomic symptoms result from activation of the parasympathetic facial nerve.

During a cluster headache, abnormal hypothalamic activity is visible on positron emission tomography. The hypothalamus functions as an internal clock for many physiological functions and explains the periodic nature of the symptoms in cluster headache.

> **Cluster headaches are usually more painful than migraines or tension-type headaches.** The pain is so severe that some patients refer to them as 'suicidal headaches'.

Clinical features

The pain is characteristically excruciating and unilateral, making patients very agitated and restless. The hallmark of cluster headache is its periodicity; headaches occur in clusters of daily headaches for weeks or months with prolonged periods of remission in between. The headaches usually occur at night and can be triggered by alcohol during a cluster.

Core features from the ICHD classification are:

- episodes of severe unilateral orbital, supraorbital or temporal pain
- duration of 15–180 min
- frequency from one every other day to eight per day
- during headache, at least one cranial autonomic symptom on the same side as the headache:
  - conjunctival injection or lacrimation
  - miosis or ptosis
  - nasal congestion or rhinorrhoea
  - forehead or facial sweating
  - eyelid oedema
- restlessness or agitation

Diagnostic approach

The clinical picture is usually characteristic, enabling a clinical diagnosis. Rarely, these headaches are secondary to a lesion in the hypothalamus. Therefore an MRI scan is indicated for all newly diagnosed patients.

Management

Cluster headaches may continue for life or go into remission, even after many years of recurrent attacks.

Acute attack

High-flow 100% oxygen through a face mask and subcutaneous sumatriptan can be very effective in acute attacks. Patients can be supplied with home oxygen to use during bouts. How oxygen helps is unknown.

Preventive therapies

Given the severity of cluster headaches, preventive therapy is crucial. It usually includes either verapamil or lithium.

Temporomandibular joint dysfunction

Temporomandibular joint dysfunction is the term for pain and discomfort around the face and mandible of the jaw from muscle spasm or dysfunction of the temporomandibular joint. There is often joint stiffness, clicking or popping on chewing. The condition is common, especially in people with migraine or tension-type headache. There is rarely any serious underlying pathology, but a full dental assessment is required for chronic cases.

Aetiology

Mechanical dysfunction of the temporomandibular joint, deformities of the jaw, stress, anxiety and muscle spasm can all cause temporomandibular joint dysfunction. Teeth clenching, chronic chewing, other jaw movements and degenerative joint changes lead to myofascial and muscle pain and spasm.

Clinical features

Patients experience jaw and facial pain, temporalis and masseter muscle pain and tenderness, restriction of jaw movements, mandibular clicking and crepitus.

Diagnosis of temporomandibular joint dysfunction is usually based on a typical history. A full dental assessment is usually done to exclude a structural cause.

Management

Patients are often worried about the possibility of an underlying disease. Therefore explanation and reassurance that the condition is benign is often helpful.

Temporomandibular joint dysfunction usually settles with simple analgesic drugs, such as paracetamol (acetaminophen) or ibuprofen, along with jaw exercises. Dental splints can limit nocturnal chewing and grinding.

Trigeminal neuralgia

Trigeminal neuralgia consists of severe paroxysms of facial pain. The condition affects about 3 per 100,000 people annually, generally those older than 40 years. Its incidence increases with age.

Aetiology

Trigeminal neuralgia is usually idiopathic. However, it occasionally develops secondary to central lesions of the trigeminal nucleus or nerve root, for example as a result of multiple sclerosis, stroke or other lesions.

A more common cause is compression of the dorsal root entry zone of the trigeminal nerve by the superior cerebellar artery. This irritates and demyelinates the nerve, leading to abnormal neuronal discharges in response to normal stimulation.

Clinical features

Patients have shooting, stabbing or electric shock-like sensations over the face in the distribution of the 2nd and 3rd divisions of the trigeminal nerve. The eyes are usually spared. The pain is short-lasting but can occur in prolonged, unrelenting bouts. It is usually triggered by sensory stimulation of the affected face or mouth.

Patients with trigeminal neuralgia learn to avoid the physical stimulation that triggers their pain. They may leave a section of their face unshaven or unclean, or avoid tooth brushing.

There are usually no physical signs of trigeminal neuralgia. However, sensory loss, weakness or muscle wasting may be present if the trigeminal ganglion is damaged.

Either MRI or CT is used to exclude compression of the dorsal root entry zone.

Management

Carbamazepine, gabapentin or lamotrigine are effective for most cases.

If medications are ineffective, surgery may be indicated. Surgical options include gamma knife or radiofrequency ablation or, in cases of dorsal root compression, microvascular decompression.

Giant cell arteritis

Giant cell arteritis, also known as temporal arteritis, is an uncommon but serious headache that affects elderly patients. It is a systemic vasculitis that can ultimately cause blindness. Diagnosis can be difficult, because the condition lacks specific clinical features.

Epidemiology

Annual incidence is 5–18 per 100,000 people over the age of 55 years and increases with age. Giant cell arteritis is very uncommon in people younger than 55 years. The condition affects four times as many women as it does men.

Aetiology

Giant cell arteritis is an immune-mediated arteritis involving extracranial large arteries, particularly the superficial temporal artery. The vasculitic lesions are focal or multifocal (as opposed to diffuse), and consist of a cellular infiltrate forming the so-called giant cells. B cells direct an antibody attack against vascular proteins, which causes vessel inflammation and stenosis. The pain arises from vessel inflammation and vasodilation.

Clinical features

The characteristic features of giant cell arteritis are headache (75%) and symptoms of systemic vasculitis (**Table 4.6**). The headache is often non-specific. The superficial temporal artery is tender, and systemic symptoms are present, including fever, myalgia, malaise, lethargy and weight loss.

Patients often have a history of polymyalgia rheumatica, an inflammatory connective tissue disease causing a syndrome of pain and stiffness in the neck, shoulders and hips.

There may be jaw claudication (pain on chewing), scalp tenderness and loss of pulsation in the affected artery. Transient monocular visual loss (amaurosis fugax) is the most serious symptom, because it can lead to permanent blindness and both eyes can be affected. In giant cell arteritis, amaurosis fugax is caused by retinal ischaemia from arterial inflammation, occlusion or embolism with reduced blood flow.

Diagnostic approach

Erythrocyte sedimentation rate and C-reactive protein level are increased in most cases. Temporal artery biopsy is necessary for diagnosis. Biopsy shows intimal proliferation and luminal stenosis along with the characteristic giant cells.

> Normal erythrocyte sedimentation rate and C-reactive protein level are strong evidence against giant cell arteritis. If there is doubt, the best diagnostic test is a biopsy of inflamed tissue.

Management

Giant cell arteritis carries a risk of blindness, so treatment is started immediately on clinical suspicion while awaiting biopsy.

Systemic symptoms of giant cell arteritis	
Symptom	Frequency (%)
Headache	75
Polymyalgia rheumatica	60
Malaise	55
Jaw claudication	40
Fever	35
Amaurosis fugax	10

Table 4.6 Systemic symptoms of giant cell arteritis

Corticosteroids are started at high dose (e.g. prednisolone 60 mg/day) and titrated down while monitoring erythrocyte sedimentation rate and C-reactive protein level. Treatment is for several years, so there is a significant risk of adverse effects from steroids, especially in the elderly.

Headache of increased intracranial pressure

Headache can be a sign of increased intracranial pressure (page 192). Such 'high-pressure headaches' can be idiopathic or secondary to a tumour, venous thrombosis or hydrocephalus.

An excess of cerebrospinal fluid results in meningeal stretching and the activation of pain-sensitive structures such as the dura.

Clinical features

The headache is dull and generalised. It is worsened by anything that temporarily increases intracranial pressure:

- lying down (so the headache is typically worse on awakening)
- coughing
- straining
- sneezing
- bending forwards

Patients may also have vomiting, papilloedema, reduced visual fields and visual obscurations (transient changes in vision). Loss of visual acuity occurs late.

Diagnostic approach

Urgent neuroimaging is indicated, especially if focal neurological signs suggest a mass lesion (**Table 4.7**). CT reveals any mass lesions, whereas a CT or magnetic resonance venogram show any venous thrombosis. Specific investigation depends on what cause is suggested by the history and examination.

Red flags for urgent neuroimaging in new headache		
Additional finding	First-line imaging	When
Papilloedema	CT	Same day
Altered consciousness	CT	Same day
Confusion	CT	Same day
New seizure	CT or MRI	Same day
Change in memory or personality	CT	Urgent outpatient appointment
History of cancer	CT	Urgent outpatient appointment
New cluster headache	MRI	Non-urgent outpatient appointment

CT, computerised tomography; MRI, magnetic resonance imaging.

Table 4.7 Red flags for urgent neuroimaging in patients with a new headache

Management

Treating the underlying cause is paramount. In selected refractory cases, lumbar puncture, extraventricular drain, or lumbar– or ventricular–peritoneal shunts can reduce the intracranial pressure. Idiopathic intracranial hypertension is treated with weight loss or acetazolamide.

Other headache syndromes

There are more than 80 types of headache in modern classification systems. Some of the commoner or life-threatening types include the following.

Thunderclap headache

A thunderclap headache has a near-immediate onset and rapidly reaches peak severity. The pain is usually very severe, and there is associated nausea or vomiting and photo- or phonophobia. Thunderclap headache is a symptom of both benign, non-life threatening conditions and life threatening ones (**Table 4.8**).

The key feature is not the severity of the headache but the time from onset to peak severity. In a true thunderclap headache, this takes seconds rather than minutes. Thunderclap headache is treated as potential subarachnoid haemorrhages (see page 258) until proven otherwise, and warrants immediate clinical assessment and neuroimaging studies.

Low-pressure headaches

This type of headache is dull or throbbing and diffuse. It is aggravated by upright posture and improved by lying down. Patients may have severe nausea and vomiting.

Low-pressure headaches are uncommon. They are usually caused by dural tears with leakage of cerebrospinal fluid and consequent reduction in cerebrospinal fluid volume. Lumbar puncture or spinal anaesthetics are the commonest causes. Spontaneous dural leaks also rarely occur.

Medication overuse headache

Opioids, paracetamol (acetaminophen), caffeine, triptans and many other analgesic drugs used to treat headaches can lead to medication overuse headache. This type of headache is surprisingly common but often underdiagnosed and mistreated with additional analgesia.

Causes of thunderclap headache		
Cause	Key investigation(s)	Prognosis
Subarachnoid haemorrhage	Plain CT	Life-threatening
Venous sinus thrombosis	MR or CT venogram	Life-threatening
Arterial dissection	MR or CT angiogram	Life-threatening
Meningitis	CT and lumbar puncture	Life-threatening
Pituitary apoplexy	CT with contrast	Life-threatening
Ischaemic or haemorrhagic stroke	Plain CT	Life-threatening
Reversible cerebral vasoconstriction syndrome	MR or CT angiogram	Non-life-threatening
Spontaneous intracranial hypotension	MR with contrast and lumbar puncture	Non-life-threatening
Exertional headache	Plain CT and lumbar puncture	Benign
Sexually induced headache	Plain CT and lumbar puncture	Benign
Idiopathic recurrent thunderclap headache	Repeated negative neuroimaging and lumbar punctures	Benign
Sinusitis	History; requires exclusion of above	Benign
Idiopathic thunderclap headache	Diagnosis of exclusion	Benign
Migraine		Benign

Table 4.8 Causes of thunderclap headache. The range of causes and neuroimaging choices mandate thorough history and examination

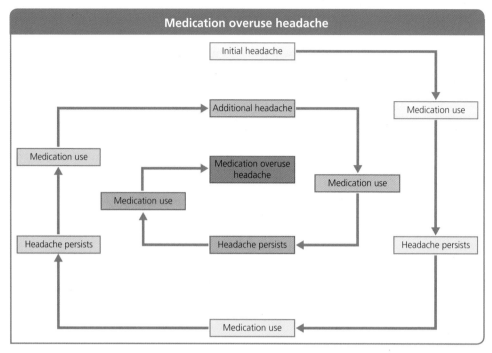

Figure 4.6 Frequent use of medications commonly used to treat headaches can lead to worsening of the headache or to a new type of headache.

A vicious cycle develops of headache, medication use, then further headache and further medication use (**Figure 4.6**). The condition is managed by patient education and the slow or rapid withdrawal of the medication. Headaches may initially worsen, and improvement can take several months.

Answers to starter questions

1. Migraines are often attributed to specific triggers such as chocolate, wine, caffeine and stress, but there is little evidence to support this. Current evidence suggests that people who experience migraines have a genetic predisposition to episodes of abnormal brain stem neuronal activity that activates pain centres and trigeminal nuclei.

2. The trigeminal nerve is central to the pathogenesis of migraine. This nerve mediates sensation from the face, nose and scalp. It also includes autonomic nerve fibres to the eye; their activity controls pupil function, lacrimal gland function and nasal watering. Therefore abnormal activation of the trigeminal system produces autonomic symptoms as well as pain.

3. Chronic headaches cause severe suffering and distress. Patients may often have to take days off work, and may even lose their job. They may withdraw from their family or social life for days at a time, and experience depression and anxiety because of the frequent attacks or fear of their recurrence. Despite a lack of serious secondary causes such as tumours or strokes, primary headache disorders are a real disability to the patients who endure them.

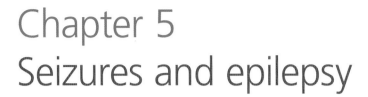
Chapter 5
Seizures and epilepsy

Starter questions

Answers to the following questions are on page 238.

1. Can anyone have a seizure?
2. Can epilepsy be cured?
3. How does epilepsy affect patients' lives?

Introduction

Seizures are spontaneous, episodic, abnormal discharges of electrical activity in the brain. About 10% of people have a seizure at least once in their life. Features include:

- abnormal motor, sensory or autonomic symptoms
- changes in behaviour and emotion
- altered consciousness

These occur in isolation or in combination.

Primary seizures have no detectable structural or metabolic cause. In contrast, provoked or secondary seizures are caused by underlying disease, such as a tumour, stroke or a metabolic problem.

Epilepsy is the tendency to have recurrent seizures with stereotypical (characteristic and repeated) features. It is one of the commonest serious neurological conditions and a major cause of disability and social stigma.

Status epilepticus is a neurological emergency (see page 448). The patient has continued or recurrent seizures lasting over 30 min or fails to regain consciousness between seizures.

Case 4 Blackout

Presentation

Harry Fraser, aged 19 years, is brought to the emergency department after being seen to suddenly lose consciousness, fall to the ground and 'shake all over'. On arrival, he is disoriented in time and place and unable to give an account of events.

Initial interpretation

The sudden loss of consciousness, 'shaking' and subsequent recovery with confusion suggest a seizure. Syncope can also present with limb jerking and remains a possibility. Identifying any prodromes (premonitory symptoms) and obtaining a clear description of events before, during and after the collapse are key to making a diagnosis.

History

Harry's brother witnessed the event and provides information. Harry has no notable medical history and appeared well until immediately before the collapse. He had been talking when he suddenly stopped speaking, turned his head and eyes to the right, raised and straightened his right arm and flexed his left arm at the elbow for about 10 s. He did not respond to his brother during this time.

Harry then 'stiffened all his muscles' and fell over 'like a log'. He lay stiff on the ground, breathing slowly, for another few seconds before his arms and legs began rhythmic, synchronised contractions. This phase lasted 1 min, during which Harry turned slightly blue. He then went limp and his breathing normalised, but he was unresponsive

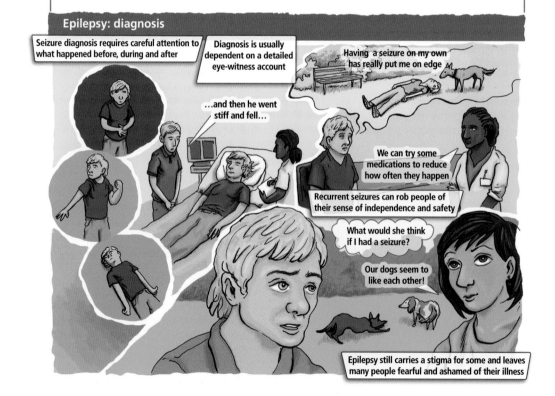

Epilepsy: diagnosis

Seizure diagnosis requires careful attention to what happened before, during and after

Diagnosis is usually dependent on a detailed eye-witness account

Having a seizure on my own has really put me on edge

...and then he went stiff and fell...

We can try some medications to reduce how often they happen

Recurrent seizures can rob people of their sense of independence and safety

What would she think if I had a seizure?

Our dogs seem to like each other!

Epilepsy still carries a stigma for some and leaves many people fearful and ashamed of their illness

Case 4 *continued*

for another 2 or 3 min. After this, he began to look around, mumble and slowly regain awareness but was very disoriented.

Interpretation of history

There are no prodromes, such as light-headedness, nausea, visual clouding, tinnitus and palpitations, to suggest syncope.

The description of the episode correlates well with the typical sequence of events of a focal seizure progressing to a generalised one. The sudden loss of awareness, head and eye turning and arm posturing are typical of a left frontal lobe seizure (**Figure 5.1** and **Table 5.6**). The subsequent 'stiffening' of the muscles describes the generalised tonic phase of continuous muscular contraction, and the rhythmic, synchronised limb contractions represent a generalised clonic phase, in which muscles rapidly contract and relax. The period of limpness and unresponsiveness is the postictal recovery phase. The ongoing disorientation is typical and should resolve within an hour or so.

Further history

Once Harry becomes fully oriented, he provides more detail. He remembers talking with his brother and suddenly experiencing an unusual 'rising' sensation in his abdomen. His next memory is of regaining consciousness in hospital. He had a few febrile convulsions as a baby but has otherwise been well. He is fit and active and does not smoke, drink or misuse drugs. His sleeping pattern has been regular recently. He drives and is studying economics at university. He has never experienced this type of episode before. No one in the family has epilepsy.

Examination

Neurological and general examinations are completely normal. Harry is systemically well, and a few minutes after regaining consciousness his vital signs have normalised.

Interpretation of findings

The history is sufficient to diagnose a seizure.

- A rising epigastric sensation suggests focal onset in the temporal lobe
- The head and eye deviation to the right with a straightened right arm and flexed left arm (the 'fencer' position) indicates spread to the left frontal lobe

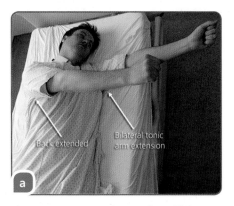 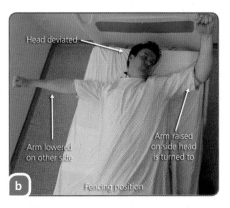

Figure 5.1 Posturing during a frontal lobe seizure. Frontal lobe seizures can result in seemingly bizarre behaviours and postures that are often interpreted as 'non-organic'.

Case 4 continued

- The subsequent tonic and clonic phases indicate secondary generalisation of the epileptic activity spreading throughout the cerebral hemispheres

Patients usually recover quickly from a frontal lobe seizure. However, the postictal confusion in this case suggests a secondary generalised seizure.

No clear provoking factors are evident, and examination has not identified any significant neurological deficit. Febrile convulsions predispose to sclerosis of the mesial temporal lobe, a recognised cause of focal onset temporal lobe seizures.

Investigations

The results of routine blood investigations are normal. Harry has fully recovered and has no neurological deficits, so an emergency computerised tomography scan is not indicated.

Before discharge, the following are arranged:

- a follow-up appointment at the first seizure clinic
- an outpatient magnetic resonance imaging (MRI) scan to identify any structural lesion
- an electroencephalogram (EEG) to identify any characteristic epilepsy syndrome

The MRI shows left-sided mesial temporal sclerosis, and the interictal EEG is normal.

Diagnosis

Before the follow-up appointment 2 weeks after the initial presentation, Harry has another, identical episode. The neurologist reviews the history and gives a diagnosis of epilepsy using a patient-oriented seizure classification as shown in **Table 5.1**.

The diagnosis is discussed with Harry, and with evidence of a temporal lobe lesion on MRI and history of multiple seizures, he is counselled that further episodes are likely. After discussing medication options, it is agreed to start treatment with levetiracetam, because it is effective for partial onset seizures and has a favourable adverse effect profile.

Harry is also informed that he cannot drive and must make the Driver and Vehicle Licensing Agency aware of his diagnosis. The neurologist arranges a follow-up appointment in 6 months to keep his case under review.

Epileptic seizure classification system	
Classification tier	**Description**
Epileptogenic zone	Left temporal lobe focal onset with secondary generalisation
Semiology	Temporal: rising epigastric sensation
	Left frontal: eye and head deviation and fencing posture
	Generalisation: tonic-clonic phase
Aetiology	Mesial temporal sclerosis
Seizure frequency	Unclear at present but appears infrequent
Related medical condition	Febrile convulsions as child

Table 5.1 Epilepsy description using patient-oriented seizure classification

Case 5 Recurrence of seizures

Presentation

Jane Stone is 32 years old and has a long history of secondary generalised epilepsy, which started in childhood. Until 2 months ago, she had not had a seizure in 20 years. However, she has recently developed a new type of seizure that is occurring up to six times daily; this is greatly interfering with her work, social life and sense of well-being.

Initial interpretation

The sudden development of very frequent attacks in a patient with previously well controlled epilepsy is unusual. Causes include:

- stopping or changing medication
- pregnancy
- new central nervous system pathology
- psychogenic non-epileptic attacks

The history must exclude these causes and in particular establish a detailed description (semiology) of previous and current seizures as well as her personal and social history.

Further history

Jane is not pregnant. She takes her medications daily, including carbamazepine for her epilepsy, and has no other neurological symptoms. She describes the sequence of her childhood seizures as follows:

- a sudden arrest of awareness
- some clonic movements on the right side of her face
- a few seconds of whole-body stiffness and altered breathing
- clonic arm and leg movements
- a period of being unresponsive and floppy
- drowsy confusion for 30 min

She describes the order and features of the current seizures as:

- suddenly feeling 'not quite there'
- standing up and walking in circles
- falling to the ground
- jerking movements of the entire body for 5–20 min, during which her eyes are closed tight
- stopping and becoming tearful but quickly returning to her normal self

Four months ago, she separated from her long-term partner and had to take up new employment. She works as an administrator in a prison and finds the job stressful.

Examination

Examination is normal.

Interpretation of findings

The normal examination is reassuring, because it suggests no underlying pathology. The new events strongly suggest a psychogenic non-epileptic attack. The abrupt onset of very frequent events, the non-specific vague depersonalisation at the onset, the unusual circling behaviour, the very prolonged shaking, the tearfulness and the rapid recovery all point towards a non-epileptic attack rather than a seizure.

Investigations

Jane undergoes a short video EEG, during which she has a typical attack. During the attack, her EEG is normal. No other investigations are organised.

Diagnosis

A normal EEG taken during an attack enables confident diagnosis of a non-epileptic attack. Non-epileptic attacks are common in people with epilepsy and frequently occur in the context of significant life stress.

Case 5 *continued*

The diagnosis is discussed with Jane, and it is explained that the attacks are likely to be a physical manifestation of psychological stress. A clinical neuropsychologist meets with her to discuss coping strategies and self-awareness techniques to help avoid further attacks. At first, she struggles to accept and understand the diagnosis. However, she engages well with therapy and the attacks subside.

Seizures and epilepsy

Seizures are a common neurological problem. They occur as a primary disease or as a result of damage to the central nervous system. Epilepsy is the tendency to have recurrent seizures.

Frequent seizures can have significant negative effects on work and social life, and much stigma is attached to the diagnosis of epilepsy. Treatment is often lifelong and includes medications with potentially severe adverse effects.

Epidemiology

Epilepsy has a prevalence rate of 0.5–1%, and an annual incidence of 20–50 per 100,000 in the UK. About 450,000 people in the UK have epilepsy, and there are about 30,000 new diagnoses each year. Worldwide around 50 million people have epilepsy.

- There is a peak in first presentations in children because of primary idiopathic epilepsies and developmental abnormalities
- A second peak incidence is in the elderly, because of acquired brain diseases such as stroke and dementia

Aetiology

Seizures can be symptomatic, idiopathic or cryptogenic (**Table 5.2**). Virtually any insult to the brain can lead to a single seizure or recurrent ones (**Table 5.3**). Focal structural brain lesions are likely to produce focal onset seizures rather than generalised onset seizures.

Idiopathic epilepsy usually has a strong genetic basis, with subtle differences in neurotransmitter receptors, neuromodulators and neural network formation conferring a predisposition to seizures.

Aetiological classification of seizures	
Category	Description
Symptomatic	A cause or provoking factor is identified
Idiopathic	No cause is identified
	There is often a strong inherited predisposition
Cryptogenic	A structural abnormality is suspected but not proven

Table 5.2 The aetiological classification of seizures

Pathogenesis

Electrical discharges between neurones are normally restricted and controlled by inhibitory interneurons and recurrent synaptic connections (see page 12). During an epileptic seizure, there is sudden and uncontrolled repetitive and synchronous activation of networks of neurones.

Structural brain lesions, such as a stroke, can cause abnormal neuronal connections and physiology that generate seizure activity.

The abnormal discharges can then lead to one of two types of seizure (**Table 5.4**).

Congenital and acquired causes of seizures		
Origin	Categories	Examples
Acquired	Infectious	Meningitis, encephalitis and brain abscess
	Neoplastic	Intracranial tumours
	Vascular	Scarring secondary to strokes or arteriovenous malformations
	Trauma	Cortical scarring after head injury
	Inflammatory	Vasculitic syndromes and autoimmune encephalitis
	Inherited	Tuberous sclerosis
	Degenerative	Alzheimer's disease
	Metabolic	Hypoxia, hypoglycaemia, electrolyte abnormalities, renal failure and liver failure
	Drugs and toxins	Alcohol and drug misuse or withdrawal
Congenital	Developmental anomalies	Cortical dysgenesis or dysplasia
	Prenatal factors	Intrauterine infections and maternal drug misuse
	Perinatal factors	Birth trauma and cerebral hypoxia

Table 5.3 Congenital and acquired causes of seizures

Seizure subtypes		
Type of seizure	Origin	Features
Partial onset	Focal brain region	Seizure aura or initial focal motor movements (e.g. initial hand jerking)
Primary generalised	No clear focus at onset	Sudden loss of consciousness without warning or aura, followed by tonic–clonic movements of arms and legs
Secondary generalised	Focal brain region, evolving to generalised	An initial partial seizure followed by a generalised seizure
Simple	Focal brain region	Preservation of awareness
Complex	Focal or generalised	Altered awareness

Table 5.4 Common seizure types

- A **partial seizure** is generated if the abnormal activity remains restricted to the area of onset or spreads to other anatomically connected areas of cortex
- A **generalised seizure** is produced if the abnormal activity becomes generalised to involve large areas of cerebral cortex

In primary generalised seizures, there is no clinical or EEG evidence of a focal area of onset. However, one or several areas of abnormal neuronal physiology or connection probably act as a focus, leading to an almost instant activation of widely distributed neuronal networks across the brain (**Figure 5.2**).

Clinical features

The sequence of events and experiences the patient has during each of their episodes are carefully assessed. Seizure semiology is a combination of the observed behaviour and the patient's subjective description. It allows seizures to be classified and the underlying lesion to be localised.

Seizures have three distinct phases: before, during and after the seizure (Latin: ictus). The details of these phases are elicited in the history (**Table 5.5** and **Figure 5.3**).

They are also characterised by whether they are focal or generalised, and simple or complex (**Table 5.4**).

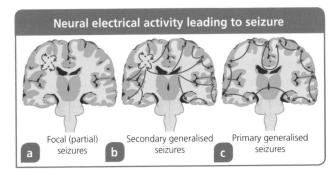

Neural electrical activity leading to seizure

Focal (partial) seizures | a
Secondary generalised seizures | b
Primary generalised seizures | c

Figure 5.2 (a) Focal (partial) seizures result from abnormal uncontrolled electrical activity in a localised region of the brain. (b) In secondary generalised seizures, the initial electrical activity originates in a focal region but spreads throughout the cortex to cause the generalised seizure. (c) In primary generalised seizures, the abnormal activity seems to occur without any initial focus, with the near simultaneous activation of widespread neural networks.

Phases of a seizure

Phase	Description
Preictal	A prodrome, lasting a few hours to days, precedes the seizure, varying from a few hours to days
	Dizziness, change in mood (e.g. irritability) or change in personality
Ictal	The seizure or attack itself
	The seizure may include an aura, which is the initial seizure
Post-ictal	The period after the seizure ends
	Drowsiness, headache, confusion and myalgia
	Possible secondary trauma

Table 5.5 The temporal course of a seizure

Urinary incontinence and tongue biting are not specific to seizures. They also occur in cases of collapse from other causes, such as syncope.

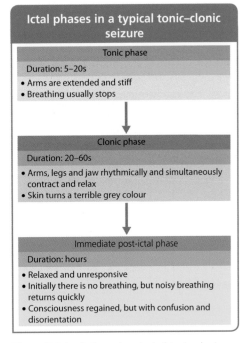

Ictal phases in a typical tonic–clonic seizure

Tonic phase
Duration: 5–20s
• Arms are extended and stiff
• Breathing usually stops

Clonic phase
Duration: 20–60s
• Arms, legs and jaw rhythmically and simultaneously contract and relax
• Skin turns a terrible grey colour

Immediate post-ictal phase
Duration: hours
• Relaxed and unresponsive
• Initially there is no breathing, but noisy breathing returns quickly
• Consciousness regained, but with confusion and disorientation

Figure 5.3 Ictal phases in a typical tonic–clonic seizure.

Auras

These stereotyped abnormal sensations (smell, taste, vision, etc.) or perceptions (fear, change in body size, etc.) are often experienced before more overt clinical seizure activity such as loss of consciousness. Auras are partial seizures; they represent abnormal activity in a relevant part of the brain. For example, rising epigastric sensation is an aura in temporal lobe epilepsy.

Localisation based on clinical features

Some clinical features suggest that a particular part of the brain is involved in a given seizure (**Table 5.6** and Figure 2.1). Therefore these features are asked about specifically.

Primary generalised seizures usually have few distinct clinical features, because they involve large areas of cortex. However, certain features characterise several distinct types of

Location and features of partial seizures		
Site of origin	Typical features	Examples
Temporal lobe	Memory disturbance	Déjà vu (feeling of familiarity)
		Jamais vu (feeling of non-familiarity)
	Psychic and emotional disturbance	Pain, terror, anger and elation
	Hallucinations	Olfactory (abnormal smells)
		Gustatory (abnormal tastes)
	Dysphasia	Receptive dysphasia
	Automatisms	Complex motor phenomena (e.g. lip smacking and chewing)
	Auditory dysfunction	Complex auditory hallucinations (e.g. the patient hears other people speaking to them, or abnormal music)
	Abdominal sensation	Rising epigastric sensation
Frontal lobe	Motor dysfunction	Usually involves contralateral face, trunk or limbs
		Abnormal motor movements (e.g. of head and eye, and postures)
	Dysphasia	Expressive dysphasia (inability to express speech)
	Behavioural dysfunction	Subtle changes in behaviour
Parietal lobe	Sensory dysfunction	Usually contralateral face, trunk or limbs
		Abnormal sensations (e.g. numbness and tingling)
	Motor symptoms	Usually caused by spread to motor cortex in frontal lobe
Occipital lobe	Visual dysfunction	Visual hallucinations (e.g. flashing lights)

Table 5.6 Typical clinical features associated with partial seizures originating from each of the major lobes

primary generalised seizure, including absence seizures, myoclonic seizures and atonic seizures (**Table 5.7**).

> Absence seizures are a type of generalised idiopathic epilepsy common in children younger than 10 years. Features include multiple daily seizures, an ictal phase in which the patient stares blankly into space for about 10–20 s, eye blinking and myoclonic jerks, and an EEG with 3 Hz (three per second) symmetrical spike-and-wave complexes in all leads.

Diagnostic approach

The diagnosis of epilepsy depends on an accurate and detailed eyewitness account. Most investigations are done to exclude certain causes, and the results are usually normal.

Differential diagnoses need to be excluded. Conditions that may mimic seizures include:

- other neurological disorders (e.g. transient ischaemic attacks, migraine, hyperventilation and panic attacks)
- cardiac syncope (loss of consciousness from a cardiovascular cause) as a result of arrhythmias or vasovagal attacks
- metabolic causes, including hypoglycaemia and electrolyte abnormalities (e.g. altered sodium level)
- psychogenic non-epileptic attack (seizure-like episodes occurring with normal EEG activity, often as a physical manifestation of psychological distress or trauma)

Syncope is a key differential diagnosis to exclude in seizure presentation, because its causes can be life-threatening. If syncope is suspected, investigations include:

- 12-lead electrocardiography, to exclude prolonged QT syndrome, Brugada's syndrome, ischaemic heart disease and arrhythmia

Clinical features of specific primary generalised seizures	
Phenotype	Description
Generalised tonic-clonic	Preictal: dizziness or irritability
	Ictal: loss of consciousness and fall to the ground
	■ Tonic phase: limbs stiffen with generalised muscle spasms ■ Clonic phase: repetitive muscle jerks Post-ictal: drowsiness, confusion and retrograde amnesia
Absence	Preictal: no warning
	Ictal: brief pause, during which the patient stops talking (usually 10–20 s), stares blankly into space and blinks their eyes; myoclonic jerks may occur
	Post-ictal: patient immediately resumes previous activity without any residual symptoms
Myoclonic	Myoclonic movements
Atonic (akinetic)	Ictal: sudden loss of muscle tone causing patient to fall to the ground; usually no loss of consciousness

Table 5.7 Clinical features typical of certain types of primary generalised seizure

- prolonged electrocardiographic monitoring, to exclude paroxysmal arrhythmias
- echocardiography, to exclude structural heart disease
- lying and standing blood pressure, to exclude postural hypotension

History

The exact nature and time course of events before, during and after the potential seizure should be established (**Table 5.8**). It is essential to distinguish seizures from syncope and non-epileptic attacks (**Table 5.9**).

A detailed medical and family history may reveal risk factors or causes of seizures. These include febrile convulsions, previous stroke and epilepsy in family members.

Social history is crucial, because the diagnosis may have implications for fitness to drive or employment.

Investigations

In the acute setting, in cases of first seizure, prolonged seizure in a patient with known epilepsy, or status epilepticus, a battery of investigations are required to exclude serious secondary causes. In the outpatient

Key questions to ask after a suspected seizure		
Preictal (leading up to the event)	Ictal (during the event)	Post-ictal (after the event)
What were they doing?	Did they lose awareness?	Did they go limp?
How or what did they feel?	Did they respond to a voice or other stimulation?	Did their colour change?
Did they get any warning?		How quickly did they start to become responsive?
Did they do anything strange?	Did they let out a scream or grunt?	
Did they make any movements or postures?	Did they fall to the ground?	Were they tearful?
	Did they make any movements?	Were they disoriented, tired or confused?
	Which body parts moved, how did they move and for how long?	How quickly did they get back to normal?
	Did they change colour?	
	How were they breathing?	

Table 5.8 Key questions to ask relating to the nature and time course of a suspected seizure

Distinguishing between seizures and non-epileptic attacks					
Feature	Epileptic seizure	Syncope			Psychogenic non-epileptic attack
		Cardiogenic	Vasovagal	Postural	
Aura or warning:	None, or olfactory, gustatory or gastrointestinal	Often none	Nausea, sweating, light-headedness or palpitations		Variable
Onset:	Sudden	Variable			
Duration:	Seconds to minutes	Seconds to minutes; protracted if sat upright after onset			Minutes to hours
Triggers:	Hyperventilation, sleeplessness, alcohol withdrawal and drugs	None or exertion	Cough, micturition or Valsalva's manoeuvre	Standing	None, or stress, anxiety or traumatic life events
Associated symptoms:	Sometimes autonomic symptoms	Palpitations, chest pain or breathlessness	Tunnelling of vision, dulling of hearing or tinnitus		Tearfulness or variable symptoms
Post-event confusion:	Variable, but often 10–30 min	Nil	Very brief		Variable; may be gradual offset, often short duration
Eyes:	Often open and deviated	Variable			Often held tightly closed

Table 5.9 Clinical features helpful in distinguishing epileptic seizure, syncope and psychogenic non-epileptic attacks

setting, the patient is generally medically well and there is less immediate concern about life-threatening causes. Nonetheless, secondary causes need to be excluded.

Blood tests

Routine biochemical and haematological tests are done to exclude a significant electrolyte disturbance or other serious cause. These tests include:

- full blood count (to identify any evidence of infection)
- measurement of urea and electrolytes, magnesium and calcium (to detect major electrolyte abnormalities)
- glucose measurement (to detect hypo- or hyperglycaemia)
- screening for drug misuse

Patients receiving antiepileptic medication require measurement of serum concentration of the drug to check adherence (if there is any doubt from the history) and if there are signs of drug toxicity. Measuring serum concentrations to guide doses is rarely helpful because therapeutic levels vary greatly from person to person. Phenytoin is an exception; measurement of levels of this drug is necessary to guide dosing.

Imaging

An acutely unwell patient presenting with new seizures or in status epilepticus first requires computerised tomography of the brain, because it is quick, widely available and can be carried out on an intubated and ventilated patient, if needed. The results can usually identify major pathology such as haemorrhage, tumour and abscess.

In an otherwise well patient, MRI is used to exclude any congenital or acquired brain lesion that may be a trigger. The results also inform prognosis and the selection of medical or surgical treatment.

Electroencephalography

A routine EEG is usually unhelpful, because 0.5% of the general population have epileptic abnormalities on an EEG, and 10% of people with epilepsy have a normal interictal (between seizure) EEG. However, this investigation is useful to:

■ identify a specific epilepsy syndrome, such as juvenile myoclonic epilepsy
■ assess and record interictal activity if seizures are very frequent (e.g. several per day) or reliably triggered
■ assess and record interictal activity over a few days in cases of diagnostic uncertainty or treatment resistance, or if surgery is being considered

> **Juvenile myoclonic epilepsy is a generalised idiopathic epilepsy syndrome.** Onset is typically in the teens, with a clinical triad of generalised myoclonic jerks (often on waking), daytime absence seizures and generalised tonic-clonic seizures.
>
> Photosensitivity is also common. EEG shows generalised spike-and-wave complexes. Remission is rare, and without medication the risk of recurrence is high.

Management

The aim of management is to prevent seizures with minimal medication and tolerable adverse effects.

Starting antiepileptic drugs after a single seizure does not reduce the proportion of people who go on to have further seizures. Half of all people who have a single unprovoked seizure never have another, so antiepileptic drugs are usually indicated only after a second unprovoked seizure.

Lifestyle changes

Patients should abstain from or reduce alcohol consumption and smoking, because these can precipitate seizures in patients with epilepsy. Sleep deprivation can also precipitate seizures and should be avoided.

Driving restrictions are a major difficulty for many patients. They must inform the Driver and Vehicle Licensing Agency or equivalent authority of their diagnosis. In the UK, restrictions last for at least 6 months and depend on the type of licence and other factors.

Medication

A wide range of anticonvulsant medications are available (**Table 5.10**). The decision on which to prescribe is based on:

■ the clinical pattern of the seizure, epilepsy syndrome or both
■ age and gender
■ comorbidities (e.g. renal or liver failure)
■ concurrent medication (e.g. warfarin or other anticoagulants, or the oral contraceptive pill)
■ preference in terms of adverse effects

Drugs used to manage seizures and epilepsy			
Seizure type		First-line drugs	Second-line drugs
Generalised	Tonic-clonic	Sodium valproate Lamotrigine	Levetiracetam Topiramate Clobazam
	Absence	Sodium valproate Ethosuximide	
	Myoclonic or atonic	Sodium valproate Lamotrigine	Levetiracetam Topiramate
Partial with or without secondary generalisation		Carbamazepine Sodium valproate Lamotrigine	Levetiracetam Topiramate Clobazam

Table 5.10 Pharmacological management of epileptic seizures, based on the clinical pattern of the seizure

Starting antiepileptic drugs

About 70% of patients achieve seizure remission with the first or second antiepileptic drug that is tried. Some of the remaining patients will not become seizure-free until a third or fourth antiepileptic drug is tried, or they may or need multiple antiepileptic drugs.

The general principles are to:

- use the minimum effective dose
- start at a low dose and build up slowly
- increase to maximally tolerated dose if the patient is still having seizures
- reduce slowly and stop before trying another first-line medication

Dual or triple therapy is required in a small proportion of patients.

Stopping or switching antiepileptic drugs

Patients or clinicians may want to stop or change antiepileptic drugs because of intolerable adverse effects, lack of benefit, or prolonged remission from seizures. This should be done only under expert supervision after consideration of seizure type and epileptic syndrome, personal circumstances and the likely impact of seizure recurrence (e.g. on employment and driving), adverse effects and duration of remission.

Antiepileptic drugs usually need slow titration down rather than sudden cessation; severe rebound seizures are a risk after withdrawal of some drugs, especially barbiturates and benzodiazepines.

> Some antiepileptic drugs induce liver enzymes, such as those in the cytochrome P450 system, that metabolise drugs. Enzyme induction can decrease the efficacy of other drugs, including contraceptive and anticoagulation medication. Always check for drug interactions before starting antiepileptic drug therapy.

Managing epilepsy in women

Consider the following points when treating female patients.

- Antiepileptic drugs interact with the contraceptive pill

- Antiepileptic drugs can have teratogenic effects and can cause intellectual disability in the patient's child
- Pregnancy often alters seizure frequency in women with epilepsy

Status epilepticus

The emergency management of status epilepticus is discussed on page 448.

Surgery

Some patients with medically refractory focal onset epilepsy benefit from surgical removal of the epileptogenic zone. This is indicated when a structural abnormality is shown by the EEG and clinical features to be the site of origin of the seizures, and functional MRI testing confirms that this zone is not required for essential cognitive function (e.g. language).

Surgery can reduce seizure frequency, allow drug dosage to be reduced and improve quality of life. Risks include central nervous system infection, haemorrhage, stroke, intellectual disability and death.

> Hemispherectomy is surgery to remove one half of the cerebral hemisphere or disconnect it from the other half. It is used in rare instances when predicted to stop seizure spread from one hemisphere to the other.

Prognosis

Half of patients who have a single seizure never have another. Of those who have multiple seizures, 70% achieve remission after trying one or two antiepileptic drugs; for most patients, epilepsy is a very treatable condition.

Patients with epilepsy have a mortality rate up to 3 times that of people without epilepsy. Mortality is higher even when deaths from accidental injury as a result of the seizure (e.g. drowning), the higher suicide rate, and other direct complications of seizures are taken into account. The reason for this is unknown.

Sudden unexpected death in epilepsy (SUDEP) is a fatality in a patient with epilepsy when no other cause is identified, despite a post-mortem. At 0.09 per 1000 patient-years, the risk is low but increases with epilepsy severity.

Answers to starter questions

1. Everyone has a seizure threshold, the level at which some form of neuronal insult will result in a clinical seizure. This threshold is lower in patients with epilepsy.

2. The risk of having a seizure cannot be removed but is lowered by treatment for epilepsy. Treatment through lifestyle changes, medications and sometimes surgery increases the threshold at which a seizure is triggered.

3. Epilepsy affects each patient differently. For some patients, it is a rare and inconvenient occurrence without significant effect on their life. For others, the prospect of a seizure haunts them and restricts their daily activities. For some, seizures occur daily but do not prohibit them from engaging with life. Always consider the effects of seizures on patients as individuals.

Chapter 6
Neurovascular disease

Starter questions

Answers to the following questions are on page 268.

1. Do people have 'silent strokes'?
2. Why does a stroke need rapid treatment?
3. Why is it important to treat transient ischaemic attacks?
4. Can rehabilitation reverse brain tissue damage?

Introduction

The term neurovascular disease encompasses all disorders affecting the vessels of the central nervous system. Neurovascular diseases arise as a result of:

- pathological changes affecting the vessels, e.g. acute and chronic occlusions of arteries or veins leading to ischaemia and ultimately, if blood flow does not normalise, infarction (death of brain tissue), or
- acquired or congenital structural abnormalities that increase the likelihood of vessels haemorrhaging intracranially or causing mass (or pressure) effect, e.g. arteriovenous malformations (which can cause any of these effects)

Stroke is the rapid onset of focal neurological deficits corresponding to dysfunction in specific vascular territories of the brain. It is the most common manifestation of neurovascular disease. Most strokes are due to cerebral ischaemia and infarction, almost always arterial rather than venous, but about a fifth are the result of intracranial arterial haemorrhage.

Stroke is the third most common cause of death after cardiac disease and cancer, and the commonest cause of neurological disability. Outcomes are greatly improved by immediate recognition and transfer for early treatment. Therefore the ability to recognise the more common presentations of stroke is essential for all doctors. 'Cerebrovascular' disease refers to vascular diseases affecting the cerebrum or cerebral hemispheres, but is used interchangeably with 'neurovascular' in practice.

Case 6 Blackout

Presentation

James Lau, a 38-year-old accountant, presents to the emergency department having collapsed at work.

Initial interpretation

Neurological and cardiac pathologies are very high on the list of causes of collapse (**Table 6.1**). The acute nature of James's symptoms suggests a vascular insult to the brain or heart.

History

James is drowsy and unable to provide a history. However, a colleague witnessed the event. James complained to him of a severe headache after going to the

Causes of sudden onset collapse	
System	Cause
Nervous system	Acute intracranial haemorrhage: subarachnoid, intracerebral (spontaneous or caused by an underlying lesion) or intraventricular
	Acute ischaemic stroke
	Seizure
	Acute hydrocephalus
Cardiac system	Acute myocardial infarction
	Acute arrhythmia
	Aortic dissection
	Cardiac arrest
Miscellaneous	Pulmonary embolism

Table 6.1 Common causes of sudden onset collapse

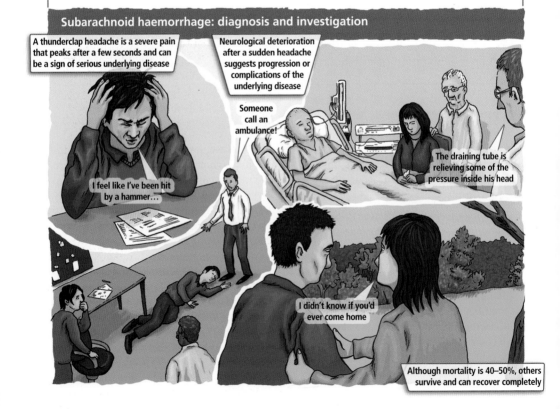

Subarachnoid haemorrhage: diagnosis and investigation

A thunderclap headache is a severe pain that peaks after a few seconds and can be a sign of serious underlying disease

Neurological deterioration after a sudden headache suggests progression or complications of the underlying disease

Someone call an ambulance!

The draining tube is relieving some of the pressure inside his head

I feel like I've been hit by a hammer...

I didn't know if you'd ever come home

Although mortality is 40–50%, others survive and can recover completely

bathroom. He had described it as the worst headache of his life. He complained of neck stiffness and of light hurting his eyes.

Interpretation of history

There are no features, such as chest pain or shortness of breath, to suggest a cardiac cause. The presentation is very typical for acute subarachnoid haemorrhage: rapid speed of onset, 'worst headache ever' description and meningism (neck stiffness and photophobia).

Further history

An hour later, James collapsed and was unresponsive for a few minutes. However, he recovered slowly afterwards. His colleagues say he did not have a seizure. An ambulance brought him to hospital. He has no medical or family history but is a heavy smoker.

Examination

After initial Advanced Life Support resuscitation and stabilisation, James's neurological status assessed. He opens his eyes to voice (eye response, E3), is confused (verbal response, V4) and obeys commands (motor response, M6), giving a total Glasgow coma scale score of 13/15. He has weakness down his left side, his pupils are equal and respond to light, and he has meningism with neck stiffness.

Interpretation of findings

The initial clinical history is consistent with aneurysmal subarachnoid haemorrhage. James's Glasgow coma scale score was 15 at first, but his subsequent collapse an hour later suggests possible complications after subarachnoid haemorrhage. The priorities are to:

- confirm the subarachnoid haemorrhage with computerised tomography (CT) of the brain
- investigate for an underlying vascular lesion, predominantly a cerebral aneurysm and less commonly an arteriovenous malformation

Investigations

An urgent brain CT scan confirms diffuse subarachnoid haemorrhage (**Figure 6.1**). There is blood in the ventricles (intraventricular haemorrhage), which increases the risk of hydrocephalus. On the unenhanced scan is a blister, which suggests a right middle cerebral artery aneurysm as the cause.

Diagnosis

James initially had a ruptured middle cerebral artery aneurysm with subarachnoid

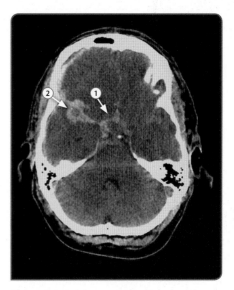

Figure 6.1 Axial computerised tomography, without contrast, at the level of the basal cisterns. Extensive subarachnoid haemorrhage is visible near the circle of Willis ①. The blister in the right Sylvian fissure suggests a middle cerebral artery aneurysm ②.

Case 6 *continued*

haemorrhage. The subsequent collapse was probably a consequence of acute complications of aneurysmal subarachnoid haemorrhage:

- rerupture and rebleeding
- acute hydrocephalus (likely in this case because of the intraventricular haemorrhage, which occludes cerebrospinal fluid pathways)
- seizures

Complications such as vasospasm (see page 261) and electrolyte abnormalities, especially hyponatraemia, usually occur few days later.

James is urgently referred to neurosurgery. CT angiography confirms the aneurysm location. Medical management measures for acute subarachnoid haemorrhage are initiated (**Table 6.2**), and he undergoes a cerebrospinal fluid diversion procedure to relieve the hydrocephalus. He subsequently undergoes interventional neuroradiological coil embolisation of the aneurysm.

Medical management of subarachnoid haemorrhage	
Therapy	Rationale
Nimodipine (60 mg every 4 h for 21 days)	Reduces risk of cerebral vessel vasoconstriction and consequent ischaemia and infarction (risk is increased after aneurysmal subarachnoid haemorrhage)
Adequate hydration (3 L/24 h with intravenous normal, 0.9%, saline)	Prevents dehydration and consequent reduced cerebral perfusion, which increases risk of ischaemia and infarction
Monitoring and regulation of blood pressure	Acutely the body autoregulates blood pressure, so optimal blood pressure targets are uncertain
	Excessive reduction in blood pressure can precipitate ischaemia and infarction due to impaired blood flow
	Excessive increased blood pressure before the aneurysm has been treated risks repeat rupture and rebleeding
	A balance between these two extremes is required
Monitoring and treatment of complications	Reduce risk of and treat:
	■ rebleeding
	■ vasospasm
	■ hydrocephalus
	■ seizures
	■ electrolyte (especially sodium) abnormalities (e.g. hyponatraemia)
	■ cardiac complications (e.g. neurogenic pulmonary oedema and myocardial infarction)

Table 6.2 Acute subarachnoid haemorrhage: medical management measures instituted as soon as haemorrhage has been diagnosed

Case 7 Sudden onset weakness

Presentation

Sheila Patterson, aged 68 years, suddenly develops right-sided face, arm and leg weakness and numbness while out shopping. The acute stroke team assess her and confirm the time of onset as 45 min ago.

Initial interpretation

Sudden onset unilateral weakness and numbness represent disruption of motor and sensory function in the left hemisphere, for which the most likely cause is an acute stroke. Further assessment is needed to identify which other brain regions are affected, and thereby classify the stroke syndrome and determine suitability for thrombolysis ('clot busting') to reopen the blocked artery.

History

Mrs Patterson has hypertension, for which she takes an angiotensin-converting enzyme inhibitor. She was otherwise well and fully independent before the event. She cannot feel her right side and denies other neurological symptoms. Her daughter, who is with her, confirms this.

Interpretation of history

Time of onset is clear from a witnessed history. Right-sided weakness and numbness without other symptoms could be from a lacunar stroke, damaging internal capsule fibres carrying motor and sensory pathways to and from the cortex, or partial anterior circulation stroke, damaging a wider area including the sensory and motor cortices. Hypertension is a risk factor for stroke, and there are no contraindications for thrombolysis in the history.

Further history

Mrs Patterson denies a hemianopia, language disturbance, diplopia, vertigo and headache. The absence of these other symptoms make partial or total anterior circulation stroke unlikely. She has had no recent surgery, rectal bleeding, haemoptysis, haematemesis or chest pain, which would have suggested occult gastrointestinal or pulmonary haemorrhage, or aortic dissection; these conditions are contraindications to thrombolysis.

Examination

Mrs Patterson has right-sided flaccid paralysis of her face, arm and leg. Her Glasgow coma scale score is 15/15, and cranial nerve function is normal. She has no visual field defect, neglect or language disturbance. There are brisk reflexes and up-going (extensor) plantar on the right. Blood pressure is 175/98 mmHg, with normal sinus rhythm on electrocardiogram.

Interpretation of findings

A clinical diagnosis of a left (side of brain lesion) lacunar stroke can be made: right-sided weakness and sensory loss of rapid onset, and absence of signs indicating involvement of other cortical or brain stem regions. This localises the stroke to the left internal capsule or basal ganglia. Hypertension is the only risk factor identified. She has no contraindications to thrombolysis (see **Table 6.7**). Her stroke is significantly disabling. She requires an immediate brain CT scan to exclude an intracerebral haemorrhage before thrombolysis.

Investigation

Computerised tomography reveals a left basal ganglia haemorrhage (**Figure 6.2**). No other imaging is required, because the location of the haemorrhage in the presence of appropriate risk factors is typical for hypertension. When the location is

Case 7 *continued*

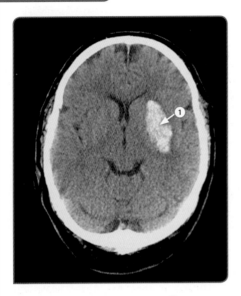

Figure 6.2 Acute hyperdense clot ① confirming left acute basal ganglia haemorrhagic stroke, probably related to hypertension.

atypical for hypertension, a CT angiogram may be done to exclude an underlying vascular malformation, or a delayed MRI (e.g. few months later) to exclude an underlying tumour.

Diagnosis

Thrombolysis is not given to Mrs Patterson, because this would worsen the underlying pathological process of haemorrhage. Her blood pressure is closely monitored during the acute phase to avoid dangerous extremes: if too high, extension of haemorrhage usually occurs; if too low, underperfusion of vulnerable tissue with subsequent infarction. She receives intensive inpatient physiotherapy, speech therapy and occupational therapy to improve her functional recovery. She is then discharged on an additional antihypertensive agent and a statin for secondary prevention.

Ischaemic and haemorrhagic stroke

Stroke describes the sudden (seconds to minutes) onset of focal symptoms or signs of brain dysfunction arising from ischaemia, infarction or haemorrhage localised to a specific vascular territory. The neurological deficits persist for ≥ 24 h.

Stroke symptoms or signs that resolve completely within 24 h represent a transient ischaemic attack, which is discussed in detail in pages 254–256. The early risk of stroke after transient ischaemic attack is high (7-day risk, 8–12%; 30-day risk, 18%).

The annual incidence of stroke is 240 in 100,000 in the UK.

Aetiology and pathogenesis

About 80% of strokes are ischaemic and usually caused by near-complete occlusion

of a cerebral vessel. The obstruction impairs the delivery of oxygen and nutrients to brain tissue, thereby causing tissue damage and neurological dysfunction. If vascular supply is not restored, infarction ('death') of brain tissue ensues.

The remaining 20% of strokes are haemorrhagic. In haemorrhagic stroke, blood vessels rupture, resulting in acute bleeding into brain substance.

Table 6.3 summarises risk factors for strokes. Identifying and targeting these for therapy remains the cornerstone of stroke management.

Ischaemic stroke

Vascular occlusion most often occurs because of thromboembolism: thrombosis (formation of a blood clot, 'thrombus') and embolisation (fragments of the blood clot travelling downstream).

Risk factors for acute ischaemic stroke	
Risk factor	Relative risk of developing stroke
Hypertension 160/95 mmHg compared with 120/80 mmHg	7
Age > 75 years compared with 55–64 years	5
Atrial fibrillation	5
Previous transient ischaemic attack or stroke	5
Ischaemic heart disease	3
Diabetes	2
Smoking	2

Table 6.3 Major risk factors for acute ischaemic stroke

Three factors precipitate thrombosis (Virchow's triad). They are:

- stasis of blood
- vessel wall changes (i.e. injury to endothelium)
- changes in blood constituency (e.g. blood hypercoagulability, an abnormal increase in blood-clotting tendency)

Any pathological process increasing these factors can lead to vascular thrombosis.

Atherosclerosis

The commonest cause of arterial thrombo-embolism is atherosclerosis, a progressive inflammatory thickening of arterial walls. Atherosclerosis begins with endothelial injury, which leads to growing 'plaques' of white blood cells, fat deposits and eventual calcification. It occurs with normal ageing but is increased by smoking, hypertension, diabetes and excessive blood cholesterol.

The atherosclerotic plaque increasingly occludes the artery as it grows. It can become unstable and rupture leading to acute clot (thrombi) formation that completely occlude the artery (thrombosis). Alternatively, a fragment (an embolus) may break off and occlude a vessel downstream of the plaque (**Figure 6.3**).

Cardioembolism

Acute clots may also form in the heart because of changes in blood flow, for example in patients with arrhythmias (such as atrial fibrillation), valvular heart disease, prosthetic heart valves and congenital defects, or after myocardial infarction. These clots may embolise to cerebral arteries, thereby causing an ischaemic stroke (cardioembolism).

Embolism

Most ischaemic strokes result from clots originating from atherosclerotic plaques (atherothromboembolism) or the heart (cardioembolism). However, rarely, other substances can embolise to the brain. These include tumour, septic (infective), air and fat emboli.

Other conditions

Various conditions increase the likelihood of ischaemic stroke, including:

- inflammatory vascular diseases (e.g. vasculitic syndromes such as polyarteritis nodosa and granulomatosis with polyangiitis, previously called Wegener's granulomatosis)
- collagen vascular diseases (e.g. rheumatoid arthritis and Marfan's syndrome)
- infection (e.g. syphilis, HIV, meningitis and tuberculosis)
- arterial dissection (rupture in the vessel wall occurring spontaneously or because of trauma or predisposed weakness)
- blood diseases predisposing to excessive clotting (thrombophilias and polycythaemia)

Haemorrhagic stroke

Most haemorrhagic strokes are intracerebral (75%); the remaining 25% are subarachnoid. Haemorrhage precipitates:

- loss of cerebrovascular autoregulation
- disruption of the blood–brain barrier
- cerebral oedema (cytotoxic and vasogenic)
- neuronal damage caused by the toxicity of blood products and mass effect of an acute blood clot
- increase in intracranial pressure
- hydrocephalus if the haemorrhage ruptures into the ventricular system

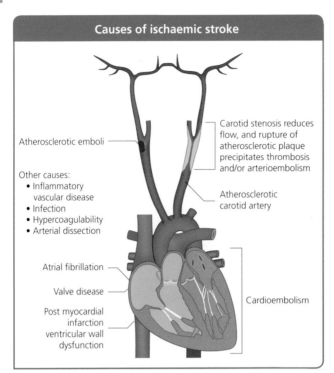

Figure 6.3 Causes of ischaemic stroke.

Causes of ischaemic stroke

Atherosclerotic emboli

Other causes:
• Inflammatory vascular disease
• Infection
• Hypercoagulability
• Arterial dissection

Carotid stenosis reduces flow, and rupture of atherosclerotic plaque precipitates thrombosis and/or arterioembolism

Atherosclerotic carotid artery

Atrial fibrillation

Valve disease

Cardioembolism

Post myocardial infarction ventricular wall dysfunction

The most common cause of spontaneous subarachnoid haemorrhage is rupture of an intracranial aneurysm.

Intracerebral haemorrhage

The commonest cause of spontaneous intracerebral haemorrhage is rupture of small cerebral vessels (perforating arteries) with walls weakened by hypertension. Other causes include:

■ arteriovenous malformations (see page 263)
■ amyloid angiopathy (degenerative blood vessel weakening as a result of amyloid deposition)
■ aneurysm (see page 257) rupture
■ tumours (haemorrhage in an intracranial tumour is sometimes its initial presentation)
■ clotting dysfunction (e.g. from the use of anticoagulant or antiplatelet drugs, or after thrombolytic therapy for ischaemic stroke)
■ haemorrhage secondary to intracranial vein thrombosis

Clinical features

History and examination are crucial to confirm signs and symptoms, identify risk factors and broadly localise the lesion. Acute stroke services are contacted in all cases of suspected stroke to arrange urgent assessment, investigation and management.

The hallmark of stroke, as with most neurovascular pathologies, is the sudden and rapid onset of neurological dysfunction.

Oxford classification of stroke

The Oxford classification divides stroke into four categories correlating the clinical features arising from dysfunction in brain regions with the main blood vessels affected (**Table 6.4**). It is the most commonly used classification in the clinical assessment of acute stroke patients, because it is easy and quick to do, and the results are highly reproducible.

Anterior circulation syndromes

These syndromes affect brain regions supplied by the internal carotid arteries and its

Oxford classification of stroke	
Syndrome	**Features**
Total anterior circulation syndrome (TACS)	All of: ■ motor or sensory deficit* (usually contralateral) ■ hemianopia (visual field deficit - usually contralateral homonymous hemianopia) ■ higher cortical dysfunction†
Partial anterior circulation syndrome (PACS)	Two of: ■ motor or sensory deficit* ■ hemianopia ■ higher cortical dysfunction†
Lacunar syndrome	One of: ■ pure motor deficit* (lesion usually in posterior limb of internal capsule) ■ pure sensory deficit* (lesion usually in thalamus) ■ sensory and motor deficit* ■ ataxic hemiparesis (ataxia and hemiparesis affecting the same side; lesion usually in ventral pons with pontocerebellar fibre disruption) ■ Without either: ■ higher cortical dysfunction† ■ posterior circulation syndrome symptoms
Posterior circulation syndrome (POCS)	Any of: ■ isolated hemianopia (lesion in occipital lobe) ■ bilateral motor and sensory deficit ■ brain stem signs and symptoms ■ cranial nerve deficits (e.g. diplopia, facial sensory loss, lower motor neurone facial nerve palsy, vertigo, hearing loss, dysphagia and dysarthria) ■ cerebellar signs and symptoms (e.g. ataxia, nystagmus, past pointing, intention tremor, dysarthria and slurred speech)

*Affecting the face, arm or leg (independently or in combination)

†Higher cortical dysfunction gives rise to various deficits that depend on whether the dominant or non-dominant hemisphere is affected.

Table 6.4 The Oxford classification system for stroke

major terminal branches i.e. the anterior cerebral and middle cerebral arteries.

Posterior circulation syndromes
These affect brain regions supplied by the vertebrobasilar vessels and their associated branches: the vertebral, basilar, posterior inferior cerebellar, anterior inferior cerebellar, superior cerebellar and posterior cerebral arteries.

Lacunar syndromes
These syndromes affect brain regions supplied by deep penetrating perforator arteries from either the anterior or posterior circulation. These arteries supply deep white matter, for example the internal capsule, or deep subcortical structures, such as the thalamus and basal ganglia. 'Lacunar' derives from 'lacunae', the

small cerebrospinal fluid–filled spaces in the deep grey matter.

Posterior circulation syndromes can present with a bewildering range of clinical findings. This variety is a consequence of brain stem involvement; many motor, sensory and cranial nuclei and nerve tracts can be affected.

Hemispheric dominance
The clinical pattern of higher cortical deficits also indicates whether the hemisphere involved is dominant or non-dominant (see page 43).

With involvement of the dominant hemisphere (usually the left):

- the patient has insight
- they may also have aphasia and difficulty reading, writing and calculating

If the non-dominant hemisphere (usually the right) is involved:

- the patient lacks insight
- they may have neglect, spatial disorientation and apraxias (e.g. difficulty dressing and constructional apraxia)

Specific vascular territories

The Oxford classification localises the lesion to a broad vascular territory. However, more specific syndromes from dysfunction of specific vessels usually present with stereotypical deficits (see **Table 6.5**).

Distinguishing between ischaemic and haemorrhagic stroke

It is difficult to differentiate between ischaemic and haemorrhagic stroke on the basis of clinical assessment alone. For example, headache is more common with haemorrhage than with ischaemia. Neuroimaging is the definitive way to distinguish between the two.

> **Some haemorrhagic strokes have a characteristic constellation of symptoms.** For example, some posterior communicating artery aneurysms compress cranial nerve III to produce a third nerve palsy. Its clinical features are ptosis, restriction of the movement of eye muscles innervated by the nerve, pain in the eye (or head) and a dilated pupil from compression of the nerve's parasympathetic fibres.

Diagnostic approach

The principles of stroke assessment are shown in **Figure 6.4**. Early referral to acute stroke services is crucial for assessment, evaluation of suitability for thrombolysis, investigation and coordinating management.

Differential diagnoses for stroke include:

- hypoglycaemia and hyperglycaemia
- complicated migraine (with prominence of atypical features for stroke: migraine

history, positive visual phenomena and paraesthesia)
- sepsis (especially in the elderly)
- seizures
- metabolic abnormalities (e.g. electrolyte disturbances and hepatic encephalopathy)
- drug overdose or effects of toxins
- other intracranial lesions (e.g. abscess, tumour, acute hydrocephalus and pneumocephalus)

Investigations

Urgent CT is used to differentiate ischaemic and haemorrhagic stroke. It is also used to identify other intracranial pathology. Acute management is then started.

Most infarcts are caused by emboli from arterial or cardiac thrombi (atherothromboembolism or cardioembolism, respectively) in a patient with significant cardiovascular risk factors such as hypertension, smoking and diabetes. Younger patients may have a rare cause of their infarct, necessitating extensive investigation after acute management.

Imaging in ischaemic stroke

The CT scan can be normal in the first few hours after an ischaemic stroke, especially in cases of posterior circulation syndromes. It can take up to 24 h for infarction to become well established on CT (**Figure 6.5**). Early subtle features of stroke to identify in an initially normal-looking CT are:

- sulcal effacement (the cortical sulci lose definition because of subtle oedema)
- loss of grey-white differentiation (oedema causes subtle loss of this distinction, especially in the basal ganglia and insular cortex)
- dense middle cerebral artery (an occluded middle cerebral artery appears hyperdense on CT)

Magnetic resonance imaging is more sensitive; it may confirm acute ischaemia in a patient whose CT scan is normal. Special sequences, such as diffusion-weighted imaging, show acute ischaemia in its earliest stages (**Figure 6.6**).

Further imaging includes:

- carotid imaging (ultrasound, CT or magnetic resonance angiography) to assess for atherosclerotic narrowing of carotid arteries

- cardiac echocardiography to assess for valvular heart disease, congenital defects and possible thrombi or embolic sources in the presence of arrhythmias
- digital subtraction cerebral angiography to assess cerebral vascular stenosis

Stroke syndromes	
Affected vessel	**Classic clinical features**
Anterior cerebral artery	Contralateral lower limb motor and sensory deficit
	Urinary or bladder sphincter disturbance (e.g. incontinence)
	Behavioural change and disinhibition
Middle cerebral artery	Contralateral motor deficit (face and upper limb affected mainly, with relative sparing of lower limb)
	Contralateral sensory deficit
	Higher cortical dysfunction
	Contralateral hemianopia
Vertebral artery*	Occlusion of one side is usually compensated by anastomoses
	If the other vertebral artery is hypoplastic (congenitally narrow), occlusion is similar to basilar artery occlusion
Basilar artery†	Total basilar occlusion:
	■ coma (midbrain damage)
	■ bilateral motor and sensory dysfunction (major tracts)
	■ cerebellar signs
	■ cranial nerve signs
	■ top of basilar occlusion is similar to posterior cerebral artery occlusion
Posterior inferior cerebellar artery	Contralateral:
	■ loss of pain and temperature sensation in body (spinothalamic tract)
	Ipsilateral:
	■ loss of pain and temperature in face (CN V)
	■ vertigo (CN VIII)
	■ nystagmus and ataxia (cerebellar tracts)
	■ dysphagia and dysarthria (CN IX and CN X)
	■ Horner's syndrome (sympathetic chain)
Posterior cerebral artery	Cortical occlusion:
	■ contralateral homonymous hemianopia (occipital lobe)
	■ memory disturbance (temporal lobe)
	Thalamic damage:
	■ chorea or hemiballismus movements with contralateral hemisensory loss
	Midbrain damage:
	■ gaze palsies
	■ pupillary abnormalities
	■ reduced consciousness level

CN, cranial nerve.

*The posterior inferior cerebellar artery is usually a branch of the vertebral artery.

†The anterior inferior cerebellar, superior cerebellar and posterior cerebral arteries are branches of the basilar artery; many perforators also originate from the basilar artery and supply the brain stem.

Table 6.5 Typical symptoms and signs associated with specific stroke syndromes

Imaging in haemorrhagic stroke

Computerised tomography rapidly localises the haemorrhage. It also visualises associated complications such as intraventricular extension of haemorrhage and mass effect.

If aneurysm or arteriovenous malformation is suspected, CT angiography, magnetic resonance angiography or digital subtraction cerebral angiography is essential. Haemorrhagic transformation (when an area of ischaemic brain becomes fragile and bleeds) can also occur after acute thrombosis, for example in sinuses or cortical veins.

An MRI scan is often done 6–8 weeks after treatment of haemorrhagic stroke, especially in younger patients. This is because acute haemorrhage may initially hide and thus prevent detection of an underlying tumour or vascular lesion such as aneurysm and arteriovenous malformation.

Electrocardiography

This is used to identify cardiac arrhythmias as either a mimic of stroke, such as heart block leading to collapse, or a cause, for example atrial fibrillation precipitating embolic stroke.

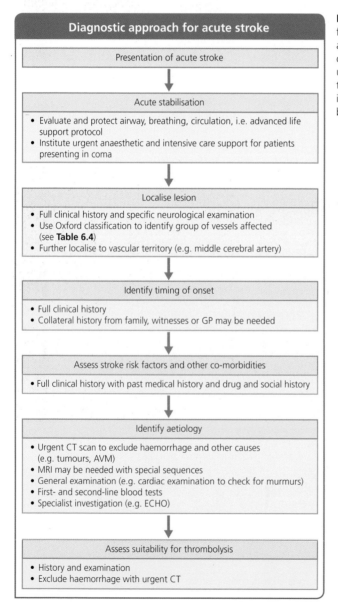

Figure 6.4 Diagnostic approach for a patient presenting with acute stroke. Identification of the cause may have to be delayed until after acute management. If thrombolysis is being considered, it is critical to exclude haemorrhage by urgent imaging.

Diagnostic approach for acute stroke

Presentation of acute stroke

Acute stabilisation
- Evaluate and protect airway, breathing, circulation, i.e. advanced life support protocol
- Institute urgent anaesthetic and intensive care support for patients presenting in coma

Localise lesion
- Full clinical history and specific neurological examination
- Use Oxford classification to identify group of vessels affected (see **Table 6.4**)
- Further localise to vascular territory (e.g. middle cerebral artery)

Identify timing of onset
- Full clinical history
- Collateral history from family, witnesses or GP may be needed

Assess stroke risk factors and other co-morbidities
- Full clinical history with past medical history and drug and social history

Identify aetiology
- Urgent CT scan to exclude haemorrhage and other causes (e.g. tumours, AVM)
- MRI may be needed with special sequences
- General examination (e.g. cardiac examination to check for murmurs)
- First- and second-line blood tests
- Specialist investigation (e.g. ECHO)

Assess suitability for thrombolysis
- History and examination
- Exclude haemorrhage with urgent CT

Blood tests

Hypoglycaemia can cause rapid onset focal neurological deficits. Therefore serum glucose concentration is always measured.

Other tests depend on the suspected cause.

- First-line tests (e.g. measurement of glucose, cholesterol and electrolytes) are carried out to guide acute management and ascertain risk factors
- Second-line tests (e.g. thrombophilia screen, blood cultures and vasculitic screen) are done to assess the rare causes of strokes

Management

Acute stroke management is divided into general principles (**Table 6.6**) and specific interventions.

Treatment is conservative in most patients with spontaneous haemorrhagic stroke not caused by aneurysm or arteriovenous malformation.

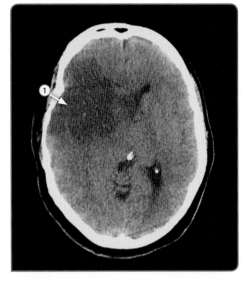

Figure 6.5 Axial non-contrast computerised tomography 24 h after symptom onset. The initial scan was normal. However, this scan shows an established right middle cerebral artery infarct ① with an extensive area of hypodensity.

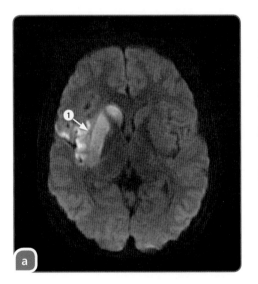

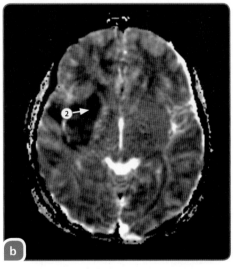

Figure 6.6 Axial magnetic resonance imaging: (a) diffusion-weighted imaging (DWI) and (b) apparent diffusion coefficient (ADC) sequences from the same patient. These were obtained immediately after normal computerised tomography (CT) and in the early stages show restricted diffusion: high bright signal on DWI ① and low dark signal on ADC ② in the right middle cerebral artery territory. Signs of ischaemia and infarction can be detected on DWI much earlier than on CT.

Medication

Medical management of stroke utilises a combination of pharmacological agents to limit the severity of ischaemic injury and mainly secondary prevention with control of risk factors.

Acute ischaemic stroke

The aim is to salvage the 'ischaemic penumbra' and limit the spread of infarction. The penumbra is the tissue surrounding the infarcted regions that has reduced blood flow and is still functional.

Thrombolysis Also called 'clot busting', thrombolysis is beneficial in patients with a major stroke and a large ischaemic penumbra. Intravenous recombinant tissue plasminogen activator (alteplase) is given within 3.5 h of onset of stroke symptoms to reperfuse ischaemic tissue. The benefit is less disability at 3 months rather than acute symptom reversal; the earlier it is given, i.e. within 90 minutes, the better the outcome.

Acute stroke management		
Principle	Aim(s)	Management method(s)
Treatment location	To improve survival (management in dedicated stroke units reduces mortality by 30%)	Admission to stroke unit or intensive care unit
Airway	To avoid hypoxia or aspiration and maintain a patent airway	Airway measures and anaesthetic support in cases of coma
BP control	Optimal management uncertain, because the brain may attempt to autoregulate Treatment of even high levels of BP may harm by compromising cerebral perfusion	Treat if complications of hypertension (e.g. hypertensive encephalopathy, aortic dissection and cardiac failure) are present If sustained, treat BP > 220/120 mmHg in ischaemic and BP > 185/115 mmHg in haemorrhagic stroke
Glucose control	In acute stroke, avoid hyperglycaemia, which is associated with poor outcome	Aim for normal levels
Hydration and nutritional support	To prevent dehydration To ensure good nutritional support	Intravenous fluids Nasogastric feeding if patient dysphagic
Deep vein thrombosis prophylaxis	Prevention of deep vein thromboses and associated pulmonary embolism as a result of immobility following stroke	Timing of initiation of prophylactic clexane following stroke is commonly debated. Most will start clexane 48–72 h following acute ischaemic stroke. Timing of clexane initiation following haemorrhagic stroke is more controversial Intermittent use of pneumatic compression stockings as mechanical prophylaxis
Seizures	To reduce risk of focal or generalised seizure (which occur in about 2% of patients)	Antiepileptic drugs as required
Physiotherapy	To prevent contractures To restore function To prevent pressure sores	Early mobilisation Early rehabilitation referral Strategies to cope with impairment
Neuropsychiatric complications	To prevent depression	Antidepressants
Communication	To ensure good communication with patients and family members	Set realistic goals
BP, blood pressure.		

Table 6.6 General principles in the management of acute stroke that apply to all types of ischaemic and haemorrhagic stroke (except aneurysmal subarachnoid haemorrhage)

> **The major complication of thrombolysis** is precipitation of acute haemorrhage in an ischaemic or infarcted region.

Thrombolysis should only be undertaken in specialised centres because of the number of contraindications (**Table 6.7**) and the potential severity of adverse events.

Antiplatelet agents These inhibit platelet activity. Unless imaging shows primary haemorrhage, antiplatelet agents are initiated after acute ischaemic stroke. Aspirin within 48 h acts as secondary prevention; it reduces mortality and recurrent stroke. It is given for 2 weeks, and then clopidogrel, another antiplatelet, is given lifelong.

Anticoagulant agents These inhibit the clotting cascade. Antiplatelet agents are replaced after 2 weeks with warfarin anticoagulation in patients with chronic non-valvular non-rheumatic atrial fibrillation or a cardioembolic cause such as prosthetic heart valve. It is superior to antiplatelet agents in reducing ischaemic stroke risk in these patients; thus it provides both primary and secondary prevention. Anticoagulation does more harm than good in other causes of ischaemic stroke.

Acute haemorrhagic stroke
There are no specific medical treatments for most causes of haemorrhagic stroke, except subarachnoid haemorrhage (see **Table 6.2**). All antiplatelet and anticoagulant drugs are stopped, and coagulation deficits are corrected. Monitoring of blood pressure and for increased ICP is needed.

Surgery

This is rarely indicated in ischaemic stroke. However, it may be life-saving in a few clinical scenarios.

Acute ischaemic stroke
Early neurosurgical referral is indicated for posterior fossa and malignant middle cerebral artery infarctions.

Posterior fossa (cerebellar) infarction
This can cause rapid neurological deterioration because of the small volume of space in the posterior fossa. It can also result in acute hydrocephalus and tonsillar herniation with brain stem compression.

Patients whose neurological examination indicates deterioration, and with hydrocephalus and brain stem compression, may benefit from surgical treatment to relieve hydrocephalus by cerebrospinal fluid diversion and subsequent decompressive surgery.

Malignant middle cerebral artery infarction
Complete occlusion of the terminal internal carotid artery or main stem of the middle cerebral artery occurs in 10% of strokes. It results in massive middle cerebral artery territory stroke.

Within 48 h, patients develop severely increased intracranial pressure with cytotoxic

Contraindications to thrombolysis	
Clinical feature	Contraindications
Presentation	Onset unclear or > 3.5 h ago
	Seizure since onset
	Invasive or surgical procedure in previous 3 weeks
	Cardiopulmonary resuscitation
	Pregnancy or recent obstetric delivery
	Minor symptoms or improving
	Significant premorbid dependence
Bleeding disorder	Previous intracranial haemorrhage
	Active bleeding
	Active peptic ulcer or gastrointestinal bleeding
	Current anticoagulation use or $< 100 \times 10^9$ platelets/L
	Severe liver disease or varices, or portal hypertension
Cranial disorder	Stroke in preceding 3 months
	Structural cerebrovascular disease (e.g. aneurysm or arteriovenous malformation)
	Major infarct or haemorrhage on computerised tomography
Cardiac disorder	Aortic dissection
	Severe hypertension (blood pressure > 220/130 mmHg)

Table 6.7 Contraindications to thrombolysis

oedema. Untreated, mortality is 80% with malignant cerebral oedema leading to intractable ICP elevation with subsequent brain herniation.

The results of a few studies have shown that decompressive hemicraniectomy (removal of part of the skull on the side of the infarction) decreases mortality, excess intracranial pressure and herniation (**Figure 6.7**). However, the effect on patients' quality of life is unclear.

Acute haemorrhagic stroke

All cases of haemorrhagic stroke require urgent discussion with a neurosurgeon.

In intraventricular haemorrhage, supportive measures such as cerebrospinal fluid diversion may be required. Patients with cerebellar haemorrhage may be treated conservatively or with surgery (either cerebrospinal fluid diversion via external ventricular drainage in isolation, or in combination with decompressive surgery). The choice depends on the degree of hydrocephalus and brain stem compression, and the patient's neurological status.

Patients with ruptured aneurysms or other intracranial arterial tears, ruptures and dissections urgently require surgical clipping, or endovascular intervention (e.g. coiling, stenting, vascular flow-diversion) (see page 259).

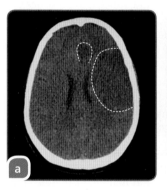 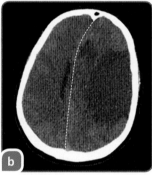 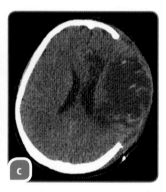

Figure 6.7 Malignant ischaemic infarction with subsequent decompressive craniectomy. (a) The initial computerised tomography scan demonstrates very early features that suggest an ischaemic event has occurred and there is a high risk of infarction. Note the subtle low density changes occurring in the left cerebral hemisphere in comparison to the right side. The patient was alert at this point. (b) Only 36 h later, the patient's consciousness level deteriorated, they became obtunded and seizures developed. Repeat CT showed a more established infarct, with swelling and midline shift to the right (dotted line) and compression of the left lateral ventricle. (c) After decompressive hemicraniectomy, the midline shift had resolved, the ventricle was visible again and the swollen tissue has space to expand and protrudes from the skull defect. The decompression helps prevent life-threatening cerebral herniation from intractable intracranial pressure in elevation.

Transient ischaemic attack

In a transient ischaemic attack, the acute symptoms and signs of neurological dysfunction from a vascular occlusion resolve completely within 24 h. However, the occurrence of a 'mini stroke' suggests systemic atherosclerotic vascular disease and a high risk of major stroke:

- 15% of first strokes are preceded by transient ischaemic attacks
- 8–12% is the 7-day stroke risk after a transient ischaemic attack

- 18% is the 30-day stroke risk after a transient ischaemic attack

Prompt investigation and intervention are essential. The latter includes secondary prevention, which reduces the 90-day stroke risk to:

- 10% if started within 3 weeks of a transient ischaemic attack
- 2% if started within 72 h

Epidemiology

The annual incidence of transient ischaemic attack is 35 per 100,000 in the UK.

Aetiology

The causes of transient ischaemic attacks are identical to those of 'ischaemic' strokes. The commonest causes are atherothromboembolism and cardioembolism.

Clinical features

As in a stroke, the features depend on the vascular territory affected. Most features resolve within 20 min. Systemic clinical examination is crucial to identifying aetiology. Listen for cardiac murmurs, assess for arrhythmias (especially atrial fibrillation) and auscultate for carotid bruit.

Amaurosis fugax is a common transient ischaemic attack syndrome caused by embolism occluding the retinal artery. A rapid, painless loss of vision in one eye is often described as 'a curtain coming down'.

Diagnostic approach

The aims of investigation are to identify the cause of the transient ischaemic attack and to define the degree of vascular risk. The ABCD2 score guides the urgency of investigation and implementation of secondary preventative measures against future TIAs and ischaemic strokes (**Table 6.8**).

Patients with suspected transient ischaemic attack should see a stroke specialist within 7 days. Those with ABCD2 score ≥ 4 are assessed ideally within 24 h. A score of ≥ 6 indicates a 35.5% risk of stroke within the next 7 days.

Transient ischaemic attacks are investigated identically to an ischaemic stroke, with:

- imaging of the brain
- imaging of blood vessels (including the carotid arteries to assess for atherosclerosis)
- imaging of the heart (to assess for sources of cardiac emboli)
- blood tests

Management

Management aims to reduce the risk of stroke (secondary prevention).

Medication

Control of risk factors reduces not only stroke but also the risk of coronary and peripheral vascular disease:

- smoking cessation, weight loss, exercise and reduction in alcohol consumption
- control of hypertension (aiming for blood pressure < 140/90 mmHg)
- optimisation of diabetes control
- control of hyperlipidaemia

ABCD2 stroke risk criteria		
ABCD2	Criteria	Score
A	**A**ge ≥ 60 years	1
B	**B**lood pressure ≥ 140/90 mmHg	1
C	**C**linical features	2 if there is weakness
		1 if there is a speech defect but no weakness
D	**D**uration of symptoms	2 if lasting ≥ 60 min
		1 if lasting 10–59 min
D	**D**iabetes	1

Table 6.8 ABCD2 risk score in the assessment of transient ischaemic attacks. The highest possible score is 7

The second step is initiation of antiplatelet therapy.

- Aspirin 300 mg daily for 2 weeks, and then 75 mg of clopidogrel daily for life, reduce by 15–18% the risk of death associated with vascular disease
- Warfarin is indicated if the transient ischaemic attack was caused by cardioembolism and risk factors for cardioembolism are present (e.g. chronic non-valvular atrial fibrillation, metallic prosthetic cardiac vavles and acute left ventricular wall motion impairment).

Warfarin is an extremely effective anticoagulant that significantly reduces stroke risk from cardiac embolism. However, it also increases the risk of haemorrhage (especially intracranial). Careful risk–benefit analysis, for example with the HAS-BLED prediction algorithm, is done before warfarin is started.

Surgery

In cardioembolism, surgery may be:

- cardiac electrophysiological ablation for atrial fibrillation
- valve repair or replacement for valvular disease

Atheroma at the carotid bifurcation is the commonest cause of atherothromboembolism. If symptomatic, carotid endarterectomy may be indicated to remove the plaque. Carotid artery stenting is an alternative, but its long-term efficacy has yet to be established.

Prevention

Table 6.9 summarises the measures implemented in the primary prevention of stroke, i.e. preventing a first incidence of transient ischaemic attack or stroke.

Stroke and transient ischaemic attack: primary prevention		
Risk factors	Rationale for intervention	Preventive measure(s)
Hypertension Smoking Diabetes Hyperlipidaemia	Precipitate atherosclerosis (by injury to vascular walls) and increase risk of atherothromboembolism	Lifestyle measures (e.g. smoking cessation, weight loss and exercise) Medical treatment of hypertension, diabetes and hyperlipidaemia
Cardiac embolism risk factors (e.g. non-valvular atrial fibrillation)	CHADS2 VASC score helps calculate this risk: **C**ongestive heart failure **H**ypertension **A**ge (< 65 or > 75 years) **D**iabetes Prior **S**troke or transient ischaemic attack **S**ex Other **VASC**ular disease	Aspirin alone may suffice for low-risk patients (i.e. those with atrial fibrillation, aged < 65 years and with no other risk factors) In the absence of contraindications, warfarin is indicated in high-risk patients (e.g. those aged > 75 years, with diabetes or with hypertension in association with atrial fibrillation)
Carotid artery atherosclerosis and stenosis	Carotid artery stenosis may be asymptomatic Stroke risk in asymptomatic stenosis is significantly lower than in symptomatic stenosis	Consideration for surgery (often a multidisciplinary team decision)

Table 6.9 Primary prevention of ischaemic stroke and transient ischaemic attack

Cerebral aneurysms

An aneurysm is an abnormal localised 'ballooning' of a blood vessel. Rupture results in intracranial haemorrhage with significant morbidity and mortality. They are mostly in the anterior circulation (80–90%).

Types

Aneurysms consist of a neck and fundus, and are characterised by size, location and aetiology (**Figure 6.8**). They may be small (< 1 cm in diameter), large (1–2.5 cm in diameter) or giant (> 2.5 cm in diameter).

Epidemiology

The prevalence of intracranial aneurysms worldwide is approximately 6% with particularly higher prevalences in Asian and Finnish populations, and those who harbor significant risk factors (e.g. smoking, family history, hypertension).

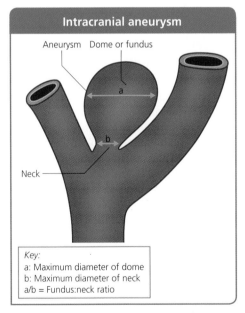

Intracranial aneurysm

Aneurysm   Dome or fundus

a

b

Neck

Key:
a: Maximum diameter of dome
b: Maximum diameter of neck
a/b = Fundus:neck ratio

Figure 6.8 Structure of a typical intracranial aneurysm: the vessel wall is thinner where it has ballooned outwards to form an aneurysm at the branching point of two vessels. The fundus:neck ratio is often used, to evaluate the suitability of the aneurysm for interventional radiological treatment (endovascular coiling).

Aetiology

Aneurysms can be developmental, inherited, infectious or traumatic.

- Developmental ('berry') aneurysms are the most common type; risk factors include hypertension, atherosclerosis and family history (up to 10% of people with two or more affected first-degree family members may have a developmental aneurysm)
- Aneurysms can develop in inherited diseases in which abnormal collagen (the key component of arterial walls) is formed (e.g. polycystic kidney disease, Marfan's syndrome and Ehlers–Danlos syndrome)
- Infectious ('mycotic') aneurysms are a rare complication of vessel wall inflammation resulting from infection
- Traumatic intracranial aneurysms (< 1%) occur as a result of penetrating head injury

> **The risk of aneurysm rupture** is related to its size and is higher in smokers and patients with hypertension.

Pathogenesis

Multiple factors are implicated in the pathogenesis of cerebral aneurysm. They include a genetic predisposition to vessel wall weakness, for example in collagen deficiency, and precipitation by haemodynamic and metabolic stresses such as hypertension, smoking and diabetes.

Clinical features

Aneurysms usually present in one of three ways: rupture leading to haemorrhage, or focal neurological deficits secondary to compression of neural structures. Rarely, aneurysms may precipitate episodes of ischaemia as a result of vascular steal (blood flow diversion) or precipitating thromboembolic events (**Table 6.10**).

Clinical features of cerebral aneurysms		
Mechanism of presentation	Classification by location	Clinical features
Aneurysm rupture	Subarachnoid haemorrhage	Sudden onset headache and meningism
	Intracerebral haemorrhage	Rupture can cause bleeding within a cerebral hemisphere with clot formation and focal neurological deficits
	Intraventricular haemorrhage	Acute hydrocephalus if aneurysm ruptures into ventricles causing obstruction to cerebrospinal fluid flow within
Focal neurological deficits (caused by compression)	Posterior communicating artery aneurysm	Fixed, dilated pupil unresponsive to light and accommodation as a result of CN III (oculomotor nerve) compression
	Aneurysm of segment of internal carotid artery in cavernous sinus	Cavernous sinus syndrome: eye movement abnormalities caused by compression of CNs III, IV and VI Facial pain and abnormalities of forehead sensation caused by compression of ophthalmic segment of CN V
	Anterior cerebral artery or anterior communicating artery aneurysm	Field defects caused by CN II (optic nerve) compression; the pituitary stalk may also be compressed with pituitary dysfunction from hypopituitarism
	Basilar artery aneurysm	Compresses brain stem structures with cranial nerve and long-tract signs/symptoms

CN, cranial nerve.

Table 6.10 Clinical features associated with cerebral aneurysms

Diagnostic approach

Subarachnoid haemorrhage (**Figure 6.9**) is discussed on page 443. Cerebral aneurysms, either symptomatic with rupture and subarachnoid haemorrhage or incidental, require non-invasive and invasive imaging to confirm diagnosis and define location and architecture.

- Non-invasive imaging techniques include CT angiography (**Figure 6.10**) and magnetic resonance angiography with three-dimensional reconstruction (**Figure 6.11**)
- Cerebral angiography with digital subtraction is invasive but is the gold standard and can be both therapeutic and diagnostic (**Figure 6.12**)

Management

Management of cerebral aneurysms depends on whether they are ruptured ('hot' aneurysm) or unruptured ('cold' aneurysm) and discovered incidentally or as a result of symptoms from mass effect.

Patients presenting with subarachnoid haemorrhage after aneurysm rupture

Patients with subarachnoid haemorrhage after aneurysmal rupture require immediate resuscitation and haemodynamic and neurological stabilisation, often in intensive care (see **Table 6.2**). Control of intracranial pressure and prevention of complications are critical (**Table 6.11**). The definitive form and timing of intervention to treat the cerebral aneurysm to prevent rebleeding is decided by taking into consideration the morphology and anatomical features of the aneurysm (fundus: neck ratio), its location, the patient's age and comorbidities and if possible, the patient's own preference.

Any patient presenting with aneurysmal subarachnoid haemorrhage is at high risk of:

- rebleed
- vasospasm
- seizures
- hydrocephalus
- electrolyte disturbance

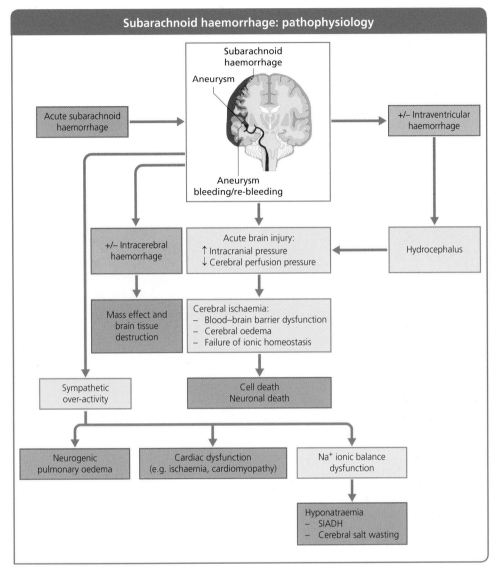

Figure 6.9 Pathophysiology of subarachnoid haemorrhage.

If consciousness deteriorates, these must be excluded.

Patients with unruptured aneurysm

In these patients, the risk of future rupture and death is balanced against the risks of aneurysm repair in considering whether to intervene. Patient factors (age, comorbidities and current neurological symptoms) and aneurysm factors (size, morphology, location, operative difficulty and rupture risk) are considered. The decision is made jointly by the neurosurgeon, neuroradiologist and patient.

Definitive treatment of aneurysms

This requires neurosurgical clipping (**Figure 6.13**) or endovascular coiling (**Figure 6.14**) to block blood to the aneurysm and thereby prevent rupture and bleeding.

Clipping is associated with higher procedural morbidity than coiling; however, successful clipping usually provides a permanent cure.

Coiling has a higher incidence of aneurysm regrowth and possible late recurrence with risk of rerupture and subarachnoid haemorrhage.

Prognosis

About 15% of patients with subarachnoid haemorrhage from a ruptured aneurysm die before reaching hospital; 25% die within 24 h. Up to 40% die within the first month. Between 50 and 80% of patients who rebleed die within the first 24–48 hours.

Screening is recommended for people with two or more first-degree relatives with confirmed aneurysms. Counselling on the risks and benefits of identifying unruptured aneurysms is provided before screening. Diagnosis raises difficult decisions about relatively high-risk treatments, pregnancy (which increases the risk of rupture), life insurance, etc.

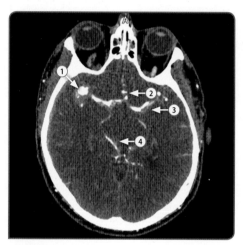

Figure 6.10 Computerised tomography (CT) angiogram obtained after unenhanced CT had confirmed subarachnoid haemorrhage. CT angiography shows vasculature and is often the initial screening tool used to identify aneurysm as a cause of subarachnoid haemorrhage. ①, right middle cerebral artery aneurysm; ②, left anterior cerebral artery; ③, left middle cerebral artery; ④, terminal branches of the right posterior cerebral artery.

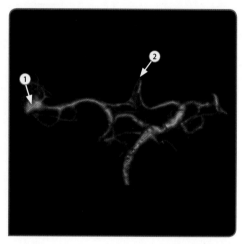

Figure 6.11 Three-dimensional reconstruction based on CT angiograms, showing a right middle cerebral artery aneurysm. These reconstructions are useful for measuring three-dimensional diameters of the aneurysm and for further planning of neurosurgical or neuroradiological intervention. ①, right middle cerebral artery aneurysm; ②, left anterior cerebral artery.

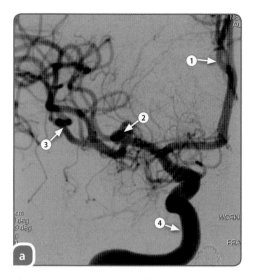
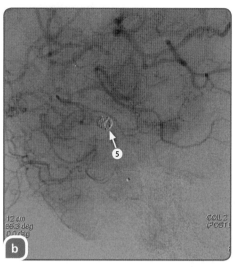

Figure 6.12 Antero-posterior (AP) cerebral catheter angiography (digital subtraction cerebral angiography) images before (left) and after (right) coil embolisation of an aneurysm. ①, anterior cerebral artery; ②, right middle cerebral artery aneurysm; ③, middle cerebral artery branches distal to the aneurysm; ④, right internal carotid artery; ⑤, coils occluding the aneurysm.

Complications of aneurysmal subarachnoid haemorrhage		
Complication	**Pathogenesis**	**Management and prevention**
Rebleeding (30% risk on days 1–28 after untreated subarachnoid haemorrhage; 70% of patients die after rebleed)	It is unclear which ruptured aneurysms are risk of early rebleeding Factors such as uncontrolled hypertension can precipitate re-rupture, as can a change in transmural pressures across the aneurysm wall (e.g. excess cerebrospinal fluid drainge following external ventricular drainage to relieve acute aneurysmal subarachnoid associated hydrocephalus)	Definitive intervention to secure the aneurysm
Cerebral vasospasm or delayed ischaemic neurological deficit	Possibly a consequence of blood irritating cerebral vessels to cause vasospasm, with subsequent ischaemia and infarction	Reduce risk with nimodipine (60 mg every 4 h) for 21 days If symptomatic, increase blood pressure with intravenous fluids and inotropic and vasopressor agents (e.g. noradrenaline) – this is called 'triple H' therapy (hypertension, hypervolaemia and haemodilution); cerebral vessel dilating agents, e.g. intra-arterial papaverine, may be utilised along with endovascular intervention
Hydrocephalus	General subarachnoid haemorrhage obstructing arachnoid villi (communicating)	Initially amenable to lumbar punctures and cerebrospinal fluid drainage May require long term cerebrospinal fluid shunting
	Blood in ventricular system (non-communicating)	Requires external ventricular drainage of cerebrospinal fluid with external ventricular drain May require long term cerebrospinal fluid shunting
Seizures	Disruption of normal neuronal electrical activity	Anticonvulsant drugs
Hyponatraemia	Syndrome of inappropriate antidiuretic hormone secretion or cerebral salt wasting	Immediate discussion with intensive care and neurosurgeons

Table 6.11 Complications associated with aneurysmal subarachnoid haemorrhage

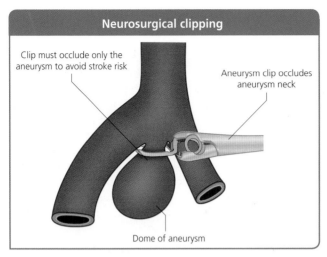

Neurosurgical clipping

Clip must occlude only the aneurysm to avoid stroke risk

Aneurysm clip occludes aneurysm neck

Dome of aneurysm

Figure 6.13 Principles of neurosurgical clipping. Craniotomy to open the skull facilitates exposure of the affected vessels. This allows a titanium clip to be passed around the aneurysm neck to occlude it. The clip is left in place permanently.

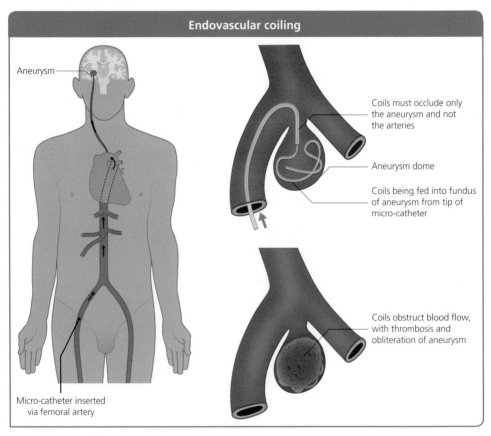

Endovascular coiling

Aneurysm

Coils must occlude only the aneurysm and not the arteries

Aneurysm dome

Coils being fed into fundus of aneurysm from tip of micro-catheter

Coils obstruct blood flow, with thrombosis and obliteration of aneurysm

Micro-catheter inserted via femoral artery

Figure 6.14 Endovascular coiling. A catheter tube is inserted, usually through the femoral artery, and passed via the aorta and carotid arteries to the neck of the aneurysm under radiographic guidance. Several platinum coils are delivered through the catheter to the aneurysm to occlude it.

Arteriovenous malformations

Arteriovenous malformations are intracranial vascular anomalies of tangled masses of pial blood vessels (nidi). They have feeding arteries and draining veins. Blood is shunted directly from arteries to veins, bypassing the normal arteriole–capillary–venule network and thus causing complications. Many patients are asymptomatic, but symptomatic arteriovenous malformations are associated with high morbidity and significant mortality.

Epidemiology

Arteriovenous malformations have an annual incidence of 1 per 100,000. Therefore, they are less common than aneurysms.

Aetiology

Most arteriovenous malformations are congenital. They are multiple in some inherited syndromes, such as hereditary haemorrhagic telangiectasia.

Clinical features

Arteriovenous malformations may remain asymptomatic throughout life or manifest as intracranial haemorrhage, seizures or focal neurological deficits (**Table 6.12**).

Risk of haemorrhage is further increased if a patient has an aneurysm associated with arteriovenous malformation; this type of aneurysm can arise as a result of the increased pressure caused by shunting. The two types of arteriovenous malformation-associated aneurysm are:

■ intranidal (in the arteriovenous malformation nidus)
■ extranidal (in arteries feeding the arteriovenous malformation)

Diagnostic approach

Computerised tomography or MRI angiography and cerebral angiography aid diagnosis.

Clinical presentations of arteriovenous malformations		
Feature	Symptoms	Natural history
Haemorrhage (intracerebral or intraventricular)	Symptoms are variable and range from mild headache to focal neurological deficits to sudden collapse and death (depending on haemorrhage location, severity and associated complications, e.g. obstructive hydrocephalus)	Annual risk of 2–4% (if no previous haemorrhage history)
Epilepsy	Generalised or partial seizures	Risk higher after haemorrhage and in cortical AVMs
Focal neurological deficit	Symptoms depend on AVM location	Deficits result from mass effect, 'vascular steal' (diminished blood flow to non-AVM areas) or haemorrhage
Venous hypertension	Symptoms are those of increased intracranial pressure	Direct shunting from arteries increases venous pressure
Aneurysm formation	May result in subarachnoid haemorrhage	Caused by high pressures in blood vessels as a result of direct arterial–venous shunting. Can present in a similar manner as aneurysms without associated AVM (see **Table 6.10**)

Table 6.12 Clinical features associated with symptomatic arteriovenous malformations (AVMs). Many patients remain symptom-free for life

They also define arteriovenous malformation architecture for planning management (**Figures 6.15** and **6.16**).

Management

Management depends on patient factors, i.e. symptoms, age and comorbidities, and arteriovenous malformation architecture, including nidus size, location relative to eloquent structures, pattern of venous drainage (superficial or deep) and presence of associated intra- or extranidal aneurysms (which potentially have an impact on risk of haemorrhage). The Spetzler-Martin grading system is used to stratify the operative risk associated with an arteriovenous malformation, based on its architecture.

Indications for intervention include expanding haemorrhage caused by arteriovenous malformation, progressive neurological deficits and high risk of haemorrhage (e.g. in a young patient with many years at risk).

Surgery

Three interventions are used, alone or in combination.

- Operative neurosurgical excision offers the best chance of cure after a single operation; small peripheral arteriovenous malformations < 3 cm in size in non-eloquent areas are ideal targets
- Stereotactic radiosurgery uses focused beams delivered in a single dose to obliterate small arteriovenous malformations; obliteration takes up to 3 years, during which haemorrhage risk persists
- Interventional neuroradiology with embolisation occludes feeding vessels to reduce vascularity, and is a useful stand-alone treatment or pre- or postoperative adjunct to surgery or stereotactic radiosurgery; complications include haemorrhage and glue extravasation

Treatment for arteriovenous malformation is extremely risky. Input from a multidisciplinary team, including a neurosurgeon and an interventional neuroradiologist, is critical in planning the optimal management strategy.

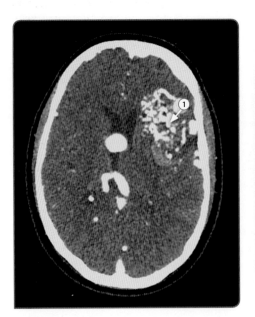

Figure 6.15 Axial post contrast computerised tomography images showing an irregular hyperdense area in the left frontotemporal regions after haemorrhage. The 'serpiginous' structures ① filling up homogeneously with contrast represent dilated vessels and strongly suggest an underlying arteriovenous malformation.

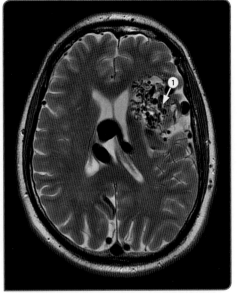

Figure 6.16 T2-weighted magnetic resonance imaging showing multiple focal and serpiginous flow voids ① (caused by flowing blood in the vessels) in the corresponding left frontotemporal regions. This finding confirms the arteriovenous malformation.

Cerebral venous sinus thrombosis

Superficial and deep cerebral veins and dural venous sinuses drain blood from the brain. Thrombosis in any of these venous structures precipitates infarction or haemorrhage in the territories they drain.

Epidemiology

The annual incidence of cerebral venous sinus thrombosis is 2 per 1 million people. Venous thrombotic infarction accounts for 1% of all strokes: 85% of these affect dural sinuses (superior sagittal sinus and transverse sinus), 10% affect deep cerebral veins and 5% affect the cavernous sinus.

Aetiology

The pathogenesis, and therefore the aetiology, is identical to that of arterial thrombosis and centres on Virchow's triad – any pathological process that affects a component of Virchow's triad can precipitate cerebral venous sinus thrombosis (see page 37; **Table 6.13** provides examples of disorders that can precipitate venous sinus thrombosis classified according to the component of Virchow's triad they affect).

Clinical features

Headache, papilloedema, increased intracranial pressure, focal neurological deficits (e.g. hemiparesis and dysphasia) and seizures may occur.

Site-specific symptoms relate to underlying anatomy. For example, cavernous sinus thrombosis presents with defects of cranial nerves III, IV and VI as well as the ophthalmic division of cranial nerve V.

Diagnostic approach

Cerebral venous sinus thrombosis is a difficult diagnosis to make, because its clinical features are non-specific and it mimics other pathologies. A high index of suspicion is required. Cerebral venous sinus thrombosis must be confirmed or excluded through imaging. Potential causes are then explored and treated.

Investigations

Computerised tomography and MRI scans can be normal, but they may show infarction in a region atypical for a specific arterial occlusion; the infarction is caused by increased venous pressure from the venous clot. The venous clot is occasionally visible with non-contrast CT, but it usually requires confirmation by the finding of filling deficits in the venous structures on CT or magnetic resonance venography (**Figure 6.17**).

Causes of intracranial venous sinus thrombosis		
Abnormalities in blood constituents	Abnormalities in blood flow	Abnormalities in vessel wall
Drugs (e.g. combined oral contraceptive pill and hormone replacement therapy)	Venous stasis	Vasculitis (e.g. polyarteritis nodosa)
Infection or malignancy affecting face, eye, ear or nose	Dehydration	Intracranial infection (e.g. meningitis, HIV and abscess)
Malignancy (intra- or extracranial)	Pregnancy and puerperium	Inflammatory disorders (e.g. superficial lupus erythematosus and sarcoidosis)
Haematological disease (e.g. inherited thrombophilias and polycythaemia)		Iatrogenic venous injury during neurosurgery

*These can be remembered easily based on the three principles of Virchow's triad, which underlies the pathogenesis of thrombosis and thrombus formation in any vessel.

Table 6.13 Examples of the causes of central venous sinus thrombosis, classified according to Virchow's triad. These can be remembered easily based on the three principles of Virchow's triad, which underlies the pathogenesis of thrombosis and thrombus formation in any vessel.

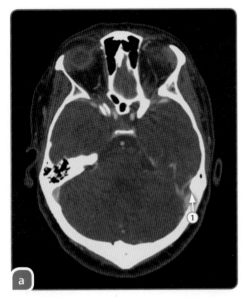
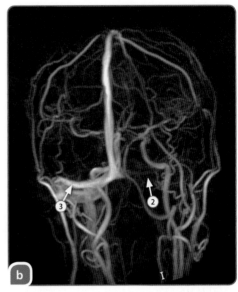

Figure 6.17 Venous thrombosis. (a) Computerised tomography venogram, with arrow showing filling defect (dark hypodensity) in the left transverse sinus (empty delta sign) ① consistent with thrombosis in the left transverse sinus. (b) Magnetic resonance venogram showing absent flow in the left transverse and sigmoid sinuses, caused by occlusive thrombus ②, compared to the normally filling right transverse sinus ③.

Management

Treatment regimens vary and can be controversial.

Medication

The cause is treated, for example by immunosuppression for vasculitis, or cessation of precipitating drugs such as the combined oral contraceptive pill. Cerebral venous sinus thrombosis requires anticoagulation with heparin initially, followed by long-term warfarin. The duration of anticoagulation depends on the precipitating factor. The timing of anticoagulation initiation in the presence of a venous thrombosis associated haemorrhage is debated.

Surgery

This may be needed for intractable increases in intracranial pressure. Procedures include external ventricular drainage of cerebrospinal fluid and decompressive craniectomy.

Prognosis

Outcome varies according to severity of infarction and presenting consciousness level. Death is mainly the result of brain herniation from the increased intracranial pressure caused by diffuse infarction associated oedema, or haemorrhagic mass lesions.

Cavernous sinus syndromes

The cavernous sinuses (see page 267) are a pair of 2 cm venous blood-filled spaces either side of the pituitary gland. Critical structures traverse through each cavernous sinus, including cranial nerves (III, IV, VI and part of V) and the internal carotid artery. Diseases affecting the cavernous sinus produce a stereotypical clinical syndrome arising from compression and damage to these structures (**Figure 6.18**); permanent dysfunction may result.

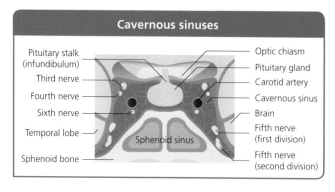

Figure 6.18 Coronal section through the cavernous sinuses, showing relationship to critical structures.

Clinical features

A variety of diseases can affect the cavernous sinus including cavernous sinus venous thrombosis (due to infection, malignancy or idiopathic), infiltration by pituitary tumour, pituitary apoplexy and carotico-cavernous fistulae (**Table 6.14**).

The following clinical features are common to and can occur with any pathological process that affects the cavernous sinus.

Painful eye movements and double vision may develop after palsies of cranial nerves III, IV and VI, and loss of forehead sensation when the ophthalmic division of cranial nerve V is affected. Eyeball protrusion (proptosis) and periorbital tissue oedema (chemosis) are common.

Ophthalmic vein dilatation and subsequent pressure–compression can lead to papilloedema, retinal haemorrhage, optic nerve atrophy and eventually loss of vision.

Pulsatile eyeball and cranial bruit (a 'whoosh' sound on eyeball auscultation) are often pathognomonic of a caroticocavernous fistula, an abnormal fistulous communication between the intracavernous portion of the internal carotid artery and the cavernous sinus.

Complications include spread of infection or malignancy to other intracranial sites in cavernous sinus thrombosis caused by infection or malignancy, respectively. Acute pituitary failure is a complication of pituitary apoplexy.

Management

Management is tailored to the cause (**Table 6.14**). Untreated, septic cavernous sinus thrombosis has 80% mortality from meningitis. This decreases to < 20% with the

Causes of cavernous sinus syndrome		
Disease	**Aetiology**	**Management**
Cavernous sinus thrombosis	Idiopathic	Anticoagulation
	Ophthalmic or facial infection with intracranial spread	Antibiotics
	Extracranial malignancy from eye or facial region with intracranial spread	Referral to specialists
Pituitary apoplexy	Acute haemorrhage, usually associated with a pituitary tumour, and subsequent infarction of pituitary gland	Refer to neurosurgeon
	Idiopathic (e.g. anticoagulant use and Sheehan's syndrome*)	
Caroticocavernous fistula	Trauma to skull base	
	Rupture of aneurysm of intracavernous portion of internal carotid artery	

*Sheehan's syndrome is pituitary failure associated with postpartum haemorrhage causing pituitary necrosis.

Table 6.14 Causes and management of cavernous sinus diseases

use of appropriate antibiotics and occasion- ally surgical drainage.

The underlying aetiology often requires emergency intervention to prevent perma- nent damage to structures traversing the cav- ernous sinus, particularly:

- infections or malignancies near the eye, which require antibiotics and ophthalmological referral
- pituitary apoplexy, which warrants urgent neurosurgical referral for consideration of decompression to prevent visual failure

Answers to starter questions

1. By definition, stroke requires the presence of neurological signs and symptoms. However, many people with risk factors for stroke (e.g. hypertension and diabetes) have evidence of damage to the brain but no symptoms. It is likely that this damage arose from the same process that occurs in clinical strokes. The brain may be so adaptable that in these people areas of it may be damaged without any clinical manifestation.

2. Treatments for stroke need to be given quickly to be as effective as possible. Intervention to restore circulation to ischaemic regions of brain is critical to limiting the size of the infarcted (dead) zone and saving the maximum amount of brain. This need for speed has led to national education programmes to educate the public on recognising stroke symptoms as early as possible.

3. Transient ischaemic attacks can precede future strokes and indicate the presence of systemic atherosclerotic disease. Initiation of secondary prevention after a transient ischaemic attack greatly reduces the risk of subsequent strokes.

4. In adults, the regenerative capability of the brain is limited. Rehabilitation cannot reverse brain damage. However, it can help patients develop alternative strategies and techniques, such as the use of prostheses and occupational therapy aids, for carrying out their day-to-day activities. Rehabilitation is also crucial for maximising brain plasticity and avoiding complications following brain damage, such as treating contractures and spasticity. In children, the developing brain has an enormous amount of plasticity. After damage, it can develop new, different connections to replace lost brain function.

Chapter 7
Neurological tumours

Starter questions

Answers to the following questions are on page 286.

1. Why is genetic analysis of brain tumour specimens important?
2. If most neurones are non-dividing cells, how can they become cancerous?
3. Does the 'immune privileged' status of the central nervous system mean that it has less surveillance of precancerous cells?

Introduction

Neurological tumours are abnormal growths of cells that arise in the central and, less commonly, the peripheral nervous systems:

- Primary tumours (e.g. gliomas) arise in the nervous system and associated structures (e.g. the pituitary gland)

- Secondary tumours originate elsewhere (e.g. lung or breast) and have metastasised to the central or peripheral nervous system

The aim for clinicians is early recognition of a potential tumour and referral for rapid specialist diagnosis and management.

Case 8 Morning headache

Presentation

Rachel Harvey is a 48-year-old right-handed accountant. She presents to her general practitioner with an 8-week history of difficulties with expression of speech.

Initial interpretation

Characterising the type of speech difficulty helps localise the pathology.

- Dysphasia (abnormal speech comprehension or expression) suggests cerebral hemispheric pathology
- Dysphonia (abnormal speech volume) suggests vocal cord pathology
- Dysarthria (abnormal speech coordination) suggests cerebellar or lower brain stem pathology

Further history

Rachel has difficulty 'finding her words' and describes recent headaches, which are worse in the morning and when coughing. She has recently had episodes of nausea and vomiting.

Examination

The general practitioner notes that Rachel has expressive dysphasia and some right arm weakness with increased reflexes. Fundoscopy reveals papilloedema (optic nerve swelling) in her left eye.

Interpretation of findings

Rachel has focal neurological deficits (specific abnormalities localised to a

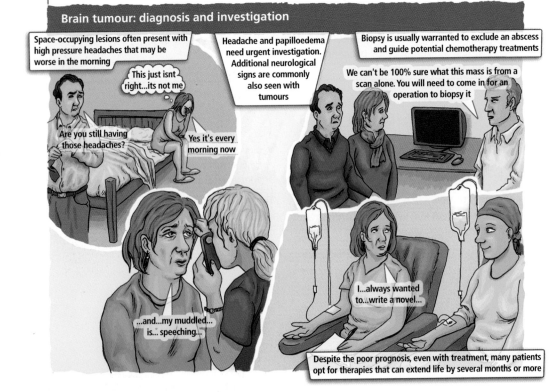

Case 8 *continued*

specific part of the brain): expressive dysphasia and right arm weakness. This suggests a lesion in the left cerebral hemisphere affecting the motor cortex and expressive speech centre (Broca's area) in the left frontal lobe. Key causes are distinguished by speed of onset (**Table 7.1**).

Rachel's symptoms suggest a chronic cause. Given the absence of features to suggest infection, and presence of features of increased intracranial pressure (headaches, vomiting and papilloedema), a tumour is likely.

> A space-occupying lesion is any mass occupying intracranial space. Non-tumour causes include infection, vascular problems (e.g. giant aneurysm and blood clot), cysts and inflammatory lesions (e.g. sarcoidosis).

Investigations

Contrast-enhanced computerised tomography (CT) of Rachel's brain shows a large left-sided space-occupying lesion (**Figure 7.1**). The results of magnetic resonance imaging (MRI) suggest a highly aggressive brain tumour. No primary extracranial tumours are visible on a CT scan of her chest, abdomen and pelvis, which suggests that the brain tumour is a primary one.

Diagnosis

Rachel is referred to a consultant neurosurgeon. A neuro-oncologist and a specialist nurse in the clinic provide support. The decision is made to proceed with surgery, with the aims of reducing the size of the tumour and obtaining a histological specimen for diagnosis. After surgery, she will probably receive radiotherapy and possibly chemotherapy.

Causes of focal neurological deficit

Speed of symptom onset	Causes
Acute (minutes)	Vascular event (e.g. ischaemic or haemorrhagic stroke)
	Seizure
	Acute metabolic abnormality (e.g. acute hypoglycaemia and hypocalcaemia)
Subacute (minutes to hours)	Migraine
	Acute demyelination (e.g. multiple sclerosis)
Chronic (days to weeks)	Infection (e.g. encephalitis and cerebral abscess)
	Space-occupying pathologies (e.g. tumour)

Table 7.1 Causes of focal neurological deficit

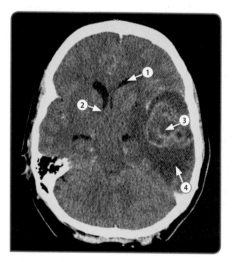

Figure 7.1 Contrast-enhanced axial CT scan of the brain demonstrating a large left frontotemporal space-occupying lesion that appears to look like a glioblastoma with mass effect, oedema and midline shift. ① Effacement of left lateral ventricle due to mass effect. ② Midline shift from right to left. ③ Space-occupying lesion likely to be GBM. ④ Surrounding cerebral oedema.

Intracranial tumours: general principles

Because the brain sits within the rigid skull, any growth of abnormal tissue can destroy surrounding structures. Therefore the terms 'benign' and 'malignant' are less relevant here than in other parts of the body.

Epidemiology

The annual global incidence of primary intracranial tumours is 10 per 100,000 persons.

Aetiology

The definitive cause of most primary brain tumours is unknown. Most patients probably have a genetic predisposition and are then exposed to one or more environmental factors that precipitate tumour development (**Figure 7.2**).

> **Cancer is a genetic disease in which a cell loses the normal behaviour of controlled cell growth, division and death.** Multiple mutations in its DNA precipitate growth, uncontrollable division and evasion of cell defence mechanisms. Predisposition is influenced by various inherited or acquired mutations. Mutagenic agents include carcinogens, such as tobacco smoke, or oncogenic ('cancer-causing') viruses.

Various inherited genetic syndromes are associated with increased risk of intracranial tumour development.

Environmental factors include immune suppression, for example in cases of primary central nervous system lymphoma. Systemic

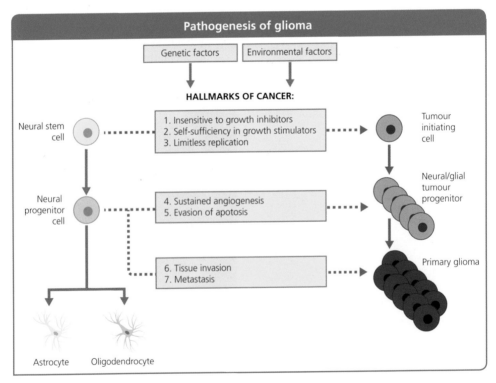

Figure 7.2 Pathogenesis of a primary brain glioma.

immune suppression can be caused by certain drugs and HIV infection. Whole-brain irradiation, as used to treat childhood leukaemia, may increase the risk of developing intracranial tumours (especially meningiomas).

Pathogenesis

Intracranial tumours are described as benign or malignant. Despite the name, a 'benign' intracranial tumour can be very destructive and even lethal, often because of its location (see page 41). Intracranial tumours with features of 'malignancy' rarely metastasise to sites outside the nervous system.

The brain comprises eloquent and non-eloquent areas. The eloquent areas are responsible for critical functions, so damage to these areas would cause significant disability (see page 41).

Clinical features

A tumour, like any space-occupying lesion, can cause:

- increased intracranial pressure, brain herniation or both (see page 190)
- acute or chronic onset of focal neurological deficits (**Table 7.2**)
- seizures
- headache
- changes in mental status
- hydrocephalus

Intracranial tumours and focal neurological deficits		
Compartment	Location	Common symptoms
Supratentorial	Frontal lobe	Contralateral weakness of face, arm or leg
		Personality change
		Expressive speech dysfunction (if dominant hemisphere affected)
	Parietal lobe	Contralateral sensory deficit in face, arm or leg
		Visual field defect
	Temporal lobe	Receptive speech dysfunction (if dominant hemisphere affected)
		Visual field defect
	Occipital lobe	Visual field defect
		Cortical blindness
	Sellar region (pituitary or hypothalamus)	Cavernous sinus syndrome (CN III–VI deficits)
		Endocrine dysfunction
		Optic chiasm compression
Infratentorial	Brain stem	Cranial nerve lesions (CN III–XII)
		Decline in level of consciousness
		Abnormalities in descending or ascending white matter tracts (e.g. corticospinal tract)
	Cerebellum	Dysdiadochokinesis
		Ataxic gait and impaired balance
		Slurred speech and dysarthria
		Intention tremor
		Nystagmus

CN, cranial nerve.

Table 7.2 Focal neurological deficits associated with intracranial tumours

Headaches caused by brain tumours are usually a consequence of increased intracranial pressure. Such headaches are classically:

■ worse in the morning

■ exacerbated by coughing, straining or bending forwards

■ associated with nausea and vomiting

In the elderly, brain tumours often present later and at a larger size. This is because the brain atrophy of ageing leaves more room for the tumour to grow before it becomes clinically evident.

The timing of presentation and the progression of clinical features can indicate the location and speed of tumour growth. Clinical features are usually chronic and develop over weeks to months or even years. However, acute presentations also occur, with rapid onset of focal neurological deficits or a decline in consciousness caused by:

■ a brain herniation syndrome (see page 193)
■ an acute haemorrhagic event within the tumour
■ acute cerebrospinal fluid obstruction, causing acute hydrocephalus (e.g. colloid cyst) (**Figure 7.3**)

A 'benign' intracranial tumour may:

■ cause blindness by compressing the optic nerves
■ cause paralysis by compressing the primary motor cortex
■ cause life-threatening hydrocephalus by obstructing pathways for the flow of cerebrospinal fluid

The timing of and size at presentation of an intracranial tumour differ depend on whether it is in an eloquent or non-eloquent area of the brain.

■ A tumours in a highly eloquent area, even if it is small, can present early
■ A tumour in a non-eloquent area may become quite large before becoming evident clinically

Diagnostic approach

Intracranial tumours are diagnosed using radiological imaging. The diagnosis can be confirmed using a biopsy of the tumour if required.

Investigations

Radiological imaging is the key investigative tool when a brain tumour is suspected (**Figure 7.4**). It provides essential information on:

■ location
■ likely aggressiveness
■ degree of mass effect and oedema

Plain CT initially confirms the presence of a space-occupying lesion. Subsequent contrast-enhanced CT often shows tumours as 'ring-enhancing' (**Figure 7.5**). Specialist imaging may be required to exclude other causes; for example, diffusion-weighted MRI can better differentiate between a tumour

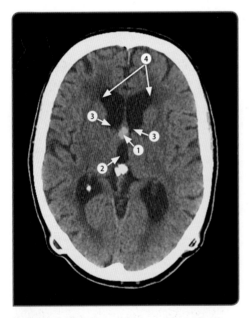

Figure 7.3 Axial CT scan demonstrating colloid cyst ① at the roof of the 3rd ventricle ② with obstruction of both inter-ventricular foramina of Monroe ③ causing ventriculomegaly and hydrocephalus ④.

Intracranial tumour diagnosis

Suspected intracranial tumour

↓

Initial imaging to confirm/exclude space-occupying lesion

- CT scan with and without contrast
- Note location of lesion, number of lesions, features of raised intracranial pressure and effect of contrast enhancement

↓

Blood tests

- Basic blood tests (e.g. FBC, U&E, LFTs)
- Inflammatory markers (e.g. CRP, ESR)
- Identify general fitness for surgery
- Exclude intracranial abscess as a cause for space-occupying lesion on imaging

↓

Further investigation to determine cause

- Staging CT scan of chest, abdomen or pelvis (to search for a primary tumour elsewhere if metastasis is suspected)
- Tumour marker for systemic malignancy (e.g. CEA for colon, CA-125 for ovarian, CA-19-9 for pancreas, PSA for prostate)

↓

Referral to brain tumour MDT and/or for other specialist investigations

- Specialist blood tests (e.g. intracranial tumour markers)
- Specialist imaging (e.g. whole spine MRI, angiography with CTA or MRA, functional MRI, magnetic resonance spectroscopy)

Figure 7.4 Diagnostic approach for a suspected intracranial tumour. CA, cancer antigen; CEA, carcino-embryonic antigen; CRP, complement reactive protein; CTA, CT angiography; ESR, erythrocyte sedimentation rate; FBC, full blood count; LFT, liver function tests; MRA, MR angiography; MRI, magnetic resonance imaging; PSA, prostate specific antigen; U&E, urea and electrolytes.

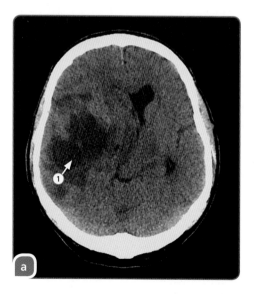

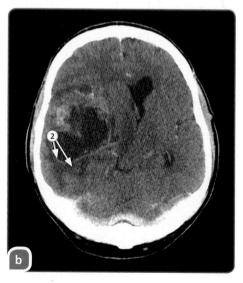

Figure 7.5 Axial CT appearances of a tumour ① with and without contrast. (a) On plain CT it is seen as a space-occupying lesion with a central hypo-dense region. (b) CT with contrast shows it as a ring-enhancing lesion ②.

and an intracranial abscess. If the tumour seems likely to be secondary, further imaging (e.g. a CT scan of chest, abdomen and pelvis) may be carried out to exclude a primary tumour elsewhere.

Table 7.3 summarises the specialist radiological imaging techniques used in the diagnosis of intracranial tumours.

The World Health Organization grading system for intracranial tumours is shown in Table 7.4.

Intracranial tumours: WHO grading

Conventional oncological grade	WHO grade	Criteria
Low (i.e. more 'benign')	1	Well circumscribed
		Often curable by surgical resection
	2	Cellular and nuclear atypia
High (i.e. more aggressive or 'malignant')	3	Grade 2 features and: ■ anaplasia ■ significant mitotic activity
	4	Grade 3 features and: ■ significant vascular proliferation ■ occluded or thrombosed vessels ■ significant necrosis

Although WHO grade 2 tumours are 'low' grade, their infiltration can be too extensive to allow complete surgical resection.

Table 7.4 The World Health Organization (WHO) grading system for intracranial tumours. Although WHO grade 2 tumours are 'low' grade, their infiltration can be too extensive to allow complete surgical resection

Tumours are graded histologically. Grading is based on levels of the following. The mnemonic 'AMEN' helps remember these key features.

■ **Atypia (cellular or nuclear):** how abnormal the cells or nuclei look

■ **Mitoses:** replication rate

■ **Endothelial and vascular proliferation:** the presence of a blood supply

■ **Necrosis:** the presence of dead tissue

■ High-grade tumours have increased levels of these features, rapid growth rates and poor differentiation (i.e. they poorly resemble their tissue of origin).

Management

Intracranial tumours are managed by a multidisciplinary team. The priority is to quickly choose the best treatment. Definitive interventions include surgery, radiotherapy and chemotherapy, either individually or in combination.

Management is guided by:

■ presenting symptoms

Intracranial tumours: specialist imaging techniques

Technique	Description
MRI of whole spine	Identifies tumours that spread through cerebrospinal fluid to the spinal cord (e.g. paediatric medulloblastoma)
Angiography (CT angiography, magnetic resonance angiography or DSA)	Shows tumour's relationship with blood vessels, to aid in surgical planning
	During invasive angiography (DSA), vessels can be blocked (embolised) to reduce tumour size and vascularity
Functional MRI	Used to assess eloquence of area involved; the results are used to aid planning to minimise damage during surgery
Magnetic resonance spectroscopy	Determines chemical constitution of a mass to differentiate between tissue types (e.g. tumour, normal or abscess) (**Figure 7.10**)

CT, computerised tomography; DSA, digital subtraction angiography; MRI, magnetic resonance imaging.

Table 7.3 Imaging techniques used in the diagnosis of intracranial tumours

- the degree of pressure on brain tissue
- tumour location (in relation to critical structures)
- likely radiological diagnosis
- the patient's clinical status (e.g. the presence of comorbidities)

Medication

The main role of non-chemotherapeutic medication is to control symptoms.

Steroids

These drugs, for example dexamethasone, are usually started if oedema is causing clinical symptoms. Steroids dramatically reduce the oedema but have no effect on tumour growth, except in the case of lymphomas.

Antiepileptic drugs

Phenytoin is often used to control acute seizures and status epilepticus in neurosurgical patients. Some liver enzyme–inducing antiepileptic drugs, for example carbamazepine, may reduce the efficacy of subsequent chemotherapy. Therefore non-liver enzyme-inducing antiepileptic drugs, such as levetiracetam, are preferred.

Surgery

The type and timing of surgery depend on various factors, including the following:

- Tumour location: accessibility and risks of post-operative morbidity
- Tumour histology: biopsy may be required for histological typing
- Presenting clinical features: whether the tumour is asymptomatic (i.e. incidental) or presents with seizures, focal neurological deficits, or life-threatening features of increased intracranial pressure and brain herniation
- Treatment aims: cure by resection, reduction of tumour load, palliation (e.g. relieving symptoms of increased intracranial pressure) or treatment of associated hydrocephalus

Intrinsic tumours in dominant hemispheric eloquent regions cannot be removed completely, because of the associated morbidity. For example, complete removal of tumours in the areas of the brain responsible for speech and language would result in loss of ability to communicate with dysphasia and therefore unacceptable neurological morbidity.

Radiotherapy

Radiation is used to destroy tumour cells. Unfortunately, radiotherapy can also damage adjacent tissue. Dosage is optimised to maximise the effect on the tumour while minimising irradiation of normal brain.

Radiation helps inhibit primary tumour growth and reduces recurrence of both benign and malignant tumours. In some circumstances, for example in cases of medulloblastoma, whole brain and spine radiation is used to minimise the risk of distant recurrence.

> **Adverse effects of radiotherapy include oedema, demyelination, radiotherapy-induced necrosis and radiation-induced tumours.** Meningioma is an example of a tumour that can be induced by radiation.

Chemotherapy

High doses of chemotherapeutic drugs are often needed to cross the blood–brain barrier, but they can lead to systemic toxicity such as life-threatening bone marrow suppression. Therefore chemotherapy is usually reserved for tumour recurrence after surgery and radiotherapy. Routes of delivery include:

- oral administration (e.g. temozolomide)
- insertion of chemotherapeutic drug 'wafers' into the cavity created in the brain by tumour resection [e.g. carmustine (Gliadel) wafers]
- intravenous

> **A brain tumour diagnosis is devastating for a patient and their family.** Cure is usually impossible for malignant and infiltrative brain tumours. Patients eventually succumb to their tumour within years, despite maximal therapy. Palliative care specialists and clinical nurse specialists are crucial in supporting patients and their families during this difficult time.

Gliomas

Gliomas are tumours that originate from neuroepithelial glial cells (see page 21): astrocytes, oligodendroglia and ependymal cells.

Over 70% of primary brain tumours are gliomas, most commonly astrocytomas. Glioblastoma multiforme is the most common high-grade tumour (see page 279).

Types

Gliomas are classified histologically as:

- low grade (World Health Organization grade 1 or 2)
- high grade (World Health Organization grade 3 or 4)

Glioblastoma multiforme is grade 4.

Pilocytic astrocytomas (grade 1) are well-circumscribed low-grade gliomas. They grow slowly, if at all, and are often cured by surgical resection. In adults, they arise in the optic pathway or hypothalamus in association with neurofibromatosis type 1.

Grade 2 tumours such as diffuse astrocytomas often lack a definitive margin between tumour and non-tumour tissue, making surgical resection and cure more difficult. They are also more likely to evolve into a high-grade tumour.

Ependymal and oligodendrocytic tumours are less common than astrocytomas. However, the principles of investigation and management are similar.

Clinical features

Gliomas present in a similar way to other intracranial tumours (see page 273). However, seizures as a presentation are more common with low-grade tumours.

Management

In addition to being managed according to general principles (see page 276), symptomatic grade 1 gliomas, depending on location, are usually surgically removed. Management options for grade 2 gliomas are:

- a conservative 'watch and wait' policy, with serial imaging and clinical assessment used to monitor the tumour closely
- surgery
- radiotherapy
- chemotherapy
- a combination of surgery, chemotherapy and radiotherapy

No well-designed study has provided results to confirm a single best approach. Most surgeons feel that tumour removal, if possible, results in a better prognosis. However, partial removal can prove useful by minimising neurological deficit, for example speech deficit and hemiparesis. This benefit is especially important considering that patients with low-grade tumours may live for many years after diagnosis.

> **Biopsy grading provides information on the histology of only the specimen and not necessarily all parts of the tumour.** Detailed imaging helps determine targets for biopsy by identifying areas of the tumour that appear to be of the highest grade. This enables specimens to be obtained whose analysis is most likely to lead to an accurate diagnosis.

Prognosis

Generally, the lower the grade, the better the median survival rate for patients with gliomas.

Glioblastoma multiforme

Glioblastoma multiforme is a high-grade (World Health Organization grade 4) glioma of astrocyte origin. It is the most common malignant primary brain tumour, accounting for 12–15% of all primary brain tumours, and most frequently presents in people in their fifties and sixties. Glioblastoma multiforme tumours usually arise in the cerebrum but may develop anywhere in the central nervous system.

Types and aetiology

Glioblastoma multiforme can be primary or secondary.

- Primary glioblastoma multiforme (> 90% of cases) develops as de novo tumours in elderly patients, with no evidence of a previous low grade precursor
- Secondary glioblastoma multiforme tends to develop in younger patients, progressing from a previous low-grade precursor (e.g. grade 2 diffuse astrocytoma)

The two types of glioblastoma multiforme are histologically the same but genetically different. Secondary glioblastoma multiforme carries a slightly better prognosis; patients survive for longer.

Clinical features

The clinical features of glioblastoma multiforme develop rapidly. The commonest presenting features are increased intracranial pressure and focal neurological deficits.

Management

Like most high-grade gliomas, glioblastoma multiforme is diffusely infiltrative; the tumour rapidly infiltrates surrounding brain tissue, without a clear margin. Tumour cells also spread far along white matter, making surgical resection and cure nearly impossible. The best treatment is to resect as much tumour as safely possible, followed by postoperative radiotherapy and chemotherapy.

Prognosis

Median survival is < 18 months. Less than 3% of glioblastoma multiforme patients are alive 5 years after diagnosis.

Meningiomas

Meningiomas are primary tumours that probably originate from the arachnoid cell layer of the meninges (see page 27). They can develop at any site where meningeal layers are present, and may grow near dural venous sinuses. This can make surgical removal difficult, because of the high risks of haemorrhage and infarction as a result of dural venous sinus injury.

Epidemiology

Meningiomas account for 15% of primary brain tumours. They are twice as common in women than in men, probably because of hormonal influences. Incidence peaks in the mid-forties.

Aetiology

The definitive cause of meningiomas is unknown. However, both low- and high-dose radiation have been associated with subsequent meningioma formation, especially if exposure occurred during childhood.

Clinical features

Presentation is as for any intracranial tumour (see page 273). However, slow growth rates mean that even a very large tumour can be asymptomatic, especially if it is in a non-eloquent area of the brain.

Management

Decision making is determined by:

- patient age
- tumour size
- tumour location
- clinical features and presentation

Meningiomas are frequently benign low-grade tumours that can be resected successfully.

More malignant high-grade forms, such as anaplastic meningioma, usually require post-operative radiotherapy to reduce the risk of recurrence.

Only monitoring is required for small meningiomas with no associated brain oedema and that present only with seizures that are easily controlled with antiepileptic drugs. They may even stop growing.

Nerve sheath tumours

Nerve sheath tumours are rare tumours that arise from nerves or nerve sheaths. They occur in any cranial, spinal or peripheral nerve.

Types

There are two main types of nerve sheath tumour.

- Schwannomas originate from Schwann cells (see page 14); the most common intracranial form is a vestibular schwannoma (acoustic neuroma) (**Figure 7.6**)

- Neurofibromas originate from Schwann cells and other components of nerves

The presence of bilateral vestibular schwannomas is diagnostic of neurofibromatosis type 2 (see Chapter 15). Patients with neurofibromatosis type 1 or 2 are at increased risk of developing neurofibromas and schwannomas, probably because of defects in genes of nerve development.

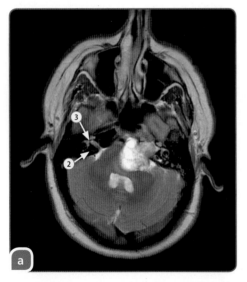
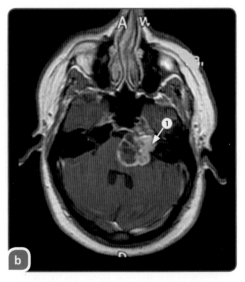

Figure 7.6 Axial MRI scans with T2W (a) and post-contrast T1W (b) sequences demonstrating a left sided Schwannoma tumour ① arising from 7th/8th cranial nerve complex in the cerebello-pontine angle and extending into the left auditory canal. The right sided cerebello-pontine (CP) angle is also shown ② with the right 7th/8th cranial nerve complex entering the right internal auditory canal ③.

Clinical features

Nerve sheath tumours present with symptoms or signs related to dysfunction in a specific nerve. They can also compress local structures, including:

- the spinal cord, causing features of cord compression
- the brain stem or other cranial nerves; for example, a vestibular schwannoma may compress cranial nerve VII, causing facial weakness, and the cochlear part of cranial nerve VIII, causing deafness and tinnitus

Management

Nerve sheath tumours can be managed conservatively (watch and wait) or treated with surgery or stereotactic 'radiosurgery' (high dose highly localised stereotactically planned and placed radiotherapy).

Pituitary tumours

Pituitary tumours can cause serious hormonal derangements and local damage to critical structures, including the optic chiasm, cavernous sinuses, internal carotid arteries and multiple cranial nerves (cranial nerves III, IV, VI and parts of cranial nerve V).

Types

Most pituitary tumours are benign adenomas arising from epithelial cells of glandular origin in the anterior pituitary (adenohypophysis). Classification is based on:

- size (microadenomas are < 1 cm and macroadenomas are larger)
- whether or not they are functional (hormone-secreting)
- the hormone or hormones predominantly secreted, and therefore the secretory cell type, if the tumour is functional

The commonest pituitary tumour types, in order of descending frequency, are:

- prolactin-secreting (prolactinoma)
- non-functional
- growth hormone–secreting
- Adrenocorticotrophic hormone–secreting

Epidemiology

Pituitary tumours account for 10% of primary intracranial tumours. They most commonly occur in people in their thirties and forties, and affect men and women equally.

> **Pituitary apoplexy is a rare feature of a pituitary tumour.** Sudden haemorrhage causes headache, vomiting and loss of consciousness. Extension into the cavernous sinus causes sudden onset of ocular movement abnormalities. Immediate treatment is with fluid resuscitation, replacement of steroids and correction of electrolyte abnormalities.

Clinical features

Pituitary tumours tend to present in one of three ways:

- excessive secretion of a hormone (**Table 7.5**)
- decreased or absent secretion of all pituitary hormones (panhypopituitarism) as a consequence of gland compression
- compression of adjacent structures (e.g. optic nerve chiasm compression causes bitemporal hemianopia; see **Figure 7.7**; with extension into the cavernous sinus, cranial nerves III, IV and VI can also be affected, causing diplopia and ophthalmoplegia)

Functional tumours of the pituitary gland: hyperpituitarism	
Pituitary tumour type	Clinical manifestation
Prolactinoma	Men: loss of libido and infertility
	Women: excessive lactation, infertility and loss of libido
Growth hormone secretory	Acromegaly in adults
	Gigantism in children
ACTH secretory	Cushing's syndrome
Follicle-stimulating hormone or luteinising hormone secretory	Infertility
Thyroid-stimulating hormone secretory	Secondary hyperthyroidism

ACTH, adrenocorticotrophic hormone.

Table 7.5 Classic clinical syndromes associated with functional tumours of the pituitary gland, in descending order of frequency

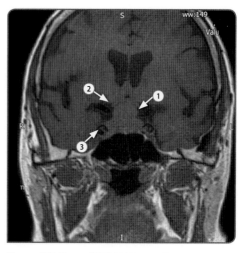

Figure 7.7 Coronal T1W MRI scan demonstrating large pituitary lesion ① compressing the optic chiasm ② and displacing it upwards. There is lateral extension into the cavernous sinuses bilaterally with encasement of the internal carotid arteries ③ within the cavernous sinuses.

Diagnostic approach

All suspected pituitary tumours are investigated with pre- and post-contrast MRI. An endocrinologist is consulted to measure all pituitary hormones. Referral to an ophthalmologist is also required for assessment of visual fields and the degree of optic nerve compression.

Management

Non-prolactinomas, and prolactinomas unresponsive to dopamine agonists, usually require surgical resection.

> **Measurement of prolactin level is essential in cases of pituitary tumour.** Prolactin level determines whether the patient requires medical or surgical intervention in the first instance. A significant increase suggests a prolactin-secreting adenoma (prolactinoma), which is highly responsive to medical therapy.

Metastatic tumours

Any malignant tumour in the body can metastasise to the brain and spine; metastatic tumours of peripheral nerves are extremely rare. Spinal metastases (see page 284) develop mostly in bony elements rather than the spinal cord or spinal nerves.

In adults, metastases to the brain (secondary brain tumours) are more common than primary brain tumours. Secondary brain tumours usually spread through the blood (haematogenously) (**Table 7.6**). The final outcome depends on finding and successfully treating the original primary tumour.

Epidemiology

Between 15 and 30% of cancer patients develop brain metastases. Of these patients, half have multiple brain metastases. Most brain metastases are supratentorial.

Sources of brain metastases	
Primary tumour site	Proportion of brain metastases (%)
Lung	45
Breast	10
Kidney	7
Gastrointestinal	6
Melanoma	5

Table 7.6 Common sources of brain metastases in adults

Clinical features

Presentation is as for any intracranial tumour (see page 273). Cerebral oedema is common, leading to mass effect and features of increased intracranial pressure. Hydrocephalus develops with infratentorial metastases, and usually results from cerebrospinal fluid obstruction at the 4th ventricle.

Diagnostic approach

The priority is finding the primary cancer. This is achieved through a thorough clinical history and examination to exclude common and uncommon primary tumours, for example lung, breast, prostate and renal cancers, and melanoma. Radiological imaging includes staging CT scans of the chest, abdomen and pelvis.

Metastatic tumours look very similar to abscesses on CT. Blood tests, including measurement of inflammatory markers (e.g. C-reactive protein), and MRI with diffusion-weighted imaging can help differentiate the two.

Management

Management of metastatic brain tumours relies not only on management of the metastasis to the brain, but more importantly identifying and appropriately treating the primary tumour or origin. Specific strategies for the brain metastasis include a combination of medication, surgery and radiotherapy.

Medication

Steroids are given to control symptoms of cerebral oedema.

Surgery

Resection is indicated for solitary, surgically accessible, symptomatic or life-threatening tumours, especially if the primary tumour is resistant to radiotherapy.

Radiotherapy

Whole-brain radiotherapy is used:

- for cases of multiple metastases
- to decrease local recurrence rates after surgical resection of a single cerebral metastasis
- in patients deemed anaesthetically unfit for surgery

This treatment option is most effective when the primary tumours are sensitive to radiotherapy (e.g. small-cell lung carcinoma and lymphoma) and least effective for radiotherapy-resistant tumours (e.g. melanoma and thyroid carcinoma).

Prognosis

This depends on disease burden from the primary tumour and the patient's age, comorbidities and level of fitness.

Spinal tumours

Several types of tumour affect the spine (**Figure 7.8**).

- Extradural tumours are outside the meninges, and include metastases as well as primary bone tumours (e.g. osteoma and osteosarcoma)

- Intradural extramedullary tumours are inside the dura but outside the spinal cord itself; they include meningiomas and nerve sheath tumours arising from spinal nerve roots (e.g. schwannoma and neurofibroma)

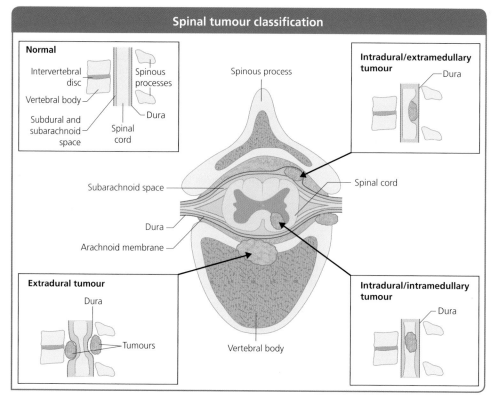

Figure 7.8 Classifying spinal tumours

- Intradural intramedullary tumours are inside the spinal cord and include gliomas (e.g. astrocytomas, ependymomas, oligodendrogliomas and ganglioglioma)

Epidemiology

The spine is the most common site of bone metastasis. Between 30 and 90% of patients with terminal cancer have spinal metastases.

Aetiology

The rich blood supply of the spine (see page 72) means that most metastases arrive haematogenously. The valveless veins of Batson's venous plexus connect to all the major venous systems of the body, enabling tumour cells to easily infiltrate the spine.

Tumours may also infiltrate by direct extension. For example, lung cancer may directly invade the thoracic segment of the spine.

Clinical features

The clinical features of spinal tumours depend on their location and speed of progression (see page 344).

Diagnostic approach

Early diagnosis and treatment of spinal tumours is essential. Urgent spine MRI is used to exclude a compressive lesion, visualise spinal cord integrity and locate any lesions. CT of the spine to assess bone integrity is indicated if mechanical stability is a concern. Total body imaging is required if metastatic spread is suspected.

Management

The aims of management are to:

- preserve neurological function and relieve spinal cord or nerve compression
- obtain a histological diagnosis

- control the tumour locally
- provide mechanical stability and correct any deformity

Medication

Steroids and prompt neurosurgical referral are indicated in cases of acute cord compression.

Palliative measures to relieve pain are essential for patients who are unfit for major treatment, such as surgery or extensive radiotherapy.

Surgery

Surgical procedures include a combination of spinal cord or nerve decompression, biopsy or resection, and stabilisation.

Surgical decompression for extradural lesions, particularly metastases, is indicated in the following cases (**Figure 7.9**):

- when disease is confined to a single spinal level
- when the tumour is radiotherapy-resistant
- when the patient is ambulant or only recently paralysed (within 24–48 h), is fit to undergo anaesthesia and has a life expectancy of over 3 months

Surgery to stabilise the spine with screws, rods and plates is carried out simultaneously if mechanical instability is a concern.

Radiotherapy

This may be given to relieve pain in patients with spinal metastases.

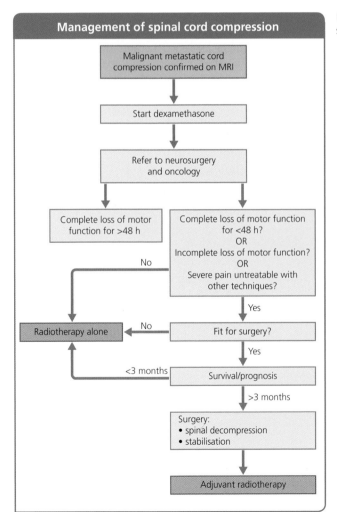

Figure 7.9 Managing metastatic spinal cord compression.

Prognosis

In cases of spinal metastases, prognosis depends on the nature and control of the primary tumour.

Most disability results from compression of neurological structures by the tumour or from iatrogenic damage during surgery.

Answers to starter questions

1. Genetic analysis of brain tumour specimens is vital, because the results are used to optimise treatment and inform prognosis. In some tumours, such as oligodendrogliomas, the presence or absence of a specific mutation indicates the effectiveness of a drug or radiotherapy. Therefore treatment can be tailored to individual patients.

2. All cells in the body have the potential to become cancerous. Cells become cancerous by adopting abnormally high growth rates, evading growth rate controls and mechanisms that target abnormal cells, and developing an increased vascular and lymphatic supply that allows cancerous cells to spread. These factors accumulate progressively through inherited mutations and new mutations that arise during a person's life.

3. The central nervous system is considered 'immune privileged' because the blood–brain barrier regulates the entry of immune cells. Therefore in the central nervous system there is less surveillance by peripheral immune cells. However, equivalent cells within the central nervous system, microglia, compensate for this deficit by killing abnormal cells.

Chapter 8
Neurological infections

Starter questions

Answers to the following questions are on page 308.

1. How does the immune response in the brain differ from that in the rest of the body?
2. How do immune cells 'know' to cross the blood–brain barrier to interact with infectious agents in the brain?
3. Steroids suppress the body's immune response, so why are they useful for treating infection?
4. Does inflammation damage the brain permanently?

Introduction

The nervous system can be infected by bacteria, viruses, fungi, spirochaetes and prions. Devastating infections such as bacterial meningitis and herpes simplex virus encephalitis are rare. In contrast, nervous system infection due to enteroviruses such as coxsackie viruses is common and less serious.

Opportunistic infections become pathogenic in cases of immunosuppression, for example in people with HIV infection. The causative agents include fungi and latent viruses.

Infection can involve one or more of the following: meninges, in cases of meningitis; brain parenchyma, in encephalitis; spinal cord, in myelitis; nerve roots, in radiculitis; dorsal root ganglia, in ganglionitis; peripheral nerves, in neuritis; arteries, in arteritis; and veins, in phlebitis.

The central nervous system's immune system is unique because:

- the brain has no lymphatic system
- B cell-mediated defences predominate over T cell-mediated ones
- the blood–brain barrier tightly controls immune cell access

Together, these properties limit oedema and secondary damage during inflammation of the central nervous system in response to infection.

Case 9 Fever and confusion

Presentation

Michael Breckford, a 19-year-old student, is brought into the emergency department confused, drowsy and feverish. He has an abdominal rash comprising small purple macules coalescing into larger patches. The rash does not disappear with pressure.

Initial interpretation

Confusion, drowsiness and fever suggest central nervous system infection, so meningitis, encephalitis and abscesses are possible diagnoses. The non-blanching purpuric rash may indicate systemic meningococcal septicaemia causing impaired coagulation, capillary leakage and haemorrhage. This is an alarming combination of symptoms that warrant urgent assessment with treatment for potential bacterial meningitis.

Even without the rash, a central nervous system infection is likely. Therefore empirical treatment to cover for both viral and bacterial infection would be initiated.

Non-central nervous system infections causing systemic sepsis with metabolic disturbance can produce a similar picture of septic encephalopathy.

History

Michael's flatmates give a collateral history. He was well until 24 hours ago, when he became increasingly sleepy and missed lectures. At first he had headache, but he became progressively less coherent over the course of the day. An hour ago, they found him feverish and confused so called an ambulance.

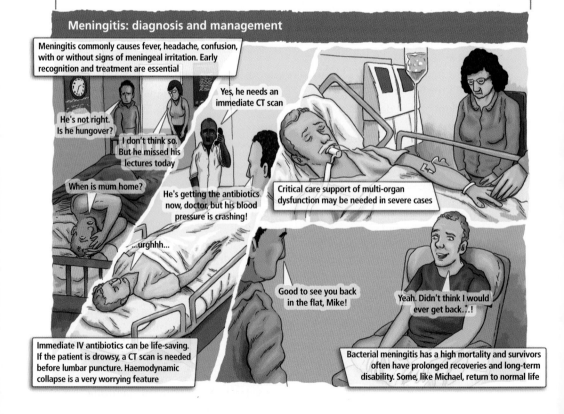

Meningitis: diagnosis and management

Meningitis commonly causes fever, headache, confusion, with or without signs of meningeal irritation. Early recognition and treatment are essential

He's not right. Is he hungover?

When is mum home?

Yes, he needs an immediate CT scan

I don't think so. But he missed his lectures today

He's getting the antibiotics now, doctor, but his blood pressure is crashing!

...urghhh...

Critical care support of multi-organ dysfunction may be needed in severe cases

Good to see you back in the flat, Mike!

Yeah. Didn't think I would ever get back...!

Immediate IV antibiotics can be life-saving. If the patient is drowsy, a CT scan is needed before lumbar puncture. Haemodynamic collapse is a very worrying feature

Bacterial meningitis has a high mortality and survivors often have prolonged recoveries and long-term disability. Some, like Michael, return to normal life

Interpretation of history

Patients with central nervous system infection are usually unable to provide a history. In cases of haemodynamic instability caused by sepsis, the priority is treatment of the most serious potential causes, including bacterial meningitis. Every effort should be made to contact the patient's family, friends and other contacts as early as possible. This is essential to obtain a collateral history regarding the patient's condition and because the patient's contacts may also be affected.

Immediate treatment for bacterial meningitis, an acutely life-threatening cause of this presentation, is mandated. Further investigation can continue after initial treatment.

Key differential diagnoses for bacterial meningitis are shown in **Table 8.1**.

Concomitant treatment with aciclovir is started empirically in cases of suspected central nervous system infection, because herpes simplex virus encephalitis can be missed, potentially leading to severe neurological disability and/or death.

> **Fever, headache and cognitive changes raise the suspicion of infective meningitis.** This presentation triggers immediate assessment, investigation and initiation of empirical antibiotics or antiviral drugs based on local treatment policies.

Bacterial meningitis: differential diagnosis	
Disease	Differentiating feature(s)
Bacterial meningitis	Acute onset
	Patients often have severe sepsis
Viral meningitis	Usually less severe
	Onset acute (hours to days) or subacute (days)
Tuberculous meningitis	More gradual onset: subacute or chronic (days to weeks)
	Cranial nerve palsies
Fungal meningitis	Usually slower onset (subacute or chronic)
	Immunocompromise is a risk factor
Autoimmune meningitis (e.g. systemic lupus erythematosus)	Slower onset (subacute or chronic)
	Less severe
Septic encephalopathy	Cerebrospinal fluid is normal
Acute subarachnoid haemorrhage	Usually apyrexial
	Sudden onset severe headache ('worst headache ever')
Septic venous sinus thrombosis	Confirmed by neuroimaging
Carcinomatous or malignant meningitis	History of malignancy
	Usually apyrexial

Table 8.1 Bacterial meningitis and its key differential diagnoses. All present with one or more of the major symptoms of bacterial meningitis (headache, fever, meningism and altered mental status)

Further history

Michael has no history of recurrent infections to suggest a primary immunodeficiency. He is not known to be HIV-positive or to have risk factors for HIV.

He has not travelled abroad in years. He has no contact with animals to suggest exposure to an uncommon infectious agent.

Examination

Michael's Glasgow coma scale score is E2 (eye opening to pain) V3 (verbal responses: inappropriate words) M5 (movement localised to stimulus) (see page 453). The non-blanching purpuric rash over his abdomen and limbs persists. His neck is stiff to passive movements.

Case 9 *continued*

He does not cooperate with neurological examination but can spontaneously move each limb in response to a painful stimulus. His pupils are equal and reactive. He is tachycardic, with a blood pressure of 90/60 mmHg and a temperature of 40.1°C.

Interpretation of findings

Michael's tachycardia, low blood pressure and fever indicate systemic sepsis; a large release of inflammatory mediators causes systemic vasodilation, hypotension and tachycardia. Neck stiffness and drowsiness indicate meningeal inflammation and global brain dysfunction. These findings suggest meningococcal septicaemia. Immediate sepsis treatment is required:

- high-flow oxygen
- blood cultures
- broad spectrum antibiotics
- intravenous fluid challenges
- measurement of serum lactate and haemoglobin
- accurate measurement of hourly urine output

Once his condition has stabilised, he needs a lumbar puncture to confirm diagnosis and guide antibiotic therapy.

His drowsiness may indicate increased intracranial pressure. Therefore computerised tomography (CT) to exclude a space-occupying lesion must be done before lumbar puncture.

Investigations

The CT scan excludes a mass lesion (**Table 8.2**). Lumbar puncture and the results of cerebrospinal fluid analysis show a high opening pressure (45 cm of H_2O), white cell count >10,000 and low cerebrospinal fluid:serum glucose ratio. Gram stain contains Gram-negative diplococci, which are identified as *Neisseria meningitidis*.

Contraindications for lumbar puncture	
Type	Contraindications
Neurological	Glasgow coma scale score reduced or fluctuating (< 13) or decreasing by 2
	Focal neurological signs, including pupil abnormalities
	Abnormal posture or posturing
	Papilloedema
	After seizure, before stabilisation
	Abnormal 'doll's eye' movements
Systemic	Bradycardia with hypertension
	Immunocompromise
	Systemic shock
	Coagulation abnormalities
	Respiratory failure
Infective	Suspected meningococcal septicaemia
	Local infection at site for lumbar puncture

Table 8.2 Contraindications for immediate lumbar puncture before neuroimaging . Cerebrospinal fluid analysis is essential for diagnosis and to guide management in central nervous system infection; it is delayed pending neuroimaging only in the conditions listed in this table.

Diagnosis

The Gram stain confirms a diagnosis of bacterial meningitis. In many cases, the initial Gram stain can be negative, but a very high white cell count and low cerebrospinal fluid:serum glucose ratio still indicate bacterial meningitis. Culture of cerebrospinal fluid requires a few days to grow and identify an organism.

Michael is given intravenous ceftriaxone based on cerebrospinal fluid culture sensitivities. After 5 weeks on the intensive care unit, he ultimately makes a full recovery.

Bacterial meningitis

Meningitis is inflammation of the meninges, which envelop the brain and spinal cord (see page 27). Bacterial meningitis is the most serious form: untreated, it commonly progresses to overwhelming brain infection, which carries a high mortality.

Patients require early, aggressive resuscitation and treatment. Bacterial meningitis is suspected in any patient presenting with meningism and features of sepsis (a severe bloodstream infection with fever and non-blanching petechial or purpuric rash).

Epidemiology

The annual incidence of bacterial meningitis is 4 per 100,000 in the UK, with peaks in infants and adolescents. Vaccinations against the common causes, *Haemophilus influenzae* type B and *N. meningitidis* type C, have significantly reduced the rate of new cases.

Aetiology

The pathogens responsible for bacterial meningitis vary depending on patient age, immune status and clinical setting (**Table 8.3**). These associations predict the most effective initial broad spectrum antibiotic therapy if meningitis is suspected.

Pathogenesis

Common bacteria in community-acquired meningitis, i.e. *H. influenzae*, *Streptococcus pneumoniae* and *N. meningitidis*, all normally colonise nasal cavities and skull sinuses.

Invasion of intracranial compartments is more likely in the context of immunodeficiency or a breach in structural defences, for example after trauma or surgery.

Bacterial invasion precipitates an acute inflammatory response with aggregation of polymorphonuclear cells. Spread through the subarachnoid space causes local and systemic complications (**Table 8.4**).

Clinical features

Meningitis classically presents with fever and meningism (the triad of headache, photophobia and neck stiffness or rigidity). The condition is usually be preceded by a prodrome, such as respiratory tract or ear infection. It is also associated with risk factors depending on the cause, for example traumatic skull fracture with cerebrospinal fluid leak.

The presence of a purpuric non-blanching rash strongly suggests meningococcal septicaemia. The pathogenesis is a systemic inflammatory response with likely disseminated intravascular coagulopathy, causing a combination of severe vasodilation, capillary leakage, haemorrhaging into skin and microvascular thromboses.

Neurological complications include:

- increased intracranial pressure (depressed level of consciousness, headache, nausea and vomiting)
- seizures (in 20%)
- focal neurological deficits (in 10%) and cranial nerve deficits

> **Aseptic meningitis is diagnosed in cases of increased cerebrospinal fluid white cell count with no organisms identified on Gram stain or standard cultures.** Causes include viruses, spirochaetes, parasites, *Brucella* species, *Mycoplasma* species, use of certain drugs (e.g. intravenous immunoglobulin and non-steroidal anti-inflammatory drugs) and meningeal tumour metastases.

Diagnostic approach

The diagnostic approach is identical for any suspected nervous system infection (**Table 8.5**).

The clinical history, presentation and examination form the initial basis of the diagnostic

Age-related bacterial causes of meningitis		
Clinical setting	Age	Common organism(s)
Immunocompetent	< 3 months	Group B *Streptococcus* *Escherichia coli* *Listeria monocytogenes*
Immunocompetent	3 months to 18 years	*Neisseria meningitidis* (meningococcus) *Strep. pneumoniae* (pneumococcus) *Haemophilus influenzae*
Immunocompetent	18–50 years	*Strep. pneumoniae* *N. meningitidis*
Immunocompetent	> 50 years	*Strep. pneumoniae* *L. monocytogenes* Gram-negative bacilli
Immunocompromised	Any	*L. monocytogenes* Gram-negative bacilli *Strep. pneumoniae* *H. influenzae*
Head trauma	Any	*Strep. pneumoniae* Staphylococci Mixed
After a neurosurgical procedure	Any	Staphylococci *Pseudomonas aeruginosa*
Epidemics	Usually 18–50 years	*N. meningitidis*
Others	Any	*Mycobacterium tuberculosis* *Brucella* species

Table 8.3 Prediction of the commonest bacterial causes of meningitis from the clinical setting and patient's age. Empirical antibiotic therapy is started to cover these organisms, based on local bacterial sensitivities and policies

Complications of bacterial meningitis		
Distribution	Complications	Pathogenesis
Local	Arteritis and phlebitis	Blood vessel inflammation
	Ischaemia	Vessel occlusion and thrombosis
	Cranial neuritis	Cranial nerve inflammation
	Hydrocephalus	Obstruction of cerebrospinal fluid outflow from inflammation
	Abscess	Inflammation spreading into focal brain region
	Increased intracranial pressure	Generalised inflammation and oedema
Systemic	Cardiovascular shock	Hypotension from vasodilation
	Renal failure	Renal hypoperfusion and nephrotoxic injury from inflammatory mediators
	Disseminated intravascular coagulation	Platelets and coagulation factors consumed in acute thromboses that cause ischaemia and infarction; state of low platelet and coagulation factor levels then leads to widespread haemorrhage
	Waterhouse-Friderichsen syndrome	Adrenal failure from adrenal gland hypoperfusion and infarction

Table 8.4 Complications of bacterial meningitis

approach. If there is any suspicion of bacterial meningitis on this initial assessment, broad spectrum antibiotics are commenced immediately prior to investigation, as any delay increases the mortality risk.

Bloods are then obtained for microbiological assessment (cultures) and severity of systemic (e.g. full blood count, renal and liver function) and inflammatory responses (e.g. CRP, white cell count).

Approach to suspected central nervous system infections	
Clinical assessment	Assess risk factors: HIV, recurrent bacterial infections, head trauma and neurosurgical intervention
	Determine haemodynamic and respiratory status
Investigations	Full blood count, urea and electrolytes, liver function tests, coagulation profile, glucose and C-reactive protein
	Blood cultures, throat swabs and serology titres
	CT, CT with contrast and MRI
	Lumbar puncture and cerebrospinal fluid analysis (see **Table 8.6**)

Table 8.5 Approach to suspected central nervous system infections (of all causes). If bacterial infection is suspected, aggressive empirical antibiotic therapy is started immediately (see page 294)

Definitive confirmation of intracranial infection is usually made on identification of a microbial organism on cerebrospinal fluid assessment (e.g. bacterial culture, fungal staining and culture, viral polymerase chain reaction). Cerebrospinal fluid is normally obtained following lumbar puncture but this is contraindicated in certain situations (**Table 8.2**).

In this day and age, rapid access to computed tomography scanning is available as an initial diagnostic tool to exclude a space-occupying lesion and is usually performed prior to lumbar puncture.

Cerebrospinal fluid assessment can be rapidly performed within a short period of time (usually < 1 h) to give an initial idea as to the nature of infection (see **Table 8.6**) but definitive culture to identify an organism takes at least 48–72 h (if not longer).

Nonetheless, when suspecting intracranial infection, the severity of complications including severe neurological disability and risk of death, means that treatment is commenced as soon as possible before awaiting results of tests.

Bacterial meningitis is confirmed by identification of an organism on cerebrospinal fluid culture. However, empirical antibiotic treatment is started immediately (see page 294).

Investigations

Lumbar puncture to obtain cerebrospinal fluid is key to confirming infection, but the procedure is contraindicated in certain

Cerebrospinal fluid findings in neurological inflammation						
Type of agent	Opening pressure	White cell count	Protein	CSF:serum glucose ratio	Lactate	Oligoclonal bands
Bacterial	Very high	1000 s (mainly polymorphonuclear cells)	Very high	< 50%	High	Paired, unpaired or polyclonal
Viral	Mildly increased	100 s (mainly mononuclear cells)	Mildly increased	> 50%	Normal	Normal
Tuberculous	Very high	10 s to 100 s (mainly mononuclear cells)	Very high	< 50%	Very high	Paired, unpaired or polyclonal
Autoimmune	Mildly increased	< 100	Mildly to very increased	> 50%	Normal	Paired, unpaired or polyclonal

Table 8.6 Typical cerebrospinal fluid findings for bacterial, viral, tuberculous and autoimmune causes of neurological inflammation

circumstances (see **Table 8.2**). Cerebrospinal fluid tests for investigation of neurological infection include the following:

- opening pressure, which indicates intracranial pressure
- white cell count, including the differential test, to help delineate whether the cause is bacterial, viral, fungal or aseptic meningitis
- glucose to distinguish between bacterial, viral and tuberculous causes
- protein to identify hypercellularity and inflammation
- Gram stain to visualise any organisms
- definitive culture for diagnosis and antibiotic sensitivity
- special tests to identify specific pathogens
- oligoclonal bands (OCBs)
  - Paired OCBs (matched immunoglobulin peaks in serum and cerebrospinal fluid) indicate a systemic immune response
  - Unpaired OCBs mean immunoglobulin synthesised in the nervous system
  - Polyclonal OCBs indicate a non-specific immune response in the central nervous system

In **Table 8.6**, typical cerebrospinal fluid findings in neurological inflammation resulting from bacterial infection are contrasted with findings in other neurological infections. Common organisms visualised by Gram staining of cerebrospinal fluid are:

- Gram-positive cocci (e.g. *Staphylococcus aureus* and *Strep. pneumoniae*)
- Gram-negative cocci (e.g. *N. meningitidis*)
- Gram-negative bacilli (e.g. *Haemophilus influenzae and Escherichia coli*)
- Other agents (e.g. *Listeria monocytogenes*)

Management

When there is suspicion of a bacterial cause for meningitis-like clinical features, antibiotics are not delayed until diagnosis. Broad spectrum antibiotics, chosen on the basis of the likely species and local sensitivities,

are started immediately. Antibiotic choice is adjusted later, when the species has been identified. The definitive choice is usually a third-generation cephalosporin such as ceftriaxone. An aminoglycoside, for example gentamicin, is usually added for neonates, and ampicillin for neonates and the elderly . The principles of treatment are:

- aggressive early resuscitation with oxygen and intravenous fluid therapy
- intravenous antimicrobial therapy for ≥ 2 weeks

Additional measures are usually required, including one or more of the following:

- Addition of aciclovir if encephalitis is suspected
- Steroids (e.g. dexamethasone 10 mg/6 h), which are usually given for 4 days, to improve morbidity and mortality in the treatment of bacterial meningitis
- Treatment of the precipitating factor (e.g. if meningitis is secondary to cerebrospinal fluid leakage following trauma or iatrogenically following surgery, this must be repaired to prevent future episodes)
- Supportive treatment for shock and increased intracranial pressure (see page 190)
- Management of complications, such as cerebrospinal fluid diversion in hydrocephalus, and abscess evacuation

Prophylaxis

Public health authorities require notification of confirmed cases to enable the tracing of contacts; oral rifampicin prophylaxis is then offered to close contacts.

Prognosis

Mortality of bacterial meningitis varies depending on the pathogen involved and the patient's age and comorbidities. It is highest in neonates (40–75%) and varies from 7% (in cases caused by *H. influenzae* or *N. meningitidis*) to 20% (in those caused by *Streptococcus* species).

Viral meningitis

Viral meningitis is more common than bacterial meningitis. However, it is usually self-limiting, and patients generally recover without major neurological complications.

Epidemiology

In the UK, 3000 cases of viral meningitis are reported annually. However, the true incidence is thought to be far higher.

Aetiology

Many viral species cause meningitis, the most commonly identified ones being echovirus, coxsackievirus B, HIV and herpes simplex virus type 2. However, in many cases no organism is identifiable by culture or polymerase chain reaction (PCR) detection.

Pathogenesis

A virus can enter the body through a skin lesion or the respiratory, gastrointestinal or urogenital tract, then replicates locally (primary replication). It may then enter the nervous system haematogenously or through a cranial or peripheral nerve, as in cases of poliomyelitis. This often happens after secondary replication at other sites, for example fat and muscle. There is localised cell death and inflammation comprising mononuclear cells, ependymal destruction and meningeal inflammation.

Clinical features

Viral meningitis presents similarly to bacterial meningitis but is usually less severe. Seizures, focal neurological deficits and profound changes in level of consciousness are rare. If such features are present, parenchymal involvement, i.e. encephalitis, is suspected.

Diagnostic approach

Viruses are difficult to culture from cerebrospinal fluid. However, PCR for viral nucleic acids identifies many common viruses, including herpes simplex virus, varicella-zoster virus and enteroviruses. A diagnosis of viral meningitis can be made confidently when the results of cerebrospinal fluid PCR are positive for viral nucleic acids. However, the organism is often not identifiable on PCR, so the diagnosis is based on a typical clinical history of fever, headache and lack of significant neurological deficit, together with cerebrospinal fluid with mildly increased white cell count and other characteristics that differentiate viral from bacterial infection (**Table 8.6**).

Imaging

Meningeal enhancement is usually visible on contrast-enhanced magnetic resonance imaging (MRI) or CT (**Figure 8.1**). However, it may also be present in other infective (e.g. bacterial and tuberculous) or non-infective (e.g. autoimmune) causes of meningitis.

Management

Viral meningitis is usually benign and self-limiting. Treatment is symptomatic.

Persistence of headache for several weeks or progressive visual impairment may indicate impaired cerebrospinal fluid reabsorption as a result of meningeal inflammation and increased intracranial pressure (see page 190). Cerebrospinal fluid diversionary procedures, such as lumbar punctures or shunting, may be indicated to prevent pressure from causing permanent visual loss.

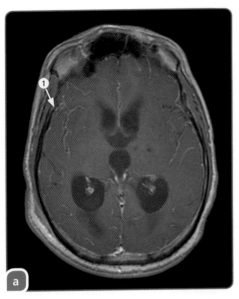
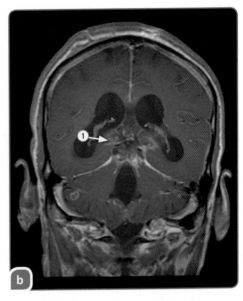

Figure 8.1 Axial (a) and coronal (b) post-gadolinium contrast-enhanced magnetic resonance imaging scan showing the non-specific features of meningitis. Diffuse leptomeningeal enhancement ① suggests meningitis, and the dilated ventricles are in keeping with communicating hydrocephalus as its result.

Encephalitis

Encephalitis is inflammation of the neuronal and glial substance of the brain (parenchyma), and can be caused by any infectious agent or autoimmune process. Herpes simplex virus is the most serious viral cause. Early treatment with the antiviral drug aciclovir reduces mortality from 70% to 20–30%.

Encephalitis can co-occur with inflammation of the:

- meninges (as meningoencephalitis)
- spinal cord (as encephalomyelitis)

Epidemiology

The annual incidence of encephalitis is 1 per 100,000.

Aetiology

The commonest identified viral cause is herpes simplex virus type 1. Others include herpes simplex virus type 2 in neonates, Epstein–Barr virus, varicella–zoster virus and the mumps virus, and in patients with immunodeficiency, cytomegalovirus, HIV and JC viruses. Most epidemics are caused by arboviruses, such those responsible for tick-borne encephalitis and Japanese encephalitis.

Herpes simplex virus enters the body through inhalation. It gains access to the central nervous system through the initial sites of exposure: the olfactory mucosa and cranial nerve (the anterior cranial fossa) and the trigeminal nerve and associated ganglion (the middle cranial fossa). This leads to diffuse inflammation in the basal frontal and medial temporal lobes. Autoimmune causes of encephalitis include:

- sarcoidosis (chronic granulomatous inflammation)
- systemic lupus erythematosus (vasculitis of the meningeal vessels)
- anti–voltage-gated potassium channel complex
- anti-*N*-methyl-D-aspartate receptor autoantibodies (in anti-NMDA receptor autoantibody-mediated encephalitis)

Clinical features

Encephalitis presents with headache, fever, seizures, focal neurological deficits and significant deterioration in mental status. **Table 8.7** lists the key differential diagnoses for viral encephalitis.

There may be a prodrome with some causes: parotitis for mumps; rash for measles virus, rubella virus and parvovirus; and myalgias for arboviruses. Herpes simplex virus encephalitis usually has no prodrome; it often presents with seizures and memory and behavioural dysfunction, resulting from temporal lobe inflammation.

In autoimmune encephalitis, there is often a history of other autoimmune conditions. The time course of onset is often days to weeks rather than hours. There is often no fever or laboratory evidence of systemic infection.

Diagnostic approach

The diagnosis of encephalitis is made when both of the following are found:

- evidence of inflammation from the results of cerebrospinal fluid analysis (e.g. increased white cell count, increased protein concentration and oligoclonal bands)
- clinical (e.g. memory loss) and/or radiological evidence (e.g. high signal changes indicating oedema in the temporal lobes) of focal brain involvement

Cerebrospinal fluid analysis

In viral encephalitis, the cerebrospinal fluid findings are similar to those in viral meningitis (see page 295).

Imaging

Nearly 30% of patients with encephalitis have a normal brain CT. However, 90% have an abnormal brain MRI (**Figure 8.2**).

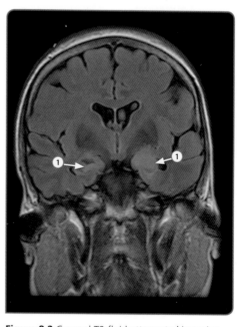

Figure 8.2 Coronal T2 fluid-attenuated inversion recovery (FLAIR) magnetic resonance imaging scan showing typical features of herpes simplex virus encephalitis. There is increased signal intensity with oedema of the medial temporal lobes ①. In severe cases, focal haemorrhage may be visible in these regions.

Differential diagnosis of viral encephalitis	
Differential diagnosis	Underlying cause
Space-occupying lesion	Tumour
	Intracranial abscess
Non-viral infectious encephalitis	Bacterial: tuberculosis, and *Mycoplasma* and *Listeria* species
	Spirochaetal: syphilis and leptospirosis
	Fungal: *Candida* and *Aspergillus* species
	Parasitic: *Toxoplasma* species, African human trypanosomiasis
Metabolic encephalopathy	Liver failure
	Kidney failure
	Drug-induced
Paraneoplastic encephalitis	Subacute inflammation of brain parenchyma, triggered by a tumour
Acute disseminated encephalomyelitis	Diffuse autoimmune white matter inflammatory process, often with spinal cord involvement

Table 8.7 Differential diagnosis of viral encephalitis. These resemble each other because they present with seizures, focal neurological deficits and deteriorating mental status

In herpes simplex virus encephalitis, electroencephalography (see page 172) shows non-specific features in the frontotemporal regions.

Management

Without treatment, herpes simplex virus encephalitis has high morbidity and mortality. Therefore most clinicians start empirical antiviral treatment in any patient presenting with suggestive features.

Medication

Intravenous aciclovir (10 mg/kg every 8 h) is administered for a minimum of 14 days (21 days in cases of immunodeficiency). The use of corticosteroids to control intracranial pressure and cerebral oedema is controversial. Supportive adjuncts may be needed, for example to control seizures.

Encephalitis with an autoimmune cause often responds to immunosuppression: intravenous steroids followed by intravenous immunoglobulin, plasma exchange and other therapies, if needed.

Prognosis

Outcome depends on the infective pathogen. Untreated herpes simplex virus has the poorest outcome, with mortality at 70%; this figure decreases to 20% with early treatment. Most survivors are left with persistent neurological deficits.

Untreated autoimmune encephalitis can cause cognitive impairment, dementia or death. Aggressive immunosuppressive treatment enables partial or full recovery.

> **Prion diseases (e.g. Creutzfeldt–Jakob disease, see page 402) are a group of unique neurodegenerative diseases caused by abnormally folding proteins.** These proteins act like infectious agents (see page 402), triggering other proteins to fold abnormally. This process is pathogenic, because the amount of abnormal protein produced ultimately becomes sufficient to cause neuronal damage and cell death.

Brain abscess

An abscess is a localised collection of pus (dead tissue, bacteria and white cells) surrounded by a capsule of fibrotic and granulation tissue; it usually results from bacterial infection. Intracranial abscesses occur at:

- extradural sites (as extradural empyema)
- subdural sites (as subdural empyema)
- intracerebral sites (in brain parenchyma)

Epidemiology

The annual incidence of brain abscess is 2–3 per million. It can occur at any age.

Aetiology

An initial infective process spreads to an intracranial compartment, either haematogenously or locally from adjacent structures. The latter process can be:

- direct (e.g. in a penetrating injury, through direct contact with the dura)
- indirect via contiguous structures (e.g. from a middle ear infection)

The infection provokes an immune response. This causes tissue necrosis and the formation of a collection of pus encased in scar tissue generated by fibroblasts.

Identification of the site and source of infection often indicates the likely pathogen (**Table 8.8**).

Clinical features

The classic triad of features, which occurs in < 50% of cases, comprises:

- fever
- headache
- focal neurological deficits (depending on location)

Causes of intracerebral abscesses		
Mode of spread	Infective sources or underlying pathologies	Likely microorganisms
Haematogenous	Chronic lung infections	Streptococci and Staphylococci
	Infective cardiac endocarditis	
	Congenital heart disease	
	Pulmonary arteriovenous malformations	
	Systemic sepsis	
Local	Trauma (e.g. penetrating brain injury)	Staphylococci
		Other contaminant organisms (e.g. clostridial spores from farmyards or soil)
	Sinus infection	Streptococci
	Facial infections	Streptococci
	Middle ear infections, including mastoiditis	Streptococci
		Enterobacteriaceae
		Pseudomonas species
		Anaerobic bacteria
	Iatrogenic (e.g. after neurosurgery)	Staphylococci
Immunodeficiency	Infection (e.g. HIV)	Any of the above organisms
	Use of certain drugs (e.g. steroids and chemotherapy drugs)	Fungi
		Parasites
	Malignancy	Others (e.g. *Listeria* and *Nocardia* species)

Table 8.8 Causes of intracerebral abscesses. The site and source of the initial infective process suggests which pathogen is implicated

Seizures occur in 30% of patients, and features of increased intracranial pressure may also be present. An intracranial abscess is part of the differential diagnosis for any space-occupying lesion visible on imaging. Features of the original infective source, for example sinusitis, pneumonia and endocarditis, may be evident.

Diagnostic approach

The diagnostic approach is as for other infections (see page 293). Urgent imaging with contrast-enhanced CT is indicated (see Figure 17.6a and b), with MRI to clarify the diagnosis (**Figure 8.3**). The source of the infection is investigated, for example echocardiography is used to assess for endocarditis, and CT sinuses for sinusitis.

Investigations

Contrast-enhanced CT shows a ring-enhancing lesion, comprising of a central area of low density surrounded contrast-enhancing ring of proliferating fibroblasts. There is usually oedema surrounding the contrast-enhancing ring lesion. Causes of a ring-enhancing lesion include:

- abscess
- tumour (primary brain or metastatic)
- cyst (e.g. in toxoplasmosis)
- tuberculosis
- lymphoma
- resolving haematoma
- demyelination plaque (e.g. in multiple sclerosis)

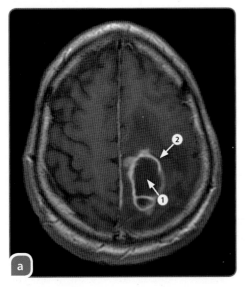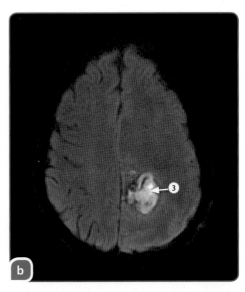

Figure 8.3 Differentiation between an abscess and a tumour. (a) Magnetic resonance imaging enhanced by contrast shows a thin-walled 'ring-enhancing' lesion. The hypodense centre ① correlates with the central zone of necrosis and inflammation, whereas the enhancing ring is the capsule of fibroblasts, collagen and vascular proliferation ②. (b) Diffusion-weighted imaging (DWI) (image shown) and associated apparent diffusion coefficient (ADC) maps help differentiate between abscess and tumour. Abscesses have restricted diffusion ③ on DWI: high signal (bright) on DWI and low signal (dark) on ADC. Tumours (not demonstrated here) usually do not: low signal (dark) on DWI and high signal (bright) on ADC.

Management

The aims of surgery are to obtain microbiological samples for identification of the causative pathogen and its antibiotic sensitivities, and to decompress any mass effect. Empirical antimicrobials are started according to the suspected pathogen, with conversion to targeted therapy once the pathogen is identified through culture and its sensitivities are confirmed.

Surgery

Extradural and subdural empyemas are neurosurgical emergencies. They require urgent surgical evacuation to prevent thrombosis and inflammation of veins and arteries on the surface of the brain. These effects of empyemas can precipitate ischaemic injury and seizures.

Medication

Common regimens include a third-generation cephalosporin, such as ceftriaxone, and metronidazole, to target anaerobic bacteria. In immunosuppressed patients, additional agents may be indicated, for example pyrimethamine, which targets toxoplasmosis; amphotericin B, an antifungal; and ampicillin, which is effective against listeria.

Supportive treatment is also required: anticonvulsants for seizures and eradication of the source to prevent recurrence.

> Ideally, tissue and abscess samples are obtained for microbiological diagnosis before antibiotics are started. This may be possible if the patient is clinically well, but antibiotics are not delayed in situations of severe or life-threatening sepsis.

Prognosis

Complications of brain abscess include focal neurologic deficits, seizures, cortical vein thrombosis and hydrocephalus. Subdural empyema has a mortality of between 10–20%, and > 50% of survivors have seizures, hydrocephalus or neurological deficits. The overall mortality of intracerebral abscesses is about 10% with treatment.

HIV and associated infections

Human immunodeficiency virus (HIV) is a blood-borne retrovirus that attacks and weakens the immune system, making patients susceptible to a range of opportunistic pathogens that do not usually cause disease. This state is referred to as acquired immunodeficiency syndrome (AIDS).

HIV-associated neurological disease is considered in patients presenting with either viral meningitis, polyneuritis or with one of the less common bacterial, fungal or viral infections. A late complication is progressive multifocal leucoencephalopathy, in which reactivation of a common latent central nervous system virus (specifically the JC virus) causes progressive central nervous system inflammation, focal signs and ultimately death.

Epidemiology

HIV and AIDS are global pandemics. An estimated 40 million people are affected; 30–80% suffer neurological dysfunction.

Aetiology

HIV infection causes profound immunodeficiency by infecting the CD4 subset of T cells (helper cells), which coordinate the entire adaptive immune response. Patents become prone to common and opportunistic infections normally subdued by a healthy immune system. Immune surveillance is also compromised, such that HIV is associated with certain malignancies caused by oncogenic viruses.

Neurological complications are summarised in **Table 8.9**; they differ depending on the stage of disease.

- **Early stage (CD4$^+$ > 500/mm):** this stage encompasses two phases: acute infection with HIV and the seroconversion phase. Neurological manifestations are due to

Stages of HIV infection and neurological complications	
Stage	Neurological complications
Early stage	
Acute infection with HIV: usually asymptomatic or with features similar to glandular fever (fever and lymphadenopathy)	None
Seroconversion of HIV	
Virus starts to infect cells and replicate over 4–12 weeks; symptomatic or asymptomatic	Viral meningitis, myopathy, neuropathy and encephalopathy
Middle stage	
Latent phase: lasts months to years; progressive destruction of CD4 T cells, with weakening of immune system and increase in viral load	Minor opportunistic infections, and immune-mediated destruction (e.g. mononeuritis multiplex)
Late stage	
AIDS phase: infection with a variety of opportunistic pathogen precipitates complications	
Cryptococcus species, fungi, *listeria* and tuberculosis	Meningitis
Cytomegalovirus, varicella-zoster virus and herpes simplex virus	Encephalitis and meningitis
Fungi (e.g. aspergillus, nocardia) and toxoplasmosis	Abscess
Cytomegalovirus and toxoplasmosis	Retinopathy
	CNS lymphoma (e.g. triggered by Epstein–Barr virus), AIDS–dementia complex, progressive multifocal leucoencephalopathy

Table 8.9 Stages of HIV infection and neurological complications

complications from HIV infection itself (e.g. HIV meningitis)

■ **Middle stage (CD4$^+$ 200–500/mm):** this stage encompasses the latent phase of HIV infection. Neurological manifestations are due to infections and complications from immune-mediated damage (e.g. mononeuritis multiplex)

■ **Late stage (CD4$^+$ < 200/mm):** this stage is the development of AIDS with complications from opportunistic pathogens (e.g. cryptococcal meningitis)

Clinical features

Primary HIV infection and viraemia can cause a seroconversion illness that is clinically similar to Guillain-Barré syndrome, with fever, lymphadenopathy and neuropathy. Indirect effects arise from opportunistic infection and adverse effects of the highly active antiretroviral therapy (HAART) used to treat HIV. Other peripheral neuropathies in many people with HIV/AIDS are listed in **Table 8.10**.

Diagnostic approach

Demonstration of anti-HIV antibodies confirms diagnosis of HIV. Most HIV-related neurological disorders are usually diagnosed in patients for whom the diagnosis of HIV is already known. Nowadays, it is rare for neurological complications to be the initial presentation of HIV.

Management

The aims of management are to:

■ treat acute neurological complications (e.g. opportunistic infection and malignancy)
■ treat HIV infection with HAART
■ assess the efficacy of treatment and monitor for development of drug resistance
■ decrease HIV viral load to < 50 copies/mL and increase CD4 T cell count to > 500/mm^3

Medication

HAART is the standard triple therapy for HIV infection. It consists of two nucleoside reverse transcriptase inhibitors and either a protease Inhibitor or a non-nucleoside reverse transcriptase inhibitor. All these block viral replication enzymes.

Specific opportunistic infections require specific treatments:

■ cytomegalovirus infection requires antiviral drugs (e.g. ganciclovir)
■ *Toxoplasma* infection requires pyrimethamine
■ cryptococcal infection requires antifungal drugs (e.g. amphotericin B)
■ primary central nervous system lymphoma requires steroids for oedema, initiation of HAART and chemoradiotherapy

Surgery

Neurosurgery may be required if patients develop mass lesions, such as abscess, metastatic deposits and primary central nervous system lymphoma, with associated increase in intracranial pressure, or if there is diagnostic uncertainty requiring tissue sample for analysis.

HIV-related peripheral neuropathy	
Tissue affected	**Causes**
Nerve roots	Seroconversion illness
	Varicella zoster virus infection
	Cytomegalovirus infection
Peripheral nerves	Polyneuropathy similar to Guillain-Barré syndrome
	Antiviral therapy-induced
Muscle	Myopathy related to zidovudine (azidothymidine, AZT) antiretroviral therapy
	Polymyositis

Table 8.10 HIV-related peripheral nervous system disorders

Specialist imaging can help differentiate lesions in patients with AIDS. For example, thallium single-photon emission computerised tomography distinguishes between a lymphoma and a *Toxoplasma* abscess.

Tuberculosis

Tuberculosis primarily affects the lung but neurological involvement does occur, most commonly in immunosuppressed patients.

> **The efficacy of antituberculous drug therapy is progressively being limited by increases in multidrug-resistant and extremely drug-resistant strains of *Mycobacterium tuberculosis*.**
> The reduction in efficacy is caused by resistant strains surviving in immunosuppressed patients treated with standard therapy.

Epidemiology

One third of the world's population is thought to have been infected by mycobacterium tuberculosis, and new infections are thought to occur in 1% of the population each year. The central nervous system is involved in 10% of patients. In the UK, the annual incidence of tuberculosis is 14 per 100,000; 40% of these cases are in London.

Aetiology

Most tuberculosis infection in humans is caused by *M. tuberculosis*, a slow-growing aerobic bacillus with a lipid-rich membrane that helps it evade the immune response. It spreads from person to person through inhalation of aerosol droplets.

Pathogenesis

The hallmark of tuberculosis is caseating (cheese-like) granulomatous lesions: tuberculomas. The initial infection is usually pulmonary, but uncontrolled infection can cause bacteraemia and haematogenous spread to the central nervous system.

Immune inflammatory responses usually control primary pulmonary infection, instigating a latent phase. Reactivation occurs after immunodeficiency or spontaneously with subsequent bacteraemia and haematogenous spread. The nervous system usually becomes affected following reactivation. Three syndromes occur, each with similar incidences:

- tuberculous meningitis after rupture of foci of tuberculosis from surrounding structures or haematogenous spread
- tuberculous abscess (tuberculoma) of the parenchyma (cerebral hemisphere, cerebellum or brain stem) or the spinal cord
- vertebral osteomyelitis (Pott's disease) or discitis

Other neurological syndromes include encephalitis, spinal cord myelitis and radiculitis (inflammation of the nerve roots).

Clinical features

Between 90 and 95% of tuberculosis infections are latent, i.e. asymptomatic. Neurological manifestations of tuberculosis depend on the site affected.

- Meninges: an acute fulminant meningitis or chronic, less severe meningitis, with systemic prodromal symptoms and meningism
- Parenchyma: the symptoms typical of any space-occupying lesion and, in 50% of patients with tuberculomas and tuberculous encephalitis, syndrome of inappropriate antidiuretic hormone
- Spine: back pain, fever, malaise and spinal tenderness
- Spinal cord: features of spinal cord and nerve root compression (see pages 344–348)

Complications depend on the site of the pathology, e.g. in meningeal infection the complications that develop in bacterial meningitis (see **Table 8.4**) also can occur. A parenchymal tuberculoma rarely can rupture into the subarachnoid space to cause meningitis.

Diagnostic approach

Culture of *Mycobacterium* species from cerebrospinal fluid is diagnostic of neurological infection, but the results are negative in over half of cases. In most cases, diagnosis is made when there is a typical clinical picture, known history of tuberculosis, tuberculosis exposure or tuberculosis risk factors, and suggestive cerebrospinal fluid analysis results (**Table 8.6**).

Investigations

Neuroimaging and cerebrospinal fluid analysis usually establish diagnosis, but these can be non-specific in central nervous system tuberculosis infection. Up to 30% of patients have normal imaging but the rest have meningeal enhancement, hydrocephalus or the characteristic tuberculoma (**Figures 8.4** and **8.5**).

In addition to the usual cerebrospinal fluid analyses (**Table 8.6**), cerebrospinal fluid is sent specifically for staining and culture of *M. tuberculosis*.

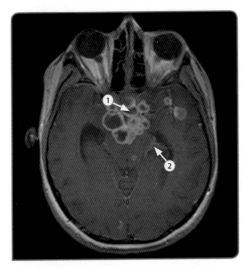

Figure 8.4 T1-weighted post-contrast magnetic resonance imaging scans showing tuberculomas ① in the basal cisterns and left temporal lobe, and meningeal enhancement ②.

Management

Treatment of the underlying tuberculosis infection is prolonged, with a combination of antibiotics used concurrently and chosen according to the strain of tuberculosis and sensitivities. Patients need frequent monitoring for adverse effects and to ensure improvement and that there's no development of resistance.

Medication

Antitubercular drug treatment is indicated for central nervous system tuberculosis infection. First-line drugs include combination therapy with isoniazid, rifampicin, pyrazinamide and ethambutol. Second-line drugs may be required for multidrug-resistant or extremely drug-resistant strains. Steroids decrease morbidity and mortality in central nervous system tuberculosis. Significant adverse effects of tuberculosis therapy include:

- hepatotoxicity from rifampicin
- peripheral neuropathy from isoniazid
- hepatotoxicity from pyrazinamide
- optic neuritis from ethambutol

Surgery

In cases of tuberculosis, surgical treatments are used to:

- aspirate tissue for microbiology analysis

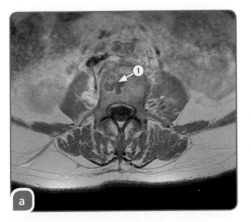
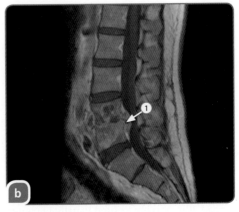

Figure 8.5 Axial (a) and sagittal (b) post-intravenous contrast magnetic resonance imaging scans showing tuberculous granuloma ① in L4, with subligamentous spread and vertebral body and disc destruction.

- evacuate tuberculoma to relieve mass effect
- treat hydrocephalus
- decompress the spinal cord and nerve roots and stabilise the spine with insertion of metalwork

Prognosis

The outcome of tuberculosis with neurological complications depends on the patient's age, the site affected and the severity of presenting neurological deficits. Even with early antitubercular drug treatment and surgical decompression, up to 30% may have persistent neurological deficits.

Spinal infections

Infections may involve the vertebral bodies, intervertebral discs or neural elements (spinal cord, nerve roots, etc.). There are three main pathologies:

- osteomyelitis (infection or inflammation of bony elements, including marrow)
- discitis (infection or inflammation of intervertebral discs and/or disc space)
- epidural abscess (pus in the spinal epidural space) or extremely rarely subdural empyema (pus in the spinal subdural space)

Epidemiology

The annual incidence of vertebral osteomyelitis is 3 per 100,000 in high-income countries.

Aetiology

Spinal infections arise from local (direct) or haematogenous spread. Common bacterial pathogens are:

- *Staph. aureus* (especially post-operative or iatrogenic)
- *Pseudomonas aeruginosa*
- *M. tuberculosis* (Pott's spondylitis)
- *Salmonella* (especially in immunodeficiency and sickle cell anaemia)

Fungal infection is usually caused by:

- *Candida* species
- *Aspergillus* species

Haematogenous spread occurs through the arterial supply or spinal epidural vertebral venous plexus (Batson's plexus) (see page 72). Possible sources that spread in this way are infective endocarditis, pulmonary infection or generalised septicaemia.

Clinical features

Neurological deficits depend on which structure is compressed, and at which level:

- spinal cord (myelopathy; see **Tables 11.2** and **11.4**)
- nerve roots (radiculopathy; see **Table 11.3** and pages 347 and 345)
- cauda equina (cauda equina syndrome; see **Table 11.3** and pages 348 and 345)

There is initially severe localised back pain, with paravertebral muscle spasm and focal spinal tenderness on palpation, all resulting from local inflammation. This develops into radicular pain in a belt- or band-like distribution in the dermatome at the level of compression. Next are signs and symptoms of spinal cord dysfunction with weakness and sensory loss, depending on the segmental level affected.

These neurological deficits are summarised in **Table 8.11.** There may be associated fever and malaise, and increased inflammatory markers. The presentation can be acute (over days to weeks) or chronic (over months).

Diagnostic approach

Systemic signs of infection (fever, malaise and increased inflammatory markers) and local signs (back pain, and focal spine tenderness on palpation) suggest spinal infection. Urgent imaging with CT, MRI or both (**Figures 8.6** and **8.7**) is required. Possible primary sites of sepsis, for example heart murmur in infective endocarditis, must be investigated.

Neurological features of compression from spinal infection

Structure compressed	Clinical features
Spinal cord	Radicular pain in belt- or band-like distribution in dermatome
	Motor deficit: LMN pattern at compression level, and UMN pattern below it
	Sensory deficits below compression level
Nerve root	Motor deficit: LMN pattern corresponding to muscles supplied by nerve root
	Sensory deficits in dermatome supplied by nerve root
Cauda equina	Bilateral sciatic pain
	Motor deficit, usually distal leg weakness in LMN pattern
	Deficits in S2–S4 distribution
	■ Sensory: perianal and saddle anaesthesia
	■ Motor: loss of anal and bladder sphincter function and tone
	■ Autonomic: bowel and bladder incontinence or retention

Table 8.11 Summary of neurological features of types of compression caused by spinal infection. LMN pattern of weakness is flaccid weakness, absence of reflexes and reduced tone; UMN pattern of weakness is spastic weakness, hyper-reflexia and increased tone

Management

Principles of treatment include:

- tissue samples for microbiological diagnosis and sensitivities
- empirical then targeted antibiotics to treat infection
- surgical decompression if needed (e.g. abscess evacuation)
- spinal stabilisation, if needed

In the absence of compressive lesions, conservative management is preferred: bed rest and 8 weeks of intravenous antibiotics is followed by 8 weeks of oral antibiotics. Serial MRI is used to evaluate resolution.

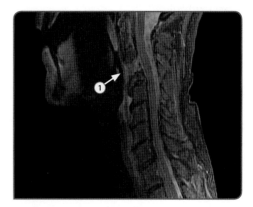

Figure 8.6 Sagittal T2W MRI showing osteomyelitis with discitis and probably vertebral body destruction at C3–C4 level ①.

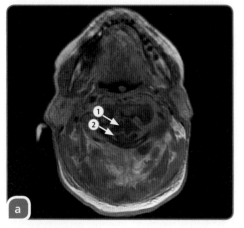
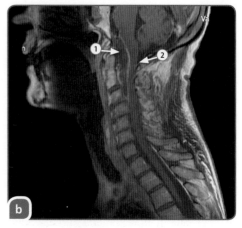

Figure 8.7 Axial (a) and sagittal (b) post-contrast magnetic resonance imaging scans of the cervical spine showing a large extradural abscess ① with associated compression of the spinal cord ②.

Surgery

Indications for surgery include:

- lesion with compression of neural tissue (e.g. epidural abscess)
- failure of medical therapy
- mechanical instability of the spine as a result of bone destruction

- intractable pain
- diagnostic purposes, if other measures have failed

Spinal cord compression secondary to abscesses requires urgent decompression (<24h) to prevent permanent neurological injury, spinal instability and spread to other structures.

Herpes zoster and post-herpetic neuralgia

Primary varicella zoster virus infection causes varicella (chickenpox) or a non-specific flu-like prodrome. During this infection, spread to the nervous system occurs haematogenously or via cranial or peripheral nerves, resulting in long-term latent infection.

Herpes zoster (shingles) arises when the virus is reactivated in the sensory nerve root or dorsal root ganglia, causing a vesicular eruption and pain in the associated dermatome.

Some, but not all people with shingles develop post-herpetic neuralgia. In this condition, fibrosis and myelin loss in the dorsal root ganglia precipitate persistent neuropathic pain.

> **Varicella zoster encephalitis is a vasculopathy.** Small- and medium-sized blood vessels develop inflammation, and the damage precipitates multiple infarcts and cerebral haemorrhages. Multifocal narrowing of blood vessels may be visible on arterial CT or MRI.

Clinical features

In shingles, the severe acute pain and vesicular rash (**Figure 8.8**) most commonly affect a truncal dermatome, but they can occur in any dermatome and elsewhere (**Table 8.12**). Patients have usually developed the problem on a background of reduced immunity, for example as a result of recent illness, advanced age, chemotherapy and HIV infection.

Dermatomal pain persisting for >30 days after a shingles attack is pathognomic of post-herpetic neuralgia. Paraesthesias and burning sensations may also be felt in the same dermatomal distribution. Increasing age and more severe pain during the shingles

attack make post-herpetic neuralgia more likely to occur.

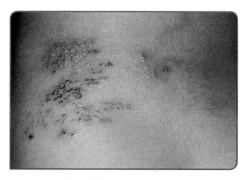

Figure 8.8 Skin vesicles in a dermatomal distribution in herpes zoster infection.

Varicella zoster virus encephalitis usually occurs only in immunocompromised people and causes multiple focal neurological deficits and cognitive impairment. Diagnosis is confirmed by PCR to identify varicella zoster virus in the cerebrospinal fluid.

> **Zoster ophthalmicus is involvement of the ophthalmic division of cranial nerve V (the trigeminal nerve).** It is an emergency requiring urgent ophthalmological assessment and treatment to prevent permanent visual impairment.

Management

Aciclovir or famciclovir is prescribed to settle the rash of shingles; it reduces the risk of post-herpetic neuralgia. Ophthalmic shingles requires close ophthalmological monitoring to treat any corneal involvement.

Clinical features of herpes zoster

Affected nerve(s)	Clinical feature(s)
Peripheral nerve ganglia and peripheral nerve	Eruption in dermatome supplied by that nerve
Cranial nerve (CN) V (trigeminal nerve)	Involvement of gasserian ganglion (CN V ganglion) and eruption in distribution of the ophthalmic division of the nerve (CN V_1)
	Risk of corneal ulceration
Cranial nerve VII (facial) nerve	Ramsey Hunt syndrome: vesicles in external auditory meatus associated with ipsilateral facial weakness due to infectious spread through the geniculate (CN VII) ganglion

Table 8.12 Clinical features of herpes zoster (shingles)

Someone who has not had chickenpox can catch it from exposure to live varicella-zoster virus released by the blisters of a person with shingles. However, they cannot catch shingles because it occurs only when latent virus is reactivated.

Varicella zoster virus encephalitis and myelitis are treated with intravenous aciclovir or famciclovir until cerebrospinal fluid analysis yields negative results with viral PCR. Identification of any immunodeficiency, especially HIV infection, is required.

Antineuropathic medications for postherpetic neuralgia include amitriptyline, pregabalin, gabapentin and carbamazepine. Transcutaneous electrical nerve stimulation is a non-pharmacological adjunct. Most patients recover within a year, but a small proportion have permanent nerve damage.

Answers to starter questions

1. Inflammation is a major part of most immune responses but is dangerous within the confined space of the skull. Therefore the brain's immune response relies less on T cell–mediated inflammation and more on antibody-mediated defences that attack specific pathogens. Usually (if well regulated) this causes less collateral damage to the brain.

2. Only a small percentage of lymphocytes and other immune cells cross the blood–brain barrier and pass through the central nervous system routinely as part of normal immune surveillance. Special transport systems allow certain cells to cross but impede the passage of others. If cells that have been allowed through the blood–brain barrier then encounter an antigen in the central nervous system, they are programmed to stay within the system, replicate and trigger an immune response.

3. Steroids reduce inflammation and oedema during an immune response, hindering the body's ability to fight infection but limiting damage caused by the response. This effect is particularly helpful in infections of the brain, because the soft nervous tissue is encased in a rigid skull and therefore susceptible to damage from swelling.

4. Different components of the immune system cause different levels of damage. Antibodies can cause receptor cross linking that blocks them from being activated by their normal stimulating transmitters, which impairs neuronal functioning, activates complement and inhibits neuronal activity but causes minimal or reversible neuronal damage. On the other hand, phagocytic and cytotoxic T cells cause extensive and largely irreversible neuronal loss. Which aspect of the immune system is dominant determines the amount of damage to the brain.

Chapter 9
Movement disorders

Starter questions

Answers to the following questions are on page 326.

1. How does neuronal degeneration in Parkinson's disease differ from that in normal ageing?
2. How can a bacterium make someone dance 'like St Vitus'?
3. How does deep brain stimulation ease the signs and symptoms of Parkinson's disease?

Introduction

Movement disorders are associated with dysfunction in pathways of the extrapyramidal system. This system is located in the base of the brain and modulates body movements. It comprises:

- the basal ganglia, which modulate fine motor planning and sequencing
- the thalamus, which processes information between the basal ganglia and the cerebral hemispheres
- brain stem nuclei, which form descending spinal pathways responsible for maintaining posture, muscle tone and reflexes

Secondary to neurogeneration, changes occur in the levels of neurotransmitters in these pathways, mainly dopamine, acetylcholine and γ-aminobutyric acid (GABA). Abnormalities in dopamine production are implicated in most movement disorders. Generally, a deficiency leads to reduced movements (hypokinesis), such as the rigidity of Parkinson's disease. Conversely, an excess leads to increased movements (hyperkinesis), as in the chorea of Huntington's disease.

Case 10 Tremor

Presentation

Graham Busby, aged 69 years, has been referred to the neurology clinic by his general practitioner. He has worsening tremor in his left hand, generalised slowing in movement and increasing stiffness in his arms and legs.

Initial interpretation

The case has features of a parkinsonian syndrome (parkinsonism), a constellation of symptoms that include bradykinesia (or akinesia), tremor and rigidity.

Idiopathic Parkinson's disease is a diagnosis of exclusion (see **Table 9.3**). Key differential diagnoses to exclude are:

■ drug-induced parkinsonism, which would be indicated by a history of antidopaminergic medications and usually causes symmetrical symptoms

■ vascular parkinsonism, which is a consequence of cerebrovascular disease and has an abrupt onset and stepwise progression

■ Parkinson's plus syndromes (see page 318)

History

Mr Busby's symptoms started with a tremor in his left hand. The tremor worsened over the past year and now affects his left leg. It is more severe at rest. He complains of left-sided stiffness and difficulty in walking and initiating movements. His general practitioner prescribed levodopa to increase the level of dopamine in the central nervous system; the drug has improved some of his symptoms.

For a long time, Mr Busby has had sleep problems; he has restless legs and acts out his dreams. He also mentions a loss of his

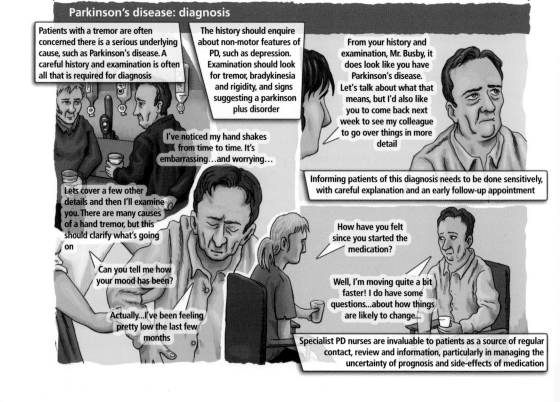

Parkinson's disease: diagnosis

Patients with a tremor are often concerned there is a serious underlying cause, such as Parkinson's disease. A careful history and examination is often all that is required for diagnosis

The history should enquire about non-motor features of PD, such as depression. Examination should look for tremor, bradykinesia and rigidity, and signs suggesting a parkinson plus disorder

From your history and examination, Mr. Busby, it does look like you have Parkinson's disease. Let's talk about what that means, but I'd also like you to come back next week to see my colleague to go over things in more detail

I've noticed my hand shakes from time to time. It's embarrassing...and worrying...

Informing patients of this diagnosis needs to be done sensitively, with careful explanation and an early follow-up appointment

Lets cover a few other details and then I'll examine you. There are many causes of a hand tremor, but this should clarify what's going on

Can you tell me how your mood has been?

How have you felt since you started the medication?

Actually...I've been feeling pretty low the last few months

Well, I'm moving quite a bit faster! I do have some questions...about how things are likely to change...

Specialist PD nurses are invaluable to patients as a source of regular contact, review and information, particularly in managing the uncertainty of prognosis and side-effects of medication

Case 10 *continued*

sense of smell (anosmia) and feeling very low in mood.

Interpretation of history

The asymmetrical onset of Mr Busby's motor symptoms, prominent tremor and progressive symptoms that respond well to levodopa point to idiopathic Parkinson's disease. The age of onset suggests that this is idiopathic Parkinson's disease rather than young onset or familial Parkinson's disease (**see Tables 9.1 and 9.2**). Loss of smell is common in Parkinson's disease.

In restless legs syndrome, the patient has an irresistible urge to move their legs in bed. Patients with Parkinson's disease often have this symptom many years before they develop the others. Disorders of sleep, including having vivid dreams and acting out movements during sleep, are also common in Parkinson's disease. Depression affects many patients as a non-motor manifestation of the disease.

Other pathologies, particularly drug-induced parkinsonism and Parkinson's plus syndromes, still need to be excluded with further detailed history and clinical examination.

Further history

Mr Busby has no history of stroke or risk factors for vascular disease. Neither does he have a history of repeated head injury or neurological infection. There are no systemic symptoms such as weight loss or night sweats to suggest a malignancy. He is not on any medications associated

Clinical features of idiopathic Parkinson's disease	
Symptom group	Features
Motor – hypokinetic	Bradykinesia or akinesia
	micrographia
	Rigidity (including cogwheeling)
	Postural instability
Motor – hyperkinetic	Resting tremor
Non-motor	Anosmia
	Sleep disorders
	Dementia, depression and psychosis
	Mild autonomic features (earlier and more severe in multiple systems atrophy): postural hypotension, and bladder and bowel dysfunction
	Dystonia

Table 9.1 Clinical features of idiopathic Parkinson's disease. Motor features are usually asymmetrical in onset, unlike the Parkinson's plus disorders

Differentiating between types of parkinsonism			
Feature	Idiopathic Parkinson's disease	Young onset or familial Parkinson's disease	Parkinson's plus syndrome
Age at onset (years) and family history	> 50	< 50; family history	> 50
Pattern of onset	Asymmetrical	Asymmetrical	Symmetrical
Tremor	Predominant	Predominant	Less pronounced
Typical non-motor features	Present	Present	Less common
Features of Parkinson's plus syndromes	Absent	Absent	Present
Response to levodopa	Good	Good	Usually poor

Table 9.2 Differentiating features of the main types of parkinsonism

Case 10 *continued*

with impairment of dopaminergic activity in the brain. He does not have a family history of similar neurological symptoms. Furthermore, there are no symptoms, such as established liver disease, to suggest Wilson's disease.

Examination

Clinical examination shows no upper motor neurone pattern of weakness, cerebellar signs or features of autonomic dysfunction such as severe postural hypotension. Mr Busby has normal eye movements and no postural instability. He does not have any features of liver disease, and slit lamp examination is normal.

His left arm has increased tone with cogwheeling (a racheting movement of the muscles felt by the examiner when moving the patient's limb). The tremor is worse at rest and is reduced by movement; it occurs at a frequency of four to seven per second. Mr Busby is slow at rising from his chair, and has a slow, shuffling gait with reduced arm swing and slow turning. He speaks with a low, monotonous voice, and his face is expressionless. He is asked to tap his hand against the table; the speed of his tapping decreases progressively.

Interpretation of findings

The tremor is a typical resting tremor. The slow movements, shuffling gait, reduced arm swing, slow turning and progressively slowing tapping are all signs of bradykinesia. The increased tone and cogwheeling indicate stiffness.

The lack of early postural instability and the absence of postural hypotension or other autonomic dysfunction, along with

the normal eye movements, are evidence against a Parkinson's plus syndrome.

The lack of previous strokes or exposure to antidopaminergic drugs, along with the normal liver function and normal eye examination, make vascular parkinsonism, drug-induced parkinsonism and Wilson's disease unlikely.

Overall, the history and examination are typical of idiopathic Parkinson's disease. The improvement of symptoms with levodopa reinforces this as a diagnosis.

Diagnosis

The working diagnosis is idiopathic Parkinson's disease. Dr Symons explains the diagnosis to Mr Busby, adjusts his levodopa prescription, and after further discussion prescribes an antidepressant.

A week later, Dr Symons discusses the case with a multidisciplinary team. The team includes the Parkinson's disease clinical nurse specialist, a physiotherapist, an occupational therapist and a social worker. Mr Busby returns 1 month later for review and formal neuropsychological testing to provide baseline data and aid long-term assessments (for example in monitoring for symptom improvement with medication).

Parkinsonism is a common clinical presentation. A careful detailed history and neurological examination are central components of the meeting with the patient, because idiopathic Parkinson's disease is a clinical diagnosis. Investigations are done to look for other causes of the patient's symptoms.

Parkinson's disease

Parkinson's disease is a complex neurodegenerative disease with several different causes. Its incidence in the UK and worldwide is increasing as the population ages, and it is the commonest neurodegenerative disease after Alzheimer's disease. The key pathological feature is loss of dopaminergic neurones in the substantia nigra pars compacta of the basal ganglia.

In about 80% of patients with parkinsonism, no specific cause can be identified. They are considered to have idiopathic Parkinson's disease.

Epidemiology

The annual incidence of Parkinson's disease is 20 per 100,000. Men are slightly more likely than women to develop the disease. The prevalence increases with age, with a peak in the mid seventies.

Aetiology

The cause of Parkinson's disease is probably multifactorial: a mix of genetic and environmental factors that ultimately lead to loss of dopaminergic neurones in the substantia nigra pars compacta. Most cases are sporadic, but first-degree family members are affected in about 15% of cases, and recognised mutations are present in about 5%. In patients with onset before the age of 50 years, about half have mutations in the *PARK2* gene. Many environmental factors have been identified as potential risk factors for Parkinson's disease, but conclusive evidence is lacking.

> In 1982, several heroin users in California rapidly developed severe parkinsonism after injecting synthetic heroin contaminated with MPTP (1-methyl-4-phenyl-1,2,3,6-tetrahydropyridine). MPTP is metabolised to the neurotoxic MPP+ (1-methyl-4-phenylpyridinium). The ability of MPTP to produce parkinsonism suggests that environmental toxins may contribute to idiopathic Parkinson's disease.

Pathogenesis

The key lesion of idiopathic Parkinson's disease is the degeneration of dopaminergic neurones in the substantia nigra pars compacta of the basal ganglia. The remaining neurones often accumulate the protein α-synuclein in Lewy bodies, which are visible in their cytoplasm.

α-Synuclein is involved in vesicles releasing neurotransmitter into synapses. Lewy bodies, the abnormal collections of α-synuclein, are present throughout the brain in Lewy body dementia (also known as Lewy body disease) as well as in Parkinson's disease. This combination of degeneration of dopaminergic neurones in the pars compacta and the accumulation of abnormal collection of α-synuclein (as Lewy bodies), cause, or are associated with, a decrease in nigrostriatal dopamine levels that leads to increased basal ganglia inhibitory output, clinically evident as the hypokinetic motor features of bradykinesia (or akinesia) and rigidity.

In Parkinson's disease, degeneration also occurs in the striatum and globus pallidus of the basal ganglia. This may explain the hyperkinetic tremor in the condition. Furthermore, changes in non-dopaminergic brain stem nuclei may explain the non-motor features of Parkinson's disease and why these do not respond to dopamine replacement therapy. However, current research suggests that the disease starts in the olfactory bulb and progresses to the basal ganglia and cortex through the brain stem.

Clinical features

Parkinson's disease presents with hyper- and hypokinetic motor features, as well as non-motor features (**Table 9.1**). Motor signs usually start asymmetrically, often as a resting tremor in the arm. They then progress to whole-body slowing (bradykinesia), rigidity and a shuffling gait. Non-motor symptoms such as hyposmia often precede motor ones.

Diagnostic approach

Diagnosis is clinical. It requires the presence of bradykinesia (or akinesia) with at least one of:

- tremor
- rigidity
- postural instability

Idiopathic Parkinson's disease usually has an asymmetrical onset of motor features (**Tables 9.1** and **9.2**). Tremor occurs in 70% of patients but is not necessary for diagnosis.

Initially, the clinical features are subtle and highly variable, and the priority is to exclude other causes of parkinsonism (**Table 9.3**). Test results are not diagnostic, but they help support or exclude other diagnoses that present with parkinsonism (**Table 9.4**).

> **Rigidity is increased tone in all muscles.** It is associated with extrapyramidal system dysfunction and upward plantar reflexes. In contrast, spasticity is increased tone in upper limb flexors and lower limb extensors, and is associated with pyramidal system or upper motor neurone dysfunction.

Investigations

Magnetic resonance imaging (MRI) can be used to try to visualise neurodegeneration in the basal ganglia. Single-photon emission computed tomography (SPECT) can be used to assess dopamine levels in these areas.

MRI usually identifies specific patterns of degeneration in Parkinson's plus syndromes:

- midbrain atrophy in progressive supranuclear palsy (**Figure 9.1**)
- parietal cortex atrophy in corticobasal degeneration
- pontocerebellar tract atrophy in multiple systems atrophy

In SPECT, radiolabelled ligands are used to visualise and thus assess dopaminergic activity by binding to presynaptic dopamine transporters in the striatum. The pattern of neurodegeneration can also help differentiate causes of parkinsonism and tremor.

- Patients with idiopathic Parkinson's disease and Parkinson's plus syndromes have asymmetrically reduced signal in the striatum
- Those with drug-induced Parkinson's disease or essential tremor have normal symmetrical uptake

Causes of parkinsonism		
Category	Causes	Examples or details
Parkinson's disease	Idiopathic	Mutations in genes such as *PARK2* in young onset and familial Parkinson's disease
	Young onset or familial Parkinson's disease	
Parkinson's plus syndromes (which mimic Parkinson's disease)	Multiple systems atrophy	
	Progressive supranuclear palsy	
	Corticobasal degeneration	
	Lewy body dementia (also known as Lewy body disease)	
Secondary Parkinson's disease	Vascular	Cerebrovascular disease affecting basal ganglia
	Drug-induced	Use of dopamine receptor antagonists (e.g. antipsychotic drugs) or dopamine function inhibitors (e.g. metoclopramide)
	Post-traumatic	Repeated head trauma
	Infectious	Encephalitis, HIV infection and Creutzfeldt–Jakob disease
	Hydrocephalus (rare)	
Genetic	Wilson's disease	Inherited disorder of copper metabolism

Table 9.3 The causes of parkinsonism

Investigations in patients with parkinsonism		
Modality	Tests	Purposes
Blood tests	Full blood count, and urea and electrolytes	To establish baseline levels to guide future management
	Liver function tests, serum copper, 24-h urine copper excretion and serum caeruloplasmin	To exclude Wilson's disease
Clinical examination	Slit lamp examination of eyes	To exclude Wilson's disease, if suspected
	Neuropsychological testing	To establish baseline functional status
	Bedside cognition testing	To exclude dementia
	Psychiatric assessment	To assess for mood disturbance
Imaging	Computerised tomography and magnetic resonance imaging	To exclude structural lesions
	Positron emission tomography scans	To differentiate drug-induced parkinsonism from idiopathic Parkinson's disease

Table 9.4 Investigations in patients presenting with parkinsonism

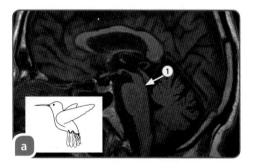 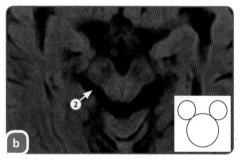

Figure 9.1 Magnetic resonance imaging appearances of progressive supranuclear palsy. (a) Sagittal and (b) axial sequences showing the ① 'hummingbird' and ② 'Mickey Mouse' signs of midbrain atrophy.

Management

Patients with Parkinson's disease require treatment for both hypokinetic and hyperkinetic motor symptoms, as well as for non-motor complications such as mood and psychotic disturbances, dementia and sleep disturbances.

Management is highly individual and requires a multidisciplinary team including neurologists, nurse specialists, physiotherapists, occupational therapists, social workers and occasionally neurosurgeons. As Parkinson's disease evolves over time (**Table 9.5**), so do the needs of the patient.

Key case-by-case decisions are when to start medication and which to use. Previously, treatment was delayed because efficacy wanes over time. More recently, there has been a tendency for earlier treatment, because evidence suggests that earlier treatment has long-term benefits such as delaying the onset of treatment-related side effects.

> **Dopamine itself cannot be used as a drug to treat Parkinson's disease.** It is unable to cross the blood–brain barrier to increase levels of dopamine in the central nervous system.

Medication

Drugs improve motor symptoms by increasing dopaminergic activity in the brain (**Table 9.6**).

Progression of Parkinson's disease			
Features	Early disease	Moderate disease	Advanced disease
Non-motor features	Sleep disorders Restless legs syndrome Cognitive impairment Depression	Social withdrawal Apathy Impulse control disorders (e.g. gambling and hypersexuality)	Dementia Psychosis
Motor features	Usually asymmetrical onset of symptoms Tremor Rigidity Bradykinesia	Progression of severity of all symptoms including progression to involve other limbs Tremor Rigidity Bradykinesia (with progression to akinesia)	Progression of severity of all symptoms including progression to involve other limbs Tremor Rigidity Bradykinesia (with progression to akinesia) Postural instability
Response to levodopa	Good	Fair	Limited
Treatment-related adverse effects	Few	Motor fluctuations (dyskinesia during wearing-off periods)	Severe motor fluctuations (dyskinesia occurs with more frequency for longer periods during the day and not just during wearing-off periods)
Other			Urinary incontinence

Table 9.5 Progression of Parkinson's disease

- Dopamine precursors such as levodopa are the most widely used treatment
- Dopamine receptor agonists (e.g. ropinirole and pramipexole) mimic dopamine
- Monoamine oxidase B inhibitors (e.g. selegiline and rasagiline) prevent the breakdown and reuptake of dopamine

Towards end-stage disease, continuous apomorphine infusions can be used to help control significant motor fluctuations. Anticholinergic medications are generally avoided, because their efficacy is minimal and they cause cognitive impairment.

Anticholinergic medications are generally avoided, because their efficacy is minimal and they cause cognitive impairment.

Levodopa

This is usually effective for only 5–10 years before it has either minimal effects or dyskinesias develop. Therefore younger patients are often started on dopamine agonists instead.

Most levodopa does not cross the blood–brain barrier, so it can accumulate to cause peripheral adverse effects such as stiffness, nausea and dyskinesia. It is often given in combination with dopa decarboxylase inhibitors, such as carbidopa, to increase the amount of levodopa that reaches the central nervous system and thereby minimise peripheral adverse effects.

> **The effects of Parkinson's disease are variable and difficult to predict in individual patients.** Drug regimens are often complex and tailored to each patient's needs – increasingly so as the disease progresses.

Surgery

For deep brain stimulation, a fine stimulating electrode is inserted under local anaesthetic through a burr hole into a carefully targeted region of the brain. These targets are often the subthalamic nuclei as well as other sites in the basal ganglia.

This is a very effective treatment for some motor symptoms. Deep brain stimulation is particularly effective in younger patients who have had some response to levodopa but remain disabled by their symptoms.

Drug treatments for Parkinson's disease					
Drug	Mechanism of action	Indication	Benefit	Adverse effects	Details
Levodopa	Precursor metabolised to dopamine in the brain	First line in elderly patients with idiopathic Parkinson's disease	Improves bradykinesia and rigidity Poor effect on tremor and non-motor symptoms	Involuntary movements (dyskinesias) Fluctuations in response Psychiatric effects (e.g. confusion and visual hallucinations)	Administered in combination with dopa decarboxylase inhibitor: inhibits peripheral breakdown, thereby increasing CNS dopamine levels
Dopamine receptor agonists	Act directly on dopamine receptors	First line in young patients	As above	Postural hypotension Psychiatric effects (hallucinations and psychosis) Impulse control disorders (e.g. gambling and hypersexuality)	Can lower dose of levodopa required in patients with levodopa-related motor adverse effects
Inhibitors of dopa breakdown	Inhibit catechol-O-methyltransferase, monoamine oxygenase B1 or dopa decarboxylase enzymes to increase dopamine levels	Used to decrease 'off' time (i.e. period of time when medication wears off and symptoms return) in patients on other medications	As above	Dyskinesias Insomnia	Usually combined with levodopa to prevent peripheral metabolism
Amantadine	Glutamate antagonist	Advanced disease	Reduces dyskinesias and motor fluctuations	Anxiety Agitation Seizures	Given orally
Apomorphine	Potent dopamine agonist acting on D_1 and D_2 receptors	Refractory motor fluctuations Rescue therapy for severe 'off' periods in patients on maximal therapy	As above	–	Poor oral bioavailability; given subcutaneously

Table 9.6 Drugs used to treat the motor manifestations of Parkinson's disease

Complications

Patients with Parkinson's disease are at risk of other general medical complications. Regular screening is required for the following.

- Infections: urinary tract infection may develop because of autonomic bladder disturbance, and respiratory tract infection because of aspiration secondary to dysphagia (difficulty swallowing) from bradykinesia
- Myocardial infarctions and strokes: Parkinson's disease patients are susceptible to these, for reasons that remain unclear
- Traumatic injuries: these are a consequence of motor control and falls

Drug-induced parkinsonism

Parkinsonism, i.e. bradykinesia (or akinesia), tremor and rigidity, results from depletion of dopaminergic activity in the basal ganglia. Unsurprisingly, the condition can be caused by drugs with antidopaminergic action (**Table 9.7**).

In contrast with idiopathic Parkinson's disease, in parkinsonism:

- the symptoms are often symmetrical rather than asymmetrical
- the tremor is more postural than resting

Antipsychotic medications are the commonest cause; drug-induced parkinsonism may limit the dose or preparation used. The condition occasionally takes weeks to months to resolve once the patient stops taking the medication.

> **Domperidone is an antidopaminergic drug used to treat nausea.** However, it does not cross the blood–brain barrier to act on the central nervous system, so is safe for use by patients with Parkinson's disease.

Drugs that cause parkinsonism		
Mechanism of action	Indications or uses	Drug or drug class
Depletion of presynaptic dopamine stores	Hyperkinetic movement disorders , e.g. Huntington's disease	Reserpine
		Tetrabenazine
Inhibition of post-synaptic dopamine receptors	Neuroleptic and antipsychotic drugs	Phenothiazines (e.g. chlorpromazine)
		Butyrophenones (e.g. haloperidol)
		Thioxanthenes (e.g. flupentixol)
		Benzamide (e.g. sulpiride)
	Antiemetic drugs	Metoclopramide

Table 9.7 Drugs that cause parkinsonism: their modes of action and indications for use

Parkinson's plus syndromes

Parkinson's plus syndromes are a group of neurodegenerative disorders causing parkinsonism. Their management usually differs from that of Parkinson's disease, as does their prognosis.

There are four major Parkinson's disease mimics:

- multiple systems atrophy
- progressive supranuclear palsy
- Lewy body dementia (also known as Lewy body disease)
- corticobasal degeneration

Most patients present in their fifties or sixties. The cause is unknown in most cases.

Clinical features

Clinical features that usually differentiate Parkinson's plus syndromes from Parkinson's disease include the following (**Figure 9.2**):

- symmetrical onset of motor symptoms
- less prominent tremor
- poor response to levodopa
- cerebellar or autonomic dysfunction in multiple systems atrophy
- vertical gaze palsy in progressive supranuclear palsy (**Figure 9.3**)
- early dementia in Lewy body disease
- myoclonus, dyspraxia and 'alien hand'

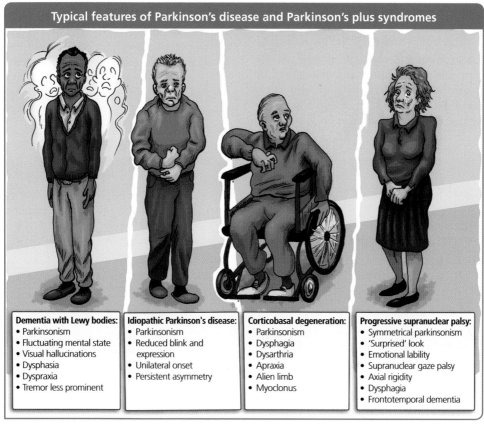

Typical features of Parkinson's disease and Parkinson's plus syndromes

Dementia with Lewy bodies:
- Parkinsonism
- Fluctuating mental state
- Visual hallucinations
- Dysphasia
- Dyspraxia
- Tremor less prominent

Idiopathic Parkinson's disease:
- Parkinsonism
- Reduced blink and expression
- Unilateral onset
- Persistent asymmetry

Corticobasal degeneration:
- Parkinsonism
- Dysphagia
- Dysarthria
- Apraxia
- Alien limb
- Myoclonus

Progressive supranuclear palsy:
- Symmetrical parkinsonism
- 'Surprised' look
- Emotional lability
- Supranuclear gaze palsy
- Axial rigidity
- Dysphagia
- Frontotemporal dementia

Figure 9.2 Typical features of Parkinson's disease and Parkinson's plus syndromes, both of which present with parkinsonism (a variable degree of rigidity, tremor and bradykinesia or akinesia). Symptoms overlap significantly, but the conditions can often be distinguished clinically.

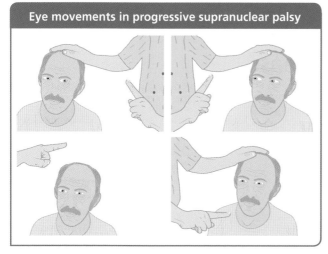

Eye movements in progressive supranuclear palsy

Figure 9.3 Limited upward eye movements are common in progressive supranuclear palsy.

phenomenon (involuntary movement of and feeling of estrangement from a hand) in corticobasal degeneration

Each syndrome is associated with distinct signs of neurodegeneration on MRI (**Table 9.8**). For this reason an MRI of the head should be performed in all patients with suspected Parkinson's plus syndromes.

Management

These syndromes have a relentlessly progressive course. They typically respond very poorly to levodopa. However, some patient's symptoms do respond (especially motor features in Lewy body disease), so levodopa should be tried. Most management is supportive (see **Table 9.8**).

Parkinson's plus syndromes: investigation and management			
Syndrome	Subtype	Investigations and findings	Response to levodopa and prognosis
Multiple systems atrophy	Parkinsonian form	MRI: hypointense signal in putamen	Poor response to levodopa compared with in Parkinson's disease; progressive course over 5–10 years
	Cerebellar form	MRI: loss of volume in cerebellum, middle cerebellar peduncle and pons	
	Autonomic failure (in both parkinsonian and cerebellar forms)	Autonomic function tests confirm clinical findings	Poor response to levodopa. Management is mainly symptom control (e.g. fludrocortisone for postural hypotension, and oxybutynin for urinary incontinence)
Progressive supranuclear palsy		MRI: midbrain atrophy and frontotemporal atrophy	Poor response to levodopa Relentlessly progressive course, with death in 3–5 years
Lewy body dementia (also known as Lewy body disease)		MRI: generalised atrophy with absence of significant temporal atrophy	Exquisitely sensitive to neuroleptic medication Motor features often respond well to levodopa
Corticobasal degeneration		MRI: asymmetrical generalised atrophy of affected regions	Poor response to levodopa
MRI, magnetic resonance imaging.			

Table 9.8 Investigation and response to levodopa of Parkinson's plus syndromes

Huntington's disease

Huntington's disease is a hereditary neurodegenerative disorder associated with progressive chorea: hyperkinetic, brief, irregular and arrhythmic movements. It is also associated with progressive dementia, psychosis, anxiety and depression.

Epidemiology

Huntington's disease has an estimated prevalence of 10 per 100,000. Disease onset is usually in the patient's thirties to fifties.

Aetiology

Huntington's disease is an autosomal dominant disorder: only one copy of a mutated gene needs to be present to lead to its development. The mutation is a repeat of CAG trinucleotides in the *Huntingtin* gene on chromosome 4. The gene encodes a protein that is cleaved abnormally, leading to a toxic accumulation of protein fragments. These interact with numerous normal proteins to form aggregates in the cell, which disrupt cellular function.

The number of CAG repeats tends to increase over generations. This phenomenon, known as genetic anticipation, occurs because the repeats tend to induce a 'slippage' error of replication. This is an error occurring during the genetic replication of DNA which precipitates addition of further repeats to the gene. More repeats result in more accumulations. Huntington's disease is associated with 36 or more repeats, and a greater number correlates with earlier onset and greater severity.

Neuronal loss occurs in the striatum, especially the caudate nucleus, along with a decrease in the neurotransmitters acetylcholine and GABA. These changes result in a relative excess of dopamine and excessive movement.

Further neuronal loss occurs in the deep layers of the frontal and parietal lobes, which project to the basal ganglia. This effect probably contributes to the neuropsychiatric and cognitive features of Huntington's disease.

> **Parkinson's disease and Huntington's disease have converse pathogenic mechanisms.** Parkinson's disease arises from dopamine deficiency in the basal ganglia, which leads to a reduction in movement. Huntington's disease is associated with excess dopamine levels and excessive movement.

Clinical features

Patients typically present with chorea, subtle cognitive changes and a family history of either Huntington's disease or an uncertain neurological or psychiatric disease (**Table 9.9**). The psychiatric manifestations of Huntington's disease, such as personality change and psychosis, may precede the movement abnormalities.

Diagnostic approach

Diagnosis is straightforward in patients with neuropsychiatric symptoms and an established family history, and is considered in all patients with neuropsychiatric changes and chorea. Huntington's disease is the commonest cause of hereditary chorea, but drug-induced chorea is always considered.

Clinical features of Huntington's disease	
Pathological site of dysfunction	Clinical features
Loss of nuclei in the caudate nucleus	Hyperkinetic (choreiform) movements
Loss of deep nuclei of the frontal and parietal regions	Dementia Psychiatric features: ■ psychosis ■ personality change ■ mood disorders Persistence of primitive reflexes: grasp, snout and palmomental reflexes reappear

Table 9.9 Clinical features of Huntington's disease

Investigations

Tests are considered following clinical history, family history and examination which raise the suspicion of hereditary chorea. The diagnosis is confirmed following genetic testing. Imaging supports the diagnosis but usually the changes are non-specific.

Blood tests

Genetic testing is cheap, reliable, and diagnostic and usually takes a few weeks. Pre-test counselling is essential, and covers the implications of diagnosis and what support is available. Assuming individual informed consent, first-degree relatives are also approached about screening for Huntington's disease. Less than 10% of people with a family history choose to pursue testing.

Imaging

Magnetic resonance imaging is often done while the result of genetic testing is awaited. MRI can show selective atrophy of the head of the caudate.

Management

No disease-modifying treatments are available for Huntington's disease. Multidisciplinary teams, including psychiatrists, help support the patient and their family throughout disease progression. The team are an experienced group of people who provide advice, practical support and connection to physical and occupational therapy services.

Medication

Symptomatic control, according to the needs of the individual patient, comprises pharmacological treatment for the following.

- **Hyperkinesis**: tetrabenazine is used to increase the breakdown of dopamine precursors
- **Severe bradykinesia**, which can be prominent in childhood cases: dopaminergic agents can be used
- **Depression**: selective serotonin reuptake inhibitors can be used to treat this symptom

Essential tremor

Essential tremor is tremor that is not associated with neurological disease. Between 15 and 50 people per 1000 over the age of 60 years have essential tremor; many are initially concerned that they may have Parkinson's disease or Huntington's disease, but most do not. The cause is unknown, but there is a strong hereditary component.

> **Tremor has a wide differential diagnosis.** The two main pathological causes are parkinsonism and cerebellar disease.

Clinical features

Essential tremor may be sporadic or inherited in an autosomal dominant manner and is associated with multiple genetic loci. It usually:

- is an action tremor (postural or kinetic) and absent at rest
- has a fast rate, at 6–12 Hz (cycles per second)
- is fine in character and amplitude
- is symmetrical, bilateral and in the upper limbs (95% of cases)
- has no features suggesting a pathological syndrome

It may also be associated with head tremor (titubation), voice tremor or both.

Diagnostic approach

Essential tremor is diagnosed when there is a stereotypical tremor with no other symptoms or signs to indicate a neurological disease.

A thorough neurological assessment, including careful characterisation of the tremor, is necessary to differentiate essential tremor from pathological tremors (**Figure 9.4**).

In cases of diagnostic doubt, specialist SPECT can be used to differentiate essential tremor and idiopathic Parkinson's disease.

- Dopamine uptake is normal in essential tremor, drug-induced parkinsonism and vascular parkinsonism
- It is reduced in idiopathic Parkinson's disease and the Parkinson's plus syndromes

Management

Once all key differential diagnoses have been excluded, the patient can be reassured that their tremor poses no risk.

Medication

If the tremor is disabling, various medications may be tried:

- beta-blockers (propranolol), usually as first-line therapy
- anticonvulsants (e.g. topiramate) as a second-line treatment
- antineuropathic agents (e.g. gabapentin) as a second-line treatment

Surgery

In extremely severe cases, intervention with surgical ablation or deep brain stimulation of the ventral intermediate nucleus of the thalamus may be considered to decrease motor symptoms.

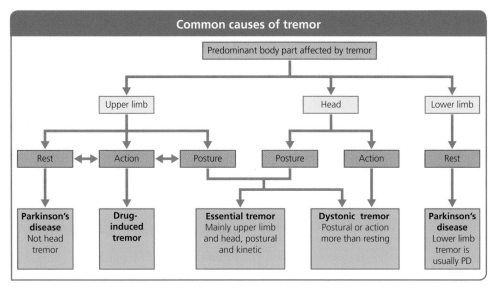

Figure 9.4 Differentiation of common causes of tremor by location and whether it is worse at rest, in action or when maintaining a particular posture.

Wilson's disease

Wilson's disease (hepaticolenticular degeneration) is an autosomal recessive disorder of copper metabolism, which leads to its deposition in organs, especially the liver. Up to half of patients present with central nervous system signs and symptoms, including parkinsonism, tremor, dystonia (abnormalities in muscle tone with sustained muscle contractions causing twisting and repetitive movements or abnormal postures) chorea, seizures and psychiatric symptoms. Wilson's disease occurs in 1 to 4 per 100,000 people worldwide

Pathogenesis

Copper is absorbed by the small intestine; 98% binds to the blood transport protein caeruloplasmin. Caeruloplasmin then transports it to the hepatocytes of the liver, from which it is excreted in the bile.

Mutation of the *ATP7B* gene on chromosome 13 impairs the incorporation of copper into caeruloplasmin. This effect increases the amount of free unbound serum copper, which is deposited in the liver, basal ganglia, eyes and kidneys. Copper deposition damages cells and tissues directly, as well as increasing damage from free radicals.

Clinical features

Presentation can be acute or chronic. The constellation of features depends on the sites of copper deposition.

- In the liver, cirrhosis causes progressive hepatic failure
- In the eye, golden-brown Kayser–Fleischer rings are visible on slit lamp examination
- In the basal ganglia, copper deposition causes bradykinesia, dyskinesias, dystonia (**Figure 9.5**), chorea, athetosis and rigidity

Dementia, psychosis and behavioural disturbance can also develop in patients younger than 50 years. Of those with neurological involvement, almost all have Kayser–Fleischer rings.

Wilson's disease is considered in patients, especially young patients, presenting with

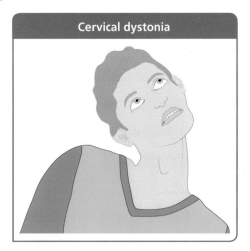

Cervical dystonia

Figure 9.5 Cervical dystonia in Wilson's disease: the head is pulled to the ear (laterocollis) and backwards (retrocollis).

- increased free unbound serum copper concentration
- decreased caeruloplasmin concentration (< 20 mg/dL)
- increased urinary copper excretion
- increased copper deposition on liver biopsy
- hyperintensity in the putamen on MRI

> **Caeruloplasmin levels vary for reasons other than Wilson's disease.** It is an acute phase protein that is increased in cases of trauma, infection and generalised inflammation.

both hepatic and neurological features. The initial neurological symptoms are usually dysarthria (difficulty coordinating speech) (60% of cases), dystonia (40%), abnormal gait (35%), tremor (35%) and parkinsonism (15%).

Diagnostic approach

More than 300 mutations can cause Wilson's disease, making routine genetic testing impractical. Diagnosis is made clinically, with supportive biochemical and imaging features including:

Management

Patients often require lifelong therapy with a low copper diet and copper-chelating agents such as d-penicillamine, which 'collect' free copper in the blood. Other treatments include trientine, a chelator, and zinc, which competes with copper for absorption, thereby limiting its initial uptake.

Liver transplantation is usually necessary in patients with severe hepatic failure and cirrhosis.

Untreated acute disease often results in death within 2 years, as a result of hepatic and renal failure. In the more chronic form, hepatic involvement is often less severe.

Restless legs syndrome

Restless legs syndrome is a chronic neuropsychiatric condition of uncomfortable sensations in a body part that lead to an uncontrollable urge to move the affected part. Nearly 10% of people are affected. The condition has a spectrum of severity ranging from minor annoyance to severe disruption of sleep and reduction of quality of life. It is usually idiopathic but can be caused or exacerbated by:

- iron deficiency
- neuropathy
- pregnancy
- thyroid disease
- renal impairment
- Parkinson's disease

The mechanism is poorly understood but may originate from dysfunction in brain stem or spinal cord nuclei.

Clinical features

The legs are most commonly affected, but any body part may be involved, including the arms, trunk and even 'phantom limbs' in amputees. Abnormal sensations vary from tingling to burning and pain. Symptoms worsen at rest, during the evening or night, and are relieved by movement.

Restless legs syndrome is classed as early or late onset depending on whether it develops before or after the age of 36 years.

- Patients with early onset restless legs syndrome typically have a strong family history of the condition, and their symptoms are more severe than in those with later onset

- Patients with later onset restless legs syndrome lack a family history of the condition and has a rapidly progressive course over 2–3 years

Management

Correction of iron deficiency often eases or completely relieves symptoms.

Other treatment is pharmacological: dopamine agonists and gabapentin. If these are ineffective, opioids may be needed.

Tics

Tics are irregular, repetitive, sudden, brief movements or sounds. They are often triggered by stress or boredom. Voluntary suppression is possible but creates internal tension within the patient.

The commonest types of tic are:

- motor, such as winking, blinking, grimacing, sniffing and throat clearing
- vocal, for example coprolalia (foul utterances) and repeating sounds or words (echolalia)

Clinical features

Patients with Gilles de la Tourette syndrome have multiple tics and vocalisations. They often also have obsessive–compulsive behaviour and reduced impulse control. The syndrome is often inherited; it is considered a genetic condition although no associated gene mutations have yet been identified.

Management

Parents of children with tics require education and counselling by physicians to inform them that it is very difficult for the child to suppress these tics, and that support groups for both patients and parents can be helpful in helping developing coping strategies. Comprehensive behavioural intervention for tics is not a cure, but it can help patients learn ways to gain more control in social situations.

Social stigma is often the greatest burden and may warrant the use of medication. This is usually in the form of drugs that antagonise dopamine receptors in the basal ganglia.

Answers to starter questions

1. In Parkinson's disease, degeneration in the dopaminergic neurones in the substantia nigra pars compacta is the primary pathological abnormality. The subsequent loss of dopaminergic input results (via a variety of complex interconnections) in an excess in the inhibitory output from the basal ganglia leading to the predominant hypokinetic motor features of Parkinson's disease. This pathologic and dramatic loss of dopaminergic neurones is not usually seen in normal ageing.

2. St Vitus's dance, now known as Sydenham's chorea, is irregular, repetitive, rapid jerking and writhing movements that primarily affect the face, hands and feet. It results from infection with group A β-haemolytic streptococci, and affects about a third of patients with acute rheumatic fever. B cells respond to the infection by producing an antibody that cross-reacts with basal ganglia to cause the uninitiated movements.

3. In deep brain stimulation, electrodes inserted into the brain send electrical impulses to the subthalamic nucleus. These inhibit the function of the subthalamic nucleus, thereby decreasing inhibitory basal ganglia output and increasing movement. The degree of stimulation can be altered depending on the patient's response and is a balance between pharmacological treatment and deep brain stimulation. Deep brain stimulation is also effective in some cases of essential tremor, dystonia, chronic pain and severe depression.

Chapter 10
Multiple sclerosis and other central nervous system demyelinating diseases

Starter questions

Answers to the following questions are on page 339.

1. In what ways can a diagnosis of multiple sclerosis affect a patient's life?
2. How is it possible to tell if a medication for multiple sclerosis is working?
3. Why does the risk of developing multiple sclerosis vary according to the place a person grew up?

Introduction

Multiple sclerosis is an immune-mediated inflammatory disease associated with multiple areas of myelin loss (demyelination) and subsequent axon loss in the central nervous system. It has a wide clinical spectrum, ranging from isolated, non-disabling symptoms to aggressive, disabling disease causing significant physical and social disability. In high-income countries, multiple sclerosis is second only to trauma as a cause of disability in young adults.

Rare conditions mimic multiple sclerosis, for example neurosarcoidosis and vitamin B12 deficiency. There are also autoimmune demyelinating diseases other than multiple sclerosis. However, in the UK, northern Europe and North America most patients with demyelination have multiple sclerosis.

Case 11 Rapid loss of visual acuity in one eye

Presentation

Greg Peters, a 37-year-old teacher, is admitted to the neurology ward from an ophthalmology clinic, with rapid loss of visual acuity in his left eye. Furthermore, the eye is painful when moved, and the ophthalmologist thinks the optic disc is swollen. Greg is also ataxic (uncoordinated).

Initial interpretation

Rapid loss of visual acuity in one eye can be caused by disease in the retina, optic disc or optic nerve (see Table 2.7). With ischaemic causes, the loss develops over seconds to hours. With metabolic or toxic causes, it normally develops over weeks or months.

Eye pain and swollen optic disc are common signs of optic neuritis. The ataxia suggests a lesion elsewhere, perhaps the brain stem or cerebellum, probably as a result of the same pathological process.

History

The visual changes started 6 days ago. They started with reduced colour sensitivity in the left eye; this was followed by loss of acuity. Greg has had pain behind the eye on extremes of gaze since his vision changed.

Interpretation of history

The visual symptoms described are typical of optic neuritis. This is a consequence of multifocal central nervous system inflammation, and multiple sclerosis is the likeliest cause. However, the optic neuritis could be a very unusual presentation of multiple cerebral metastases or central nervous system infection.

Further history

Greg has had a feeling of being off balance. This sensation, which he described

Multiple sclerosis: diagnosis

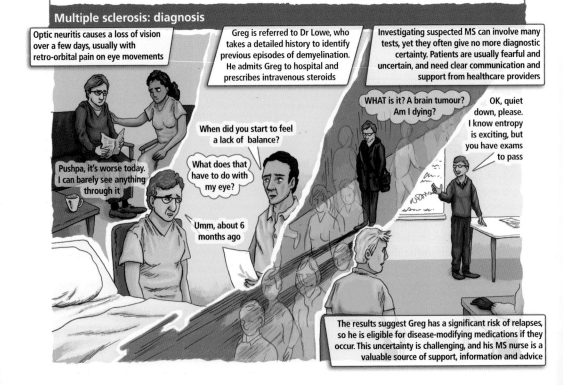

Optic neuritis causes a loss of vision over a few days, usually with retro-orbital pain on eye movements

Greg is referred to Dr Lowe, who takes a detailed history to identify previous episodes of demyelination. He admits Greg to hospital and prescribes intravenous steroids

Investigating suspected MS can involve many tests, yet they often give no more diagnostic certainty. Patients are usually fearful and uncertain, and need clear communication and support from healthcare providers

WHAT is it? A brain tumour? Am I dying?

OK, quiet down, please. I know entropy is exciting, but you have exams to pass

When did you start to feel a lack of balance?

Pushpa, it's worse today. I can barely see anything through it

What does that have to do with my eye?

Umm, about 6 months ago

The results suggest Greg has a significant risk of relapses, so he is eligible for disease-modifying medications if they occur. This uncertainty is challenging, and his MS nurse is a valuable source of support, information and advice

as 'feeling drunk', started 6 months ago and progressed over 4 days. The balance disturbance was very severe for the first 3 weeks; he struggled to walk and had several falls. However, it then eased to settle at a static level. His sense of balance has never completely returned to normal.

In answer to direct questions, Greg describes an episode of foot drop that occurred 2 years ago; he was unable to dorsiflex the ankle of his right foot. Again, this problem progressed over a few days. He required crutches for 3 months until it resolved fully.

Examination

Greg cannot read the Snellen chart but can count the number of fingers the doctors holds up in front of his affected left eye. Acuity is normal in the right eye.

The optic disc of the left eye is swollen. However, eye movements are normal, and Greg has no nystagmus. His gait is mildly ataxic, in that he wobbles when standing on one foot, and he leans on furniture for support. He has brisk reflexes on the right leg, with an up-going plantar reflex.

Interpretation of findings

The swollen disc is a consequence of the local oedema and cellular infiltration that are part of the optic neuritis. The gait disturbance on examination is consistent with the history of balance disturbance. The brisk reflexes and up-going plantar reflex suggest an upper motor neurone cause for the previous foot drop.

Together, the history and examination results suggest multiple sites of central nervous system damage that occurred at separate times. Multiple sclerosis is the most likely cause.

Investigations

Greg undergoes magnetic resonance imaging (MRI) of the head and spine. The

scan shows oedema of the optic nerve, as well as several small ovoid lesions in the brain stem and spinal cord when fluid-attenuated inversion recovery sequence is used. Several similar small lesions are present in the corpus callosum; the corresponding areas enhance when contrast is used, showing that they are actively inflamed. Analysis of cerebrospinal fluid obtained through lumbar puncture shows a white blood cell count of 20 lymphocytes per mL and unpaired oligoclonal bands.

Diagnosis

The MRI findings of multiple non-enhancing ovoid lesions in the brain stem and spinal cord are probably old demyelinating lesions. The enhancing lesions represent areas of active demyelination. The optic nerve oedema also confirms active inflammation in these areas.

The results of cerebrospinal fluid analysis are typical for an active relapse of multiple sclerosis. The white cell count is increased, but not dramatically so (i.e. it is not in the hundreds or thousands of cells per mL as would be the case with an infection). Furthermore, the unpaired oligoclonal bands indicate that the inflammation is restricted to the central nervous system, and is not secondary to a systemic infection.

Greg meets with his consultant as well as a multiple sclerosis nurse specialist, who discuss the diagnosis of optic neuritis in the context of relapsing–remitting multiple sclerosis. He has many questions about how he got the condition, how it will progress and whether any treatments are available. His questions are answered fully, and he is given patient information and the nurse specialist's contact details. The nurse specialist will act as a point of contact.

Greg is concerned about his ability to continue working. The nurse specialist explains that many people with multiple sclerosis are very active and able to work full time.

Case 11 *continued*

An often neglected symptom of multiple sclerosis is extreme fatigue. During a relapse, this can be more disabling and difficult to treat than other neurological deficits such as weakness or ataxia. Patients are advised that their fatigue will lessen as the relapse settles.

For this relapse, Greg receives 3 days of intravenous methylprednisolone therapy (1 g intravenously once per day). He has now had two disabling relapses in a year. Therefore, after detailed discussion about the risks and benefits of treatment, he is started on natalizumab as a disease-modifying therapy. He will have regular follow-up appointments as an outpatient.

Multiple sclerosis

Multiple sclerosis is an idiopathic immune-mediated disease of the central nervous system. It is characterised by central nervous system demyelination and associated loss of axons in discrete areas, called plaques (see **Figure 10.3**). Clinically, multiple sclerosis presents as recurrent bouts of neurological deficits that come and go, producing variable degrees of long-term disability.

Disruption of neuronal function from the demyelination and axonal degeneration results in a wide range of symptoms and signs. These include visual or oculomotor dysfunction, motor deficits, sensory deficits, bladder and bowel sphincter dysfunction, speech and swallowing dysfunction and cognitive impairment.

The sclerosis (Greek, 'hardening') of multiple sclerosis refers to the plaques ('scars') formed in the brain and spinal cord as a consequence of demyelination and subsequent damage. Histologically, the plaques are areas of myelin loss, with lymphocytes and macrophages.

Epidemiology

In the UK, around 100,000 people have multiple sclerosis; it has a prevalence of 100–150 per 100,000 and an annual incidence rate of 7 per 100,000. Peak incidence is between 20 and 40 years of age, and twice as many women than men are affected. Worldwide about 2.5 million people have multiple sclerosis. It is rare in countries near the equator and much more frequent in countries further from the equator.

The increased incidence of multiple sclerosis in more northern latitudes is inversely proportional to the reduction in the amount of ultraviolet light at the wavelength needed for the skin to synthesise vitamin D. This has led to the hypothesis that low vitamin D levels trigger multiple sclerosis.

Diet also influences vitamin D levels. Scotland and Norway are at similar latitudes, but Norwegians have higher vitamin D levels and roughly half the incidence of multiple sclerosis because of a diet that includes more oily fish rich in vitamin D.

Aetiology

The inflammation in multiple sclerosis is mediated by a T-cell immune response. The trigger is probably a complex interplay between multiple genetic predispositions and environmental factors, such as vitamin D deficiency and infectious agents (**Table 10.1**).

Pathogenesis

The three main pathological characteristics of multiple sclerosis are:

- demyelination (destruction of the myelin sheath and oligodendrocytes)
- acute inflammation around the demyelinated regions
- plaque formation after incomplete healing

T cell acute inflammation

First, an unknown trigger disrupts the blood–brain barrier, which normally regulates the entry of T cells into the central nervous system. Autoreactive T cells primed against myelin antigens then attack myelin-containing oligodendrocytes, thereby causing acute inflammatory demyelination and some destruction of axons.

Healing

When the inflammation subsides, incomplete healing creates plaques around damaged axons. Cycles of acute inflammation and healing constitute the relapsing–remitting phase of multiple sclerosis.

Progressive inflammation

Years later, recurrent attacks (relapses), poor remyelination and other factors result in axonal loss and a degenerative phase of progressive neurological dysfunction without remission. These are the progressive phases of multiple sclerosis.

Clinical features

The features of multiple sclerosis depend on the site of the lesion (**Table 10.2**), but visual, motor, sensory and autonomic (bladder and bowel sphincter) symptoms and signs predominate. Between 75 and 85% of patients present with one major symptom or deficit:

- 45% have motor symptoms (e.g. limb weakness) or sensory symptoms (e.g. numbness, tingling and paraesthesias)
- 20% experience spasticity (increased muscle tone) at some point
- 20% have optic neuritis
- 10% have symptoms of brain stem dysfunction (e.g. double vision) or cerebellar dysfunction (e.g. ataxia and nystagmus)
- 25% have a combination of the above

Other common but non-diagnostic features include the following.

- Lhermitte's sign: neck flexion causes paraesthesia or tingling down the spine because of cervical spinal cord plaques
- Uhthoff's phenomenon: worsening of symptoms with an increase in body temperature (e.g. visual loss with strenuous exercise in a patient with optic neuritis)

Some patients develop mild cognitive problems such as short-term memory lapses or word-finding difficulties. These are caused by the lesions of multiple sclerosis or the psychological stress and fatigue associated with the disease.

Possible causes of multiple sclerosis	
Aetiological group	Aetiological factor
Geography	Lifetime risk increases with distance from equator
	Risk is 'fixed' after the age of 15 years
Genetics	HLA variants (which affect the way immune cells recognise 'self' antigens) with increased risk:
	■ HLA-DR15
	■ HLA-DQ6
Infection	Epstein–Barr virus
	Human herpesvirus 6
Metabolic	Low sunlight and low vitamin D levels (see 'Geography'); vitamin D interacts with HLA-DR15
Toxins	Smoking
HLA, human leukocyte antigen.	

Table 10.1 Possible causes of multiple sclerosis. The cause is probably multifactorial. These factors are associated with increased risk.

Clinical features of multiple sclerosis	
Site or dysfunction	**Clinical features**
Optic nerve	Optic neuritis: acute visual loss, painful eye movements, impaired colour vision, decreased visual acuity, optic atrophy and relative afferent pupillary defect
Motor symptoms	
Motor cortex	Hypertonia, hyper-reflexia and spastic weakness
Spinal cord	Loss of function below lesion ■ Motor: hypertonia, hyper-reflexia and spastic weakness ■ Sensory ■ Autonomic ■ Reflex ■ Sphincter: for example urinary retention
Cerebral hemisphere	
Frontal lobes	Disinhibition
Parietal lobes	Visuospatial dysfunction
Temporal and limbic system	Poor memory and dementia
Cerebellum	
Cerebellar syndrome	Dysarthria, nystagmus, ataxia and intention tremor
Brain stem	
Oculomotor dysfunction	Diplopia
Internuclear ophthalmoplegia	Weak adduction of ipsilateral eye and nystagmus in abducting contralateral eye
Descending white matter tracts	Facial numbness, trigeminal neuralgia, etc.
Bulbar dysfunction	Dysphagia, spastic tongue movements and dysarthria

Table 10.2 Clinical features of multiple sclerosis based on the site of the lesion or type of dysfunction

Relapses

A relapse is an acute 'attack' of motor, visual, balance, bladder or bowel dysfunction which comes on over hours or days. Symptoms experienced previously or new symptoms appear with a variable degree of severity and persist for days or months before resolving.

Relapses usually occur without warning. However, stress and acute infection are known to increase the likelihood of a relapse.

> **Multiple sclerosis relapses usually occur without warning.** However, they are occasionally preceded by common triggers such as stress and viral infections. Pregnancy decreases the risk of relapse, but the risk increases in the first few months after delivery; this may be a consequence of the effects of changing hormonal levels on immune function.

Clinical patterns

Multiple sclerosis has four clinical patterns and two further multiple sclerosis-associated isolated syndromes, (**Table 10.3** and **Figure 10.1**). The four clinical patterns are:

■ relapsing–remitting
■ primary progressive
■ secondary progressive
■ progressive relapsing

It is clinically necessary to identify the pattern of multiple sclerosis, because this information guides treatment and informs prognosis.

Isolated syndromes

Multiple sclerosis-associated isolated syndromes are either radiologically or clinically isolated (**Figure 10.2**).

■ In radiologically isolated syndromes, there is incidental radiological evidence of central

Clinical patterns of MS

Clinical pattern	Epidemiology	Features
Relapsing–remitting MS	85% of patients with MS	Relapse of acute unpredictable deterioration followed by periods of remission Less recovery as disease progresses
Primary progressive MS	10–15% of patients with MS Average age of onset is 40 years More common in men than in women	Characterised by progressive neurological disability from onset of symptoms, with no remission or resolution of symptoms
Secondary progressive MS	50–60% of patients with relapsing–remitting MS develop secondary progressive MS after 10–15 years	Patients with relapsing–remitting MS develop unremitting disease
Progressive relapsing MS	Rarest form of MS, about 5–10% of patients	Progressive disease and neurological decline from onset, with pattern of exacerbations

Table 10.3 The four clinical patterns of multiple sclerosis (MS)

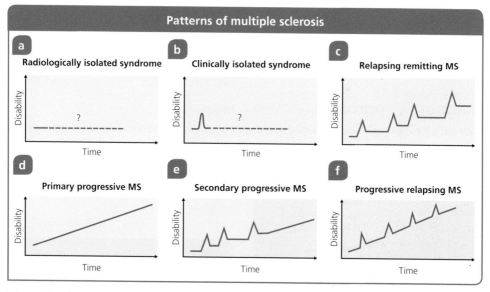

Figure 10.1 There are several different patterns of multiple sclerosis (MS). For example radiologically isolated syndrome (a) is asymptomatic but has radiological evidence of demyelinating lesions whereas in clinically isolated syndrome (b) there is one clinically symptomatic demyelinating event. The long term prognosis of both these patterns is unpredictable. In relapsing–remitting MS (c) episodes of severe disability partially or fully resolve but less fully over time. In primary progressive MS (d) there is a slow and steady progression of disability. In secondary progressive MS (e) a phase of steady progression in disability follows an initial relapsing-remitting pattern. In progressive-relapsing MS (f) there are episodes of acute deterioration on top of a continuous slow decline.

nervous system demyelination, but patients are completely asymptomatic; about 60% of patients go on to develop multiple sclerosis
- Conversely, in clinically isolated syndromes patients have a single clinical episode of one or more symptoms of central nervous system demyelination but no medical history to suggest previous episodes, and their MRI scan may be normal; 50–85% of patients go on to develop recurrent attacks and multiple sclerosis is diagnosed

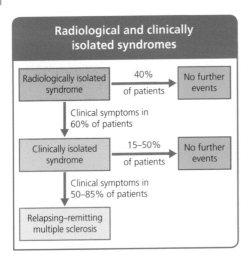

Radiological and clinically isolated syndromes

Radiologically isolated syndrome → 40% of patients → No further events

Clinical symptoms in 60% of patients

Clinically isolated syndrome → 15–50% of patients → No further events

Clinical symptoms in 50–85% of patients

Relapsing–remitting multiple sclerosis

Figure 10.2 Relationship between radiologically isolated syndrome, clinically isolated syndrome and relapsing–remitting multiple sclerosis.

Patients identified as having had an isolated syndrome should be reassessed and rescanned in 3 months.

Diagnostic approach

Multiple sclerosis is a clinical diagnosis, based on signs and symptoms. The diagnosis is supported by the results of neuroimaging and other tests, including cerebrospinal fluid analysis and evoked potentials.

Rare recurrent demyelinating diseases can mimic multiple sclerosis, including:

- vasculitides (primary central nervous system vasculitis and systemic lupus erythematosus)
- neuromyelitis optica
- neurosarcoidosis

These diseases are differentiated from multiple sclerosis by clinical symptoms and the results of imaging studies and cerebrospinal fluid analysis. For example, pyrexia or meningism, bilateral optic neuritis and markedly increased white cell counts in cerebrospinal fluid are rare in multiple sclerosis but often present in the above disorders.

Investigations

Magnetic resonance imaging, cerebrospinal fluid analysis and evoked potentials can support a clinical diagnosis of multiple sclerosis.

Imaging

Magnetic resonance imaging usually shows well-defined, homogenous, ovoid contrast-enhancing lesions in white matter, especially

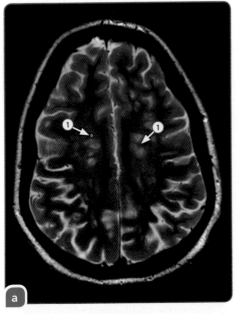

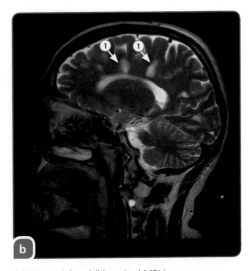

Figure 10.3 The radiological appearance of MS plaques. (a) T2W axial and (b) sagittal MRI images demonstrating ① multiple deep white matter plaques in periventricular locations involving corpus callosum – characteristic of multiple sclerosis.

the corpus callosum, periventricular regions, brain stem and cerebellar peduncles (**Figure 10.3**). It can also help differentiate a tumour or neurosarcoidosis, and can indicate the risk of a subsequent attack:

- abnormal MRI findings after an initial clinical attack are associated with a 90% chance of a further attack
- a normal MRI scan correlates to a 15% chance of a further attack

Cerebrospinal fluid analysis

Multiple sclerosis is associated with the presence of oligoclonal bands of immunoglobulin G in cerebrospinal fluid. These bands indicate increased immunoglobulin G production in the central nervous system by B cells.

The presence of oligoclonal bands is highly sensitive. They are present in most cases of multiple sclerosis but also in other central nervous system inflammatory disorders, such as sarcoidosis (i.e. it is a sensitive but non-specific test for multiple sclerosis).

Evoked potentials

Demyelination results in decreased conduction velocity along axons, which can be measured with evoked potentials (see page 173). These tests can identify a demyelinating pathology in the brain, and therefore may support a diagnosis of multiple sclerosis.

Management

There is no cure for multiple sclerosis. Treatment aims to:

- limit acute relapses
- improve function after a relapse

- prevent new relapses
- control symptoms

This requires a coordinated multidisciplinary approach, tailoring care to the individual patient. Care should be delivered by neurologists, nurses, physiotherapists and occupational therapists who are specialists in MS, liaising with the patient's GP. Other therapists are involved as required by the patient's

symptoms, e.g. speech and language therapists, incontinence therapists and psychologists. Patients should be given a single contact who helps coordinate the various aspects of their care.

Ideally a comprehensive expert review of care is carried out annually, even in the absence of relapses. As well as reviewing medical care, this includes a review of social care needs because many patients eventually require help in this respect.

Acute relapses

An acute relapse is managed with a 3- to 5-day course of oral or intravenous methylprednisolone. This reduces the severity of symptoms and speeds recovery, though it has no effect on long-term disability or relapse rate. Some people, especially those whose social and medical care needs cannot be met at home, benefit from in-patient treatment in a dedicated unit during a significant relapse and the rehabilitation phase.

Appropriate physiotherapy, occupational therapy, and speech and language therapy are essential to maximise recovery from a relapse.

Disease-modifying drugs

These are used to reduce the rate of relapses in relapsing–remitting multiple sclerosis (**Table 10.4**). With one exception (beta interferon) they are not used for other patterns of multiple sclerosis. They have broadly similar efficacies but different and significant adverse effect profiles, and different mechanisms of action (as shown for two examples in **Figures 10.4** and **10.5**). Natalizumab is the most widely used in the UK.

Choice of drug is made by a multiple sclerosis specialist and the patient after detailed discussion. Conventionally, treatment with a disease-modifying drug has often been postponed to see how a patient's disease develops. However, there is a growing consensus that starting treatment as soon as possible after diagnosis improves long-term outcomes.

Vaccinations may be contraindicated in patients receiving disease-modifying treatment. Specialist advice should be sought.

Disease-modifying drugs for multiple sclerosis

Drug	Indications	Mechanism	Route
Alemtuzumab	Active RRMS	Depletes all autoreactive T cells	Intravenous; 2 courses 12 months apart
Beta-interferon*	Active RRMS Progressive MS with relapses	Reduces traffic across BBB, inhibits antigen presentation, enhances apoptosis of autoreactive T cells, various other immune changes	Intramuscular or subcutaneous, several days per week
Dimethyl fumarate	Active RRMS that is not highly active or rapidly evolving	Promotes anti-inflammatory activity; inhibits pro-inflammatory cytokines and adhesion molecules	Oral, daily
Fingolimod	Rapidly evolving severe RRMS MS highly active despite beta interferon	Stops circulating lymphocytes from leaving lymph nodes, reducing number entering brain (see **Figure 10.5**)	Oral, daily
Glatiramer acetate*	Active RRMS	Promotes production of Th2 and Treg cells, increases immune cell release of neurotrophic factors, deletes myelin-reactive T cells	Subcutaneous, daily
Natalizumab	Rapidly evolving severe RRMS MS highly active despite beta interferon	Blocks migration of white blood cells through BBB (see **Figure 10.4**)	Intravenous, monthly
Teriflunomide	Active RRMS that is not highly active or rapidly evolving	Anti-inflammatory, blocking proliferation of stimulated lymphocytes	Oral, daily

*Not available for new prescription in the UK due to cost–benefit considerations

Table 10.4 Disease-modifying drugs for relapsing–remitting multiple sclerosis (RRMS)

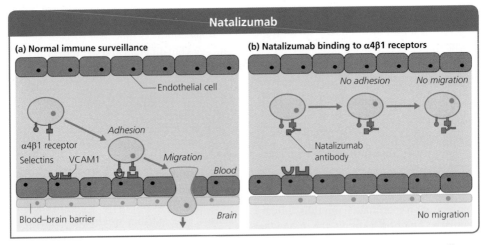

Figure 10.4 Mechanism of action of the monoclonal antibody natalizumab. In normal immune surveillance of the brain T-cells adhere to then migrate through the endothelium and blood–brain barrier to enter the brain. This requires a number of receptor–ligand interactions, including VCAM1 on endothelial cells binding to α4β1 receptors on T-cells (a). By binding to α4β1 receptors natalizumab prevents T-cells migrating into the brain (b) and so reduces relapses in MS patients.

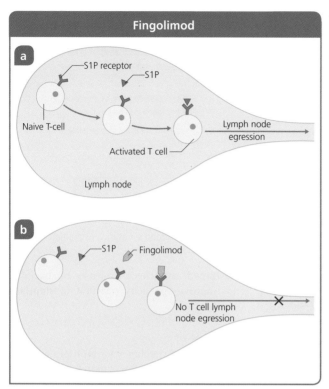

Figure 10.5 Mechanism of action of fingolimod. Normally, naive T-cells become primed against specific antigens in lymph nodes in a process requiring S1P activation of receptors and then enter circulation to find antigen (a) or migrate through the blood–brain barrier. (b) Fingolimod blocks the SP1 receptors on T cells, which prevents their egression from nodes, leading to a decreased number of circulating T cells.

> **The effects on long-term disability of the newer disease-modifying drugs for multiple sclerosis are unclear** but clinical trials show they decrease relapse rates and reduce short-term disability. Many experts now believe relapses are central to accumulation of disability, so the recently developed drugs may improve long-term outcome; however, this is not yet proven.

Symptom control

As outlined in **Table 10.5**, a wide range of pharmacological and non-pharmacological therapies are used for controlling common symptoms of multiple sclerosis, for example spasticity, fatigue, bladder dysfunction, depression and cognitive problems. **Many patients** require treatment for musculoskeletal pain secondary to mobility problems or for neuropathic pain. Exercise is important to maintain strength which can help with mobility when symptoms flare. Patients who develop chronic mobility problems require expert physiotherapy and advice on devices to assist mobility.

Alternative therapies

More than 50% of patients try complementary (alternative) symptomatic therapies, such as hyperbaric oxygen therapy or cannabis. None have evidence of a significant effect, but most are harmless and may improve quality of life, if only by a placebo effect. The autonomy these options offer can be highly valued by patients so it is worth maintaining an open, if sceptical, view. However, patients should be advised on avoiding expensive therapies that do not help, and encouraged to consult their GP about risks before starting any complementary therapy.

Symptom control in multiple sclerosis		
Symptom	Medications	Non-pharmacological therapies
Spasticity and contractions	Baclofen, gapapentin, benzodiazepines or botulinum toxin injections	Physiotherapy and hydrotherapy
Fatigue	Amantadine or modafinil, if disabling	Regular sleep patterns and relaxation techniques
Bladder dysfunction	Anticholinergic drugs such as oxybutynin Botulinum toxin injections into bladder muscle	Intermittent self-catheterisation
Depression	Selective serotonin reuptake inhibitors	Psychotherapeutic counselling and support groups
Cognitive and memory problems	–	Neuropsychiatric and occupational therapy

Table 10.5 Pharmacological and non-pharmacological therapies for common symptoms of multiple sclerosis

> **The family and carers of patients with multiple sclerosis require support** because their responsibilities can easily become overwhelming. Therefore supportive nursing and medical care are essential, especially in the advanced stages of severe disease, when patients may require nursing home and respite care.

Surgery

This is occasionally offered in severe cases to restore movement or relieve severe persistent spasms, for example if contractures prevent walking. More commonly minor surgery is done, in the form of insertion of a pump for sustained intrathecal release of baclofen to improve spasticity resistant to standard therapy.

Prognosis

Average life expectancy for multiple sclerosis patients is 5–10 years less than for the general population. Older age at presentation, male sex, progressive subtype, symptoms other than sensory or optic neuritis at onset, and multiple relapses early on are associated with poor prognosis.

Multiple sclerosis is not fatal but some of its complications are, such as urinary sepsis or aspiration pneumonia secondary to dysphagia.

Other central nervous system demyelinating diseases

Multiple sclerosis is the most common demyelinating central nervous system disorder, but other such disorders exist. These rarer conditions have distinct causes, pathogenic mechanisms (**Figure 10.6**), treatments and prognosis. They must be distinguished from multiple sclerosis so that an appropriate treatment can be selected.

Acute disseminated encephalomyelitis

Acute disseminated encephalomyelitis (ADEM) is a T cell mediated autoimmune demyelinating attack on multiple areas of the brain and spinal cord. The disease often follows an infectious illness or vaccination, is most common in

Immunopathological spectrum of CNS demyelinating diseases

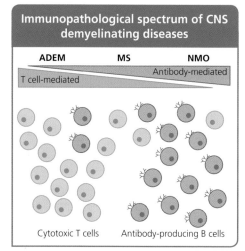

Figure 10.6 Immunopathological spectrum of CNS demyelinating diseases. Acute disseminated encephalomyelitis (ADEM) is dominated by T cell mediated cytotoxicity whilst neuromyelitis optica (NMO) is an antibody-mediated disorder. Multiple sclerosis (MS) lies somewhere in between with a combination of cell and antibody-mediated autoimmune processes

children and does not relapse. Symptoms are severe, with rapid onset, and the patient may be confused, drowsy or delirious (encephalopathic). MRI shows widespread lesions.

The prognosis is usually good. The likelihood of recovery is excellent; the likelihood of recurrence low.

Neuromyelitis optica spectrum disorder

Neuromyelitis optica (NMO, also known as Devic's disease) is a relapsing–remitting antibody-mediated central nervous system demyelinating disorder with more severe, frequent and disabling attacks than those of multiple sclerosis. Features include:

- extensive spinal cord plaques (transverse myelitis)
- optic neuritis (unlike in multiple sclerosis, both eyes are usually involved)

Neuromyelitis optica is caused by anti-aquaporin 4 antibody-mediated damage to astrocytes around the blood–brain barrier.

Patients require aggressive immunosuppression. Without treatment, half of people with neuromyelitis optica would be wheelchair-bound and blind within 5 years of diagnosis.

Answers to starter questions

1. Even mild forms of multiple sclerosis can have significant consequences for patients. In addition to dealing with the physical disability that may follow a relapse, they often feel fearful and uncertain about potential future relapses, life and travel insurance can be difficult to obtain, the ability to drive may be limited and work may become impossible. The diagnosis may also affect decisions such as whether or not to enter a long-term relationship or have children.

2. It is difficult to tell if a medication is working for an individual patient with multiple sclerosis, because relapses may occur despite treatment with even the most effective medications, and the condition may go into remission in patients who are not taking medication. The 'status of disease activity' can be assessed by using MRI to look for any new active lesions while the patient is on medication.

3. There seems to be a window during early childhood when unknown environmental factors prime or set the immune system to a level of risk for multiple sclerosis. This level does not change in later life, even if a person moves to a different environment.

Chapter 11
Spinal disorders

Starter questions

Answers to the following questions are on page 360.

1. What causes the 'shooting pains' associated with neck and back pain?
2. Why does the thoracic segment of the spinal cord have a comparatively poor vascular supply?
3. Why do spinal deformities predispose patients to pulmonary complications?

Introduction

Spinal disorders arise from pathologies affecting the following (**Table 11.1**):

- the spinal cord
- associated neural structures (spinal nerve roots) and vascular structures
- the structural framework of the vertebral column (i.e. the vertebrae, spinal ligaments and intervertebral discs)

Pathologies present as stereotypical spinal syndromes depending on lesion location. When the spinal cord itself is affected, the pathology is termed a myelopathy.

This chapter focuses on degenerative disorders of the spine. Spinal tumours, infections, congenital malformations and spinal trauma are discussed in Chapters 7, 8, 15 and 17, respectively.

The most common presentation of degenerative disorders of the spine is low back pain, which in the UK has a lifetime prevalence of 60–80% and is the most common and expensive work-related disability in people older than 45 years, as well as the second commonest cause for medical consultation after urinary tract infection.

Spinal disorders	
Type	Example(s)
Trauma	Fractures of vertebral body, pedicle, lamina or spinous process
	Spinal cord injury secondary to bony injury
Tumours	Primary: in spinal cord (e.g. glioma and meningioma), nerve roots (e.g. neurofibroma and schwannoma) or bones (e.g. osteosarcoma)
	Secondary: metastases from distant sites, such as breast, lung, prostate, blood (myeloma) and immune system (lymphoma)
Degenerative	Spinal canal and intervertebral exit foraminal stenosis (narrowing)
	Spinal spondylosis (akin to 'wear and tear' or 'arthritis' of spine)
	Spinal spondylolisthesis (slippage of one vertebra on another)
	Intervertebral disc disease (e.g. prolapse of a disc into the spinal canal)
Syringomyelia	Cystic cavity forming in the spinal cord
Vascular	Haemorrhage in the spinal cord (e.g. caused by trauma or vascular malformation)
	Ischaemic infarction of the spinal cord (e.g. caused by occlusion of the spinal cord vasculature)
Congenital	Spinal dysraphism (e.g. spina bifida)
	Scoliosis (abnormal lateral curvature of the spine)
Infection	Infection affecting the disc (discitis) or bones (osteomyelitis), or formation of abscesses compressing the spinal cord (e.g. tuberculosis)

Table 11.1 Disorders of the spine

Case 12 Arm pain worsened by coughing

Presentation

Matt Johnson, a 38-year-old left-handed builder, woke up one morning with neck stiffness and pain. Two days later, he developed severe pain radiating down his right arm.

Initial interpretation

Back and neck pain is common. It usually has a mechanical cause, such as poor posture, muscle cramps and aches. Other causes include osteoarthritis of the joints, spinal canal narrowing and disc prolapses.

A history of neck pain with radiation down the right arm suggests radiculopathy caused by irritation or compression of spinal nerve roots.

Certain features of back and neck pain suggest a sinister cause such as spinal tumour or infection. These red flags are:

- pain at night
- weight loss, which suggests malignancy
- fevers and night sweats, which suggest infection
- a history of cancer
- age < 20 or > 55 years
- acute onset pain in elderly patients
- constant or progressive pain
- bowel or bladder dysfunction, which indicates cauda equina syndrome until excluded
- history of immunosuppression

Further history

Matt gives a history of on-and-off neck pain and stiffness over many years. The pain is usually worst at the end of the day. It does not keep him awake at night, and he has not noticed other systemic symptoms such as weight loss.

His pain is 'sharp' and like an 'electric shock' running down the arm into his forearm and thumb. It is worsened by coughing or sneezing. He also has numbness in his right forearm and thumb.

Examination

Matt has a decreased range of cervical movements. Examination shows normal tone in his right arm but a very subtle decrease in elbow flexion and wrist extension, and reduced biceps reflex. There is decreased sensation to pain in his right thumb.

Interpretation of findings

The altered sensation is affecting the skin (dermatome) supplied by the 6th cervical spinal nerve root (C6). The muscle weakness and reduced reflex suggest lower motor neurone impairment in the myotome supplied by the same spinal nerve root (C6): a radiculopathy affecting the 6th cervical spinal nerve root.

The most likely cause is an intervertebral disc prolapse between C5 and C6, compressing the C6 spinal nerve root, with a background of degenerative arthritis, given Matt's long history of neck pain.

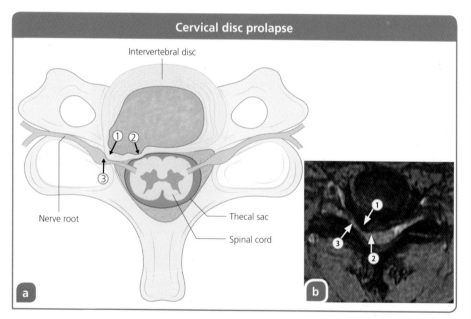

Cervical disc prolapse

Intervertebral disc

Nerve root

Thecal sac

Spinal cord

a

b

Figure 11.1 Cervical disc prolapse: (a) axial anatomical representation and (b) axial T2-weighted magnetic resonance imaging corresponding to each other. ① The intervertebral disc has prolapsed and herniated to the right side with narrowing and compromise of the neural foramen. ② Disc prolapse will also compress the spinal cord and compress the cerebrospinal fluid in the thecal sac. ③ The herniated disc compresses the spinal nerve root exiting from the spinal cord.

Case 12 *continued*

To localise spinal pathology, consider which neural structures must be affected, and at what spinal segmental level, to explain the clinical features. For example, if both arms and legs are affected, the lesion must be in the cervical segment of the spine and spinal cord. If only the legs are affected, then it must be in either the thoracic or the lumbar segment.

Investigations

Magnetic resonance imaging (MRI) of his neck is carried out (**Figure 11.1**).

Diagnosis

The MRI scan confirms a C5–C6 intervertebral disc prolapse compressing the C6 nerve root on the right. A trial of conservative management with analgesics and antineuropathic medication is agreed, with review in 6 weeks to determine if surgical intervention is required.

Spinal syndromes

Spinal injuries, and the degenerative spinal disorders described later in this chapter, present as clinical spinal syndromes that have stereotypical motor and sensory features depending on the site of the pathology in the cord, its nerve roots or both. Some of the disorders described later in this chapter can present as more than one of these syndromes. For example, spondylolysis can develop at any spinal level.

To understand the spinal syndromes, it is necessary to recall the normal anatomy of the spine (**Figure 11.2**), the normal anatomy of the spinal cord and nerve roots (**Figure 11.3**). The spine's principle functins include:

- protecting the spinal cord and spinal nerve roots (**Figure 11.3**)
- transmitting signals from the brain to the rest of the body
- supporting the weight of the head and body (page 68)

The clinical signs produced by the spinal syndromes depend on precisely how the spinal cord and nerve roots are damaged (**Table 11.2**).

The spinal syndromes that present most commonly are outlined in **Figure 11.4**, and **Tables 11.3** and **11.4**.

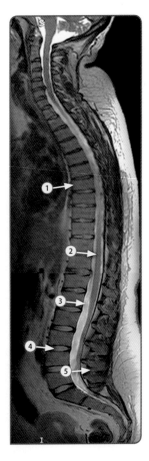

Figure 11.2
Sagittal T2-weighted magnetic resonance of the whole spine demonstrating the normal anatomy of the major structures including the vertebral body ① spinal cord ② cerebrospinal fluid within the thecal sac ③ the intervertebral disc ④ and the spinous process ⑤.

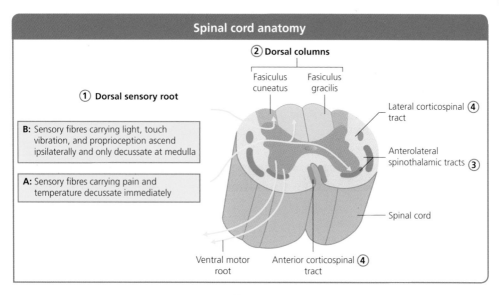

Spinal cord anatomy

② **Dorsal columns**

Fasiculus cuneatus   Fasiculus gracilis

① **Dorsal sensory root**

Lateral corticospinal ④ tract

B: Sensory fibres carrying light, touch vibration, and proprioception ascend ipsilaterally and only decussate at medulla

Anterolateral spinothalamic tracts ③

A: Sensory fibres carrying pain and temperature decussate immediately

Spinal cord

Ventral motor root   Anterior corticospinal ④ tract

Figure 11.3 The spinal cord and its major tracts. ① Dorsal sensory nerve roots carry information from the ipsilateral side of the body on sensation. Two types of fibres are present: (A) fibres carrying pain and temperature sensation (B) fibres carrying light touch, proprioception and vibration. sensation. ② Dorsal columns are ascending tracts that receive ipsilateral dorsal sensory nerve root fibres subserving light touch, proprioception and vibration sensation. The fibres decussate at the medulla. ③ The dorsal sensory nerve roots carrying pain and temperature information decussate immediately across the midline through the anterior commissure and enter the contralateral antero-lateral spinothalamic tract. This tract transmits pain and temperature information to the brain. ④ Cortical motor function is transmitted through descending anterior and lateral corticospinal (pyramidal) tracts down to the cell bodies of motor neurones in the ventral horn. Ventral motor roots transmit signals to muscles for motor function.

Signs of spinal cord lesions

Spinal cord area	Features of damage
Cauda equina or sacral nerve roots	Bowel or bladder dysfunction
Spinal cord – descending motor tracts	Upper motor neurone weakness
Spinal cord – ventral horn motor neurones	Lower motor neurone weakness
Dorsal columns	Impairment of light touch, vibration and proprioception
Spinothalamic tracts	Impairment of pain and temperature sensation
Ventral motor nerve root	Radicular motor weakness (lower motor neurone pattern)
Dorsal sensory nerve root	Radicular sensory loss

Table 11.2 Related signs from damage to neural spinal structures

Complete cord injury

Complete cord injury is the most devastating type of spinal cord injury. It is usually caused by trauma that results in transection of the entire cord, with complete loss of function from that level downwards (see **Figure 11.4**).

Unilateral cord injury: Brown–Sequard syndrome

Brown–Sequard syndrome is an injury affecting one half of the spinal cord (see **Figure 11.4**). It causes ipsilateral loss of motor function and dorsal column function and contralateral loss of spinothalamic tract function.

Anterior cord injury

Anterior cord injury affects the anterior two thirds of the spinal cord (bilateral motor function and spinothalamic tracts), with preservation of the dorsal columns (see **Figure 11.4**). The classical cause is a vascular ischaemic stroke.

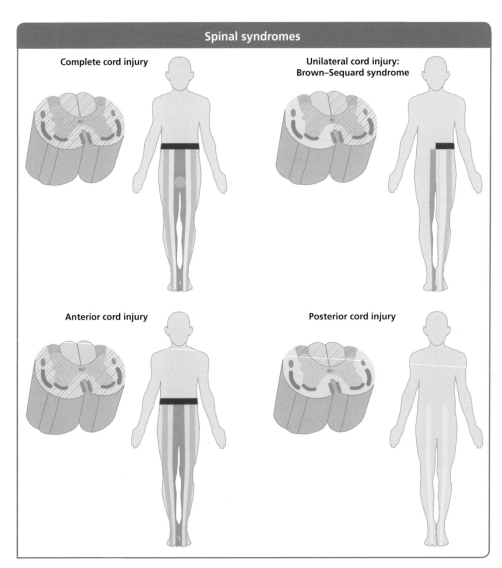

Figure 11.4 Spinal syndromes (*continued opposite*). For key see opposite. See Tables 11.3 and 11.4 for details of sensory abnormalities.

Posterior cord injury

Posterior cord injury is the opposite of anterior cord injury affecting the posterior one third of the spinal cord. It causes isolated dysfunction of the dorsal columns (see **Figure 11.4**).

Central cord injury

This is a variable clinical syndrome. Its effects depend on the extent of central cord injury (see **Figure 11.4**).

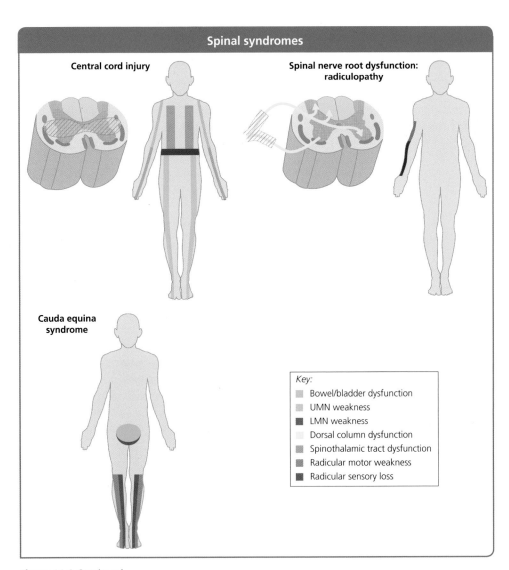

Spinal syndromes

Central cord injury

Spinal nerve root dysfunction: radiculopathy

Cauda equina syndrome

Key:
- Bowel/bladder dysfunction
- UMN weakness
- LMN weakness
- Dorsal column dysfunction
- Spinothalamic tract dysfunction
- Radicular motor weakness
- Radicular sensory loss

Figure 11.4 *Continued*

Spinal syndromes				
Syndrome (structure affected)	Motor abnormalities*			Sensory abnormalities*
	Muscles affected	Pattern of weakness†		
		At level of lesion	Below lesion	
Complete cord (**Figure 11.4**)	*Bilateral*	LMN	UMN	*Bilateral*: complete loss of all sensory modalities below level of lesion ■ Pain and temperature ■ Light touch, vibration and proprioception Bowel and/or bladder function likely to be disrupted
Unilateral cord (Brown–Sequard) (**Figure 11.4**)	*Ipsilateral*	LMN	UMN	*Ipsilateral*: complete loss of light touch, vibration and proprioception below level of lesion Contralateral: complete loss of pain and temperature sensation below level of lesion
Anterior cord (**Figure 11.4**)	*Bilateral*	LMN	UMN	*Bilateral*: complete loss of pain and temperature sensation below level of lesion
Posterior cord (**Figure 11.4**)	Not affected	–	–	Bilateral: complete loss of light touch, vibration sensation and proprioception
Central cord (**Figure 11.4**)	*Bilateral* Arms more than legs Distal muscles more than proximal	LMN	UMN	*Bilateral*: pain and temperature sensation impaired in areas supplied by segment affected

LMN, lower motor neurone; UMN, upper motor neurone.

*Ipsilateral: the effect is on the same side as the lesion. Bilateral: the effect occurs on both sides. Contralateral: the effect is on the opposite side to the lesion.

†LMN pattern of weakness is 'flaccid' weakness, decreased tone, decreased or absent reflexes and down-going plantar response; UMN pattern of weakness is 'spastic' weakness, increased tone and 'clonus', increased reflexes and extensor up-going plantar response.

Table 11.3 Clinical syndromes associated with spinal cord injury

Spinal nerve root and cauda equina syndromes			
Syndrome (structure affected)	Motor abnormalities	Sensory abnormalities	Additional abnormalities
Spinal nerve root syndromes ('radiculopathy') (**Figure 11.4**)	LMN pattern of weakness only affecting muscles innervated by that spinal nerve root (myotome)	Decreased sensation in all sensory modalities in area supplied by that spinal nerve root (dermatome)	Pain radiating into area of skin or muscle supplied by that spinal nerve root Described as 'burning', 'sharp', 'shooting' or 'electric shock-like' Aggravated by coughing, straining and movement
Cauda equina (lowest lumbar and sacral nerve roots) (**Figure 11.4**)	Usually LMN pattern of weakness affecting the most distal muscles of the leg (e.g. ankle and foot)	Decreased sensation in all sensory modalities in area supplied by the sacral spinal nerve roots (usually the perineal, perianal or genital regions)	Bladder or bowel abnormalities are always present (e.g. urinary retention, and faecal and urinary incontinence) caused by disruption of sacral autonomic fibres

LMN, lower motor neurone; UMN, upper motor neurone.

†LMN pattern of weakness is 'flaccid' weakness, decreased tone, decreased or absent reflexes and down-going plantar response; UMN pattern of weakness is 'spastic' weakness, increased tone and 'clonus', increased reflexes and extensor up-going plantar response.

Table 11.4 Clinical syndromes associated with dysfunction of the spinal nerve roots, cauda equina and bony elements of the spine

Spinal nerve root dysfunction (radiculopathy)

Radiculopathy (Latin: radix, 'root') is an abnormality that compresses or impinges on a spinal nerve root in a way that causes pain, numbness, weakness or poor control of muscles in the distribution of the affected spinal nerve root. Symptoms affect the muscle group (myotome) and area of skin (dermatome) supplied by that spinal nerve root (see **Figure 11.4**). Radiculopathy classically results from disc prolapse affecting either the cervical or the lumbar spine, and the diagnosis, investigation and management of various causes of radiculopathy is discussed in more detail on pages 352–354.

Cauda equina syndrome

The spinal cord ends level with the L1 vertebra. Below this, the lumbar (L1-L5) and sacral (S1–S4) spinal nerve roots continue down within the spinal canal, each exiting through an intervertebral exit foramen. In the canal, these spinal nerve roots are known collectively as the cauda equina (see page 71).

Pathologies that compress or irritate the cauda equina produce cauda equina syndrome. The commonest is compression caused by a lesion, usually disc prolapse (see **Figure 11.4**). Cauda equina syndrome is a medical emergency because of the potential rapid permanent loss of sphincter function, affecting the bowel and bladder.

The aetiology, investigation and management of suspected cauda equina syndrome is discussed in more detail on pages 356–357.

Spondylosis

Spondylosis (Greek: spondulos, 'vertebra'; 'osis', pathology) is a non-specific term for osteoarthritis or degenerative change affecting the spine.

Epidemiology

Cervical spondylosis affects over 50% of people aged over 50 years. However the condition becomes symptomatic in less than 20% of those it affects. It is the commonest cause of myelopathy of the cervical spine.

Aetiology

Spondylosis is akin to arthritis affecting any joint. Ageing and cumulative stress cause intervertebral disc degeneration, which reduces the ability of the disc to act as a shock absorber. Pathological changes include:

- disc rupture and prolapse into the spinal canal or intervertebral exit foramina
- abnormal bone growth (osteophytes) along joint margins
- abnormal bone thickening (hypertrophy) at the joints
- hypertrophy of spinal ligaments

These changes lead to stenosis (narrowing) of the central spinal canal and intervertebral exit foramina, compressing the spinal cord and spinal nerve roots, respectively (**Figure 11.5).**

Clinical features

The spinal cord ends at the lower border of L1 (see page 71). Beyond this point, the spinal canal contains spinal nerve roots of the lowest lumbar and sacral segments of the spinal cord: the cauda equina.

- Narrowing above L1 compresses the spinal cord, leading to features of myelopathy and/or radiculopathy in cases of concurrent nerve root compression
- Narrowing below L1 compresses nerves or nerve roots of the lowest lumbar and sacral segments, leading to features of radiculopathy, and if particularly the nerve roots supplying the bowel and/or bladder are affected, cauda equina syndrome (see page 356)

The onset of symptoms is usually gradual. Narrowing of the central spinal canal compresses the spinal cord, which in the

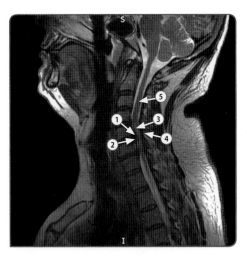

Figure 11.5 Sagittal T2-weighted magnetic resonance image of the cervical spine demonstrating cervical spondylosis affecting C5/6 and C6/7 vertebral levels. Disc prolapse at C5/6 ① and degenerative bone changes ② have caused spinal cord compression with increased signal change and myelomalacia within the cord. Hypertrophy of the posterior ligamentum flavum also adds to compression from posteriorly further compressing the cord and narrowing the spinal canal ④ Normal spinal cord free from compression in a capacious spinal canal is demonstrated at C3 vertebral body level above ⑤.

cervical or thoracic spine can cause myelopathy (see page 350). Narrowing of intervertebral exit foramina leads to radiculopathy (page 354).

Diagnostic approach

Magnetic resonance imaging shows the degree of compression of the spinal cord and nerve roots.

Management

Conservative management with analgesia is indicated if there is no significant motor deficit. A worsening neurological deficit warrants surgery.

Medication

If symptoms are mild or there is no significant motor deficit, the initial approach is usually analgesia, commonly provided by non-steroidal anti-inflammatory drugs (NSAIDs), and neck support with a cervical collar.

Surgery

Decompression surgery carries significant risks, especially in the cervical spine. Complications include permanent paralysis, leakage of cerebrospinal fluid and spinal instability. Therefore surgery is reserved for patients with progressive or persistent neurological deficits, or significant pain unresponsive to medical treatment.

Myelopathy

Myelopathies (Greek: muelos, 'marrow') are often caused by pathologies that compress or expand the spinal cord. Cervical spondylosis is the commonest cause of cervical myelopathy.

Aetiology

Three mechanisms underlie the many causes of myelopathy (**Table 11.5**):

- direct cord compression
- impairment of cord blood supply
- extensive oedema or swelling

Clinical features

The severity of compression, lesion level and speed of onset determine the clinical presentation. Onset is usually slow and insidious, with loss of reflexes and flaccid weakness at the level of the lesion, spasticity and increased reflexes below the level of the lesion.

Generalised hyper-reflexia, especially in the lower limbs, and any of the following 'pathological' reflexes are almost pathognomonic of cervical myelopathy (see page 350):

- Babinski's sign

Causes of myelopathy		
Timing of symptoms and signs*	Causes	Examples
Acute (minutes to hours)	Trauma	Acute bony injury (fracture) with spinal cord compression
		Acute disc prolapse
	Vascular	Haemorrhage into the spinal cord or compressing it from outside (e.g. trauma and vascular malformation)
		Ischaemic stroke affecting the spinal cord (e.g. spinal artery thrombosis)
Subacute (days to weeks)	Inflammation	Demyelination secondary to multiple sclerosis or infection
	Infection	Viral infection (e.g. HIV and human T-cell leukaemia virus type 1), tuberculosis or abscess
Chronic (weeks to months)	Degenerative	Cervical spondylosis
	Tumours	Primary or secondary tumours
	Syringomyelia	Idiopathic or secondary to other pathologies (e.g. tumour)
	Congenital	Congenital stenosis and spinal dysraphism
	Metabolic	Vitamin B12 deficiency

*Timing is an important differentiating factor, but all can present acutely.

Table 11.5 Causes of myelopathy

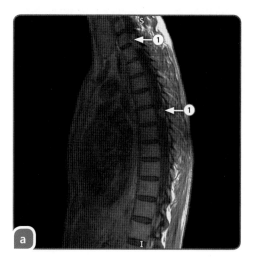 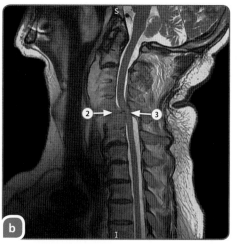

Figure 11.6 Sagittal magnetic resonance imaging (MRI) scans showing examples of possible compressive lesions that can lead to myelopathy as a result of spinal cord compression. (a) T1-weighted MRI post-contrast sequences of the thoracic spine, showing two meningiomas ① causing spinal cord compression. (b) T2-weighted MRI scan showing a complex cervical fracture at the C5–C6 vertebra ②, with resultant compression of the spinal cord and associated signal change in the cord ③.

- Hoffmann's sign
- clonus

Diagnostic approach

Magnetic resonance imaging shows most lesions that compress the spinal cord, such as tumour and fracture (**Figure 11.6**), and it may indicate non-compressive causes, including demyelination. MRI also shows spinal cord viability, for example the extent of oedema and ischaemic damage, and therefore the potential for recovery.

Management

The priority is urgent MRI to find a compressing lesion.

- If a compressing lesion is present, the patient is referred to neurosurgery for decompression surgery

- If no such lesion is detected, the patient is referred to neurology for further investigation and medical management

After definitive treatment, neurological rehabilitation, physiotherapy and occupational therapy minimise the patient's disability and maximise their quality of life.

Radiculopathy

Radiculopathy arises from compression or irritation of a spinal root. The principle causes are listed in **Table 11.6**.

Epidemiology

The commonest cause of radiculopathy is a herniated intervertebral disc. Intervertebral disc disease is most common in the lumbar spine and is symptomatic in 2% of the population.

Clinical features

Compression or irritation of a spinal nerve root produces a stereotypical pattern of neurological symptoms depending on the muscles (myotome) and area of skin (dermatome) supplied by that nerve root (see page 345). The affected spinal nerve root is localised by considering the:

- myotome affected by weakness (including the exact reflex lost)
- dermatome where sensation is disrupted
- distribution of radicular pain

Radicular pain

Acute radicular pain is described as 'sharp', 'burning', 'shooting' and 'electric shock'-like. Coughing, sneezing and movement often exacerbate it. Pathogenesis is most likely through a combination of factors, such as friction and pressure on the nerve root, leading to demyelination, ischaemia and disrupted transmission of electrophysiological signals. Any pathological process affecting spinal nerve roots can produce radicular pain, and episodes may be intermittent or persistent.

- Cervical radiculopathy presents with neck pain and brachialgia (pain radiating down the upper limb)
- Lumbar or sacral radiculopathy commonly causes low back pain and associated sciatica (radicular pain radiating down the lower limb in the sciatic nerve distribution)

Causes of radiculopathy	
Cause	Examples
Intervertebral disc prolapse	Prolapse of a lumbar, cervical or thoracic disc, usually on a background of spinal spondylosis
Nerve sheath tumour	Neurofibroma and schwannoma
Other tumours	Primary (e.g. osteosarcoma) or secondary (e.g. metastasis) spinal tumours
Infection	Viral infection (e.g. HIV, varicella zoster virus and herpes simplex virus) causing nerve root inflammation (radiculitis)

Table 11.6 Common causes of radiculopathy

> The straight leg-raising test is used to confirm irritation or compression of the lumbosacral nerve roots as the cause of a patient's symptoms. With the patient lying flat on their back, the examiner elevates the leg while keeping it straight. Elevation to 90° without discomfort is normal. However, in patients with lumbosacral radicular pain from nerve root compression pain occurs with minor elevation, for example 30°.

Intervertebral disc herniation can occur in different directions to compress different structures (**Table 11.7**).

Diagnostic approach

The priority is to exclude a compressive lesion.

Investigations

The primary modality of investigation remains radiological. Establishing congruence between the clinical and radiological features is important in deciding to purse surgical intervention.

Imaging

Spinal MRI is used to exclude compressive lesions affecting one or more spinal nerve roots.

Neurophysiology

If no lesion that could cause the clinical features is visible on MRI, nerve conduction studies and muscle examination with electromyography are done to:

- confirm the presence of radiculopathy
- assess the severity of neurological dysfunction
- detect other pathology, such as anterior horn lower motor neurone dysfunction, peripheral nerve dysfunction and myopathy

Management

For about 75% of patients with acute radiculopathy caused by disc herniation, their symptoms improve spontaneously. Initial management is usually non-operative and includes physiotherapy to strengthen muscle and improve spinal alignment. Occupational therapy includes arranging ergonomic modifications at work and home.

Medication

Both NSAIDs (e.g. diclofenac) and antineuropathic medications (e.g. pregabalin) may be used for symptomatic relief of radicular pain. Non-compressive lesions require specific treatment depending on the cause, for example infection and demyelination.

Compressive lesions such as tumours may require chemotherapy, radiotherapy or both.

Surgery

Early decompression surgery is indicated if a compressive lesion is causing:

- severe intractable pain that is unresponsive to medical management
- acute spinal cord compression with myelopathy, or cauda equina compression with cauda equina syndrome
- severe motor deficits (e.g. foot drop)

Disc herniation radiculopathy	
Site	Structure compressed
Lateral or posterolateral herniation	Exiting spinal nerve root in the intervertebral neural exit foramina (for lateral herniation) and the traversing/transiting nerve root in the lateral recess (for postero-lateral herniation)
Posterocentral herniation backwards into the spinal canal above the L1 vertebra	Spinal cord compression (myelopathy)
Large posterocentral disc herniation below L1	Cauda equina, causing cauda equina syndrome (see page 356)

Table 11.7 Disc herniation and radiculopathy

Lumbar spinal stenosis

Lumbar spinal stenosis is narrowing of the central spinal canal in the lumbar spine. It is either congenital or acquired (**Table 11.8**).

Because the spinal cord ends at L1 and the cauda equina (nerve roots L1–S4) begins at about L1, lumbar spinal stenosis can also cause cauda equina syndrome (see page 356).

Epidemiology

The incidence of lumbar spinal stenosis increases after 50 years of age.

Causes of lumbar spinal stenosis	
Category	Examples
Congenital	Achondroplasia ('dwarfism')
	Congenital spondylolisthesis
	Scoliosis
Acquired	Degenerative (e.g. caused by lumbar spondylosis)
	Iatrogenic (e.g. after spinal surgery for other causes)
	Traumatic (e.g. caused by traumatic spondylolisthesis)
	Inflammatory (e.g. ankylosing spondylitis and acromegaly)

Table 11.8 Causes of lumbar spinal stenosis

Clinical features

The clinical features of lumber spinal stenosis are caused by mechanical compression and vascular compromise of lower lumbar and sacral spinal nerve roots. Most patients are initially asymptomatic, but when symptoms develop they commonly present with:

- chronic progressive lower back and bilateral buttock and leg pain
- pain with 'radicular' features (see **Table 11.4**)

There may also be:

- leg abnormal sensations (e.g. numbness and tingling)
- leg motor weakness and 'heaviness'

Claudication

This is the term for muscular pain and weakness that worsen with exercise but improve with rest. Claudication can be vascular or neurogenic (**Table 11.9**).

Lower limb neurogenic claudication in lumbar spinal stenosis is caused by compression of lumbosacral spinal nerve roots supplying the lower limb musculature. It is important to differentiate it from the more common vascular claudication and make the correct diagnosis to

Vascular and neurogenic claudication		
Category	Features of vascular claudication	Features of neurogenic claudication
Cause	Atherosclerotic narrowing of arteries	Compression of neural structures
Pain description	'Cramping' and 'tightness'	'Tiredness' and 'heaviness'
Walking distance until onset of symptoms	Constant and often fixed ('claudication distance')	Variable
Factors improving symptoms	Rest Changes in posture do not improve symptoms	Adopting of flexed posture improves symptoms: ■ walking uphill ■ cycling ■ leaning forwards and pushing a trolley
Other features on examination	Other signs of peripheral vascular disease (e.g. absent or decreased peripheral pulses)	No signs of vascular disease (unless dual pathologies coexist)

Table 11.9 Vascular and neurogenic claudication: differentiating features

ensure the correct treatment is offered. A key difference is that neurogenic claudication is often relieved by bending forwards, which probably widens the spinal canal.

Diagnostic approach

Examination findings are often subtle: only mild sensory or motor deficits. A positive straight leg-raising test result and features of radiculopathy suggest a concurrent herniated intervertebral disc.

MRI confirms the diagnosis (**Figure 11.7**). Key differentials to exclude are:

- peripheral vascular disease (with vascular claudication)
- hip or knee joint disease (e.g. degenerative arthritis)
- other causes of back pain (e.g. tumour, infection and inflammatory arthritis)

Management

Often conservative measures are tried first. These include physiotherapy, analgesia and NSAIDs, antineuropathic agents (e.g. gabapentin), and steroid injections into the epidural space. The timing of surgery is controversial but it is usually offered if there are neurological symptoms in association with significant radiological evidence of compression.

Surgery

The aim of surgery is to prevent symptoms progressing and to preserve physical function in patients with progressive or unremitting neurogenic claudication. The method is surgical decompression, which is performed by removing parts of the posterior elements (e.g. spinous process, laminae, medial aspect of the facet joints) of the vertebrae in the affected area (lumbar laminectomy) and removing other structures that are causing narrowing, e.g. the ligamentum flavum. Development of delayed instability in the spine is one of the risks of performing decompression surgery.

In some patients, imaging suggests the spine will be at risk of instability if decompression is carried out, often when extensive amounts of the posterior elements of the vertebrae need to be removed. In these situations, decompression is accompanied by insertion of metal screws into the spine to prevent destabilisation.

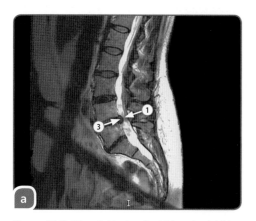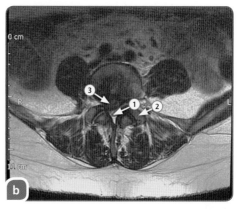

Figure 11.7 T2-weighted sagittal (a) and axial (b) magnetic resonance imaging sequences of the lumbar spine. Lumbar canal stenosis secondary to combined disc prolapse and facet joint hypertrophy has led to compression of the cauda equina and nerve roots and a decrease in the anteroposterior diameter of the spinal canal. ①, compressed thecal sac with effacement of cerebrospinal fluid and near complete effacement of cauda equina; ②, hypertrophic facet joint; ③, prolapsed disc.

Cauda equina syndrome

Cauda equina compression can lead to cauda equina syndrome, which is a medical emergency (see page 456).

Aetiology and pathophysiology

Cauda equina syndrome is rare. It is usually a consequence of a herniated lumbar intervertebral disc. Other causes include:

- spinal tumours
- fractured bone fragments after trauma
- haemorrhage (e.g. after spinal surgery)
- infective abscesses
- rarely, non-compressive causes such as viral infection and demyelination

Damage to the lower sacral nerves (S2–S4) leads to sensory, motor and autonomic dysfunction in their distribution.

Clinical features

Patients with cauda equina syndrome usually have anal and bladder sphincter disturbance (loss of function and tone), as well as altered sensation, especially anaesthesia, in the perianal or 'saddle' region (see **Figure 11.4**). Motor deficit results in distal leg weakness in a lower motor neurone pattern. Autonomic dysfunction results in bowel and bladder incontinence or retention.

If sciatica (pain radiating down the leg in a sciatic nerve distribution) is present, it is usually bilateral.

> **Bowel and bladder incontinence cause considerable morbidity, embarrassment and discomfort.** It necessitates a complete change in lifestyle. Patients often require permanent bladder catheterisation and have to wear nappies.

Management

Cauda equina syndrome is a medical emergency. Immediate spinal MRI is required to identify a compressive lesion (**Figures 11.7** and **11.8**; see page 456).

- If such a lesion is detected, surgical decompression is carried out, preferably within 24 h of symptom onset

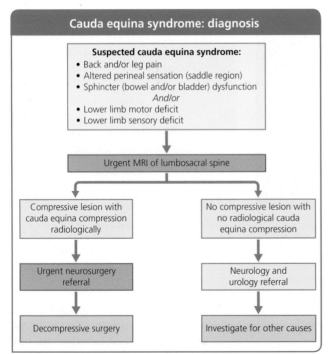

Figure 11.8 Diagnostic approach in suspected cauda equina syndrome.

Cauda equina syndrome: diagnosis

Suspected cauda equina syndrome:
- Back and/or leg pain
- Altered perineal sensation (saddle region)
- Sphincter (bowel and/or bladder) dysfunction
  And/or
- Lower limb motor deficit
- Lower limb sensory deficit

↓

Urgent MRI of lumbosacral spine

Compressive lesion with cauda equina compression radiologically → Urgent neurosurgery referral → Decompressive surgery

No compressive lesion with no radiological cauda equina compression → Neurology and urology referral → Investigate for other causes

- If no compressive lesion is found, the patient is referred to a neurologist and urologist

> **Acute onset dysfunction of bowel, bladder or both, accompanied by altered perineal 'saddle' sensation, is cauda equina syndrome until proven otherwise.** Urgent spinal MRI is essential.

Spondylolysis and spondylolisthesis

Spondylolysis and spondylolisthesis are spinal disorders affecting the bony components of the facet joints (**Figure 11.9**), which have a critical role in maintaining spinal stability.

Spondylolysis

Spondylolysis (Greek: spondulos, 'vertebra'; lysis, 'break') is a congenital defect in or absence of the pars interarticularis on one or both sides of a vertebra.

Clinical features

Spondylolysis may be asymptomatic or can cause back pain resulting from spinal microinstability. This can initiate a vicious circle of inactivity, weight gain, and loss of muscle strength and spinal alignment, further worsening the biomechanical stress on the spinal joints. Eventually, spondylolisthesis (slippage of one or more vertebrae) can occur. The vertebra above the level affected, i.e. the one with the pars interarticularis defect, is usually the one to slip forwards. Other complications include:

- lumbar spinal stenosis with neurogenic claudication (in the lumbar vertebrae)
- radiculopathy
- cauda equina syndrome (in the lumbar vertebrae)

Spondylolisthesis

Spondylolisthesis occurs when a vertebra slips forwards on the one below. The condition is graded according to the extent of slippage until complete slippage occurs, in which case it is termed spondyloptosis. The five main causes are described in **Table 11.10**.

Clinical features

Spondylolisthesis can compress spinal nerve roots, the cauda equina or the spinal cord (see **Table 11.3** and **Table 11.4**) giving rise to the stereotypical features. Associated spinal malalignment can cause back pain and postural changes.

Management

Treatment is initially non-operative. Physiotherapy strengthens the supporting core abdominal and back musculature. Patients can wear specially designed spinal orthotic braces to facilitate this. Analgesics and NSAIDs are prescribed.

Surgery can decompress compromised neurological structures, correct alignment and stabilise the spine with screws and rods (**Figure 11.10**).

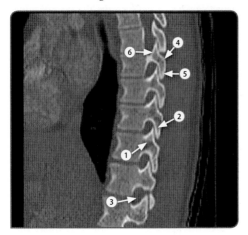

Figure 11.9 Sagittal computerised tomography scan of thoracic vertebrae, showing facet joints. The facet of the superior articular process of one vertebra ① articulates with the facet of the inferior articular process of the vertebra above ②. ③, the intervertebral neural foramen through which the spinal nerve roots exit; ④, pars interarticularis; ⑤, inferior articular process; ⑥, superior articular process.

Causes of spondylolisthesis	
Cause	Mechanism
Isthmic spondylolisthesis	Spondylolysis: the most common cause
Degenerative spondylolisthesis	Degenerative disease weakens the spinal joints in older adults
Pathological spondylolisthesis	Damage from malignancy, metabolic bone disease or infection (e.g. tuberculosis)
Traumatic spondylolisthesis	Secondary to acute fractures of the posterior spinal bone structures
Dysplastic spondylolisthesis	Congenital vertebral malformation of the lumbosacral junction, leading to facet joint incompetence

Table 11.10 Causes of spondylolisthesis

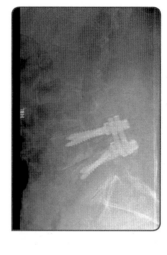

Figure 11.10 Lateral X-ray of the lumbar spine, showing screw-and-rod fixation to stabilise the spine by fusing the motion segment and preventing further spondylolisthesis at the L4–5 levels.

Syringomyelia

Syringomyelia (Greek: syrinx, 'pipe'; muelos, 'marrow') is development of a cystic fluid-filled cavity (syrinx) in the central spinal cord (**Figure 11.11**). It can occur anywhere in the spinal cord, and even in the lower brain stem (syringobulbia). However, most instances are in the middle to lower cervical segments (between C3 and C7).

Causes include craniovertebral junction malformation, arachnoid inflammation, trauma and tumours.

Pathogenesis

The exact mechanism is unknown, but the central factor is believed to be obstruction of cerebrospinal fluid flow across the craniovertebral junction between the skull and spine, for example as a consequence of a Chiari 1 malformation of the cerebellar tonsils.

The Chiari 1 malformation is congenital: the cerebellar tonsils are very low lying at the craniovertebral junction. It often associated with syrinx formation. They block the exit of cerebrospinal fluid from the 4th ventricle into the subarachnoid spaces surrounding the brain and spinal cord, thereby creating a pressure gradient across the craniovertebral junction that results in formation of a syrinx in the spinal cord.

Clinical features

Most small syrinxes cause no neurological deficit. Initially, there is disruption of the central part of the spinal cord (see **Figure 11.4**). Symptoms usually progress gradually, but acute exacerbations are possible. Features of cervical syrinxes include:

- lesion-level lower motor neurone features in the arms (e.g. flaccid weakness, wasting, decreased tone and reflexes), with features more pronounced distally in the arm
- loss of pain and temperature sensation in the arms; vibration and proprioception are usually preserved
- below the lesion, upper motor neurone features in the legs, including spasticity and increased tone and reflexes

Diagnostic approach

If syringomyelia is suspected, MRI of the brain and spine is done to identify the syrinx

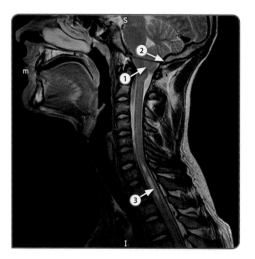

Figure 11.11 Sagittal T2-weighted magnetic resonance imaging scan showing a Chiari 1 malformation. The cerebellar tonsils ① are clearly lying > 5 mm below the foramen magnum: see red line extending anteriorly from the basion (anterior lip of foramen magnum) to opisthion (posterior lip of foramen magnum ②). No flow of cerebrospinal fluid is visible around the foramen magnum at the craniovertebral junction. The malformation has led to a fluid-filled cystic syrinx cavity in the cervical cord ③.

and confirm its level. An underlying cause, such as tumour, may also be seen. Knowledge of the cause is critical for determining management.

Management

Treatment of syringomyelia depends on the cause; for example, surgery is used to decompress the posterior fossa in cases of Chiari 1 malformation. Shunting fluid from the syrinx into the abdomen or lungs can relieve symptomatic idiopathic syringomyelia.

Spinal cord infarction

The spinal cord has several 'watershed' zones with poor blood supply (see page 72). One example is between the 4th and 9th thoracic vertebrae (see page 68), where ischaemia and infarction can develop rapidly if there is vascular disruption. Spinal cord ischaemia and infarction have several causes (**Table 11.12**) and are rare. They can result in paralysis, with the associated complications that may ensue from this including venous thrombosis (e.g. deep venous thrombosis affecting the legs and pulmonary venous thromboembolism), urinary tract infections, respiratory infections and pressure sores.

Clinical features

Onset of features is rapid. In almost 80% of spinal infarctions, sudden and severe back pain occurs in association with acute onset neurological symptoms.

Anterior infarction affects the anterior two thirds of the spinal cord, with preservation of the dorsal columns and features of anterior cord syndrome. Posterior spinal artery infarction impairs dorsal column function in the posterior third of the spinal cord only, with features of posterior cord syndrome.

Diagnostic approach

Spinal cord infarction usually presents with paraplegia or quadriplegia. Differential diagnoses such as Guillain-Barré syndrome and transverse myelitis usually have a slower evolution of clinical features.

Investigations

Urgent MRI of the spine is indicated to exclude spinal cord compression by mass lesions or transverse myelitis. Neurophysiological tests,

Spinal cord ischaemia and infarction

Cause	Examples
Spinal vascular disease	Thromboembolism in any spinal vessel
	Risk factors same as for stroke (see page 245)
Iatrogenic	Impaired vascular perfusion resulting from non-spinal surgery (e.g. cardiac operations and operations on abdominal aorta for aneurysm or dissection)
	Vascular damage during spinal surgery (e.g. thoracic spine surgery) or vascular angiography
Arterial dissection or aneurysm	Dissection of thoracic aorta can precipitate ischaemia and infarction by either direct vascular occlusion or embolic seeding into spinal vessels
	Abdominal aortic aneurysm rupture can precipitate ischaemia and infarction by global hypoperfusion caused by haemorrhage, embolic seeding into spinal vessels or direct vascular occlusion
Trauma	Direct disruption of spinal vasculature or haemorrhage-related compression

Table 11.12 Causes of spinal cord ischaemia and infarction

for example nerve conduction studies and electromyography, can differentiate spinal cord infarction from Guillain–Barré syndrome. Investigations to uncover the cause of ischaemia include:

- coagulation screen for thrombophilia
- echocardiography to exclude cardiac embolism
- angiography to exclude arterial dissection or aneurysm, or vascular malformations of the spinal cord
- blood tests for immunological blood markerws associated with vasculitides

Management

There is no specific treatment for spinal cord infarction. Secondary prophylaxis with antiplatelet agents such as aspirin and clopidogrel may be considered.

General management measures for any case of acute spinal cord injury and paralysis include:

- prevention of pressure ulceration
- prophylaxis against deep venous thromboses and pulmonary emboli
- bowel and bladder sphincter care (laxatives and urinary bladder catheterisation)

Answers to starter questions

1. 'Shooting pains' running down the arms and associated with neck pain are typical of radicular pain resulting from dysfunction of spinal nerve roots in the cervical spine. The pain is caused by any pathology that produces friction and pressure on the nerve root, which lead to demyelination, nerve root ischaemia and disrupted electrophysiological signal transmission.

2. The spinal cord is supplied primarily by three vertical arteries; it also has a secondary horizontal supply at each of the three segmental levels (cervical, thoracic and lumbar). Blood supply at each level varies according to the needs of the cord and nerves. The thoracic segment does not control limb function and therefore with few anterior horn motor neurones, requires a proportionally less metabolic and vascular supply compared to the cervical and lumbar segments. The blood vessels supplying the thoracic cord are the thinnest and this region has proportionally fewer vascular reinforcement and collateral blood supply. This property makes them most prone to ischaemic disease.

3. The thoracic spine helps regulate intrathoracic volume to enable ventilatory function. Therefore spinal curvature deformities can cause significant pulmonary complications by restricting the ability of the lungs to expand. This can significantly impair ventilatory capacity, thereby increasing the risk of pulmonary infections, pulmonary hypertension and heart failure.

Chapter 12
Systemic immune disease affecting the nervous system

Starter questions

Answers to the following questions are on page 374.

1. Why was the central nervous system considered 'immune privileged'?
2. What triggers or drives autoimmune diseases?
3. Why do some cancer patients develop paraneoplastic neurological syndromes?
4. Should every neurology patient be offered a trial of steroids?

Introduction

Immune-mediated diseases that affect the nervous system have a broad spectrum of clinicopathological features. These disorders cause often widespread and either acute or chronic destruction of neural tissue, and they are differential diagnoses in many neurological presentations.

Some immune-mediated diseases, for example myasthenia gravis and multiple sclerosis, affect nervous tissue only. Others principally affect different body systems but also have the potential for significant neurological involvement; these disorders include:

- autoimmune rheumatic diseases (also called connective tissue diseases)
- vasculitis
- paraneoplastic syndromes

Immune dysregulation is a common but poorly understood pathophysiological process precipitated by genetic predisposition, environmental insults and infection. It causes progressive disease as a consequence of inflammatory tissue damage. This leads to production of autoantibodies by B cells, or autoreactive T cells, against autoantigens (normal constituents of the body, such as DNA or phospholipids, that trigger a targeted immune response).

Management is usually limited to immunosuppressive therapies. However, these can cause liver, renal or bone toxicity.

Case 13 Generally feeling unwell with weakness

Presentation

Janet Munn, aged 76 years, is admitted by her general practitioner with suspected Guillain–Barré syndrome. She has had a recent upper respiratory tract infection and now has leg weakness.

Initial interpretation

Guillain–Barré syndrome causes acute or subacute onset weakness after an infection and is a medical emergency. Thorough history taking establishes:

- preceding 'infective' symptoms
- time course and distribution of weakness
- sensory symptoms
- presence or absence of systemic features
- medical history

Clinical examination will confirm the nature and distribution of weakness and the presence or absence of other signs. Guillain–Barré syndrome causes a bilateral, broadly symmetrical, predominantly motor polyneuropathy affecting the legs before the arms. Weakness causes flaccidity with loss of reflexes.

History

Mrs Munn has recently had 'bloody, dirty nasal discharge', which she attributed to a virus. She has been feverish and lethargic, with muscle aches. This morning, she was unable to flex her left ankle when trying to stand.

She has no other weakness, and no sensory symptoms in her legs. However, she has lost sensation over the 4th and 5th fingers of her right hand, extending up to her elbow.

Interpretation of history

The initial history is untypical of Guillain–Barré syndrome: the symptoms are asymmetrical (left foot and right arm) and started simultaneously in legs and arms. Onset in the legs with later spread to the arms is more usual in Guillain–Barré syndrome. The nasal discharge and systemic symptoms (e.g. fever and lethargy) suggest that a systemic illness is probably causing the peripheral neurological symptoms. Guillain–Barré syndrome is usually preceded by viral or diarrhoeal symptoms, but there is usually no fever or such marked systemic symptoms as in this case.

The combination of fever, lethargy and nasal discharge is more consistent with a systemic illness that has now caused neurological dysfunction. The pattern of sensory loss and ankle weakness appears to be the result of separate peripheral nerve lesions. A vasculitis is likely; it can cause systemic features and multiple mononeuropathies by occluding vascular supply to individual nerves.

Further history

Mrs Munn's only medical history is of stable autoimmune thyroiditis, for which she takes levothyroxine.

Examination

Mrs Munn has a low-grade fever (37.9°C). On neurological assessment, there is flaccid weakness of left ankle dorsiflexion, eversion and great toe extension. Foot inversion and plantar flexion are normal, as are all her reflexes. Sensory examination reveals a patch of complete sensory loss in the ulnar nerve distribution on the right arm. The results of systemic examination are normal.

Interpretation of findings

The pattern of motor weakness suggests a lesion in the left common peroneal nerve. The sensory loss indicates a lesion in the sensory branch of the right ulnar nerve, which supplies the medial forearm and hand.

The preservation of reflexes, marked asymmetry and associated systemic symptoms make Guillain–Barré syndrome unlikely. The working clinical diagnosis is of vasculitis causing the syndrome of multiple mononeuropathies. Vasculitis is suggested by the systemic symptoms and history of autoimmune disease.

Investigations

Initial blood tests show mild eosinophilia, normocytic normochromic anaemia, increased C-reactive protein concentration (244 mg/L normal range, <3 mg/L), increased erythrocyte sedimentation rate (119 mm/h, 1–7 mm/h) and mild new renal impairment. In addition, the result of the antineutrophil cytoplasmic antibody (ANCA) test is positive. Nerve conduction studies confirm multiple mononeuropathies.

Diagnosis

Neurophysiological tests confirm that several specific nerves are affected, and that Mrs Munn's condition is not a widespread polyneuropathy. She has 'mononeuritis multiplex'; this is a type of neuropathy usually caused by occlusion of blood vessels supplying the affected nerves, as a result of vasculitis.

The high C-reactive protein concentration and erythrocyte sedimentation rate provide evidence of systemic inflammation, and increased eosinophil count is common in vasculitis. In systemic vasculitis, renal function is usually impaired because small renal vessels and glomeruli are often affected by inflammation. ANCA positivity is highly suggestive of a vasculitic process being an autoantibody against a common autoantigen involved in vasculitis.

Mrs Munn is treated first with high-dose corticosteroids (usually 1 g intravenous methyl-prednisolone) and then cyclophosphamide (an immunosuppressive agent). Her symptoms stabilise, her renal function eventually normalises and she slowly regains all her motor function.

Systemic lupus erythematosus

Systemic lupus erythematosus (SLE) is a multisystemic autoimmune rheumatic disease with many presentations (see **Table 12.1**). The autoantigen is usually DNA or the histone proteins that package DNA.

Epidemiology

The disease is more common in women than in men. African-Caribbeans, South Asians and people aged 20–40 years are also more commonly affected.

The prevalence of SLE is 40 per 100,000 in the UK.

Aetiology

The cause of SLE is not known. Precipitating factors are thought to include Epstein–Barr virus infection, ultraviolet light, certain drugs (e.g. the anti-hypertensive hydralazine and the anti-tubercular isoniazid) and genetic factors such as complement protein gene deficiencies.

Pathologically, there is a vasculopathy with endothelial proliferation and oedema but without florid vascular inflammation. About half of patients have large vessel cerebral infarction or microinfarction. Haemorrhage occurs in up to 40% of these patients, making antiplatelet and anticoagulant therapy for infarctions difficult to initiate. Benefits of starting blood thinning medications must be balanced against the risk of precipitating and/or worsening acute haemorrhage, and these risks should be discussed with the patient before starting medication.

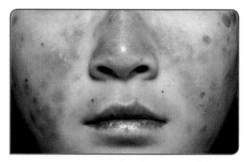

Figure 12.1 A typical butterfly, or malar, rash seen in systemic lupus erythematosis (SLE).

Clinical features

SLE is characterised by fever, skin rashes (**Figure 12.1**), arthritis, pleurisy and kidney dysfunction. The systemic features of SLE are described in **Table 12.1**. Neuropsychiatric manifestations occur in 75% of patients:

- mood disturbance
- cognitive slowing
- headaches

Systems affected by systemic lupus erythematosus		
System affected	Patients affected (%)	Diagnostic criteria
Dermatological	80	Erythematous malar (butterfly) rash, i.e. over cheeks and bridge of nose
		Discoid rash leading to scaling and eventually scarring (affects ears, cheeks, scalp, forehead and chest)
		Photosensitive rashes on sun-exposed skin (e.g. forehead and upper chest)
		Ulceration, either oral or nasopharyngeal and usually painless
Musculoskeletal	90	Non-erosive arthritis in two or more peripheral joints, which is associated with tenderness, swelling and effusion
Cardiopulmonary (inflammation of cardiac and pulmonary serosal surfaces)	65	Pleuritis presenting with chest pain; pleural effusions may be present
		Pericarditis presenting with chest pain; pericardial effusions may be present
Renal	40	Glomerulonephritis: nephritic syndrome,† nephrotic syndrome‡ or rapidly progressive renal failure can develop
Neurological	60	Seizures or psychiatric complications if other reversible causes (e.g. metabolic factors) have been excluded
Haematological	85	Bone marrow suppression in absence of other causes (e.g. drug use): anaemia, leucopenia and thrombocytopenia
Immunological	98	Diagnostic autoantibody positivity: ANA (positive test in > 90%), anti-dsDNA, anti-Sm and antiphospholipid

ANA, antinuclear autoantibody; anti-dsDNA, anti-double-stranded DNA autoantibody; anti-Sm, anti-Smith autoantibody (an autoantibody against extractable nuclear antigens and associated with autoimmune rheumatic diseases).

†Blood and protein in urine.

‡Persistent proteinuria and oedema.

Table 12.1 Systems affected by systemic lupus erythematosus (SLE). SLE is diagnosed if 4 of the 11 criteria are present

Other neurological manifestations are rare but include:

- seizures
- ischaemic or haemorrhagic stroke
- demyelination induced neural injury (e.g. weakness and/or sensory dysfunction due to demyelinating neuropathy)

Diagnostic approach

Systemic lupus erythematosus is considered as part of the differential diagnosis in many neurological presentations. The clinical history and examination findings (**Table 12.1**) are usually suggestive of the diagnosis. A battery of tests are then conducted to confirm or refute the diagnosis as well as simultaneously evaluate the effect of the disease process on the rest of the organ systems.

In clinical practice, a variety of blood tests ranging from routine [e.g. full blood count, urea and electrolytes (renal function)] to special immunological tests are all sent for evaluation simultaneously (**Table 12.2**). Broadly speaking the investigative tests fall into three major categories:

1. Immunological tests assaying for the presence of specific autoantibodies and serum markers to confirm the diagnosis (anti-dsDNA)
2. Detecting the degree of disease activity (e.g. C-reactive protein, ESR, complement levels)

Test results in systemic lupus erythematosus		
Type	Examples	Description
Markers of disease activity	Anti-dsDNA titre	Higher titres correlate with higher disease activity
	Complement levels	Disease activity correlates with consumption of complement ■ C3 and C4 (complement subtypes) are low ■ C3d and C4d (complement breakdown products) are high
	Inflammatory markers	Erythrocyte sedimentation rate is high* C-reactive protein is normal†
Immunological tests for associated autoantibodies	ANA titre	> 90% have a positive result
	Anti-dsDNA titre	> 60% have a positive result, and this is highly specific
	Antibodies against extractable nuclear antigens [e.g. anti-Ro (SSA), anti-La (SSB) and anti-Sm]	20–30% have a positive result
	Antihistone titre	Usually positive result in drug-induced systemic lupus erythematosus
Other tests to ascertain key organ involvement and for complications	Biochemistry and haematology	Full blood count, urea and electrolytes and renal function assessment, and liver function tests
	Computerised tomography or magnetic resonance imaging	May show multiple haemorrhages or ischaemic infarctions caused by small vessel disease
	Electroencephalography	Diffuse abnormalities
	Cerebrospinal fluid sampling	May show increased protein
	Renal biopsy and skin biopsy	Histological diagnosis from other involved systems

ANA, antinuclear autoantibody; anti-dsDNA, anti-double-stranded DNA autoantibody; anti-La (SSB); anti-Ro (SSB); anti-Sm, anti-Smith autoantibody.

*Erythrocyte sedimentation rate is a non-specific marker for chronic inflammation.

†C-reactive protein is an acute phase protein; an increase in C-reactive protein concentration usually indicates an inflammatory process.

Table 12.2 Test results in suspected systemic lupus erythematosus

3. Routine haematological and biochemical tests to ascertain the degree of reversible or irreversible organ destruction

> **The spectrum of autoimmune rheumatic diseases is wide, and clinical features and serum autoantibodies overlap.** For example, anti-Ro (SSA) is detected in 40–60% of cases of systemic lupus erythematosus and 60–90% of primary Sjögren's syndrome. Positive autoantibody test results are helpful but not essential in diagnosis.

Management

The aims of immunosuppression are to preserve renal function and to minimise central nervous system manifestations. Disease activity markers are measured to identify flare-ups and relapses and to monitor clinical remission.

Medication

Most patients with minor joint symptoms respond to non-steroidal anti-inflammatory drugs. Neurological exacerbations and systemic autoimmune disease require high-dose corticosteroids and immunosuppression (e.g. cyclophosphamide, azathioprine and mycophenolate mofetil). If immunosuppression is ineffective, monoclonal antibodies (e.g. rituximab), which deplete the B cells producing the pathogenic autoantibodies, can be tried.

Close monitoring is essential, because immunosuppressive drugs can cause:

- increased susceptibility to infection
- bone marrow suppression (anaemia, thrombocytopenia and leucopenia)
- increased risk of malignancies (B cell lymphoma)

Prognosis

Neurological disease in systemic lupus erythematosus is a source of significant morbidity. However, mortality is usually a consequence of renal disease or occlusive vascular disease (coronary artery or cerebrovascular disease).

Sjögren's syndrome

Sjögren's syndrome is an inflammatory autoimmune disorder affecting up to 3% of the population in the UK. It can present in isolation as primary Sjögren's syndrome but is more often associated with systemic lupus erythematosus or other autoimmune rheumatic diseases (i.e. as secondary Sjögren's syndrome). Symptoms are mostly mild, but about 5% of patients develop non-Hodgkin's lymphoma from altered lymphocyte turnover.

Pathogenesis involves B cell–mediated destruction, infiltration and fibrosis of exocrine glands, especially the salivary and lacrimal glands, and other organs. The central nervous system is involved in up to 15% of cases.

> **Benign does not mean that everything is fine for the patient.** Disease can continue to disrupt, disturb and dominate the patient's life.

Clinical features

Systemic and neurological clinical features are listed in **Table 12.3.**

Diagnostic approach and management

The aims of investigations in suspected cases of Sjögren's syndrome are to establish the diagnosis and to identify associated autoimmune conditions. Invasive tests are shown in **Table 12.4.** The classic non-invasive test is Schirmer's test for lacrimal hyposecretion. In this test, a strip of paper is placed under the lower eyelid and the distance that consequent tears travel is estimated:

- 15 mm in 5 min is normal
- < 5 mm in 5 min is hyposecretion

The initial tests performed are blood tests (invasive) and the non-invasive lacrimal

Clinical features of Sjögren's syndrome	
Type	Feature (% of patients, if known)
Systemic (present in 85% of patients)	Dry eyes (keratoconjunctivitis sicca), (c. 100%)
	Dry mouth (xerostomia) (c. 100%)
	Polyarthritis or arthralgia (60%)
	Lung involvement (15%)
	Kidney involvement (10%)
	Non-Hodgkin's B-cell lymphoma (5%)
Neurological (present in 15% of patients)	Peripheral neuropathy
	Myelopathy
	Polymyositis
	Meningoencephalitis

Table 12.3 Clinical features of Sjögren's syndrome

hyposecretion test. The combination of these along with clinical features on examination are sufficient to confirm the diagnosis. Invasive histological assessment with salivary gland biopsy is rarely performed.

Other associated autoimmune conditions that are tested for are: autoimmune rheumatic diseases (rheumatoid arthritis, systemic

Key investigations for Sjögren's syndrome	
Type	Findings
Salivary gland biopsy	Focal lymphocytic aggregates on histology
Autoantibodies	Anti-Ro (SSA)
	Anti-La (SSB)
	Antinuclear antibody

Table 12.4 Key investigations for suspected Sjögren's syndrome

lupus erythematosus, systemic sclerosis, vasculitis and polyarteritis nodosa), autoimmune hepatitis, primary biliary cirrhosis and autoimmune thyroid disease.

If neurological manifestations are present, appropriate investigations (e.g. computerised tomography or magnetic resonance imaging, and neurophysiological tests) should exclude other common causes before the manifestations are attributed to Sjögren's syndrome and the diagnosis confirmed.

Treatment of the neurological manifestations of Sjögren's syndrome is the same as that for systemic lupus erythematosus (see page 366).

Vasculitis and polyarteritis nodosa

Vasculitic syndromes (of which polyarteritis nodosa is one example) are rare multisystemic conditions associated with immune complex deposition, immune-mediated inflammation and blood vessel necrosis. Vessel wall inflammation can cause:

■ haemorrhage, as a result of vascular aneurysm formation, weakening and rupture
■ ischaemic infarction, as a result of acute thrombosis, embolisation, stenosis and occlusion

Any organ can be affected, so these conditions have a wide range of clinical features.

Vasculitic syndromes are classified by size of vessel affected and association with other systemic disease (**Tables 12.5** and **12.6**).

Antineutrophil cytoplasmic antibodies (autoantibodies are commonly found in systemic vasculitis. ANCA-positive vasculitis is associated with glomerulonephritis, which can lead rapidly to renal failure.

Epidemiology

Vasculitis is rare, with an annual incidence of 10 per 100,000 in the UK. However, vasculitis is a differential diagnosis for neurological symptoms in patients with known autoimmune rheumatic diseases, multisystemic involvement and typical patterns of neurological dysfunction.

Classification of vasculitic syndromes by vessel size

Vessel size	Vasculitic syndrome
Large	Giant cell (temporal) arteritis
	Takayasu's arteritis
Medium	Polyarteritis nodosa
	Kawasaki's disease
Small	ANCA-positive
	Microscopic polyangiitis
	Granulomatosis with polyangiitis
	Eosinophilic granulomatosis with polyangiitis (previously known as Churg–Strauss syndrome)
	ANCA-negative
	Henoch–Schönlein purpura
	Goodpasture's syndrome
	Cryoglobulinaemia

ANCA, antineutrophil cytoplasmic antibody.

Table 12.5 Classification of vasculitic syndromes by size of affected vessels

Classification of vasculitic syndromes by association with systemic disease

Associated systemic disorder	Vasculitic syndrome
Autoimmune rheumatic disease and connective tissue disorders	Rheumatoid arthritis
	Systemic lupus erythematosus
	Sjögren's syndrome
Infections	Bacterial: Lyme disease, tuberculosis and syphilis
	Viral: HIV, cytomegalovirus, hepatitis B virus, hepatitis C virus and varicella zoster virus
Hypersensitivity vasculitis	Drug induced
	Malignancy associated
Systemic necrotising vasculitis	Polyarteritis nodosa
	ANCA-positive vasculitides

ANCA, antineutrophil cytoplasmic antibody.

Table 12.6 Classification of vasculitic syndromes by aetiological association with systemic diseases

Clinical features

Symptoms and signs vary considerably, depending on the specific cause of the vasculitis. Common systemic features are:

- fever
- malaise
- joint and muscle aches
- weight loss

Features suggesting vasculitis, include:

- palpable purpura
- pulmonary infiltrates and microscopic haematuria
- chronic inflammatory sinusitis
- mononeuritis multiplex
- glomerulonephritis

Neurological involvement is common, present in 80% of cases. Any part of the nervous system can be affected.

> **Acute vasculitis is a medical emergency, because irreversible organ damage can develop rapidly,** e.g. critical renal failure can occur within 24 h. Vasculitic specialists, often nephrologists or rheumatologists, should be consulted

Diagnostic approach

Vasculitic patients require screening and treatment for associated diseases, including HIV and hepatitis C virus. Specific blood tests include:

- vasculitis and autoimmune rheumatic disease-associated autoantibody screens (ANCA, antinuclear antibody and anti–double-stranded DNA autoantibody)
- disease activity markers (C-reactive protein and erythrocyte sedimentation rate, and complement levels C3 and C4)
- markers used to evaluate critical organ complications (e.g. renal function)

Other investigations are:

- CT and MRI for vasculitic complications (infarction and haemorrhage)
- angiography for vessel irregularities and

microaneurysm formation (polyarteritis nodosa classically causes renal vasculature microaneurysms)

- biopsy (nerve, muscle and renal) for histological confirmation

Management

Generally, the degree of immunosuppression increases with the severity of symptoms and organ dysfunction. Significant neurological complications include haemorrhage and infarction of the brain or spinal cord.

Medication

Intravenous corticosteroids and cyclophosphamide are frequently used, with plasma exchange in severe cases.

> **Autoantibodies are not all pathological.** Some probably have housekeeping functions, such as removing waste proteins and surveying for cancer cells. They become pathological in large numbers, when a dysregulated immune response amplifies the attack against self-antigens.

Paraneoplastic syndromes

Paraneoplastic syndromes are clinical manifestations associated with malignancy but not explained by the direct effects of an active tumour or metastases. Neurological paraneoplastic syndromes develop in 0.1% of cancer patients and represent central or peripheral nervous system dysfunction. The dysfunction is precipitated by immune responses against a tumour; the tumour antigens cross-react with neuronal antigens. This 'molecular mimicry' disrupts and results in immune-mediated destruction of nervous tissue, and the clinical features of paraneoplastic syndromes are a consequence of this.

Aetiology

Common malignancies associated with neurological paraneoplastic syndromes include small-cell lung carcinoma, gonadal malignancies (of testis, ovary and breast) and Hodgkin's lymphoma. These tumours are usually derived from cells with neuroendocrine features and expressing neuronal antigens, which could account for the antitumour response cross-reacting with nervous tissue.

Paraneoplastic syndromes are usually a T cell-driven inflammation against specific tissues. Half of patients have non-pathogenic paraneoplastic or antineuronal antibodies; the presence of these antibodies helps confirm the diagnosis, but they do not cause any symptoms themselves.

Clinical features

Paraneoplastic syndromes have many clinically distinct syndromes, but their features usually overlap (**Table 12.7**). The clinical picture is usually one of a subacute slowly progressive syndrome. However, rarely the condition has a rapidly progressive or even relapsing–remitting course.

Paraneoplastic syndromes are classic or non-classic. Patients with classic syndromes more frequently have underlying tumours than those with non-classic syndromes.

> **Paraneoplastic syndromes are often the initial presentation of a malignancy.** Cases of these syndromes must be investigated exhaustively to find the precipitating malignancy. Successful treatment of the underlying malignancy is often the only hope for improvement.

Diagnostic approach

The syndromes are initially diagnosed by their stereotypical features which are suspected based on the clinical presentation and examination findings. A detailed exposition

Paraneoplastic syndromes affecting the nervous system

Classic (stronger association with a known or occult tumour)	Non-classic (weaker association with a known or occult tumour)
Limbic encephalitis: memory disturbance, confusion and psychiatric disturbances, and complex partial temporal lobe seizures	Brain stem encephalitis
	Paraneoplastic retinopathy
	Stiff person syndrome
Subacute cerebellar degeneration: rapidly developing ataxia and cerebellar syndrome, nystagmus and vertigo because of brain stem involvement	Necrotising myopathy
	Paraneoplastic myelopathy
Opsoclonus–myoclonus: 'dancing eyes and dancing feet' (involuntary chaotic and repetitive eye movements)	Autoimmune autonomic ganglionopathy
	Myasthenia gravis
Lambert–Eaton myasthenic syndrome	Neuromyotonia
Dermatomyositis: associated with arthropathy, typical rashes on hands (Gottron's papules)	
Chronic gastrointestinal pseudo-obstruction	
Subacute sensory neuropathy	
Encephalomyelitis	

Table 12.7 Paraneoplastic syndromes affecting the nervous system

of the clinical features of each other paraneoplastic syndromes is beyond the scope of this book and the remit of neuro-immunological and neuro-oncological specialists given their rarity and complexity. The presence of anti-neuronal antibodies strengthens suspicion of malignancy. Brain imaging usually confirms the presence of nervous system lesions (**Figure 12.2**), and cerebrospinal fluid analysis may confirm an inflammatory response through the detection of oligoclonal bands and increased protein levels (**Figure 12.3**).

Patients require either testicular ultrasound or breast imaging followed by computerised tomography of the chest, abdomen and pelvis. If no tumour is identified, positron emission tomography is necessary. Imaging is repeated at 6-monthly intervals, often for several years, to fully exclude tumour.

Management

Curative surgical treatment of the primary malignancy is considered, if possible. Earlier tumour removal stabilises or halts paraneoplastic syndrome progression in many cases.

Immunosuppression (often of little benefit) includes corticosteroids, ciclosporin, intravenous immunoglobulin and plasma exchange.

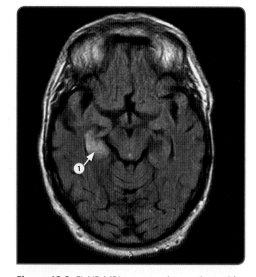

Figure 12.2. FLAIR MRI sequence in a patient with paraneoplastic limbic encephalitis. The patient had an acute onset of partial seizures, confusion, and memory loss ①. The MRI shows high signal in the right temporal lobe. The patient had a small-cell lung tumour.

Intriguingly, there is some evidence that patients with a neurological paraneoplastic syndrome have a better prognosis than others. The aggressive (auto-) immune response of the syndrome may correspond with a more successful antitumour immune response.

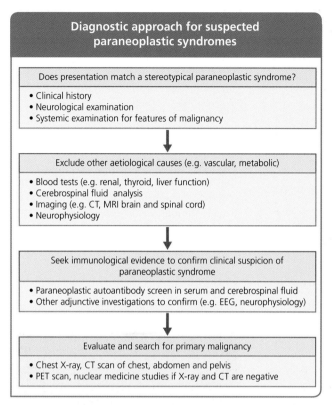

Figure 12.3 Diagnostic approach and investigations for suspected paraneoplastic syndromes.

Neurosarcoidosis

Sarcoidosis is a multisystemic disorder associated with formation of non-caseating granulomatous lesions (in contrast to caseating granulomas in tuberculosis). The lesions of sarcoidosis consist of focal accumulations of epithelioid cells, macrophages and T cells. Only 10% of patients develop clinically significant neurological involvement, but it may be the only manifestation of the disease in this group.

Epidemiology

Sarcoidosis is commonest in northern European countries including the UK, with a prevalence of 40 per 100,000. Women are more likely than men to be affected. The condition typically affects people aged less than 50 years.

Aetiology

The cause of sarcoidosis is unknown. However, an exaggerated T-cell response to self-antigens is understood to drive autoimmunity in the condition. Possible risk factors include infection with atypical mycobacterial species, fungi and Epstein–Barr virus, as well as varying occupational, genetic, social and other environmental factors.

> **An 'idiopathic' disease may have discernible factors that influence its course in an individual patient.** The immune system is influenced by many factors, including hormones, the nervous system and mental state. Learning which factors are involved takes time but can help patients better manage their condition.

Clinical features

Common systemic features are:

- bilateral hilar lymphadenopathy (> 90% patients)
- hypercalcaemia
- increased serum immunoglobulin G
- fatigue
- weight loss
- fever
- lymphadenopathy

Cranial neuropathies are common. Particularly affected are cranial nerves II, VII (often causing bilateral palsies) and VIII, because the meninges around the skull base is vulnerable. Myelopathy, basilar meningitis, diabetes insipidus, pituitary failure, peripheral neuropathy, focal mass lesions and many other manifestations are possible.

Red/purple cutaneous lesions (**Figure 12.4**) and uveitis (**Figure 12.5**) are also common in patients with sarcoidosis.

Diagnostic approach

Definitive diagnosis follows histological analysis (biopsy of affected tissue). A working diagnosis is based on suggestive history, clinical and radiological evidence of multisystemic disease and laboratory findings.

Investigations for suspected sarcoidosis are listed in **Table 12.8**. They are done to seek recognised biochemical and radiological features of sarcoidosis, and to identify tissue suitable for biopsy (e.g. lymph nodes). Magnetic resonance imaging may show meningeal

inflammation or diffuse, patchy white matter lesions (**Figure 12.6**).

Management

Sarcoidosis is treated by immunosuppression to minimise parenchymal lung disease, renal involvement and neurological involvement.

Medication

Intravenous methylprednisolone is used during exacerbations. Oral prednisolone, methotrexate, azathioprine or cyclophosphamide is used in the long term. Monoclonal antibodies such as anti-tumour necrosis factor (tumour necrosis factor is an immune mediator) may be required in highly refractory cases.

Surgery

Intracranial or intraspinal lesions causing

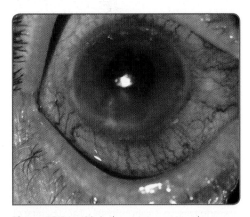

Figure 12.5 Uveitis is the commonest ocular finding in sarcoidosis.

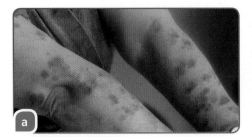 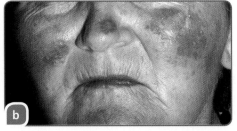

Figure 12.4 Skin changes are seen in approximately one third of patients with systemic sarcoidosis, due to a complex process of immune-mediated inflammation and destruction. (a) Sarcoid skin plaques on the forearm. (b) Lupus pernio appears as shiny, swollen red or purple lesions on the cheeks, lips, nose or ears, and is specific to sarcoidosis.

Investigations for sarcoidosis		
Non-neurological	Neurological	Invasive

Biochemical:
 	
  Calcium increased
 	
Immunological:
 	
  Angiotensin-converting enzyme increased in 60% (non-specific)
 	
  Immunoglobulins increased
	Cerebrospinal fluid:
	
	  Angiotensin-converting enzyme increased
	
	  Cell count increased
	
	  Oligoclonal bands (non-specific)
		Biopsy of tissue from involved organs (lung, liver, lymph nodes and lacrimal glands)
		
		Histological investigation shows non-caseating granulomas

Imaging:
 	
  Chest X-ray abnormal in 90% (e.g. bilateral hilar lymphadenopathy)
 	
  High-resolution CT of lungs (to assess severity of pulmonary disease)
	Imaging:
	
	  CT and MRI for intracranial or intraspinal lesions
		Bronchoalveolar lavage: fluid collected from bronchial aspirates shows increased white blood cells in active disease

Table 12.8 Investigative techniques to confirm diagnosis of sarcoidosis

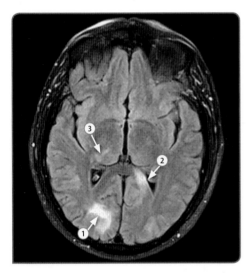

Figure 12.6. FLAIR MRI sequence in a patient with neurosarcoidosis. There are white matter lesions in the right occipital white matter (1), left corpus callosum (2) and right thalamus (3).

mass effect may require surgical intervention. The surgery often includes the removal of tissue for biopsy to confirm diagnosis.

Prognosis

Neurological disease can be disfiguring, for example by causing facial palsies. It can also be disabling, for example through neuropathy. Common causes of death are respiratory failure and cor pulmonale (right-sided heart failure) resulting from severe lung disease.

Spontaneous remission occurs in half of patients. In about a third, sarcoidosis has a steadily progressive course and immunosuppression is required.

Answers to starter questions

1. The central nervous system used to be considered 'immune privileged' because there is less inflammation and immune response in the brain and spinal cord. However, it is actually highly immunologically active, with different key cellular immune system components and more persistent antibody responses than the rest of the body. The innate immune system is very active in the brain and has a role in neurodevelopment. Some neurodegenerative conditions, such as Parkinson's and Alzheimer's diseases, also have inflammatory components.

2. The triggers for autoimmune diseases remain unknown. However, it is likely that people who develop autoimmune diseases have an immune system genetically predisposed to autoimmunity, which is then triggered by an infection or other environmental agent.

3. Patients with paraneoplastic neurological syndromes have a better overall prognosis for their cancer than similar patients without these syndromes. The syndromes probably prime the immune system to produce a stronger 'anti-self' response, which results in more aggressive and successful tumour clearance. However, this immune response also increases vulnerability to pathological autoimmunity, which damages nervous tissue.

4. Most neurologists would agree that many patients should be offered a trial of steroids in case their condition has an inflammatory cause. Because inflammatory neurological conditions have a wide range of clinical presentations a useful question to ask is, 'is there any evidence for an inflammatory cause for this patient's symptoms?'

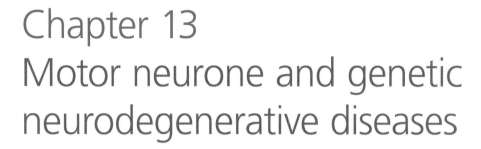

Chapter 13
Motor neurone and genetic neurodegenerative diseases

Starter questions

Answers to the following questions are on page 386.

1. Why do neurones degenerate?
2. Is a cure for neurodegeneration theoretically possible?
3. Should people be offered genetic tests for incurable diseases?

Introduction

Neurones generally cannot divide and regenerate. Therefore cumulative damage to their genes and proteins more easily leads to disordered cellular metabolism, with:

- gradual accumulation of toxic intracellular proteins
- abnormal or excessive activation of intracellular cascades, resulting in oxidative stress
- ultimately, cell death and neuronal loss (degeneration)

Such acquired damage is the cause of 'normal' ageing. However, it is also more likely to precipitate neurodegeneration in cells with a genetic predisposition, such as those with mutations causing abnormal protein production, function or degradation. The syndromes associated with such mutations can be clinically asymptomatic, cause a generalised neuronal degeneration and dementia (see Chapter 14) or lead to degeneration of specific cells or areas of the nervous system, as discussed in this chapter. These localised neurodegenerative conditions, the most common of which is motor neurone disease, present with slowly progressive weakness or mobility problems.

Neurodegenerative disease is incurable. However, a multidisciplinary team of specialist nurses, physiotherapists, neurologists, occupational therapists and social workers has much to offer patients in terms of support and improving quality of life.

Case 14 Tendency to fall over

Presentation

David Gilroy, a 53-year-old accountant, is referred to the neurology clinic with a history of an increasing number of falls and difficulty walking over the past year.

Initial interpretation

Problems with walking and balance that increase over a year suggest a progressive disorder; this makes diagnoses such as transient ischaemic attack, strokes and seizures unlikely. Neurological causes of such symptoms include lesions in muscle, nerve, spine, the basal ganglia, the vestibular system or the cortex. Non-neurological causes for falls include cardiac conditions such as orthostatic hypotension and cardiac dysrhythmias.

History

Until a year ago, David was an active squash player with no medical problems. He then noticed that he was unable to move around the court as quickly as he used to. About 4 months later, he began to trip over his right leg when walking, particularly by catching it on the edge of stairs. Over the past 2 months, he has started falling while walking.

Interpretation of history

There has been a gradual progression of motor symptoms over the preceding year, without any sensory symptoms. Tripping over stairs suggests a foot drop (see page 426). Such a slow deterioration is unusual for cerebrovascular disease.

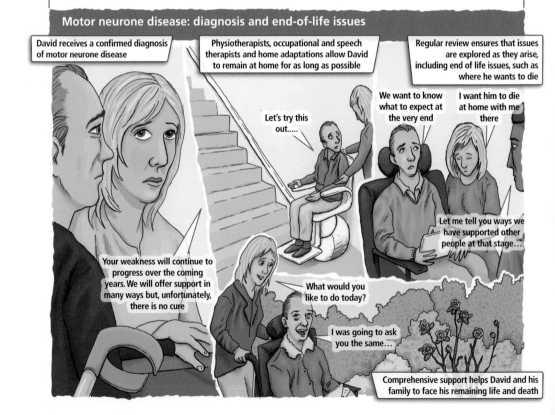

Motor neurone disease: diagnosis and end-of-life issues

David receives a confirmed diagnosis of motor neurone disease

Physiotherapists, occupational and speech therapists and home adaptations allow David to remain at home for as long as possible

Regular review ensures that issues are explored as they arise, including end of life issues, such as where he wants to die

We want to know what to expect at the very end

I want him to die at home with me there

Let's try this out.....

Your weakness will continue to progress over the coming years. We will offer support in many ways but, unfortunately, there is no cure

Let me tell you ways we have supported other people at that stage…

What would you like to do today?

I was going to ask you the same…

Comprehensive support helps David and his family to face his remaining life and death

Case 14 *continued*

Demyelinating disorders such as multiple sclerosis and peripheral nerve disease tend to present with both motor and sensory symptoms.

Parkinsonian disorders can present with deteriorating gait and falls, but the large majority of patients also have stiffness and tremor (see page 313). Motor neurone disease very often presents with slowly progressive motor weakness without other symptoms, as is the case here.

Further history

On further questioning, David gives no history of any sensory disturbance, stiffness, bladder or bowel dysfunction, tremor or other neurological symptoms.

Examination

Fasciculations and wasting in tibialis anterior on the left leg are found on inspection. Tone is increased in both legs. David has 4/5 power in all muscles tested on the left and on hip flexion on the right. Other muscles have normal power. Ankle and knee reflexes are very brisk on both sides, and the plantars are both up-going. In the arms, power is normal but reflexes are brisk. Coordination and sensation are normal throughout. Jaw jerk is brisk, but the remainder of cranial nerve examination is normal. There are no extrapyramidal signs.

Interpretation of findings

The absence of other neurological symptoms supports localisation of the disorder to the motor system alone.

In the legs, the increased tone, up-going plantar reflexes, brisk reflexes and weakness are signs of an upper motor neurone lesion, whereas the wasting and fasciculations are lower motor neurone lesion signs (see page 136). There are upper motor neurone signs of brisk reflexes in the arms and brain stem (i.e. the brisk jaw jerk). These findings,

in the context of the history of a progressive motor syndrome, strongly suggest motor neurone disease. This possible diagnosis now needs support from the results of neurophysiological tests.

Compressive lesions in the neck (e.g. cervical myelopathy) cause upper motor neurone signs in the arms and legs but would not cause the brisk jaw jerk, nor the lower motor neurone signs in the legs (see page 379).

An HIV test is done, because there is a rare motor neurone disease-like syndrome associated with HIV infection that can improve with antiviral treatment.

Investigations

The results of nerve conduction studies and electromyography show normal sensory nerve conduction but widespread active denervation in all muscles tested. The result of the HIV test is negative.

Diagnosis

At the initial clinic visit, the diagnosis of motor neurone disease seemed highly probable from the history and examination. David was counselled then on the diagnosis of motor neurone disease.

A diagnosis of motor neurone disease is best given when the patient has family or friends present to provide support, and the health care team has time to discuss all the implications. This is possible in a dedicated clinic with longer consultation times. Alternatively, the patient could be asked to attend as an in-patient for key investigations and discussions to take place during a brief stay on the ward.

The results of neurophysiological tests show normal sensory function, but there is degeneration of motor neurones throughout David's body. Therefore a diagnosis

Case 14 *continued*

of limb-onset motor neurone disease is strengthened.

Despite the difficulty David has in learning that he has a fatal illness, he feels that 'knowing is better than not knowing', and that he can now begin to face the next phase of his life. Regular reviews are scheduled to monitor progression, review symptoms, and provide specialist motor neurone disease nursing, physiotherapy, occupational therapy, and speech and language therapy. David is started on riluzole, a medication which extends life in cases of motor neurone disease, a few weeks later.

Motor neurone disease

Motor neurone disease is a group of disorders affecting upper or lower motor neurones and sparing other systems, such as sensory neurones. It is a clinical diagnosis based on motor symptoms and signs, with motor nerve and tract lesions confirmed by the results of neurophysiological tests and magnetic resonance imaging (MRI).

The usual clinical presentation is that of amyotrophic lateral sclerosis, a pathological diagnosis of muscle wasting (Greek, amyotrophia, 'no muscle nourishment'), lower motor neurone degeneration and corticospinal tract degeneration (lateral sclerosis is hardening in the areas of the spinal cord where the affected neurones are located). Other forms of motor neurone disease include:

- primary lateral sclerosis, in which only corticospinal tract degeneration is present
- progressive muscular atrophy, which comprises isolated lower motor neurone degeneration

In this chapter, as is usual in the UK, the term motor neurone disease is used to refer to all these conditions. However, in the USA the term amyotrophic lateral sclerosis usually refers to all of them.

Motor neurone disease is usually an acquired condition. However, rare inherited forms exist, and research on these forms of the disorder has provided information on genetic factors and pathophysiological mechanisms.

Epidemiology

Motor neurone disease has an annual incidence rate of 1–2 per 100,000 people. Risk factors include age > 50 years, male sex and a family history of motor neurone disease. The reasons why motor neurone disease is slightly more common in men are unknown.

Pathogenesis

The mechanism through which motor neurone disease arises is uncertain. However, research has identified the following central pathophysiological processes.

- Abnormal ubiquination produces abnormal collections of waste proteins (ubiquitinated inclusions); the reasons why the ubiquitination process, in which old proteins are normally 'tagged' for destruction, becomes abnormal is unknown
- Abnormal glutamate signalling mediates excitotoxic damage in motor neurones through excessive intracellular calcium and mitochondrial damage
- Neurofilaments and microfilaments are damaged by oxidative stress

Ubiquination adds ubiquitin 'tags' to proteins to mark them for destruction or removal. If neither occur, the proteins accumulate, which causes cellular dysfunction and cell death. The protein TDP-43, present in the nucleus of normal cells, builds up in the cytoplasm of affected cells in patients with motor neurone disease, as well as in some patients with frontotemporal dementia. Therefore these conditions are sometimes called TDP-43 proteinopathies.

Clinical features

The characteristic feature of motor neurone disease is the presence of mixed upper and lower motor signs that cannot be caused by a single lesion. In practice, this means finding lower motor signs at a spinal level below upper motor neurone signs and without sensory involvement (see **Figure 13.1**). Few other conditions affect both upper and lower motor neurones while sparing sensory neurones.

In 90% of cases, motor symptoms start in a single limb (**Figure 13.2**). The symptoms spread over months and years, first to the other leg or arm, then to other limbs and bulbar muscles. About 10% of patients present with a bulbar or pseudobulbar palsy (**Table 13.1**), which has a poorer prognosis because of earlier complications, such as pneumonia. There are also a few less common presentations of motor neurone disease (**Table 13.2**). Sensory, bladder and bowel symptoms are minimal.

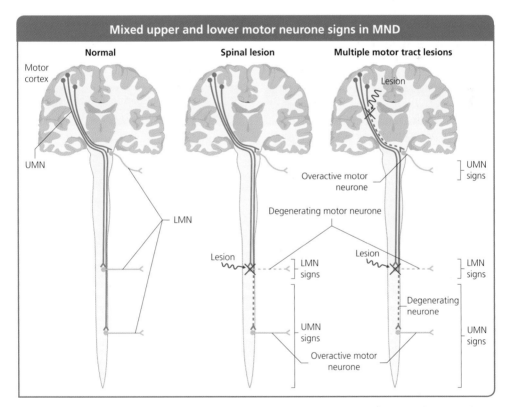

Figure 13.1 Mixed upper motor neurone (UMN) and lower motor neurone (LMN) signs in motor neurone disease (MND). The combination of clinically obvious UMN and LMN signs in combination is suggestive of MND. When there are UMN signs rostral to (i.e. higher than) LMN signs the diagnosis is very likely.

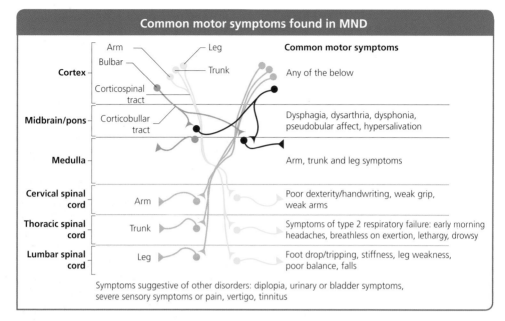

Figure 13.2 Common motor symptoms in motor neurone disease (MND) and their anatomical correlates. Other symptoms which are unusual for MND are also shown and the presence of any of these should lead to a search for an alternative diagnosis.

Bulbar and pseudobulbar palsy: clinical features

Clinical feature	Bulbar palsy	Pseudobulbar palsy
Tongue fasciculations	Present	Absent
Tongue movements	Slow (muscle wasting)	Stiff
Speech	Dysarthric	Dysarthric
Dysphagia	Present	Present
Affect	Normal	Inappropriate crying or laughter
Gag reflex	Reduced	Exaggerated ('brisk')
Jaw jerk	Reduced or normal	Exaggerated ('brisk')

Table 13.1 Clinical features of bulbar and pseudobulbar palsy

Rare presentations of motor neurone disease

Presenting feature	Pathophysiology
Respiratory failure	Intercostal and diaphragmatic muscle weakness
Wasted hand	Denervation of hand muscles
Weight loss	Dysphagia from weakness of bulbar muscles
Dropped head	Weakness of neck extensors

Table 13.2 Rare presentations of motor neurone disease

About 10% of cases of motor neurone disease are bulbar-onset. These cases often present through stroke or otolaryngology clinics, because the patient has developed dysarthria. Surprisingly, some of these patients remain fully ambulant, without significant limb involvement, despite the progression of their symptoms to complete loss of speech or swallowing.

Diagnostic approach

The diagnosis of motor neurone disease is a clinical one, supported by the exclusion of key differentials (**Table 13.3**) and the confirmation of lesions in the motor system. Structural brain or spinal cord lesions occasionally mimic motor neurone disease, so MRI of the brain and spinal cord is usually indicated (**Figure 13.3**).

Investigations

All patients with motor neurone disease require neurophysiological studies (**Table 13.4**; see page 173).

Patients with mostly upper motor neurone signs require an MRI scan of the brain and spinal cord to exclude structural lesions such as multiple cervical disc prolapses. MRI also occasionally shows a high signal in the corticospinal tracts, the site of active motor neurone degeneration (**Figure 13.3**).

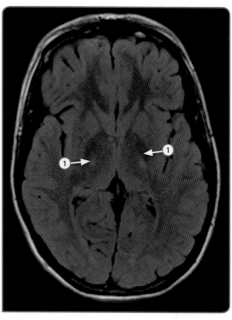

Figure 13.3 Radiological signs occasionally found in MND. There is subtle bilateral high signal in both corticospinal tracts on FLAIR sequence ①. This represents UMN degeneration.

Suspected motor neurone disease: differential diagnoses		
Condition	Clinical features	Key investigation(s)
Multifocal motor neuropathy	Multifocal LMN signs	Nerve conduction studies and anti-GM1 anti-ganglioside antibodies
Heavy metal toxicity	Variable LMN signs	Blood and urine testing
Spinocerebellar ataxia type 3	Ataxia, muscle wasting, fasciculations and extrapyramidal signs	Genetic testing
Adult Tay–Sachs disease	Proximal weakness, dysarthria, LMN signs and spasticity	Genetic testing
HIV-related motor neurone disease-like syndrome	Rapidly progressive limb-onset motor neurone disease-like syndrome	HIV testing
Kennedy's disease	LMN signs, bulbar symptoms, and gynaecomastia, with X-linked inheritance (affects men only)	Genetic testing

LMN, lower motor neurone.

Table 13.3 Rare but treatable differential diagnoses in suspected motor neurone disease

Neurophysiological investigations in suspected motor neurone disease		
Investigation	Findings	Significance
Nerve conduction studies	Normal sensory findings	Excludes a disorder involving the sensory system
	Normal motor conduction velocities: no conduction block	Excludes inflammatory peripheral nerve disorders such as multifocal motor neuropathy
Electromyography	Fibrillation and fasciculation potentials	Shows ongoing denervation of muscles
	Denervation in two or more body regions	Confirms a widespread motor neurone disorder

Table 13.4 Neurophysiological investigations in suspected motor neurone disease

Rarely, HIV can cause a motor neurone disease-like syndrome. Therefore an HIV test is required.

Management

Motor neurone disease is managed by supporting the patient through the predictable progression and complications of neuromuscular failure, by:

- maximising mobility at each stage with physiotherapy, occupational therapy and home adaptations
- helping the patient cope with the progression of dysphagia and dysarthria, through regular reviews with speech and language therapists
- regular medical reviews to identify and address new problems or questions

Nurse specialists offer an invaluable source of advice, support and information to patients. Supportive treatments include:

- percutaneous gastrostomy, inserted whilst the patient still has some swallowing function left, to manage dysphagia, a common and dangerous symptom that can otherwise prevent adequate nutrition; a feeding tube is inserted through the abdominal wall under local anaesthetic
- non-invasive ventilation for progressive respiratory failure; specialised nasal or face masks provide pressure support to the patient's own breathing efforts

Medication

Riluzole is the only approved medication shown to alter disease progression in cases of motor neurone disease. It has a modest effect, increasing survival by only a few months.

Prognosis

Sadly, the condition is relentlessly progressive. Most patients die from respiratory failure within 3–5 years of symptom onset. However, it is difficult to estimate life expectancy in individual patients.

Spinal muscular atrophy

Spinal muscular atrophy is an autosomal recessive genetic disease. Mutations of the survival motor neurone 1 (*SMN1*) gene lead to degeneration of the lower motor neurone and atrophy of the muscle it innervates from lack of trophic signalling from the nerve.

The cell bodies of all lower motor neurones are in the spinal cord. Their axons make up the peripheral nerves, but their cell bodies are in the central nervous system.

Subtypes of spinal muscular atrophy			
Subtype	Age of onset	Life expectancy	Maximum function
I	< 6 months	2 years	Sitting with support
II	6–18 months	> 25 years	Sitting independently
III	> 1 year	Normal	Walking
IV	Adult	Normal	Normal

Table 13.5 Subtypes of spinal muscular atrophy

Four clinical types of spinal muscular atrophy are recognised (I–IV). The classification is based on the severity of illness (**Table 13.5**).

Epidemiology

One in 50 people are carriers of *SMN1* mutations. About 1 in 10,000 newborn babies are affected by the disease.

Aetiology

The *SMN1* gene codes for the survival motor neurone protein 1 (SMN1), an enzyme that regulates global gene expression in cells. Its main function is in gene splicing: the editing down of longer sequences of messenger RNA (mRNA) to the shorter sequences encoding specific proteins. SMN1 mutations lead to defective splicing and therefore defective proteins, particularly those required for the normal growth, development and function of motor neurones. The result is neuronal death and spinal muscular atrophy.

SMN2 is a separate but similar gene that is spliced to produce both a short version of SMN and a normal version (**Figure 13.4**).

> Gene splicing is a mechanism by which cells can produce multiple types of protein from a single gene. This usually involves changing the sections of DNA that are transcribed to form mRNA (i.e. the exons) and which are not (i.e. the introns). The different mRNA sequences are then translated to form different proteins.

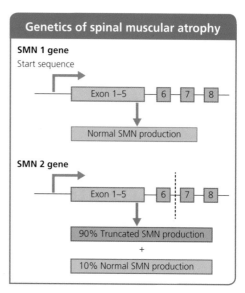

Genetics of spinal muscular atrophy

Figure 13.4 Spinal muscular atrophy (SMA) is caused by loss of functional SMN1 due to a mutation in the *SMN1* gene. The SMN1 gene normally encodes a full length functional SMN1 protein. The *SMN2* gene normally produces only 10% full length functional SMN1 protein (shortened splicing site shown by dashed line), but normal individuals may have 2–4 copies of it. In SMA the *SMN1* gene is mutated and produces no SMN1 or only a small percentage of functional SMN1. Extra copies of SMN2 are likely to modify the phenotype in SMA by increasing the amount of functional SMN1 available.

Clinical features

The main symptoms and signs of spinal muscular atrophy are:

- muscle weakness
- lack of motor development
- reduced muscle tone
- tongue fasciculations
- postural finger tremor
- loss of tendon reflexes

Adults present with progressive proximal muscle weakness, tongue fasciculations and a tremor. The legs are often affected first, with reduced reflexes. Facial muscles are usually spared.

Diagnostic approach

Genetic testing for *SMN1* mutations is widely available; it is very sensitive and specific.

Testing is required in cases of progressive proximal leg weakness, reduced tone and reflexes, and tremor.

Management

No treatments are available that significantly slow disease progression. Management of major complications includes:

- orthopaedic surgery for severe scoliosis or hip dislocation
- respiratory support with non-invasive ventilation
- nutritional support, including gastrostomy

Life expectancy depends on the type of spinal muscular atrophy (see **Table 13.5**).

Friedreich's ataxia

Friedreich's ataxia is an autosomal recessive genetic disease caused by expansion of a guanine–adenine–adenine (GAA) trinucleotide repeat, which leads to mitochondrial dysfunction. It has neurological, cardiac and endocrine manifestations.

Epidemiology and aetiology

The prevalence of Friedreich's ataxia is 3 per 100,000 in the UK. Over 98% of patients have a highly increased number, i.e. an expansion, of GAA trinucleotide repeats in the *FRDA1* gene, which encodes the protein frataxin. This protein is present in mitochondria and regulates iron transport and storage. The trinucleotide expansion results in low levels of functional frataxin (**Figure 13.5**). This deficiency leads to mitochondrial dysfunction in neurones and other high-energy cells.

FRDA1 mutations are inherited in an autosomal recessive manner. This means that two abnormal copies of the gene must be inherited for symptoms to arise, i.e. both mother and father need to be carriers of the abnormal gene. Carriers are people with only one abnormal copy of the gene; they are usually asymptomatic or have only mild symptoms.

Trinucleotide repeat disorders are a group of genetic neurological conditions characterised by abnormally high numbers of copies of three nucleotides occurring together in sections of genes. The GAA repeats in Friedreich's ataxia are an example. These sequences are prone to increasing in number (trinucleotide repeat expansion) during each round of DNA replication. The more repeats, the less functional the protein, and the earlier onset of and more severe the disease.

Clinical features

Between the ages of around 2–16 years, there is slow and progressive onset of signs and symptoms. The core features of a clinical diagnosis are:

- onset before the age of 25 years
- progressive ataxia of limbs and gait
- loss of knee and ankle reflexes
- extensor plantar response

Cardiac and endocrine complications are common, occurring in 90% and 20% of cases, respectively.

Diagnostic approach

Genetic testing is available and is diagnostic in suspected cases.

Management

Regrettably, no specific treatment is available for Friedreich's ataxia. Management is supportive, with monitoring for and treating of complications.

- Hypertrophic cardiomyopathy, which affects half of patients, is caused by cardiac muscle dysfunction and is often fatal; regular echocardiography and electrocardiography are required
- Diabetes affects a quarter of patients; regular screening is essential

Tragically, patients usually become wheelchair-bound within 15 years of symptom onset, and most die in their fifties. The usual cause of death is hypertrophic cardiomyopathy.

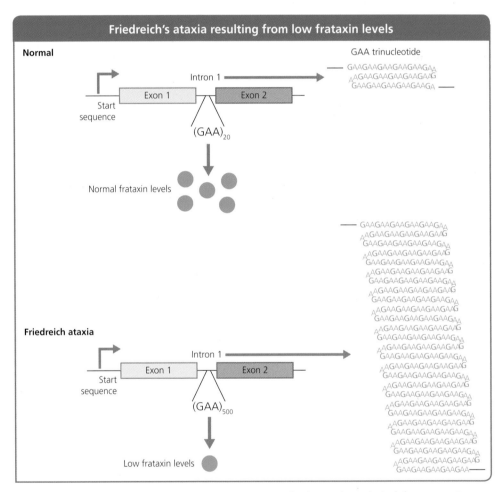

Figure 13.5 Expansion of the GAA trinucleotide repeat in Friedreich's ataxia results in failure to translate normal levels of functional frataxin protein.

Spinocerebellar ataxia

The spinocerebellar ataxias are a diverse group of autosomal dominant clinical syndromes whose core feature is progressive cerebellar ataxia (see page 142). Patients present in their twenties or thirties.

Spinocerebellar ataxia is similar to Friedreich's ataxia in that it is caused by triplet expansion mutations of CAG in specific genes. No specific treatment is available.

Answers to starter questions

1. The causes of neuronal degeneration are not completely understood. However, ageing is a major risk factor for degenerative diseases such as motor neurone disease, which suggests that degeneration results from the accumulation of toxins, metabolic stress or other cellular factors. In some conditions, such as Friedreich's ataxia, degeneration is caused by genetic mutations that lead to abnormal metabolic pathways.

2. Most patients with neurodegenerative diseases present with symptoms arising from a pathological process that started years earlier. In such cases, the aim is to halt the disease, not to cure the already established disability. There is great interest in identifying presymptomatic patients to increase understanding of the pathology of degenerative diseases and to develop more effective therapies. The downside is that the results of the tests used for early diagnosis usually carry a degree of uncertainty that some patients find difficult to live with.

3. Genetic testing should be approached with great caution, and the benefits and pitfalls fully explained to people considering them. Some prefer to have a clear diagnosis and prognosis, and so find testing helpful. However, others may be adversely affected by such information and may not want to know. Informing someone of the nature of their condition and its likely course can help them come to terms with approaching death and to live the rest of their life in light of their diagnosis.

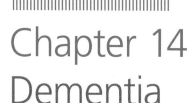

Chapter 14
Dementia

Starter questions

Answers to the following questions are on pages 403–404

1. Can dementia be prevented?
2. Is all dementia caused by neuronal degeneration?
3. How are normal age-related neuronal degeneration and dementia differentiated?
4. What is the best way to tell a patient that they have dementia?

Introduction

Dementia is a syndrome of progressive impairment in at least two domains of cognitive function (memory, language and intellect) that significantly interferes with daily life. Primary neurodegenerative diseases such as Alzheimer's disease have a significant negative impact on the lives of patients and their families, and the patient will need increasing care and support as the disease progresses.

Dementia also results from non-degenerative brain injuries, for example head trauma and encephalitis. This type of dementia differs from neurodegenerative dementia in the way it progresses but causes similar cognitive, behavioural and social disabilities.

The prevalence of dementia in people older than 60 years is 1%; it increases to 40% in those aged over 85 years.

Neuropsychiatric features such as depression, anxiety and psychosis are common in the later stages of dementia and require specialist support.

This chapter starts with the general approach to diagnosis when a patient presents with signs and symptoms of dementia and outlines general issues in dementia management. Then each of the more common types is discussed in more depth in its own section.

Case 15 Change in personality and decline in memory

Presentation

Mrs Yvonne Mathieson, aged 56 years, is admitted from the neurology clinic for urgent investigation. She has been referred by her general practitioner because of a 3-month history of incoordination, declining memory and difficulties at work.

Initial interpretation

The neurologist feels that this is a case of a rapidly progressive dementia warranting urgent investigation. The differential diagnosis includes potentially treatable conditions, such as autoimmune encephalitis, and incurable ones, for example atypical Alzheimer's disease and Creutzfeldt–Jakob disease (CJD).

History

Mrs Mathieson has no notable past medical history. Over the past 3 months, her personality has changed; she has become easily frustrated and short-tempered with family members, as well as disinhibited, talking to strangers about personal matters. She has also become forgetful. Mrs Mathieson has poor coordination, with left hand clumsiness and difficulty walking.

Interpretation of history

The history suggests progressive dysfunction of higher cognitive functions in several domains: visuospatial function, executive function and memory. Personality change and disinhibition suggest

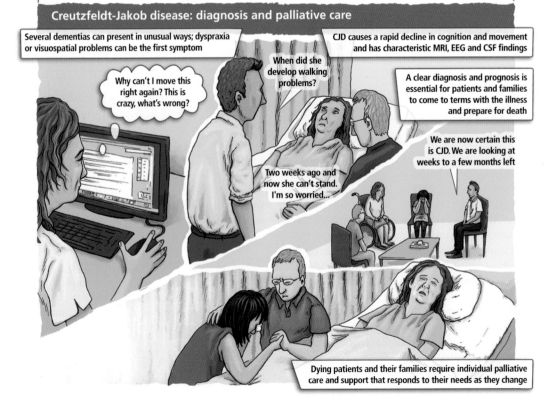

Creutzfeldt-Jakob disease: diagnosis and palliative care

Several dementias can present in unusual ways; dyspraxia or visuospatial problems can be the first symptom

CJD causes a rapid decline in cognition and movement and has characteristic MRI, EEG and CSF findings

Why can't I move this right again? This is crazy, what's wrong?

When did she develop walking problems?

A clear diagnosis and prognosis is essential for patients and families to come to terms with the illness and prepare for death

We are now certain this is CJD. We are looking at weeks to a few months left

Two weeks ago and now she can't stand. I'm so worried...

Dying patients and their families require individual palliative care and support that responds to their needs as they change

frontal lobe dysfunction, and forgetfulness suggests temporal lobe dysfunction. Difficulty with work tasks and clumsiness may represent dyspraxia from parietal lobe or cerebellar dysfunction.

Alzheimer's disease is the commonest cause of dementia. However, it is unlikely in this case for the following reasons.

- Mrs Mathieson is a younger patient (Alzheimer's disease is rare in patients younger than 65 years)
- The degree of forgetfulness is more than would be expected in Alzheimer's disease
- Mrs Mathieson's central features of the case (impairment of executive function and some dyspraxia) are uncommon in early Alzheimer's disease
- Personality and behavioural changes suggest behavioural variant frontotemporal dementia or Creutzfeldt–Jakob disease

Further history

Part of Mrs Mathieson's work is designing and arranging greeting cards. Recently, she has had difficulty visually aligning and arranging as well as creating them, despite years of experience. She admits to no longer driving because of poor visuospatial judgements, and she cannot use her computer or calculate the weekly accounts. Her husband says she has become easily startled, jumping at unexpected sounds.

Examination

Mrs Mathieson has pronator drift, increased tone and 'cogwheel' rigidity in her left arm (see page 135). She has past-pointing and dysdiadochokinesia on her left side. Her plantar reflexes are both up-going, and all reflexes are brisk. Cranial nerve examination suggests no cranial lesions. The results of bedside cognitive testing with Addenbrookes' Cognitive Examination suggest impaired memory,

visuospatial function, fluency and praxis (the ability to interact successfully with the environment in planning, organising and carrying out a sequence of unfamiliar actions successfully, which requires ideation and planning an activity, motor planning and execution). Mrs Mathieson has startle myoclonus. Myoclonus is the brief involuntary, twitching of a muscle or a group of muscles. In startle myoclonus, the entire body may spontaneously jerk just like a startle response.

Interpretation of findings

Difficulties with arranging displays at work and driving suggest visuospatial dysfunction, with which difficulties with calculation are usually associated. Being easily startled is a symptom of startle myoclonus. These are features of Creutzfeldt–Jakob disease; they are not often present in cases of early Alzheimer's disease or frontotemporal dementia.

Examination findings indicate impairment of multiple brain regions:

- the cortex and pyramidal system, as suggested by pronator drift, increased tone, up-going plantars and brisk reflexes
- the basal ganglia, as suggested by the cogwheel rigidity
- the cerebellum, as suggested by past-pointing and dysdiadochokinesia

Patients with early Alzheimer's disease or frontotemporal dementia usually have normal physical examinations, although some patients have primitive reflexes. The extent of Mrs Mathieson's extrapyramidal signs would be unusual in dementia with Lewy bodies (also known as Lewy body dementia or Lewy body disease) or Parkinson's plus syndromes.

Mrs Mathieson has rapidly progressive cognitive impairment with pyramidal, extrapyramidal and cerebellar signs and startle myoclonus. The probable diagnosis is sporadic Creutzfeldt–Jakob disease.

Case 15 *continued*

Autoimmune encephalitis occasionally presents in a similar way.

Investigations

Magnetic resonance imaging (MRI) of the brain shows high signal on diffusion-weighted images along the cortical grey matter (cortical 'ribboning') in the right parietal cortex. Electroencephalography shows periodic triphasic complexes. Cerebrospinal fluid analysis shows normal cell count, mildly increased protein concentration and increased levels of 14-3-3 proteins (an indicator of neuronal destruction). The results of tests for antibodies against voltage-gated potassium channels and N-methyl-D-aspartate (NMDA) receptors are negative.

Diagnosis

The diagnosis is sporadic Creutzfeldt–Jakob disease. The rapid speed of progression, the early involvement of so many different domains of cognitive function, and the extent of neurological signs make Alzheimer's disease, frontotemporal dementia and dementia with Lewy bodies unlikely. All these features are typical of sporadic Creutzfeldt–Jakob disease.

The abnormal MRI and high levels of 14-3-3 proteins in the cerebrospinal fluid support the diagnosis. Most types of early dementia produce no abnormalities on investigations, although generalised cerebral atrophy is visible with neuroimaging in cases of Alzheimer's disease.

Mrs Mathieson and her family are informed of the diagnosis. They are told that life expectancy is short, and that the disease will progress relentlessly, rendering her mute and bedbound within weeks. This is a profound shock for all of them. A palliative care consultant meets with Mrs Mathieson and her family to discuss the options of staying at home with support or moving to a hospice for end-of-life care. She agrees to post-mortem examination to confirm the diagnosis. She dies 4 months later in a hospice she had chosen with her family.

> **Most types of dementia do not progress as rapidly as Creutzfeldt–Jakob disease.** Many patients and their families learn to cope with the slow decline in personality and cognition, as well as the progressive dependence. Specialist geriatric units, physiotherapy and occupational therapy, psychiatrists, nurses and respite homes support patients through the challenging period after diagnosis.

Dementia

Dementia is a syndrome of progressive chronic cognitive impairment. It is not a single disease entity; rather, it is caused by different congenital and acquired neuropathologies. When a patient presents with a dementia-like syndrome, the initial task is to distinguish between irreversible dementia and the reversible causes of similar signs and symptoms (**Tables 14.1** and **14.2**). Care should be taken to exclude delirium in particular, with its acute though temporary impairment in consciousness and cognition.

Distinguishing delerium and reversible and neurodegenerative dementia		
Condition	Core clinical feature	Approach to diagnosis
Delirium	Fluctuating cognition and consciousness	Check for signs or symptoms of the many causes of delirium, e.g. fluid and electrolyte imbalances, hypoglycaemia, anaemia, hypoxia, UTI, drug side effects and alcohol withdrawal; follow up clinical suspicion with appropriate tests
Treatable dementia	Progressive cognitive decline	History and examination (with appropriate investigations) to rule out reversible causes listed in Table 14.2
Neurodegenerative dementia	Progressive cognitive decline	Diagnosed on basis of clinical features of neurodegenerative dementia or after negative results for the above investigations

Table 14.1 Distinguishing delirium, reversible causes of dementia and neurodegenerative dementia

Aetiology

Dementia results from irreversible primary neurodegeneration or develops secondary to often reversible conditions (**Table 14.2**). The most common types of primary neurodegeneration are:

- **Alzheimer's disease** (> 70% of cases), which is caused by the degeneration of neurones throughout the cortex and limbic system as a result of deposition of β-amyloid protein
- **dementia with Lewy bodies** (20%), in which α-synuclein aggregations (Lewy bodies) form in cortical and subcortical neurones, leading to cell death

Reversible causes of dementia	
Category	Examples
Neurological	Tumours, chronic subdural haemorrhage and normal pressure hydrocephalus
Infection	Syphilis, HIV, encephalitis
Inflammatory	Central nervous system vasculitis
	Autoimmune encephalitis
Metabolic	Folate (vitamin B_{12}) deficiency, hypothyroidism, renal failure, liver failure, Wilson's disease, mitochondrial diseases and thiamine deficiency (Wernicke–Korsakoff syndrome)
Psychiatric	'Pseudodementia' (depression)

Table 14.2 Reversible causes of dementia to exclude before attributing symptoms to a primary neurodegenerative disorder

- **frontotemporal lobar degeneration** (10%), in which aggregations of abnormally ubiquitinated TDP-43 protein (trans-active response DNA-binding protein-43) inclusions lead to cell death in selected cortical areas
- **vascular dementia**, in which cortical neurones die from ischaemia; it often coexists with the above

Other neurodegenerative diseases can also cause dementia. They include the extrapyramidal movement disorders (idiopathic Parkinson's disease, Huntington's disease, corticobasal degeneration and progressive supranuclear palsy) and motor neurone disease.

> Half of patients with motor neurone disease have cognitive impairment, and 5–10% have frontotemporal dementia. These conditions have a common pathological finding of TDP-43 inclusions. They are now considered different manifestations of the same neurodegenerative process.

Clinical features

The clinical features of dementia depend on the underlying pathological process. Deficits occur across five cognitive domains:

- attention and orientation
- memory
- visuospatial function and calculation

- language
- executive function

Among these, the first features of Alzheimer's disease are usually memory, visuospatial and language problems.

Dementia is often relentlessly progressive, with loss of intellect, changes in personality and social behaviour, and disinhibition. Disturbance in mood and psychosis are associated severe neuropsychiatric complications. The generalised decline in function is associated with diffuse degeneration and atrophy of both cerebral hemispheres.

The rate of cognitive deterioration in dementia depends on its cause. Cognitive deterioration is often accelerated by acute complications, for example pain, infection, surgery and vascular events such as strokes. In elderly patients, falls, hip fractures, medication changes and urinary tract infections commonly precipitate 'acute-on-chronic' deteriorations.

Diagnostic approach

Initial principles of diagnosis are to:

- exclude and treat delirium
- exclude and treat reversible causes of dementia (see **Table 14.2**)

- diagnose the primary neurodegenerative disease to guide management and inform prognosis (see pages 394–403)

The primary dementias have different spectrums of clinical features and imaging findings (**Table 14.3**) and different responses to treatment. Sometimes diagnosis is certain only after post-mortem examination.

A complete history, including from collateral sources, is critical to assess the nature and progression of cognitive impairment.

Examination is carried out to detect focal neurologic signs, such as abnormal motor features, that point to a particular neurodegenerative dementia (see **Table 14.3**). Reappearance of primitive reflexes, such as the grasp reflex, indicates frontal lobe dysfunction, and is a non-specific sign in many dementias.

Investigations

Investigations are done to screen for treatable causes of cognitive impairment, such as thyroid dysfunction, folate (vitamin B_{12}) deficiency and chronic subdural haemorrhage (**Table 14.4**). Neuroimaging findings are often non-specific; scans show generalised atrophy (**Figure 14.1**). Only when the history or examination findings point away from a typical dementia are more extensive investigations carried out using more specialised tests.

Clinical features of neurodegenerative dementias				
Dementia	Cognitive functions impaired at early stage	Other neurological signs or symptoms	Neuroimaging findings	Other
Alzheimer's disease	Memory, visuo-spatial function and language	None	Non-specific	–
Dementia with Lewy bodies	Memory and executive function	Parkinsonism	Non-specific	Fluctuating cognition and visual hallucinations
Frontotemporal dementia	Memory, executive function, behaviour and language	Progressive supranuclear palsy, corticobasal degeneration and motor neurone disease	Focal cortical degeneration	Behavioural and language variants
Vascular dementia	Executive function	Focal deficits from strokes	Cerebrovascular disease	History of strokes; fluctuating course

Table 14.3 Typical clinical features of the main neurodegenerative dementias

Dementia investigations	
Investigation	**Examples**
Clinical evaluation	Formal neuropsychological tests
Blood tests	Renal, liver and thyroid function Folate and B12 level
Specialist blood tests	Tests for: ■ metabolic disease (e.g. Wilson's disease) ■ infectious disease (e.g. syphilis serology, HIV) ■ vasculitic syndromes (e.g. polyarteritis nodosa and systemic lupus erythematosus) ■ genetic disorders (e.g. Huntington's disease and mitochondrial disease) ■ paraneoplastic disorders
Imaging	Cranial imaging with computerised tomography or magnetic resonance imaging
Cytology	Cerebrospinal fluid examination for malignant, inflammatory or infectious processes
Neurophysiology	Electroencephalography

Table 14.4 Investigations in cases of dementia

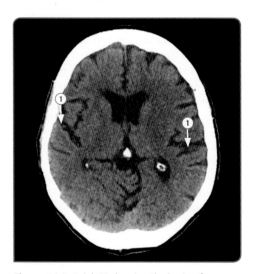

Figure 14.1 Axial CT showing the brain of a patient with dementia. Note the widespread generalised atrophy in the cortex and gyri, creating prominent sulcal and cerebrospinal fluid spaces ①.

Cognitive assessment

Bedside tests are frequently used to screen patients for cognitive impairment. They are also used to monitor cognitive change over time and response to treatments.

■ The abbreviated mental test score is a very short series of questions designed primarily to identify disoriented patients who need further cognitive testing
■ The mini mental state examination is a more detailed assessment with high sensitivity for identifying and monitoring Alzheimer's disease
■ Addenbrookes' cognitive examination is a more lengthy assessment measuring a wider range of cognitive functions

Detailed assessment by a neuropsychologist helps in cases in which there is diagnostic doubt, or when dementia is secondary to a treatable cause or from a fixed brain injury and is not expected to deteriorate. Such assessments provide details of the cognitive domains affected, and are used to aid diagnosis, monitor changes and help plan the beneficial types of support and therapy.

> **Ageing is the greatest risk factor for neurodegeneration.** The distinction between clinical dementia and normal age-related neurodegeneration is blurred. Neuroimaging findings can be surprisingly normal in severe dementia and markedly atrophic in people with no overt cognitive difficulties. People with pathological neurodegeneration are those who have clinical signs or symptoms of it.

Management

Reversible causes of dementia are addressed:

■ antimicrobial therapies are used to treat infection
■ neurosurgery is carried out for chronic subdural haemorrhage, normal pressure hydrocephalus and tumours

No treatments are available that significantly improve primary neurodegenerative disease. Symptomatic relief and psychological and social support are key. A multidisciplinary team of neurologists, psychiatrists, general practitioners, nurse specialists and community carers manage each case. They ensure that the evolving needs of the patient are met. Supportive care includes:

- counselling for the patient and their family, often through patient support groups and meeting with other people with dementia or caring for them
- occupational therapy to optimise the home environment
- respite for carers through temporary care for patients in nursing homes

Neuropsychiatric symptoms require psychiatric management. Depression may be caused by neurodegeneration or secondary to the symptoms or diagnosis of dementia.

In many patients with dementia, psychotic symptoms develop in the later stages. However, antipsychotic agents are used with caution, because they can lead to movement disorders or worsen cognitive impairment. Some of their adverse effects are more common in the elderly, including tardive dyskinesia, Parkinsonian symptoms, and hypo- and hyperthermia. There is also a small rise in the risk of stroke and TIAs in elderly patients taking antipsychotic drugs. They are not recommended for mild or moderate psychotic symptoms and require regular review. In dementia with Lewy bodies, these drugs can cause severe parkinsonism.

Towards the terminal stages of dementia, help from social services or admission to long-term residential and nursing care is usually needed.

Alzheimer's disease

Alzheimer's disease is the leading cause of dementia in high-income countries. The condition results from progressive widespread neurodegeneration of cortical neurones, especially in the hippocampus and temporal lobe, as well as protein plaques and neurofibrillary tangles in surviving neurones. It first causes memory problems but progresses to affect all cognitive functions.

Epidemiology

The annual incidence of Alzheimer's disease is 1 in 1000 people aged 65-69 years. This increases to 53 per 1000 in those over 90 years old. Women are more likely than men to be affected.

The condition is rare in people younger than 45 years, except in cases of familial Alzheimer's disease and patients with Down's syndrome. About 75% of people with Down's syndrome over 60 years old have Alzheimer's disease.

Pathogenesis

Amyloids consist of abnormally folded proteins clumped together as insoluble fibres; they resist degradation and accumulate in organs and extracellular spaces. These proteins cause various pathologies by precipitating cell disruption and necrosis. Alzheimer's disease is associated with cortical deposits (plaques) of amyloid proteins A4, β-amyloid protein and parts of the cytoskeleton. The last of these include the tau protein, which is abundant in nerves.

The accumulation of abnormal proteins leads to neuronal dysfunction, depletion of neurotransmitters (especially acetylcholine) and severe cortical atrophy. The atrophy specifically affects structures with roles in memory: the hippocampus, amygdala and temporal lobes. Some subcortical nuclei, for example the substantia nigra, are also vulnerable, hence the presence of parkinsonian features in advanced stages.

Amyloid deposition in cerebral vasculature increases the risk of stroke; a large proportion of patients with Alzheimer's disease also have vascular dementia.

Aetiology

Most cases are sporadic. However, various gene mutations may predispose to the condition, especially in earlier onset Alzheimer's disease. Numerous modifiable risk factors for Alzheimer's have been proposed, including:

- mid-life diabetes
- vascular risk factors
- cognitive disengagement
- systemic or central nervous system inflammation

The contribution of these factors to Alzheimer's disease remains unproven. However, they are potentially treatable factors, and research interest in them is growing.

Familial Alzheimer's disease is usually inherited in an autosomal dominant manner. Mutations in three genes lead to abnormal amyloid protein metabolism and generation:

- the amyloid precursor protein (*APP*) gene on chromosome 21, which encodes A4 and β-amyloid proteins
- presenilin 1 and 2
- apolipoprotein ε4

People with Down's syndrome (trisomy 21) often develop features of Alzheimer's disease between the ages of 40 and 50 years. Theoretically, this is because amyloid precursor protein accumulates as a result of the extra chromosome 21.

Clinical features

The vast majority of patients with Alzheimer's disease present with chronic and progressive decline in memory. They often have no insight and are brought to medical attention by concerned family members. First, the inability to form new memories is predominant, with patients complaining of forgetting tasks, getting lost or failing to take medications (**Table 14.5**). Distant memory remains intact until advanced disease.

Early problems in Alzheimer's disease	
Social or cognitive area	Complaint
Learning and retaining information	Repetitiveness, forgetfulness and losing objects
Everyday tasks	Difficulty preparing food and managing financial matters
Spatial awareness	Getting lost in familiar places and difficulty driving
Behaviour	Passivity, irritability, paranoia, hallucinations, and socially inappropriate speech or acts
Language	Word-finding difficulties and losing track of conversations

Table 14.5 Common early problems in Alzheimer's disease

Language problems, such as word-finding difficulties, are also common initially. Apraxia is common with disease progression, manifesting as difficulty in carrying out simple tasks such as dressing.

Personality starts to 'unravel' as many cognitive domains become affected; the patient's unique experiences and traits are lost with their memory.

Focal neurological complications such as pyramidal or extrapyramidal features are rare. The exception is seizures, which are common in the later stages.

> **Memory is a core part of our identity; when we forget our stories, we forget ourselves.** Patients in the middle stages of Alzheimer's disease often feel lost, without knowing why. They need a great deal of support to come to terms with such a deep loss of identity.

Depression, euphoria, aggression, disinhibition, irritability, hallucinations and delusions are common psychiatric manifestations in the advanced stages of Alzheimer's disease.

Diagnostic approach

Investigations are carried out to exclude reversible pathologies (see **Table 14.2**). The only definitive way to diagnose Alzheimer's disease is with neuropathological examination – this is often only possible post mortem: a clinical diagnosis must suffice during life. The following support the diagnosis in a typical case:

- progressive cognitive decline confirmed on serial neuropsychological assessment
- computerised tomography or MRI findings of diffuse temporal lobe and hippocampal atrophy (**Figure 14.2**)
- exclusion of other causes of the patient's symptoms

In atypical cases, single-photon emission computerised tomography (SPECT) shows defects in perfusion and metabolism in the temporal lobes. These findings provide further evidence of a neurodegenerative process.

Management

The aims of management are to:

- slow progression, when possible

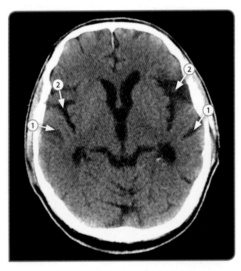

Figure 14.2 Axial computerised tomography scan showing bilateral temporal lobe atrophy ①, which suggests Alzheimer's disease. Note the prominence of Sylvian fissures ② with increased sulcal and cerebrospinal fluid spaces.

- educate and support patients and their families through the progressive decline
- provide rehabilitation to maximise independence for as long as possible
- treat comorbid conditions (e.g. depression)
- prepare for the later stages, when the patient will lack capacity and become very dependent

Management of dementia in patients with learning disabilities such as Down's syndrome is different for several reasons:

- Early symptoms are different
- Diagnosis is often delayed
- Progression is often quicker
- Families may have been expecting the condition

Medication

No curative medications are available. However, acetylcholinesterase inhibitors (donepezil, rivastigmine and galantamine) and the NMDA receptor antagonist memantine can improve cognitive function for a period of months to few years before the advanced stages (see page 395). Generally, when the patient's mini mental state examination score decreases to <12, medications are ceased because benefits are unlikely but adverse effects such as cardiac arrhythmias and worsening confusion remain.

Neuropsychiatric dysfunction requires expert management, especially because antipsychotic medications can have severe adverse effects in the elderly (see page 318).

Prognosis

Mean survival time from disease onset is about 8 years. The prognosis is poor because of the relentlessly progressive nature of Alzheimer's disease. Patients usually die from comorbid conditions such as cerebro- or cardiovascular disease, pneumonia or unrelated illnesses.

Vascular dementia

This often coexists with other causes of dementia, such as Alzheimer's disease and dementia with Lewy bodies. In vascular dementia, pathological changes occlude blood flow to cortical and subcortical areas of the brain. The occlusion causes:

- ischaemic necrosis of cortical neurones
- fibrous and hyaline degeneration of small arteries of the brain, resulting in small-vessel ischaemic disease of white matter regions

Clinically, there is a stepwise decline in cognitive function.

Epidemiology

People who develop vascular dementia usually have vascular risk factors. These include hypertension, smoking and diabetes.

Aetiology

Vascular dementia is most commonly the result of multiple infarcts, with a series of strokes causing progressive cortical and subcortical damage and neuronal loss. It affects:

- large vessel territories in the cortex
- small vessel territories in subcortical areas, deep white matter tracts and brain stem

The effects of the condition overlap with those of clinically significant ischaemic strokes, which result from blockages of larger arteries and cause acute focal or generalised neurological deficits.

Most patients have signs of systemic vascular disease caused by atherosclerosis of vessels. Many have had clinical strokes. Vascular dementia usually presents after atherosclerotic vasculopathy elsewhere.

- Vasculopathy in the cerebral and carotid arteries presents as transient ischaemic attacks and ischaemic strokes
- Heart vasculopathy causes coronary artery ischaemic heart disease, which presents with angina or myocardial infarction
- Vasculopathy of the limbs results in peripheral vascular disease presenting with vascular claudication (see page 354)
- In the kidneys, vascular disease presents with hypertension and kidney failure

Immune-mediated vasculitis, such as polyarteritis nodosa and systemic lupus erythematosus, can also cause vascular dementia. In such conditions, antibodies attack blood vessel walls, and this leads to inflammation and infarction. These immune-mediated causes of vascular dementia must be identified, because immunosuppressive therapy often improves symptoms and slows or even halts disease progression.

Clinical features

Vascular dementia usually presents in one of three patterns:

- Stepwise, slowly progressive deterioration in cognitive function (the commonest pattern): usually frontal or executive dysfunction with disinhibition, apathy and difficulty planning tasks
- Sudden decompensation in cognition after multiple insidious 'silent' strokes that are not clinically evident
- Stepwise subcortical disease (subcortical ischaemic leukoencephalopathy): small-vessel infarctions affect subcortical structures; this is similar to the first pattern but has subcortical features, including parkinsonism from basal ganglia disruption, pyramidal signs from long white matter tract disruption and pseudobulbar palsy with cranial nerve involvement (see page 380)

Diagnostic approach

Diagnosis is confirmed by a history of cognitive impairment occurring in one of the above patterns, in the context of cerebrovascular or systemic vascular disease and risk factors. The diagnosis can be supported by radiological imaging showing regions of ischaemia in large vessels, small vessels or both (**Figure 14.3**).

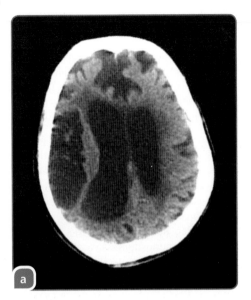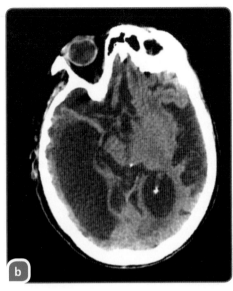

Figure 14.3 Axial computerised tomography scans at two levels, showing (a) bilateral infarcts (widespread low-density regions) and (b) cerebral atrophy. These findings are consistent with vascular dementia.

Management

Non-pharmacological management is the same as for Alzheimer's disease (see page 396), supporting the patient and family.

Once infarction has led to the death of neurones, no treatment can regenerate them. The aim of pharmacological management is to prevent further strokes by using antiplatelet, antihypertensive and lipid-lowering agents.

Stem cell therapy is a source of potential new neuronal tissue. This could be used to help regenerate the central nervous system after stroke. Stem cell therapy remains experimental but early clinical trials have started.

Dementia with Lewy bodies

Dementia with Lewy bodies accounts for 20% of cases of dementia. It is associated with deposition of Lewy body protein inclusions in the cortex and basal ganglia. Amyloid protein plaques are also present in nearly half of patients.

Dementia with Lewy bodies presents with prominent extrapyramidal features. These may initially respond to levodopa, so this type of dementia is often mistaken for idiopathic Parkinson's disease (see **Tables** 9.3, 9.8 and **14.6**).

Aetiology

Dementia with Lewy bodies is mostly sporadic. Lewy bodies are cytoplasmic deposits of α-synuclein, a protein essential in neurotransmitter release from presynaptic membranes. In dementia with Lewy bodies, Lewy bodies are present throughout the brain but particularly in the cortex and basal ganglia. They are also present in subcortical areas in idiopathic Parkinson's disease.

Distinguishing dementia with Lewy bodies from Parkinson's disease		
Feature	Dementia with Lewy bodies	Parkinson's disease
Extrapyramidal symptoms	Symmetrical	Asymmetrical
Dementia	Early prominence	Late onset
Resting tremor	No	Yes
Response to levodopa	Initially can be good	Good

Table 14.6 Distinguishing dementia with Lewy bodies from idiopathic Parkinson's disease

Why α-synuclein accumulates is unknown. The effect is neurodegeneration and disruption of neurotransmitter levels in the regions in which it accumulates.

Clinical features

Dementia with Lewy bodies develops mostly in patients over the age of 65 years. The condition presents gradually with features of Alzheimer's disease and Parkinson's disease, as well as certain unique features:

- persistent, detailed visual hallucinations (75% of cases)
- extrapyramidal features caused by Lewy bodies in the basal ganglia (60%), making patients prone to falls
- dysphasia and dyspraxia from cortical degeneration
- fluctuating attention and alertness over minutes, hours or even days
- delusions
- sleep disorders

> **Visual hallucinations associated with dementia with Lewy bodies often include frighteningly real images of people or animals.** These illusions result from dysfunction in visual association cortices. Delusions (firmly held beliefs of something untrue), such as of persecution, are often secondary to hallucinations and equally distressing for patients and their families and carers.

Diagnostic approach

Dementia with Lewy bodies can be difficult to diagnose, because its features overlap with those of Alzheimer's disease, idiopathic Parkinson's disease and vascular dementia. A rough clinical distinction from Parkinson's disease is that patients with dementia with Lewy bodies have < 1 year of parkinsonism preceding the features of dementia. Other features suggesting dementia with Lewy bodies, in addition to those listed in **Table 14.6**, are:

- typical clinical features (e.g. visual hallucinations and extrapyramidal signs)
- generalised cerebral atrophy visible on computerised tomography or MRI

In uncertain cases, SPECT scans can help show reduced dopamine uptake in the basal ganglia. This is a finding in idiopathic Parkinson's disease as well as the Parkinson's plus syndromes (**Figure 14.4**).

Management

As with all dementias, management by a multidisciplinary team is essential to arrange supportive and symptomatic treatments.

There is some evidence that rivastigmine, an acetylcholinesterase inhibitor, helps maintain or improve cognitive function in dementia with Lewy bodies. Antidopaminergic antipsychotic medications are frequently used to control difficult agitation in patients with dementia. However, they tend to worsen parkinsonism and agitation in patients with dementia with Lewy bodies and are therefore avoided. Levodopa is often tried, but its benefits may be short-lived.

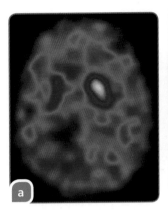
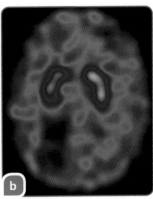

a

b

Figure 14.4 ^{123}I FP-CIT (ioflupane ^{123}I dopamine transporter – DaTSCAN) single-photon emission CTs. (a) Asymmetrical reduced dopamine uptake in the basal ganglia, supporting diagnosis of a neurodegenerative parkinsonian syndrome, including dementia with Lewy bodies, idiopathic Parkinson's disease, corticobasal degeneration and progressive supranuclear palsy. (b) Uptake is normal in essential tremor, drug-induced parkinsonism and Alzheimer's disease.

Frontotemporal lobar degeneration

About 10% of patients presenting with dementia have frontotemporal dementia. It is caused by the prominent atrophy of frontal and temporal lobes, with relative sparing of the parietal and occipital lobes. There are four subtypes, based on clinical features (**Table 14.7**).

- Behavioural variant frontotemporal dementia (70% of cases) causes personality change, poor social functioning and disinhibition
- Progressive non-fluent aphasia (15%) causes difficulty in articulation and loss of speech syntax
- Semantic dementia (10%) causes loss of understanding of the meanings of words, but speech remains fluent
- Frontotemporal dementia with motor neurone disease (5%) is associated with disinhibition

In rare cases, the clinical features of frontotemporal dementia overlap with those of progressive supranuclear palsy.

Clinical features of frontotemporal dementias				
Subtype	Language disturbance	Social appropriateness	Memory problems	Other
Behavioural variant	Normal	Sexually inappropriate behaviour, childishness, rudeness and impatience	Not prominent	Compulsive behaviour, roaming, binge eating and food preferences
Progressive non-fluent aphasia	Reduced speech output and loss of grammatical structure	Usually preserved until later	Not prominent	Difficulty recognising faces or objects
Semantic dementia	Fluent speech but word-finding difficulty and loss of understanding of words	Sexually inappropriate behaviour, childishness, rudeness and impatience	Not prominent	Compulsive behaviour and food preferences
Frontotemporal dementia with motor neurone disease	May be normal	Disinhibition	Not prominent	Signs and symptoms of motor neurone disease

Table 14.7 Clinical features of the subtypes of frontotemporal dementia

Epidemiology

Onset is usually between the ages of 45 and 65 years. The cohort of patients is younger than those with sporadic Alzheimer's disease.

Aetiology

Half of cases of frontotemporal dementia have autosomal dominant inheritance. Most mutations involve two genes:

- microtubule-associated protein tau (*MAPT*), which leads to extracellular accumulation of tau protein
- progranulin (*PGRN*), which leads to ubiquitin protein inclusions

Frontotemporal dementia with motor neurone disease is associated with chromosome 9 abnormalities.

Pathogenesis

The results of early studies showed that frontotemporal dementia is associated with deposits of abnormally phosphorylated tau protein. These deposits are also a finding in Alzheimer's disease, progressive supranuclear palsy, corticobasal degeneration and motor neurone disease, i.e. the tauopathies. Tau proteins facilitate axonal transport through microtubular protein interactions. However, the results of histological studies show that it was abnormal ubiquitin inclusions, not abnormal tau, present in most cases of frontotemporal dementia.

Ubiquitin inclusions consist of abnormal TDP-43 proteins or abnormal FUS proteins. Research linking these proteins and clinical disease is in its infancy.

> Pick's disease is an archaic term for the frontotemporal dementias in which cytoplasmic silver-staining tau protein inclusions ('Pick bodies') are visible. The term now refers to the pathological presence of Pick bodies on neuropathological examination.

Clinical features

Frontotemporal dementia tends to present with language disturbance or personality and behavioural changes (see **Table 14.7**). Unlike in Alzheimer's disease, short-term memory is usually intact.

> Frontotemporal dementia is occasionally difficult to distinguish from Alzheimer's disease. The latter tends to have an older age of onset, cause prominent memory problems and show relative sparing of frontal and parietal lobes.

Diagnostic approach

The diagnosis of frontotemporal dementia is a clinical one. It is supported by neuroimaging evidence of asymmetrical atrophy predominantly in the frontal and anterior temporal lobes.

Management

Frontotemporal dementia is relentlessly progressive; without specific treatment, average survival from symptom onset is about 6–11 years. Management by a multidisciplinary team is essential to monitor the patient's progress and needs and to provide symptomatic and supportive treatment.

Patients with frontotemporal dementia are often too young to qualify for the geriatric (elderly care) services that often support dementia patients. They often rely on help from specialist clinicians or specific support groups for people with young-onset dementia.

Wernicke–Korsakoff syndrome

Wernicke–Korsakoff syndrome is a rare dementia caused by thiamine (vitamin B_1) deficiency. It has a prevalence of between 0.5% and 2%. Causes include:

- chronic alcoholism (associated with poor dietary intake of thiamine)
- severe vomiting
- gastric band surgery
- malabsorption
- prolonged intravenous therapy without adequate thiamine supplementation

Thiamine is involved in glucose and neurotransmitter metabolism. Deficiency triggers decreased intracellular energy, increased histamine release, glutamate accumulation and neuronal cell death. Pathologically and radiologically, there is symmetrical atrophy and infarction of regions crucial in normal memory function: the mammillothalamic tracts, mammillary bodies and anterior thalamus.

Clinical features

Wernicke–Korsakoff syndrome encompasses neurological features of acute and chronic thiamine deficiency.

Wernicke's encephalopathy is an acute manifestation with a classic triad:

- ataxia
- nystagmus and ophthalmoplegia
- neurocognitive dysfunction (amnesia and stupor)

Korsakoff's psychosis results from chronic deficiency. It manifests with:

- anterograde amnesia (inability to form new memories)
- retrograde amnesia (loss of existing memories)
- confabulation (the unique feature of false perception and memories on direct questioning)

Management

Initial treatment is intravenous or intramuscular thiamine and riboflavin (vitamin B_2) for 2–7 days. This is followed by oral thiamine, usually indefinitely.

Progression to Korsakoff's psychosis with amnesia makes complete recovery unlikely.

Creutzfeldt–Jakob disease

Creutzfeldt–Jakob disease (CJD) is a rare, rapidly progressive and fatal neurodegenerative disease. It is caused by abnormal accumulation of prion-related protein in the central nervous system. This protein is part of the family of amyloid proteins, which are characterised by their β-pleated sheet structure and high resistance to degradation.

Prion-related protein accumulation results in neuronal dysfunction. Clinical features depend on the site and rate of deposition. Other prion diseases exist, but they are extremely rare. The majority of CJD cases are sporadic (i.e. arise spontaneously). However variant CJD can be transmitted in some animal products (see box) and iatrogenically. The latter has occurred via surgical instruments and contaminated human products such as blood and human-derived growth hormone prior to the advent of artificial hormone in 1985.

Clinical features

Creutzfeldt–Jakob disease presents with rapidly progressive dementia over weeks or months, eventually leading to immobility and mutism. Marked cognitive impairment occurs, with varying degrees of other features depending on the sites of prion-related protein accumulation:

- visual cortex – visual disturbances
- basal ganglia – extrapyramidal signs and symptoms
- motor cortex – pyramidal signs

- global cortex – myoclonus
- cerebellum – ataxia

Autoimmune encephalitis can mimic Creutzfeldt–Jakob disease and is potentially reversible. Therefore it must be identified quickly.

Diagnosis is by clinical history, MRI showing high diffusion-weighted imaging signal in the basal ganglia (**Figure 14.5**), electroencephalographic findings of periodic triphasic complexes (present in 60% of cases) and cerebrospinal fluid analysis results showing high levels of 14-3-3 proteins.

> **Prion diseases exist in cattle as bovine spongiform encephalopathy, and in sheep as scrapie.** In the UK, ingestion of infected nervous tissue in meat from cattle infected with bovine spongiform encephalopathy led to fears of an epidemic of new variant Creutzfeldt–Jakob disease in humans. Thankfully, this epidemic has not emerged but concern remains that it may yet do so.

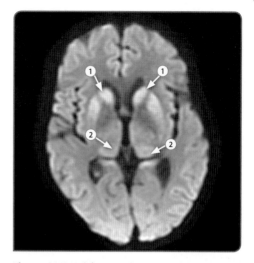

Figure 14.5 Axial magnetic resonance imaging of the brain, showing distinctive bilateral head of caudate ① and thalamus ② high signal in a patient with a rapid dementia, pyramidal and extrapyramidal motor signs, cerebellar signs and myoclonus. The final diagnosis was sporadic Creutzfeldt–Jakob disease.

Management

There is no cure for prion diseases. They progress rapidly and are fatal, with an average of 6–12 months between symptom onset and death. In the UK, patients with Creutzfeldt–Jakob disease are referred to a national surveillance unit in Edinburgh which provides specialist advice.

Answers to starter questions

1. There is no cure for dementia, but the risk of developing it can be decreased. Continuous mental activity, such as reading, can postpone the onset and slow the progression of Alzheimer's disease and vascular dementia. Physical activity and dietary factors (e.g. avoidance of saturated fats, red meat) have also been linked with a lower risk of dementia.

2. Most patients with dementia have evidence of widespread neuronal degeneration and distinct abnormal neuropathological findings and markers. However, the link between these and the underlying disease process is unclear; the degeneration may be secondary to another cause, such as chronic low-level inflammation. A minority of patients have features of dementia that are caused not by neurodegeneration but by other secondary treatable pathologies, for example chronic subdural haemorrhage and normal pressure hydrocephalus, that precipitate similar symptoms.

Answers *continued*

3. Differentiating normal age-related neurodegeneration from dementia is difficult. Ultimately, the distinction is based on dementia presenting with clinical features combined with specific patterns of neuropathology. For example, clinical symptoms of dementia with prominence of personality dysfunction, poor social functioning and disinhibition combined with the radiological appearance of anterior frontal and temporal lobe atrophy, in particular, is probably frontotemporal lobar degeneration rather than age-related changes.

4. A diagnosis of dementia is a difficult and has a significant impact on lives of both patients and their families. There is no happy way to break the news to patients and their families. However, many of them will be expecting or fearing the diagnosis, and having it confirmed and confronted is the first step in coping with it. An unrushed clinical consultation with family members present, plenty of written information to hand, and planned support and early review contribute greatly to supporting people at the point of diagnosis.

Chapter 15
Congenital and
hereditary conditions

Starter questions

Answers to the following questions are on page 420.

1. Why might a label of 'cerebral palsy' be unhelpful to a patient?
2. Are all congenital diseases genetic?

Introduction

Congenital conditions are present from birth and include hereditary diseases resulting from inherited gene mutations as well as diseases caused by pathological events during pregnancy and birth. Any part of the nervous system can be affected.

The diagnosis of many inherited disorders can now be confirmed by DNA analysis. This is a powerful tool able to identify mutations at even a single gene level. However, the decision whether or not to use DNA analysis must be considered carefully because of the effects of the results on the lives of both patients and their families.

Knowledge of family history is essential when patients present with clinical features suggesting a hereditary syndrome. If family history is negative for the syndrome, it usually has been caused by a new mutation development, a non-paternity event or even 'genetic anticipation' (the tendency for disease severity to increase with each generation).

Case 16 Partial seizure

Presentation

Maxine Edwards, who is 23 years old, is reviewed at the first seizure clinic. She had a seizure 10 days ago. It started with her left hand twitching for a couple of seconds. Then her whole arm shook, and she became stiff, lost consciousness and fell to the ground. Both arms and legs had tense contractions and relaxations for a few seconds. Her body became floppy before she slowly regained alertness.

Initial interpretation

This presentation suggests a partial seizure originating in the right motor cortex because the symptoms initially started in the left hand, which corresponds to a seizure focus in the right motor cortex; it was partial because she didn't lose awareness or consciousness. It soon spread to involve the entire cortex, i.e. secondary generalisation, and she lost consciousness.

Common differential diagnoses in potential first seizure presentations include syncope and a non-epileptic attack. However, syncope is less likely in this case because of the absence of prodromal autonomic symptoms (such as an initial feeling of light-headedness or dizziness that probably corresponds to parasympathetic over-activity) or rapid recovery. Furthermore, there are no markers of non-epileptic attacks, such as a very prolonged period of unresponsiveness, and provocation by stress. A detailed history is needed to identify other symptoms of neurological disease.

History

This is Maxine's first 'episode', and there is no family history of neurological symptoms or conditions. She is awaiting evaluation by an otolaryngologist, because of left-sided hearing loss over the past 4 months. She has been experiencing frequent headaches over the past 2 months.

Interpretation of history

Hearing loss and headaches may indicate a structural lesion, but these symptoms may be unrelated to the seizure. Differential diagnoses include focal onset epilepsy without a structural cause and with unrelated hearing loss; focal lesion from any cause, including tumour or inflammation; and mitochondrial disease causing hearing loss, seizures and headaches.

Further history

About 4 months ago, Maxine became unable to hear music through the left side of her headphones. She also has some left-sided tinnitus. Her headaches are mild and bifrontal; they are present on most days and slightly worse in the morning. No features of migraine are described.

Examination

Maxine has left-sided sensorineural hearing loss. The remainder of cranial nerve and limb examinations are normal. She has two café-au-lait spots on her back but no other neurocutaneous features.

Interpretation of findings

The skin findings may be incidental. However, together with hearing loss and tinnitus they suggest a neurocutaneous syndrome, possibly neurofibromatosis type 2. Neurocutaneous syndromes are genetic disorders causing nerve and skin tumours (Nerve and skin have shared embryological origin; they both develop from ectoderm). Magnetic resonance imaging (MRI) will confirm the site and nature of any intracranial lesions.

Case 16 *continued*

Investigations

Magnetic resonance imaging shows a left cerebellopontine angle vestibular schwannoma partially compressing the vestibulocochlear nerve. There is also a small one on the right, which does not compress the nerve. In addition, a right frontal meningioma is compressing the motor strip, and some oedema surrounds the tumour.

Diagnosis

Bilateral vestibular schwannomas strongly suggest neurofibromatosis type 2, because two simultaneous tumours are extremely unlikely to arise from any other cause. Neurofibromatosis type 2 is associated with other nervous system tumours, including meningiomas.

Maxine is told that her symptoms are the result of the development of several non-cancerous tumours, which in turn can be attributed to an uncommon condition that she was born with. At first, she is very frightened. However, her neurosurgeon explains the nature of her condition, the role of surgery in preventing symptoms, and the non-life-threatening nature of the tumours.

She is started on levetiracetam and advised of the significant risk of further seizures caused by the meningioma. She undergoes sequential surgeries to resect the meningioma and the left schwannoma. The right schwannoma is observed with regular surveillance scans due to its small size and asymptomatic nature. After these procedures, she is free from further seizures, her hearing loss on the left does not progress and her hearing on the right remains normal.

Cerebral palsy

Cerebral palsy is an abnormality of movement and posture caused by a permanent, non-progressive cerebral lesion acquired either before birth or in infancy. In addition to the musculoskeletal problems, the condition may cause neurological symptoms such as:

- epilepsy
- visual impairment
- hearing loss
- speech disorders
- behavioural disorders
- learning difficulties

Although the lesions are non-progressive, the clinical features of cerebral palsy become more apparent with growth and development. The degree of disability ranges widely, from mild (minor motor weakness and no intellectual disability) to severe (tetraplegia and intellectual disability).

Epidemiology

Cerebral palsy is the commonest cause of motor impairment in children. It has a prevalence of 2.5 in 1000 live births in the UK.

Aetiology

Causative injuries occur prenatally, perinatally or postnatally, and up to 2 years of age (**Figure 15.1**). Injuries over the age of 2 years are not classified as consequences of cerebral palsy.

Clinical features

In 90% of cases, cerebral palsy is spastic, characterised by increased muscle tone; this subtype is classified by the number of limbs involved (**Figure 15.2**).

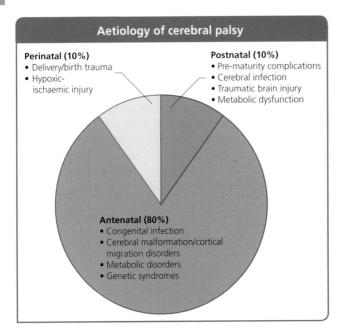

Figure 15.1 Aetiology of cerebral palsy. It is classified into antenatal, perinatal and postnatal causes.

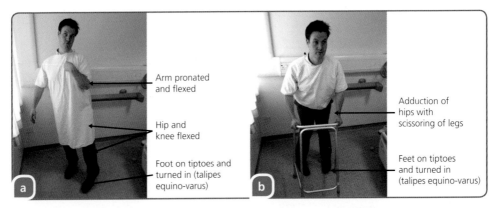

Figure 15.2 The patterns of 'spastic' cerebral palsy. (a) Hemiplegic – the arm, body and leg are usually affected on one side of the body. (b) Diplegic – both legs are involved with the arms much less affected or unaffected. In the quadriplegic subtype of spastic cerebral palsy (not represented) all extremities are affected and there is total body impairment. Patients are often wheelchair bound with severe learning disability, seizures and swallowing difficulties.

Neonatal neurological features present in virtually all cases by definition, include:

■ tone abnormalities (spasticity and abnormal posture)
■ delays in motor development (sitting, rolling and walking)
■ abnormal motor development (abnormal gait and asymmetrical hand function before 1 year of age)

■ oromotor incoordination (difficulty feeding and swallowing)

Up to half of children with cerebral palsy develop seizures in their first few years. This development usually coincides with learning difficulties becoming apparent. A fifth have problems with hearing, vision or speech. 10% of cases of cerebral palsy are the hypotonic, ataxic type. This is rarer and subtypes are:

- dyskinetic cerebral palsy (6%), with features similar to those of movement disorders (see page 309) and arising from damage to the basal ganglia or extrapyramidal pathway
- ataxic cerebral palsy (4%), with incoordination, ataxic gait and poor balance as a result of damage to the cerebellum

Diagnostic approach

Diagnosis is clinical. Computerised tomography and MRI are used to help delineate the extent of the lesion and exclude progressive or treatable causes, such as tumours.

Management

Children with cerebral palsy require treatment from a multidisciplinary team (Table 15.1). These management principles continue throughout the child's life through to adulthood. They are often born prematurely or with birth complications. At first, they are under long-term follow-up from paediatric services. Repeated assessments are done to detect deficits that become apparent with development. The aims are to:

- maximise the child's skills and independence

Support for a child with cerebral palsy	
Team member	Role(s)
Medical team	
Paediatrician	Assessment and diagnosis
	Liaison and coordination of team
	Management of medical complications (e.g. seizures and spasms)
Neurosurgeon	Insertion of shunts to treat possible complications such as hydrocephalus
	Insertion of surgical pumps intrathecally and into the spine to provide treatment of spasticity (and occasionally pain)
Orthopaedic surgeon	Treatment of hip dislocation from spasticity and contractures
Otolaryngologist	Treatment of hearing and swallowing abnormalities
Ophthalmologist	Correction of squints, if required
Psychologist	Cognitive testing
	Behavioural support
	Educational advice
Non-medical support team	
Specialist visitor	Coordination of multiagency care
Physiotherapy	Provision of exercises to relieve contractures and muscle spasms and to improve posture
Occupational therapist	Provision of mobility aids
	Arrangement of modifications to the home environment
Speech and language therapist	Improvement of feeding and swallowing difficulties
	Improvement of ability to communicate
Dietician	Provision of feeding and nutritional advice
Social services	Registration of child as one with special needs
	Arrangement of school and housing needs
	Provision of respite care for the family

Table 15.1 The multidisciplinary and multiagency support team for a child with cerebral palsy

- optimise physical and intellectual development
- medically treat complications (e.g. seizures)

> **Most children born with cerebral palsy survive into adulthood.** Those who are immobile or require feeding through nasogastric tube tend to have shorter life expectancy. Muscle contractures and joint deformities developing later in childhood lead to loss of mobility, independence and quality of life. A supportive family and specialist medical team can help patients regain some of these.

Myotonic dystrophy

Myotonic dystrophy is an inherited multi-systemic disease characterised by myotonia (failure of muscle relaxation once voluntary contraction ceases) and various muscle, eye, heart, endocrine and other complications. The condition is slowly progressive. It affects 1 in 8000 neonates in the UK.

Aetiology

Myotonic dystrophy is inherited in an autosomal dominant manner: only one copy of the mutated gene is required for the disease to manifest. The mutation is a trinucleotide repeat 'expansion' in the dystrophia myotonica–protein kinase (*DMPK*) gene.

These repeats are not translated into protein sequences. Instead, they accumulate as sections of messenger RNA in the cell nucleus. These accumulations interrupt the normal function of other intranuclear proteins that control the transcription of additional unrelated genes, such as muscle and insulin receptor genes. Disruption of the transcription of these genes underlies the multisystem manifestations of myotonic dystrophy.

The DMPK protein is an enzyme expressed mainly in skeletal muscle, where it regulates myosin phosphatase and other proteins.

> **Like all trinucleotide repeat disorders, such as Huntington's disease (see page 320), myotonic dystrophy shows genetic anticipation.** Genetic anticipation is the tendency for disease severity to increase in successive generations as the number of repeats increases. This phenomenon is a result of the repeats causing a slippage during DNA replication, which leads to more repeats in the new daughter DNA of gametes.

Clinical features

Myotonia is evident on examination: when patients are asked to grip an object and then release it, they take time to relax their hand. Other neuromuscular features are listed in **Table 15.2**. For unknown reasons, myotonic dystrophy causes distal upper limb weakness rather than the usual myopathic pattern of proximal weakness.

Patients usually present in their teens and twenties with variable combinations and severity of myotonia; dysphagia; and progressive muscle weakness of hands, feet and face. There are often abnormalities on electrocardiogram (e.g. prolonged PR interval). Patients may also

Myotonic dystrophy: clinical features		
Feature	Proportion of patients (%)	Example
Neuromuscular		
Distal muscle weakness	> 90	Limb weakness and wasting
Ocular weakness	> 90	Bilateral ptosis
Facial weakness	> 90	Wasting of muscles of temporalis and masseter, with characteristic 'myopathic' face (hollow cheeks and scalp)
Shoulder girdle weakness	< 10	Wasting and weakness of neck muscles (trapezius and sternocleidomastoid) and shoulder girdle muscles
Non-neurological features		
Ophthalmological complications	> 90	Posterior subcapsular cataracts
Cardiac complications	30–70	Conduction defects, such as heart block caused by fibrosis of sinoatrial node and conduction pathways
Intellectual disability and somnolence	33–50	Excessive daytime sleepiness caused by altered hypothalamic signalling and sleep cycles
Endocrine abnormalities	10–20	Insulin resistance, testicular atrophy and infertility, frontal balding and increased frequency of miscarriages

Table 15.2 Neuromuscular and systemic clinical features of myotonic dystrophy

have diabetes or cataracts. Patients with rare and less severe forms of myotonic dystrophy may present later in adulthood with only one or two features, for example heart block and cataracts.

Diagnostic approach

Myotonic dystrophy is diagnosed clinically, especially if there is a known family history. Genetic testing for the triplet expansion is confirmatory:

- > 37 repeats is considered a 'premutation'
- > 50 is usually clinically evident

Differential diagnoses, usually distinguished by neurophysiological testing, include motor neurone disease, neuropathies and neuromuscular junction disease.

Management

Screening for diabetes (through measurement of fasting blood glucose) and cardiac disease (through echocardiography) is essential; these conditions are common, potentially serious and treatable. Quality of life can be improved with regular physiotherapy to maximise function, use of orthoses (foot or wrist splints) and surgical treatment of cataracts.

No effective disease-modifying therapies are available for inherited myopathies, including myotonic dystrophy.

Spina bifida

Spina bifida encompasses a group of fetal developmental neural tube defects resulting from failure of formation of the posterior neural arch of the spinal column. A spectrum exists from barely perceptible and asymptomatic to severe spinal cord malformation with neurological deficits and hydrocephalus.

Epidemiology

The incidence of spina bifida is 1 or 2 in 1000 live births in the UK.

Aetiology

Spina bifida is associated with genetic and environmental factors. If one child in a family has spina bifida, subsequent children have a 5% risk of being affected. Environmental factors include:

- deficiency of folate, a B vitamin essential for DNA synthesis and repair
- use of teratogenic drugs, such as sodium valproate

The use of folate as a dietary supplement before conception and during pregnancy halves the risk of a child developing spina bifida.

Clinical features

There are three major types of spinal bifida (**Table 15.3**).

- Spina bifida occulta is the most common and mildest defect, with absence of part of the posterior neural arch but no cystic protrusion or skin defect, and usually without neurological deficit
- Meningocele is the absence of the posterior neural arch, with meninges exposed on skin
- Myelomeningocele is the absence of the posterior neural arch and maldevelopment of the dura and spinal cord; hydrocephalus affects 80% of patients with this condition

In addition to the associated abnormalities listed in **Table 15.3**, spina bifida occulta can present with a tuft of hair, dimple or other cutaneous features. This subtype is associated with additional underlying defects, including malformations of the spinal cord, e.g. diastematomyelia (**Figure 15.3**), lipomas of the cord and tethering of the cord.

Myelomeningocele and meningocele are differentiated on examination by transillumination (shining a light through the cystic protrusion).

- A myelomeningocele contains spinal cord and nerve roots, so light does not pass through it well

- A meningoceles transilluminates 'brilliantly'

Diagnostic approach

Diagnosis is often during prenatal screening. Increased α-fetoprotein in maternal serum or amniotic fluid indicates spina bifida. Fetal ultrasonography confirms the defect.

Affected newborn babies need careful clinical assessment.

- Bony deformities are most common in the lumbar spine but may occur in the cervical or thoracic spine
- Limb weakness is assessed
- Screening is required for associated congenital abnormalities, such as cardiac echocardiography for cardiac defects, orthopaedic and hip assessment for possible dislocation, and renal ultrasound for renal defects
- Increasing head circumference suggests hydrocephalus
- Magnetic resonance imaging may be required to ascertain the presence of hydrocephalus or Chiari 2 malformations

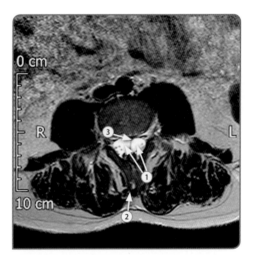

Figure 15.3 Axial scan of diastematomyelia showing lack of fusion of the posterior neural arch and spinal elements. Note the split cord malformation of diastematomyelia and the bony septum at L3 level that is causing the split. ① Split cord ② Unfused posterior elements ③ Bony septum.

Spina bifida: clinical features			
Feature(s)	Spina bifida occulta	Meningocele	Myelomeningocele
Sagittal representation of defect			
Posterior neural arch spine	Absent	Absent	Absent
Cystic protrusion (herniating sac lined by meninges)	Absent	Present	Present
Cystic contents	Not applicable	Cerebrospinal fluid	Cerebrospinal fluid, spinal cord and nerve roots
Skin covering defect	Present	Present	Absent, with cystic membrane exposed
Neurological deficit (e.g. motor weakness, sensory deficit, sphincter dysfunction)	Rare	Present in about 30%	Present in almost all patients
Associated abnormalities	Tethered cord (attached to vertebra and stretched, leading to neurological defects) Lipoma (fatty tumour attached to cord) Diastematomyelia (spinal cord 'split' in two and separated by a bony structure)	Rare	Hydrocephalus in 80% of patients Cardiac or renal defects Foot deformity or scoliosis

Table 15.3 Clinical features of spina bifida

Management

Spina bifida occulta and meningoceles not associated with other congenital abnormalities usually require no further treatment. Corrective surgery may be considered if neurological or other defects are present.

Patients with myelomeningocele require neurosurgical repair within the first day or two of birth to decrease the risk of spinal cord damage, cerebrospinal fluid leak from the exposed cavity and infection. Until surgical closure, the defect must be covered with a sterile saline-soaked swab. Patients are monitored for hydrocephalus (see page 204) and treated if there is persistent cerebrospinal fluid leak or if they are symptomatic. Assessment by orthopaedic surgeons, renal surgeons and others may be needed to manage other abnormalities.

Prognosis

Virtually all children with untreated myelomeningocele die within the first year. Those with surgical correction survive into adulthood. About half with surgically corrected myelomeningocele can walk for at least short distances, and 75% with ventriculoperitoneal shunts (for hydrocephalus) have intelligence quotients in the normal range, although 60% in this group have some form of learning difficulties.

> Between 2006 and 2013, more than 6600 cases of spinal bifida are estimated to have been prevented by folate supplementation of grains as part of international public health programmes. The number of cases prevented would probably be higher if more countries participated in supplementation.

Hereditary spastic paraplegia

Hereditary spastic paraplegia (Strümpell–Lorrain disease) is a rare cause of spastic paraparesis (worldwide prevalence is 2–6 per 100,000 people), a common neurological presentation characterised by bilateral upper motor neurone features in both legs. Compressive or inflammatory, and therefore often reversible, cranial or spinal lesions must be excluded as a priority.

Hereditary causes are grouped together under the term hereditary spastic paraplegia. Most cases are inherited in an autosomal dominant manner, with mutations in genes *SPG4, 3A* and *6* accounting for 80%.

Clinical features

Clinical features include spasticity, a pyramidal pattern of motor weakness, increased tone, increased reflexes and bilateral extensor plantar responses in both lower limbs. Hereditary spastic paraplegia is classified by:

- symptom spectrum
  - simple if only lower limb features are present
  - complex if associated with other signs (e.g. ataxia, dementia and epilepsy)

- inheritance
  - dominant
  - recessive
  - X-linked
- age of onset
  - type 1 if < 35 years
  - type 2 if > 35 years
- specific genetic mutation

Management

Only symptom relief is possible. Muscle relaxants (e.g. baclofen) and physiotherapy reduce tone and spasticity, thereby increasing the range of movements and reducing the risk of developing contractures. Surgery includes deformity correction and spinal implants that pump baclofen directly around the spinal cord (intrathecal baclofen).

> Spinal cord compression can cause spastic paraparesis and is a medical emergency. Suspect this condition if there is a short history, associated back pain and bowel or bladder symptoms. Urgent clinical assessment followed by spinal MRI is essential.

Neurofibromatosis

Neurofibromatosis is one of the neurocutaneous syndromes; these are hereditary disorders characterised by multiorgan malformations and tumours.

Epidemiology

There are two types of neurofibromatosis, with differing prevalences in the UK.

- Neurofibromatosis type 1 (von Recklinghausen's disease) affects 1 in 2500
- Neurofibromatosis type 2 affects 1 in 50,000

Aetiology

Both neurofibromatosis type 1 (caused by a defect in neurofibromin at chromosome 17) and neurofibromatosis type 2 (caused by a defect in Merlin at chromosome 22) are inherited in an autosomal dominant manner. There is overgrowth of embryological ectodermal tissue in both types, and of mesodermal tissue in type 1, resulting from loss of tumour suppressor gene function (see page 272). The tumours themselves are usually benign; they become malignant in < 1% of patients.

> The neurocutaneous syndromes include neurofibromatosis, tuberous sclerosis complex, Sturge–Weber syndrome, Von Hippel–Lindau disease and more than 100 other disorders. They are all characterised by abnormal ectodermal derivatives in nervous tissue and skin. Most have identified genetic causes.

Clinical features

The clinical features of neurofibromatosis types 1 and 2 are summarised in **Tables 15.4** and **15.5**. The classic abnormality in neurofibromatosis type 2 is the presence of bilateral vestibular schwannomas (also known as acoustic neuromas); these are tumours of myelin-forming Schwann cells surrounding the vestibulocochlear cranial nerve (cranial nerve VIII). Skeletal manifestations are often absent. Ocular manifestations include cataracts (in a posterior subcapsular location) in half of patients. Other central nervous system tumours, e.g. meningiomas, may develop.

Diagnostic approach

There are strict diagnostic criteria for both types of neurofibromatosis. A family history, careful physical examination for cutaneous features and MRI to detect optic pathway gliomas or acoustic neuromas (see **Figure 15.4**) are essential.

Neurofibromatosis type 1: clinical features	
Structure	Manifestation(s)
Skin	Café-au-lait spots
	Freckling
	Neurofibromas
Central nervous system	Intracranial neoplasms (e.g. optic nerve glioma)
	Intraspinal neoplasms (e.g. neurofibroma and glioma)
	Epilepsy
Peripheral nervous system	Peripheral nerve neurofibroma
Solid organs and other systems	Haematological (e.g. leukaemia)
	Neuroblastoma (adrenal)
	Medullary thyroid carcinoma
Eye	Lisch nodules
Meninges	Intracranial and intraspinal meningiomas
Skeleton	Scoliosis
	Bone hypertrophy and pathological fractures caused by subperiosteal neurofibromas
	Dysplasia of sphenoid wing

Table 15.4 Clinical features associated with neurofibromatosis type 1. The meningeal and skeletal features are mesodermal in origin; the rest are ectodermal.

Neurofibromatosis type 2: clinical features	
Structure	Manifestation(s)
Central or peripheral nervous system	Bilateral acoustic neuromas and vestibular schwannomas
	Other neoplasms, including neurofibromas and gliomas
Eye	Cataracts (juvenile posterior subcapsular)
Skin	Café-au-lait spots (rarely)

Table 15.5 Clinical features associated with neurofibromatosis type 2. All are ectodermal in origin

Neurofibromatosis is diagnosed if two or more of the following are present or applicable:

- six or more café-au-lait spots (**Figure 15.5a**)

- two or more nodular neurofibromas
  (**Figure 15.5b**) or one plexiform
  neurofibroma
- axillary or inguinal freckling (**Figure 15.5c**)
- optic pathway glioma
- two or more Lisch nodules

- first-degree relative with neurofibromatosis
  type 1, according to the above criteria
- a distinctive osseous lesion (e.g. sphenoid
  wing dysplasia)

The presence of bilateral acoustic neuromas is
diagnostic of neurofibromatosis type 2.

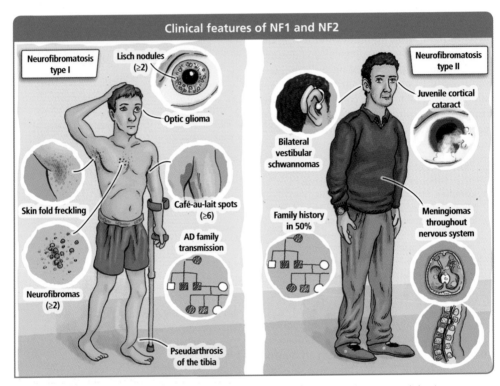

Figure 15.4 Clinical features of neurofibromatosis type 1 and 2 (NF1 and NF2). Autosomal dominant.

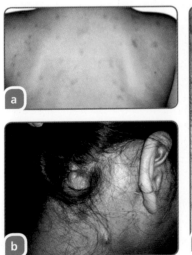

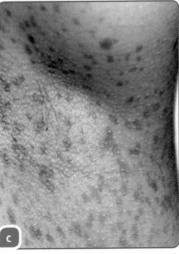

Figure 15.5
(a) Multiple café-au-lait spots seen in a patient with neurofibromatosis type 1 (NF1). (b) Nodular neurofibroma in a patient with NF1. (c) Axillary freckling in a patient with NF1.

In their absence, it may be diagnosed if the following criteria are met:

- first degree relative with neurofibromatosis type 2

and

- presence of unilateral acoustic neuroma *or* two typical lesions (i.e. meningioma, glioma, cerebral calcification, posterior subcapsular lens opacity and schwannomas)

Management

Neurofibromatosis is managed by a multi-disciplinary team of geneticists, neurologists, neurosurgeons, plastic surgeons and physiotherapists. Symptomatic treatment is often required, for example anticonvulsants for epilepsy. Intracranial and intraspinal tumours may require surgical resection, especially if associated with compressive symptoms.

Familial screening and genetic counselling are important for all patients with inherited neurocutaneous syndromes to identify and diagnose other family members at risk. Members of families affected by neurofibromatosis type 2 have audiological assessments from puberty, with MRI of the brain if any abnormality is detected. Families are also monitored for complications:

- neurofibromas, which can compress nerve roots to cause pain, weakness and paraesthesia
- hypertension, which can develop because of associated adrenal gland tumour (phaeochromocytoma)
- either intellectual disability or learning difficulty
- sarcomatous malignant change, which can occur in a neurofibroma (in 5% of patients with neurofibromatosis type 1)

Tuberous sclerosis complex

Tuberous sclerosis complex (Bourneville's disease) is an inherited neurocutaneous syndrome. Less common than neurofibromatosis, it has a prevalence of 1 in 30,000 in the UK. Tuberous sclerosis complex is associated with a classic clinical triad of intellectual disability, intractable epilepsy and facial angiofibromas (adenoma sebaceum).

Aetiology

Tuberous sclerosis complex is inherited in an autosomal dominant manner, but there is a high rate of sporadic mutation. Two tumour suppressor genes are associated with the condition: *TSC1* (hamartin, chromosome 9) and *TSC2* (tuberin, chromosome 16). Their mutations result in abnormal cell signalling, growth proliferation and migration.

Clinical features

The tumours of tuberous sclerosis complex are ectodermal in origin and affect multiple organ systems, including skin, nervous system, solid organs and skeletal structures

(**Table 15.6**). The classic triad (Vogt triad) occurs in only one third of cases.

Diagnostic approach

The diagnosis is suspected in a patient with seizures, delayed development and facial angiofibromas. Imaging, for example brain MRI, renal ultrasound, cardiac echocardiography and retinal fundoscopy, is used to assess cranial and systemic features.

Major features include facial angiofibromas, shagreen patches, subependymal giant cell astrocytoma (**Figure 15.6**) and cardiac muscle rhabdomyoma. Pitting of the teeth, cerebral white matter 'migration tracts' and bone cysts are examples of minor features. Diagnosis is based on combinations of major and minor criteria (**Figure 15.7**).

Management

Seizures are controlled with anticonvulsants. Intracranial lesions causing significant compression or obstructive hydrocephalus may need to be removed. Chemotherapeutic

Tuberous sclerosis complex: clinical features

Structure	Manifestation(s)
Skin	Adenoma sebaceum (angiofibromas) of nose and cheeks
	Ash leaf macules
	Shagreen patches
Central nervous system	Tumours:
	■ Cortical and subependymal hamartomas (tubers)
	■ Subependymal giant cell astrocytoma
	■ Obstructive hydrocephalus caused by subependymal giant cell astrocytoma
	Other manifestations:
	■ Epilepsy
	■ Intellectual disability
Solid organs and other systems	Renal cysts and tumours
	Muscle tumours
	Lung lesions (lymphangiomyomatosis)
	Intestinal cysts
Eye	Retinal hamartomas

Table 15.6 Clinical features associated with tuberous sclerosis complex

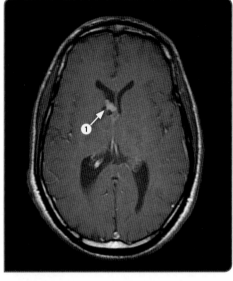

Figure 15.6 A sub-ependymal giant cell astrocytoma ① seen on axial post contrast T1W MRI images. As it is in the right lateral ventricle near the foramen of Monro it could cause CSF flow obstruction and hydrocephalus.

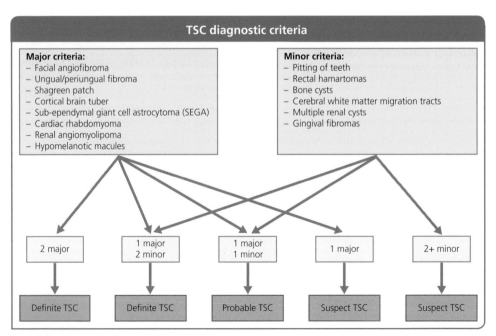

TSC diagnostic criteria

Major criteria:
– Facial angiofibroma
– Ungual/periungual fibroma
– Shagreen patch
– Cortical brain tuber
– Sub-ependymal giant cell astrocytoma (SEGA)
– Cardiac rhabdomyoma
– Renal angiomyolipoma
– Hypomelanotic macules

Minor criteria:
– Pitting of teeth
– Rectal hamartomas
– Bone cysts
– Cerebral white matter migration tracts
– Multiple renal cysts
– Gingival fibromas

2 major	1 major 2 minor	1 major 1 minor	1 major	2+ minor
Definite TSC	Definite TSC	Probable TSC	Suspect TSC	Suspect TSC

Figure 15.7 Diagnostic criteria for tuberous sclerosis complex (TSC).

agents [e.g. mammalian target of rapamycin (mTOR) inhibitors] may be indicated for subependymal giant cell astrocytoma.

Multidisciplinary management of associated conditions is required.

Sturge–Weber syndrome

Sturge–Weber syndrome (encephalotrigeminal angiomatosis) is a congenital neurocutaneous syndrome that arises spontaneously. Clinical features result from errors in ectodermal and mesodermal development.

Clinical features

The syndrome is associated with:

■ facial port wine stain, a capillary naevus of the forehead and eyelid in the distribution of the 1st and 2nd divisions of the trigeminal nerve
■ abnormally tortuous and fragile blood vessels on the brain surface, ipsilateral to the port wine stain
■ ocular disorders such as glaucoma

Vasculopathy causes atrophy of the affected hemisphere, which leads to degeneration and vascular calcification (**Figure 15.8**). These effects can manifest with seizures (75% of cases), intellectual disability (80% of cases) and variable progressive hemiparesis.

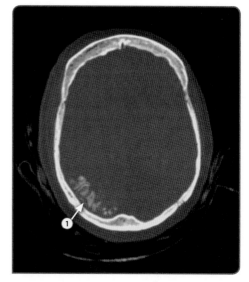

Figure 15.8 Non-contrast CT scan showing calcified blood vessels ① in a patient with Sturge–Weber syndrome. These abnormal vessels in the parieto-occipital region are on the same side as the port-wine naevus seen on the patient's face.

Management

Treatment is symptomatic. Anticonvulsants are required to control seizures. In cases of intractable epilepsy, neurosurgery may be needed: either lobectomy or even hemispherectomy (disconnection or removal of the affected part of the brain). Referral to an ophthalmologist for glaucoma management, and laser treatments for facial capillary naevus, may be needed.

Answers to starter questions

1. Cerebral palsy has a wide range of causes and clinical features, so patients may have a noticeable physical problem and normal cognitive function. However, this variety of manifestations is not widely appreciated. Patients may consider the term 'cerebral palsy' an unhelpful label that causes others, including physicians, to assume they have learning disabilities and are unable to engage with decision making. The use of specific terms for, or descriptions of, the types of associated deficits an individual patient has is more helpful to them than the single term and improves the care they receive.

2. The term 'congenital' is often assumed to indicate a disorder with a genetic basis. This is true for many conditions, such as neurofibromatosis and myotonic dystrophy, in which a distinct, identified genetic mutation produces the clinical syndrome. However, environmental factors can also have a significant role in precipitating or causing congenital disease. For example, in spina bifida low maternal folate intake is a major factor underlying maldevelopment of the spinal column and cord.

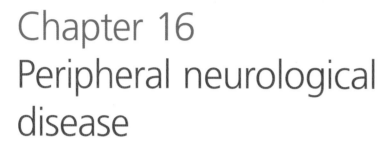

Chapter 16
Peripheral neurological disease

Starter questions

Answers to the following questions are on page 440.

1. What is it like to have Guillain–Barré syndrome?
2. Do peripheral nerves heal and regenerate better than central nerves?
3. Why do neurologists look after patients with muscle diseases?

Introduction

The peripheral nervous system comprises the nerve roots, peripheral nerves, neuromuscular junctions and muscles. It can be affected by a wide range of disorders, with congenital and hereditary disease, traumatic, compressive, infectious, inflammatory, toxic and metabolic aetiologies. These conditions vary in clinical presentation, duration, severity and outcome.

The array of rare conditions affecting the peripheral nervous system is vast. A pragmatic approach to diagnosis is to ask two central questions:

■ Where is the lesion?
■ What is the likely aetiology?

This chapter outlines the commoner or life-threatening conditions, categorised by anatomical involvement.

Case 17 Numbness and tingling in feet

Presentation

Ahktar Rhaman, aged 67 years, is admitted to his local hospital complaining of pins and needles in his leg, leg weakness and double vision. These symptoms developed over 2 days. Now he cannot stand and feels that his hands are getting weak.

Initial interpretation

Mr Rhaman has leg weakness, sensory disturbance and double vision that have progressed over a few days. Muscle or neuromuscular junction problems do not cause sensory disturbance. However, peripheral nerve disease or a brain stem central nervous system lesion can cause leg weakness, sensory symptoms and diplopia.

History

Mr Rhaman was in hospital 3 weeks ago with an atypical pneumonia. He had almost fully recovered from this illness at home when he developed tingling and pain in both feet. This was constant and crept up his legs to his knees. Over the same period, he became weak in his ankles then knees, and he now struggles to lift his leg at the hips. His hands have also now developed the same sensations, and he finds it difficult to grip things. The double vision started yesterday and is worse with distant vision. He has no bladder or bowel disturbance.

Interpretation of history

Symmetrical ascending sensory and motor symptoms starting a few weeks after

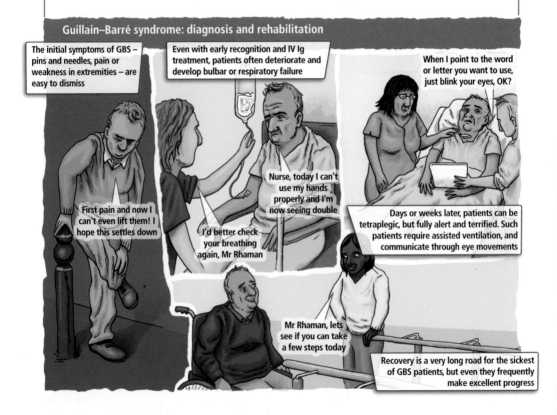

Guillain–Barré syndrome: diagnosis and rehabilitation

The initial symptoms of GBS – pins and needles, pain or weakness in extremities – are easy to dismiss

Even with early recognition and IV Ig treatment, patients often deteriorate and develop bulbar or respiratory failure

When I point to the word or letter you want to use, just blink your eyes, OK?

First pain and now I can't even lift them! I hope this settles down

Nurse, today I can't use my hands properly and I'm now seeing double

I'd better check your breathing again, Mr Rhaman

Days or weeks later, patients can be tetraplegic, but fully alert and terrified. Such patients require assisted ventilation, and communicate through eye movements

Mr Rhaman, lets see if you can take a few steps today

Recovery is a very long road for the sickest of GBS patients, but even they frequently make excellent progress

Case 17 *continued*

a lower respiratory tract infection suggest Guillain–Barré syndrome. Diplopia can be caused by cranial nerve involvement. Bladder and bowel function is typically normal in Guillain–Barré syndrome, but there can be autonomic involvement. Other causes of an acute severe polyneuropathy need to be excluded but are rarer.

Further history

Mr Rhaman has no medical history other than type 2 diabetes, which is well controlled by diet. He occasionally travels to various places in Pakistan.

Examination

He has reduced tone and absent reflexes in all limbs. He is weak in all muscles tested in the legs and in muscles supplied by distal radial, ulnar and median nerves in the hands. He has bilateral 6th nerve palsies and no gag reflex, a weak cough and bilateral facial weakness. His chest wall movement is good.

Interpretation of findings

The lower motor neurone findings of reduced tone, weakness and loss of reflexes are consistent with an acute polyneuropathy affecting the limbs and the cranial nerves. The weak cough, loss of gag reflex and bifacial weakness are concerning, because they indicate poor bulbar function and may require intubation to support the weakened airway.

> **Patients with Guillain–Barré syndrome often go from being active and independent to bedbound and dependent on others for toileting, washing, feeding and even breathing.** They have seldom heard of the condition, and it is a major psychological shock for them and their families.

Investigations

Lumbar puncture shows an acellular cerebrospinal fluid with a high amount of protein. Nerve conduction studies confirm widespread slowed conduction velocities and absent F waves in motor and sensory nerves.

Diagnosis

This demyelinating polyneuropathy confirms acute inflammatory demyelinating polyneuropathy, the commonest pathological subtype of Guillain–Barré syndrome.

Mr Rhaman is given a course of intravenous immunoglobulin over 5 days. His condition deteriorates during this period; he becomes tetraplegic and only able to move his eyes to communicate. He requires intubation and ventilation, and eventually has a tracheostomy. After 3 months in intensive care, his condition starts to improve. He eventually makes a full recovery over about 8 months.

Peripheral nerve lesions

The key clinical features of a peripheral nerve lesion are:

- reduced power or tone, or reduced or absent reflexes, in muscles supplied by a specific nerve or nerves

- sensory disturbance in the distribution of a specific nerve or nerves

Peripheral nerve lesions are divided into mononeuropathies and polyneuropathies because these have different aetiologies.

Mononeuropathies are caused mostly by local entrapment or trauma, whereas polyneuropathies have a wider range of causes.

Pathophysiology

There are four mechanisms of peripheral nerve injury common to both mononeuropathies and polyneuropathies (**Figure 16.1**).

- **Wallerian degeneration:** nerve degeneration occurs distal to an injury; regeneration is possible if Schwann cell basement membrane remains
- **Segmental demyelination:** Schwann cells are destroyed, but the axon is preserved; if the neurone cell body is preserved, regeneration can occur
- **Neuronopathy:** neuronal cell body degeneration, for example in motor neurone disease
- **Axonal degeneration:** this occurs as a primary event or secondary to chronic demyelination; it can be a progressive process preventing regeneration

The severity of neurological impairment and length of recovery depend mainly on the amount of axonal damage and wallerian degeneration. This is because it takes much longer to recover from axonal damage than from demyelination.

Mononeuropathies

Mononeuropathies are lesions restricted to individual peripheral nerves. They are mostly caused by focal compression at anatomically vulnerable sites along the nerve, or from trauma. Mononeuropathies are common; most cases are straightforward and can be managed in the community with observation. Most patients recover well.

To identify an affected nerve, the anatomical course of each nerve, including its motor and sensory innervation, must be known.

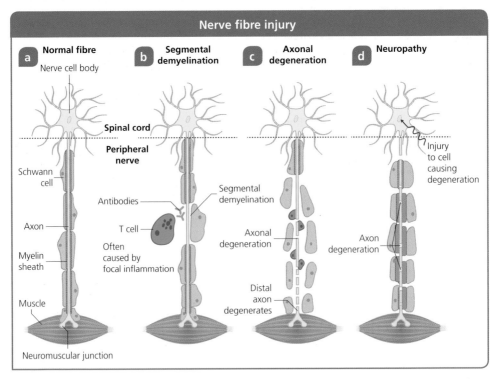

Figure 16.1 Mechanisms of nerve fibre injury. (a) Normal fibre. (b) Segmental demyelination. Compression injury or immune-mediated damage can produce focal areas of demyelination leading to impaired electrical conduction. (c) Axonal degeneration. Prolonged compression, toxic or severe inflammation can damage the axon and stop conduction. (d) Neuronopathy. Damage to the cell body results in the whole axon dying back.

The most common mononeuropathies are radial, median, ulnar and common peroneal neuropathy.

> **In mononeuritis multiplex, multiple single nerves are affected one by one.** They are usually not anatomically close to each other, so symptoms cannot be attributed to a lesion at one specific location. They usually indicate a systemic illness, such as vasculitis, rather than entrapment.

Aetiology

The most common sites of nerve entrapment are sites where the nerve goes through anatomical narrowings, for example median nerve compression in carpal tunnel syndrome in the wrist. Such tunnels can be narrowed by bony growths, fluid retention or soft tissue swelling.

> **Conditions that lead to tissue oedema or thickening, such as pregnancy, thyroid disease and amyloidosis, are associated with an increased risk of entrapment neuropathies.** This is because they cause narrowings to become even smaller.

Clinical features

Mononeuropathies present with deficits of the nerve's normal functions; see cranial nerve functions on page 100 and normal limb motor and sensory function in **Tables 2.14** and **2.15**.

Motor nerve features are used to help localise the lesion, because the muscles involved are innervated by specific branches of the nerve.

Limb mononeuropathies

Any peripheral nerve can succumb to compressive neuropathy. However, only those in **Tables 16.1** and **16.2** are sufficiently common to require detailed knowledge.

Carpal tunnel syndrome is particularly common; it is entrapment mononeuropathy of the median nerve at the wrist. The nerve passes through the carpal tunnel underneath the fibrous flexor retinaculum, and competes for space with nine tendons. Compression can occur because of pregnancy, diabetes, hypothyroidism or rheumatoid arthritis. It leads to:

- aching pain in the hand or arm at night
- numbness in the thumb, index finger or middle finger (relieved by shaking the hand)
- weakness and wasting of thumb abduction

Upper limb compression neuropathies			
Affected nerve	Site of entrapment	Cause of compression	Key clinical feature(s)
Long thoracic	Thorax	Surgery or trauma	Winging of the scapula
Median	Wrist	Carpal tunnel syndrome	Pain and paraesthesias in the first three digits
			Difficulty with fine manual tasks
Ulnar	Elbow	Leaning on bent elbow	Pain and numbness in 4th and 5th digits
			Difficulty with fine manual tasks
Radial	Axilla	Axilla: pressure from crutch in the armpit	Wrist drop
	Spiral groove		Weak triceps if in axilla
	Wrist	Spiral groove: prolonged pressure over the humerus	Numbness on dorsum of hand
		Wrist: handcuffs	

Table 16.1 Common upper limb compression neuropathies

Lower limb compression neuropathies			
Affected nerve	Site of entrapment	Cause of compression	Key clinical feature(s)
Lateral femoral cutaneous	Anterior superior iliac spine	Obesity or pregnancy	Pain on outer aspect of thigh
Femoral	Anterior thigh	Femoral artery or vein catheterisation	Weakness of hip flexion and knee extension Loss of patellar reflex
Sciatic	Pelvis	Hip surgery or fracture	Weakness of knee flexion, and ankle dorsiflexion and plantar flexion Loss of ankle jerks
Peroneal	Fibular head	Leg crossing	Foot drop

Table 16.2 Common lower limb compression neuropathies

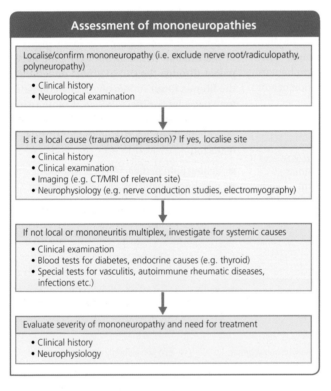

Figure 16.2 Diagnostic approach for assessment of mononeuropathies.

Treatments include splinting, local steroid injection and decompression surgery.

> **Foot drop is a neurological presentation and often comes up in examinations.**
> It is caused by a lesion in the common peroneal nerve or the sciatic nerve. In the former, ankle plantarflexion and inversion are normal.

Diagnostic approach

Three main principles apply to assessments of a patient with a suspected mononeuropathy (**Figure 16.2**):

■ exclude wider peripheral or central nervous system involvement

■ assess for common local causes such as trauma or compression

■ if there is no local entrapment, investigate for systemic causes

Neurophysiological tests (see page 173) are required if more than one peripheral nerve is involved, or if symptoms do not improve within 6 weeks. The test results can show whether there is a more widespread subclinical process, and whether there is axonal damage, which carries a poorer prognosis.

Diabetes and thyroid disease are readily treatable conditions that can cause or predispose to compression neuropathies. These conditions are screened for by measurement of serum glucose and glycated haemoglobin and by thyroid function tests.

Management

Management includes:

- analgesics (e.g. gabapentin or duloxetine)
- mechanical support with wrist or foot splints
- avoidance of behaviours that cause nerve compression (e.g. leg crossing)

In carpal tunnel syndrome, the site of entrapment can be surgically decompressed by releasing the transverse ligament. The procedure results in marked improvement in 90% of cases initially, and > 60% at 5-year follow-up. It can prevent motor weakness as well as relieving pain.

Polyneuropathies

A polyneuropathy is the dysfunction of several nerves, and usually indicates a systemic or hereditary condition. Most polyneuropathies affect longer, more distal axons first before affecting shorter, proximal ones later. This is because the longer nerves have a larger surface area over which circulating toxic, metabolic or inflammatory factors can act. A typical presentation is of motor and sensory abnormalities affecting the distal extremities of the upper and lower limbs in a 'glove and stocking' distribution.

Aetiology

The most common causes are Charcot–Marie–Tooth disease, alcohol, medication side effects, diabetes and inflammatory polyneuropathies such as Guillain–Barré syndrome (**Table 16.3**).

Toxic and metabolic polyneuropathies

Diabetes is the commonest cause of neuropathy and produces many clinical syndromes. The chronic hyperglycaemia triggers various metabolic changes that lead to a predominantly axonal neuropathy.

Nutritional insufficiency or dietary deficiency associated with alcoholism, or malabsorption resulting from gastrointestinal disease, lead to nutritional neuropathies.

Many medications and toxins cause an axonal neuropathy by interfering with cell turnover, microtubule structure and function, and mitochondrial function.

Inherited polyneuropathies

Charcot–Marie–Tooth diseases are a clinically and genetically diverse group of inherited neuropathies with similar clinical features and a hereditary basis. They are further subdivided by the specific genetic mutation present. Most Charcot–Marie–Tooth mutations are in genes encoding proteins with roles in myelin structure and function.

Inflammatory polyneuropathies

Guillain–Barré syndrome is the most common acute immune-mediated neuropathy; it affects 2 per 100,000 people annually. A less severe and relapsing form is chronic inflammatory demyelinating polyneuropathy. Both conditions are caused by dysregulation of the immune system and can have demyelinating and axonal forms.

Clinical features

Clinical features are grouped to define the clinical syndrome present and narrow the list of differential diagnoses.

- **Distribution of nerves affected:** proximal, distal, symmetrical or asymmetrical
- **Type of nerves affected:** motor, sensory or autonomic (**Table 16.4**)
- **Time course:** acute (days), subacute (weeks) or chronic (months)
- **Involvement of other organ systems:** e.g. skin or kidneys in vasculitis; haematological problems in leukaemias

Polyneuropathies: aetiology and pathogenesis			
Type of cause	Cause	Speed of onset	Pathological process
Inflammatory	Guillain–Barré syndrome	Acute	Demyelination and axonal injury
	Chronic inflammatory demyelinating polyneuropathy	Chronic	
Infection	HIV	Subacute	Inflammatory
	Lyme disease		
Vasculitis	Systemic	Acute to subacute	Fibrinoid necrosis
			Wallerian degeneration
Metabolic	Renal failure	Chronic	Axonal degeneration
	Liver failure		
	Mitochondrial		
Endocrine	Hypothyroidism	Chronic	Axonal degeneration
	Diabetes		
Malignancy	Paraneoplastic	Subacute	Axonal degeneration
Inherited	Charcot–Marie–Tooth disease	Chronic	Demyelination (Charcot–Marie–Tooth disease type 1)
			Axonal degeneration (Charcot–Marie–Tooth disease type 2)
Nutritional deficiency	Especially B vitamins	Chronic	Axonal degeneration
Drugs and toxins	Alcohol	Chronic	Axonal degeneration
	Lead		
	Medication side effects		

Table 16.3 Aetiology and pathogenesis of polyneuropathies

The signs, symptoms, family history and medical history are key to establishing the likely causes.

Systemic features, such as those of infection, toxicity, vasculitis or metabolic disorders, suggest a systemic cause.

Toxic and metabolic polyneuropathies

The commonest pattern in diabetic neuropathy is a chronic, distal, symmetrical, sensory neuropathy that can be painful. Patients often damage their feet because they have impaired pain perception. Weakness is a later feature and affects distal muscles. Autonomic features are also common. Most other toxic and metabolic neuropathies present in this way.

Vitamin B_{12} deficiency is a key cause of mixed upper motor neurone signs, for example extensor plantar response, and lower motor neurone signs, such as absent knee reflexes. This is because the deficiency causes degeneration of both descending white matter tracts in the spinal cord, leading to upper motor neurone signs, and peripheral nerve damage, resulting in lower motor neurons signs.

Inherited polyneuropathies

Charcot–Marie–Tooth disease presents with symmetrical distal muscle wasting and weakness, particularly in the legs, as well as foot deformities such as pes cavus and hammer toes. Reflexes are reduced.

Peripheral polyneuropathy		
Function	Symptoms	Signs
Sensory		
Joint position and vibration sense (large fibres)	Decreased sensation Paraesthesia*	Sensory ataxia Positive result with Romberg's test
Pain and temperature sense (small fibres)	Decreased sensation Abnormal sensations (e.g. allodynia†)	Ulceration, trauma or burns because of lack of pain sensation in skin and joints Neuropathic (Charcot) joints‡
Motor	Weakness Fasciculations Respiratory or axial muscle weakness	Lower motor neurone pattern of weakness Wasting or flaccid weakness Fasciculations Decreased tone Absent reflexes
Autonomic		
Sympathetic	Postural hypotension Ejaculatory failure Excessive or absent sweating	Postural blood pressure decrease of > 20 mmHg systolic or 10 mmHg diastolic Cardiac arrhythmias Pupillary abnormalities (small or large)
Parasympathetic	Erectile dysfunction Sphincter dysfunction (e.g. retention)	Trophic changes in skin (loss of autonomic tone), with hair loss and smooth, shiny and atrophic skin
Cranial nerves	Dysarthria, dysphagia, ophthalmoplegia and bilateral facial weakness	

*Pins and needles.

†Pain in response to non-painful stimuli.

‡Deformed but painless joints.

Table 16.4 Clinical features associated with peripheral polyneuropathy

Inflammatory polyneuropathies

Guillain–Barré syndrome usually presents with an acute to subacute flaccid weakness starting in the legs and ascending to the arms; it is often preceded by a gastrointestinal or respiratory tract infection. Bulbar weakness, with dysphagia and dysarthria, is common, as are bilateral facial nerve palsies. Respiratory muscle involvement is less common but still affects about 25% of patients. Reflexes are lost, and back pain from nerve root inflammation is common.

The four subtypes of Guillain–Barré syndrome are:

- acute inflammatory demyelinating polyneuropathy, the most common in western countries
- acute motor axonal neuropathy
- acute motor sensory axonal neuropathy
- Miller Fisher syndrome

Diagnostic approach

Clarification of the onset, distribution and potential underlying pathophysiology in each case helps identify the cause (**Tables 16.3** and **16.5**).

Investigations

Investigations are selected based on the clinical picture and likely causes. Nerve conduction studies help to confirm the types of nerve fibres involved and the extent of demyelination and axonal injury.

Nerve conduction studies

Normal nerve fibres contain many neurones whose action potentials travel at similar speeds. Therefore when normal nerve fibres are stimulated at one site during nerve conduction studies, their action potentials reach the recording electrode at about the same time (**Figure 16.3**).

- In cases of partial demyelination, the action potentials of particular neurones slow in proportion to the degree of demyelination; this leads to action potentials reaching the recording electrode at different times, i.e. a temporally dispersed recording with a lower amplitude, and slower overall conduction velocity (**Figure 16.4**)
- With axonal damage, the conduction speed is unchanged but some neurones

stop conducting; the result is an action potential with normal conduction velocity but smaller amplitude (**Figure 16.5**)

Normal and abnormal results of nerve conduction studies are compared in **Figure 16.6**.

A second, later action potential called the F wave (**Figure 16.7**) is shown in recordings from nerve conduction studies. It reflects proximal nerve root function and is often slowed or absent in nerve root disease.

Blood tests

Investigations in cases of polyneuropathy often include:

- full blood count and measurement of levels of vitamin B12, folate and other vitamins to assess for nutritional or vitamin deficiency
- liver function tests, urea and electrolytes, thyroid function tests and glucose concentration for evidence of metabolic or endocrine causes
- titres of autoantibodies, such as antineutrophil cytoplasmic antibody and antinuclear antibody, associated with autoimmune syndromes
- erythrocyte sedimentation rate and complement as markers of general inflammation in suspected vasculitis
- antiganglioside antibodies if Guillain–Barré syndrome is suspected
- less commonly HIV, hepatitis B and C and syphilis can cause an inflammatory neuropathy, so testing may be considered

In cases of suspected inherited neuropathies, specific genetic testing is available. The choice of test is determined by the clinical phenotype, pattern of inheritance and neurophysiological findings.

Cerebrospinal fluid analysis

This usually shows a slightly increased white cell count (e.g. < 20 cells/mL) and increased protein concentration. A very high white cell count suggests infection and would be a contraindication for immunosuppressive drugs such as steroids or immunoglobulins.

Assessment of polyneuropathy		
Onset	Distribution	Common causes
Acute	Distal more common than proximal	Inflammatory
	Multifocal	Vasculitis
Subacute	Distal more common than proximal	Inflammatory Infection
	Multifocal	Vasculitis
	Asymmetrical	Paraneoplastic
Chronic	Distal more common than proximal	Many

Table 16.5 Assessment of polyneuropathy to identify common causes

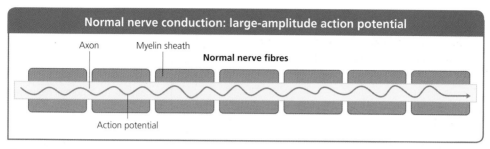

Figure 16.3 Normal nerve fibres contain multiple axons that conduct action potentials at broadly the same speed. Stimulation of the nerve fibre sends multiple action potentials to the recording electrode, which they reach at roughly the same time. The multiple action potentials summate to form a large-amplitude action potential.

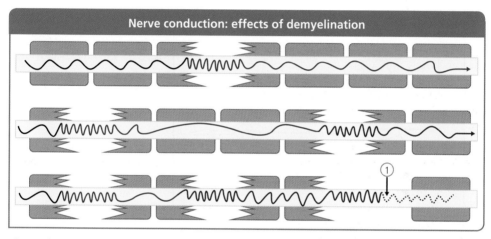

Figure 16.4 Demyelination slows action potentials in proportion to its severity. The change in colour from black, to red, to purple represents the progressively slower electrical conduction. More severe demyelination results in slower or total block of conduction ①. Therefore the action potentials reach the recording electrode at different times, producing a more dispersed action potential with smaller amplitude.

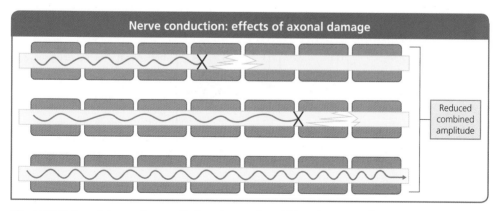

Figure 16.5 Axonal damage has no effect on the speed at which action potentials are conducted, but it stops conduction in some fibres. Therefore fewer action potentials reach the recording electrode, albeit at normal speed. The result is an action potential with smaller amplitude, representing the smaller combined action potentials from the reduced number of active fibres.

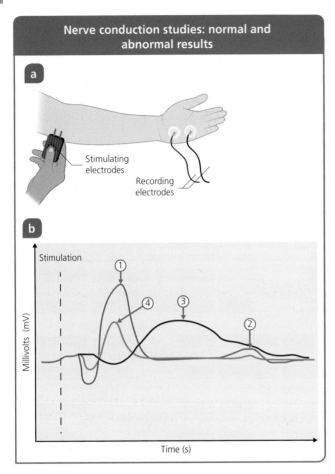

Nerve conduction studies: normal and abnormal results

a

Stimulating electrodes

Recording electrodes

b

Stimulation

Millivolts (mV)

Time (s)

Figure 16.6 Nerve conduction studies. (a) Recording electrodes are attached to distal muscles, and the supplying nerve is stimulated at various distal sites to calculate nerve conduction velocity and amplitude. (b) A normal recording (grey), with a large amplitude ①, representing multiple summated action potentials, followed by an F wave ②. A demyelinating recording (purple) has a later and smaller peak ③, and is more spread out, because the fibres conduct action potentials more slowly. An axonal recording (green) shows a peak at the same time as normal ④ but of lower amplitude because of the reduction in the number of active fibres.

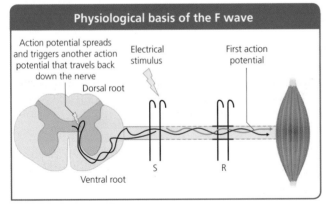

Physiological basis of the F wave

Action potential spreads and triggers another action potential that travels back down the nerve

Dorsal root

Electrical stimulus

First action potential

S   R

Ventral root

Figure 16.7 The F wave (②) in Figure 16.6) results from a backward-propagating stimulation (purple) from the stimulating electrode (S) that travels up the axon and into the spinal cord to activate another action potential back down. The recording electrode (R) then detects a later, smaller peak known as the F wave. Changes in the F wave reflect proximal nerve and root changes and are a common finding in demyelinating illnesses.

Pulmonary function tests and arterial blood gases

In cases of severe Guillain–Barré syndrome, ventilatory assessment with forced vital capacity and measurement of arterial blood gases are helpful to monitor for respiratory muscle failure.

Management

Drug- and toxin-induced neuropathies are often reversible if the causative agent is withdrawn or any vitamin deficiencies are corrected.

Inflammatory polyneuropathies

Intravenous immunoglobulin is the first-line treatment for Guillain–Barré syndrome. It is an in-patient treatment in which pooled human immunoglobulin is infused over 5 days. Plasma exchange is an alternative.

Supportive treatment includes analgesic medication for symptomatic relief, physiotherapy and occupational therapy to aid mobility and prevent contractures, and monitoring and intervention for acute respiratory failure resulting from respiratory muscle weakness.

Vasculitic neuropathies are often responsive to steroids. However, they may require more aggressive immunosuppression.

> **Despite the inflammatory aetiology of Guillain–Barré syndrome, corticosteroids are not helpful.** The reasons for this are debated. Corticosteroids have proved ineffective in clinical trials, whereas intravenous immunoglobulin and plasma exchange have been confirmed to improve outcome.

Prognosis

Patients with axonal degeneration as well as demyelination recover slowly, because the axon needs time to regenerate. If the neuronal cell body is damaged, prognosis is very poor. This is because the muscle it supplies can only be reinnervated by other nerves.

Inflammatory neuropathies usually cause demyelination. Therefore they can be reversed if the immune cause is subdued or the pathophysiology is self-limiting and burns out.

In Guillain–Barré syndrome, the mortality rate is about 5%. Death occurs primarily from secondary causes.

Many neuropathies with toxic and metabolic causes result in axonal damage and wallerian degeneration. These effects limit recovery and lead to a poorer outcome.

Most nutritional neuropathies are predominantly axonal. However, recovery can be good if early treatment is given.

Muscular disease

Muscular disorders are individually rare and highly variable, making them a diagnostic challenge. They are usually managed by a neurologist with a subspecialist interest in neuromuscular diseases.

Muscle disease (myopathy) has both hereditary and acquired causes (**Table 16.6**). Inflammation is the most common acquired cause, and myositis has an incidence similar to that of Guillain–Barré syndrome, at about 1 or 2 per 100,000 people per year. Many drugs cause mild to moderate muscle pains and cramps but only rarely a frank myositis. The dystrophies are the commonest inherited type of myopathy and include a large family of very different clinical diseases that have primary muscle wasting in common. Channelopathies are a group of very rare inherited myopathies

The myopathies	
Hereditary	Acquired
Congenital myopathies	Inflammatory myopathies
Muscular dystrophies	Drug-induced myopathies
Channelopathies	Toxin-induced myopathies
Metabolic myopathies	Endocrine myopathies
Mitochondrial disease	Infectious myopathies

Table 16.6 Hereditary and acquired myopathies

that involve mutations in the ion channels of muscle membranes, which causes episodic weakness.

Aetiology

Myopathies result from interruption of normal muscular cellular metabolic processes.

- The **channelopathies** affect the excitability of the muscle membrane
- **Limb girdle muscular dystrophy** affects the contractile mechanisms
- **Duchenne's muscular dystrophy** affects structural elements of the cell
- **Mitochondrial diseases** affect the energy supply system

Inherited myopathies

There are many types of inherited myopathies, including dozens of very rare metabolic disorders. The commonest are the muscular dystrophies:

- Duchenne's muscular dystrophy
- myotonic dystrophy (see page 410)

Much rarer dystrophies include:

- fascioscapulohumeral dystrophy
- limb girdle muscular dystrophy
- oculopharyngeal muscular dystrophy

The inherited myopathies are genetic disorders, mostly of myocyte membrane constituents, with progressive muscle fibre degeneration and replacement with fatty tissue.

Duchenne's muscular dystrophy

This X-linked recessive condition causes proximal muscle weakness and calf muscle pseudohypertrophy in boys before the age of 5 years. It is the most common childhood muscular dystrophy, affecting 1 in 3500 newborn boys. Cardiac fibrosis affects most patients and contributes to cardiac death in their late teens or twenties. Some female carriers have muscle weakness.

The mutation underlying Duchenne's muscular dystrophy causes loss of function of the dystrophin protein, a central component of the normal muscle cytoskeleton. Its absence leads to a disrupted cytoskeleton, membrane instability, abnormal ion fluxes and progressive fibrosis and loss of muscle fibres.

Other dystrophies

Myotonic dystrophy is the most common dystrophy after Duchenne's muscular dystrophy; fascioscapulohumeral dystrophy, limb girdle muscular dystrophy and oculopharyngeal dystrophy are much rarer causes of focal muscle disease.

Metabolic myopathies

These are complex inherited disorders caused by enzyme deficiencies in metabolic pathways. They usually present non-specifically with muscle fatigue, pain and weakness during exercise. They are broadly divided into abnormalities of:

- carbohydrate metabolism
- lipid metabolism
- nucleotide metabolism

Channelopathies

These are defects in myocyte ion channels and present with episodes of profound weakness when physiological changes, such as high or low potassium levels, provoke ion channel dysfunction as a result of genetic mutations in the ion channels.

Carbohydrate load, exercise and stress increase potassium cellular fluxes and are common precipitants in these patients.

Acquired myopathies

Most acquired myopathies are triggered by a drug-induced, toxin-induced, metabolic or inflammatory derangement. Generally, the chemical can be removed and the derangement or inflammation corrected. Collectively, these myopathies are a common cause of adult-onset muscle pain and weakness.

Inflammatory myopathies

Primary inflammatory myopathies are usually caused by an adaptive immune response that targets muscle antigens. They can be a presentation of systemic diseases, including malignancy, autoimmune and connective tissue diseases, and are often treated with immunosuppression.

There are three major inflammatory myopathies:

- polymyositis
- dermatomyositis
- inclusion body myositis

The pathogenesis of all three is cell-mediated immune destruction of CD8 T cells, along with antibody-mediated (B cell) immune destruction in the case of dermatomyositis. Their clinical features are summarised in **Table 16.7**.

Infectious myopathies

HIV infection can cause progressive proximal muscle weakness and pain. It can be from viral infection or as an adverse effect from antiretroviral therapy with zidovudine (azidothymidine, AZT).

Drug and toxic myopathies

Corticosteroids are a common cause of slowly progressive proximal muscle weakness. The mechanism is unknown, but histologically they cause type 2 muscle fibre atrophy without an increase in serum creatine kinase.

Statins cause myopathic changes in about 0.5% of patients, and can rarely progress to fulminant muscle necrosis and rhabdomyolysis through unknown mechanisms.

Heavy alcohol consumption can lead to an acute painful proximal myopathy or chronic painless myopathy. There is reduced muscle RNA and protein synthesis, as well as selective loss of type 2 muscle fibres.

Secondary metabolic myopathies

Low potassium and low phosphate are common findings in patients with other major medical illnesses and can lead to muscle weakness by altering muscle membrane polarisation. When these levels are corrected, the weakness rapidly resolves.

Chronic renal failure and thyroid disease are other common diseases that can lead to myopathy by altering trophic signals to the nerve endings, thereby affecting mitochondrial function and other complex mechanisms.

Diagnostic approach

Major differential diagnoses for myopathy include neuropathies, neuromuscular junction disease and anterior horn motor neurone disorders (**Table 16.8**).

Distinguishing between different myopathies can be challenging and requires a structured history and examination to elicit particular features (**Table 16.9**). Investigations also help in differentiation.

Investigations

These are used to:

- seek evidence of muscle breakdown and enzyme dysfunction
- detect treatable causes, such as thyroid or connective tissue disease
- look for complications
- monitor response to treatment

Inflammatory myopathies			
Clinical features	Polymyositis	Dermatomyositis	Inclusion body myositis
Pattern of muscle weakness	Proximal weakness Symmetrical Painful muscles	Proximal weakness Symmetrical Painful muscles Skin changes	Distal weakness (finger flexors and/or foot extensors) Asymmetrical May be painless
Associated skin rashes	Rare	Violet discoloration of sun-exposed skin Heliotrope rash (violet discoloration of eyelids) Shawl sign (erythematous scaly rash on cheeks, nose and shoulders) Gottron's papules (rash over knuckles and limb extensor surfaces)	Rare

Table 16.7 Clinical features of the major inflammatory myopathies

Myopathy and key differential diagnoses	
Disease	Features
Myopathy	Symmetrical proximal muscle weakness (inclusion body myositis is an exception in which the weakness is initially distal)
	Weakness affecting selective muscle groups in muscular dystrophies (e.g. fascioscapulohumeral dystrophy)
	Preservation of tendon reflexes
Neuropathy	Loss of tendon reflexes
	Sensory symptoms (e.g. 'pins and needles' and numbness)
	Autonomic symptoms (including bowel and/or bladder sphincter dysfunction)
Neuromuscular junction disease	Fatiguable weakness (weakness increasing with exercise)
	Improvement with anticholinesterase enzymes
Anterior horn motor neurone disease	Fasciculations and upper motor neurone features

Table 16.8 Myopathy and its key differential diagnoses

Muscle enzymes

Dermatomyositis and other inflammatory myopathies are associated with creatine kinase at >10 times normal levels. Creatine kinase is also increased in endocrine, metabolic and mitochondrial myopathies. Aspartate aminotransferase and alanine transaminase are other enzymes released from muscle. Tests for these three enzymes form the first-line assessment of muscle integrity.

Resting or exercise lactate levels are often high in muscle disorders. This is particularly so in mitochondrial diseases, because there is dysfunctional oxidative metabolism.

Muscle biopsy

Biopsy facilitates histological, muscle enzyme and mitochondrial DNA analysis and enables classification or diagnosis of the muscle disorder.

Typical findings include inflammation, necrosis and inflammatory cell infiltration in inflammatory myopathy.

Ragged red muscle fibres are degenerating muscle fibers characteristic of mitochondrial disorders.

Muscle enzyme deficiency indicates metabolic myopathy.

Molecular genetics

Genetic analysis for specific mutations confirms the diagnosis in many of the inherited myopathies, including myotonic dystrophy and Duchenne's muscular dystrophy.

Other blood tests

These include thyroid function tests for endocrine myopathy, and tests for disease activity markers and autoantibodies in inflammatory myopathies.

Neurophysiology

Nerve conduction studies can exclude neuropathy. Electromyography is carried out to confirm a myopathy.

Assessment for complications

After diagnosis, further tests are done to monitor for common or life-threatening complications associated with many myopathies:

- echocardiography and electrocardiography for cardiomyopathy, conduction defects and arrhythmias
- assessment of respiratory function to determine ventilatory capacity
- eye assessment for cataracts in myotonic dystrophy

Management

Inflammatory myopathies are treated with immunosuppression. Initially, steroids are given, then steroid-sparing agents, such as azathioprine, or intravenous immunoglobulin, in cases that are resistant to treatment. However, none of these treatments have proved effective in inclusion body myositis.

Drug- and toxin-induced myopathies are treated by avoidance of the offending agents. Secondary metabolic disorders often improve dramatically on correction of the abnormality.

Differentiating types of myopathy

Points in history taking	Examples	Likely diagnosis
Pattern of weakness	Proximal weakness (e.g. difficulty ascending stairs, sitting up from a low position and reaching up to shelves)	Drug- or toxin-induced myopathy
		Endocrine myopathy
		Inflammatory myopathy (polymyositis or dermatomyositis)
	Distal weakness (hand or foot)	Inflammatory myopathy (inclusion body myositis)
		Muscular dystrophy (distal)
	Specific muscle groups affected (e.g. facial, extraocular, facial and shoulder)	Myotonic dystrophy (facial weakness and extraocular weakness)
		Mitochondrial myopathy (e.g. chronic progressive external ophthamoplegia associated with extraocular weakness)
		Muscular dystrophy (e.g. facial and shoulder in fascioscapulohumeral dystrophy)
Other systemic complications	Cardiac complications (e.g. arrhythmias), diabetes, cataracts, testicular atrophy and subfertility	Myotonic dystrophy
		Muscular dystrophy
		Mitochondrial dystrophy
Medical history	Systemic or metabolic disease	Endocrine or inflammatory myopathy
Drug history	Drug such as statins, steroids, vincristine and zidovudine (azidothymidine, AZT)	Drug- or toxin-induced myopathy
Developmental history and family history	Family history of illness	Inherited myopathy
	Delay in acquiring developmental milestones	
	Poor performance in school (in sports or cognitive tasks)	

Table 16.9 A guide to differentiating types of myopathy in the history

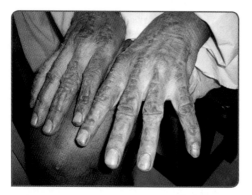

Figure 16.8 Gottron's papules are characteristic thickened plaques of discoloured skin on the dorsal hand seen in dermatomyositis.

Genetic screening and diagnosis

This allows genetic counselling for patients and their families. It has implications for the patient's family members in conditions in which genetic anticipation occurs, such as myotonic dystrophy (see page 410).

Monitoring for complications

Myopathies can fatally involve the muscles of respiration or swallowing, or cardiac muscle. Therefore these complications are screened for and addressed, if detected.

Cardiac abnormalities such as arrhythmias, conduction defects and cardiomyopathies are common in most inherited myopathies. Interventions are often required. Examples include treatment for heart failure, implantable defibrillators and pacing for arrhythmias.

Most myopathies eventually lead to respiratory failure and weakness as respiratory muscle weakens, and impaired ventilatory capacity as a result of contractures and scoliosis. There is an associated increased risk of respiratory infections. Non-invasive ventilatory support, using a tight-fitting face or nasal mask that provides pressurised delivery of oxygen, is often used in Duchenne's muscular dystrophy and prolongs survival and quality of life.

Physiotherapy and rehabilitation

These increase mobility and support the patient's independence. Surgery for correction of scoliosis and contractures may assist with mobility.

Prognosis

Outcomes are variable and depend on the type of myopathy. The inherited conditions are generally irreversible and shorten life expectancy, whereas the acquired types are potentially fully reversible.

Life expectancy in muscular dystrophies such as Duchenne's is only up to the 2nd decade of life, with death the result of respiratory failure or cardiac abnormalities. Endocrine myopathies usually respond well to treatment of the underlying pathology.

Neuromuscular junction disease

Neuromuscular junction disease is caused by either a failure of the neuromuscular junction nerve terminal to release sufficient acetylcholine, or in the muscle's response to acetylcholine. In both cases, the consequence is reduced or absent muscle contraction. The resulting muscle weakness is usually bilateral and changes with exercise. There are no sensory signs or symptoms.

Myasthenia gravis

Myasthenia gravis is an autoimmune disorder characterised by the presence of autoantibodies against acetylcholine receptors on the post-synaptic motor end plate. The binding of these autoantibodies competitively obstructs the binding of acetylcholine and leads to immune-mediated destruction and impaired synthesis of acetylcholine receptors. In this way, neuromuscular transmission and muscular contraction are impaired.

The condition is associated with other autoimmune disorders, including Addison's disease, Graves' disease (a form of hyperthyroidism), vitiligo and pernicious anaemia. Between 10 and 15% of cases are secondary to thymic tumours (thymoma); there is a cross-reaction of antitumour antibodies to the neuromuscular junction. In these cases, myasthenia gravis is often relieved or cured by thymectomy.

Epidemiology

Myasthenia gravis has an annual worldwide prevalence of about 5 per 100,000. Most patients present in their twenties and thirties or over seventy.

Clinical features

The hallmark of myasthenia gravis is fatigability: weakness of various muscle groups, worsening with repeated use and improving with rest. Onset is often in the highly active and sensitive ocular and bulbar muscles, but within 1 year it spreads to generalised muscle involvement in 80% of cases (**Table 16.10**).

Patients describe:

- feeling stronger in the morning (because they have rested overnight) than over the course of a day
- speech that becomes slurred with talking
- difficulty finishing a meal because of progressive difficulty chewing or swallowing
- eyelids that become heavy
- double vision that comes and goes

Myasthenia gravis: clinical features

Muscle region	Clinical feature(s)	Example(s)
Ocular muscle weakness	Ptosis worsening with use	Inability to keep looking up, because eye drifts to looking down and eyelids droop
	Ophthalmoplegia	Restriction in range of eye movements
Bulbar muscle weakness	Weakness of muscles involved in swallowing and speaking	Dysphonia Dysarthria
Axial muscle weakness	Weakness of central axial muscles	Trunk weakness Neck weakness
Distal muscle weakness	Weakness of upper and lower limbs on exercise or fatigue	Muscle wasting very uncommon
Respiratory muscle weakness	A result of central axial muscle weakness	Ventilatory failure with impairment of oxygenation and carbon dioxide expiration

Table 16.10 Myasthenia gravis: major muscle groups affected and clinical features

An acute myasthenic crisis is a severe acute exacerbation of myasthenic symptoms. It can be precipitated by infection, certain drugs (e.g. antiarrhythmic agents and antibiotics such as gentamicin), pregnancy and any kind of stress (e.g. surgery).

Diagnostic approach

A clinical diagnosis can be made if there is characteristic fatigable weakness in a proximal pattern, along with other typical findings, such as flaccid weakness and no sensory symptoms or upper motor neurone signs.

Autoantibodies to acetylcholine receptors are present in almost 90% of patients.

The hallmark finding in nerve conduction studies is a decreasing response of the muscle fibre action potential with repetitive stimulation.

Patients with a new diagnosis require:

- CT of the mediastinum to exclude thymic lesion; if a lesion is present, the condition often improves with surgical removal
- screening for other associated autoimmune conditions, including pernicious anaemia (with anti-intrinsic factor antibodies) and Graves' disease (with antithyroid receptor antibodies)

Management

Management includes symptomatic, immunosuppressive and surgical treatments.

Symptomatic treatment

The acetylcholinesterase inhibitor pyridostigmine prolongs the action of acetylcholine at the neuromuscular junction. Its effects last only a few hours, so repeated dosing is required throughout the day. Adverse effects include gastrointestinal upset and excess salivation from the enhanced effects of acetylcholine at autonomic nerve fibre terminals.

Patients with significant bulbar or respiratory compromise may need intubation for airway protection and ventilatory support during a crisis.

Immunosuppression

Prednisolone is used as first-line treatment in patients with more clinical features than isolated ocular symptoms.

Intravenous immunoglobulin or plasma exchange is used:

- when patients remain very symptomatic despite pyridostigmine and steroid therapy
- to rapidly improve symptoms during crises

Azathioprine is often used as a steroid-sparing agent to reduce long-term steroid use. All immunosuppressive therapies can take several weeks to reach their peak effects.

Surgery

Patients with a thymoma usually have a thymectomy. This procedure leads to clinical improvement or remission, with few adverse effects from the loss of thymic immune function, because the thymus loses much of its function after adolescence.

Prognosis

About 80% of patients develop generalised symptoms within the first year. Most have normal life expectancy and good quality of life if they receive optimal treatment. However, the adverse effects of steroids, including weight gain, cataracts and osteoporosis, can impair quality of life.

Lambert–Eaton myasthenic syndrome

Lambert–Eaton myasthenic syndrome is also an autoimmune neuromuscular junction disease. However, it differs from myasthenia gravis in that the autoantibodies target voltage-gated calcium channels on the presynaptic terminal, where they prevent calcium influx and acetylcholine release. It is also much rarer. About 60% of cases are paraneoplastic and associated with malignancy, especially small-cell lung carcinoma.

Patients present with proximal weakness affecting lower and then upper limbs. Ocular and bulbar muscles are rarely involved.

Management requires symptomatic therapy with 3,4-dipyridamine, a drug that blocks potassium channels at the nerve terminal and prolongs calcium influx and the action potential. Intravenous immunoglobulin and plasma exchange are also often used in resistant cases.

Answers to starter questions

1. Guillain–Barré syndrome is a rare autoimmune syndrome that causes previously fit people to become suddenly dependent on others. They can be completely paralysed and need every bodily function attended to. They are conscious and aware of their surroundings, and often hallucinate from the effects of sleep deprivation and medications.

2. Regeneration in the central nervous system is noticeably poorer than in the peripheral nervous system. This is because inhibitory molecules in the central nervous system prevent axonal growth. These molecules are lacking in the peripheral nervous system. Therefore although recovery from damage can often be frustratingly slow in the peripheral nervous system, it is much quicker than in the central nervous system.

3. Muscle disorders often closely mimic neuropathies and neuromuscular junction disorders, and their diagnosis requires a detailed neuromuscular examination. Neurologists assess and manage muscle disorders alongside geneticists, rheumatologists and other specialists.

Chapter 17
Emergencies

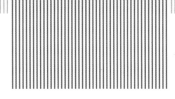

Introduction

In all emergencies, immediate resuscitation and stabilisation are ensured by use of a structured approach to evaluate the patient's ABCDE:

- Airway
- Breathing
- Circulation
- Disability, including neurological status
- Exposure, status of other organ systems (e.g. kidneys, temperature, metabolic and liver)

Once the patient's condition is stabilised, imaging is required to localise pathology and determine definitive management. For intracranial pathology, computerised tomography (CT) of the head rapidly confirms or excludes haemorrhage, obvious space-occupying lesions (e.g. tumour) and hydrocephalus.

When cerebrospinal fluid sampling is required, for example in cases of intracranial infection, CT scanning is mandatory before lumbar puncture. CT excludes any mass lesions that potentially contraindicate lumbar puncture, especially in the presence of focal neurological deficits and signs of increased intracranial pressure.

Rapid referral to neurologists and neurosurgeons is required. Remember: time is brain as the nervous system is highly sensitive to irreversible damage within minutes of suffering an insult, and its capacity of repair and regeneration is limited.

Case 18 Acute onset severe headache

Presentation

A 30-year-old man, Adam Greenspan, presents to the emergency department with a sudden onset headache described as the 'worst of his life'.

Initial interpretation

With headache described as 'the worst ever', or likened to a 'thunderclap' or 'being hit on the head with a sledgehammer', the key diagnosis to exclude is acute subarachnoid haemorrhage secondary to ruptured aneurysm.

History and examination

The headache started suddenly during sexual intercourse this morning and caused Adam to feel nauseous and vomit. The pain has now been ongoing for 2 h. He reports severe neck stiffness. He has no other medical or drug history but is a smoker. Examination shows a right-sided palsy of the oculomotor nerve and dilation of the right pupil.

Further interpretation

Sudden onset severe headache with a third nerve palsy strongly suggests aneurysmal subarachnoid haemorrhage, although other causes remain possible (**Table 17.1**).

> **Sudden onset severe headache** is assumed to be caused by subarachnoid haemorrhage until proven otherwise.

Acute onset severe headache: causes	
Mechanism	Causes
Vascular	Aneurysmal subarachnoid haemorrhage
	Cerebral venous sinus thrombosis
	Carotid or vertebral artery dissection
	Intracerebral haemorrhage [e.g. hypertensive haemorrhage, spontaneous haemorrhage secondary to underlying lesion (tumour, AVM)]
	Giant cell arteritis
Infection	Meningitis
	Encephalitis
	Cerebral abscess
Tumour	Acute haemorrhage into a tumour
	Tumour causing acute hydrocephalic attack (e.g. colloid cyst)
Primary headache syndromes	Migraine
	Acute cluster headache

Table 17.1 Causes of acute onset severe headache. AVM, arterio-venous malformation

Immediate intervention

An emergency CT head scan shows diffuse subarachnoid haemorrhage. CT angiography shows a right posterior communicating artery aneurysm. Adam is prescribed nimodipine, a calcium channel antagonist, to reduce vasospasm, and he undergoes emergency coil embolisation of the aneurysm. After 3 weeks of monitoring for complications, he recovers and is discharged.

Differential diagnoses

The speed of onset usually provides a clue as to the likely aetiology. Headache of sudden onset usually is of vascular origin and the commonest causes are described below.

Subarachnoid haemorrhage

This is the most common life-threatening cause of acute onset severe headache. Red flag signs include:

- 'worst ever headache' description
- onset with exertion (e.g. exercise, straining during defecation and sexual intercourse)
- signs of meningism

The sensitivity of CT is highest on the 1st day after a subarachnoid haemorrhage (95%) and decreases with time (74% on day 3 and 30% on day 14). If the CT scan is normal, lumbar puncture is needed to detect blood breakdown products in the cerebrospinal fluid. These products give the fluid a yellow colour, i.e. xanthochromia (Greek: xanthos, 'yellow'), which confirms subarachnoid haemorrhage (**Figure 17.1**). Definitive management requires neurosurgical and neuroradiological procedures.

Cerebral venous thrombosis

Thrombosis of cerebral veins presents with acute onset headache, focal neurological deficits, increased intracranial pressure or seizures. CT or MRI venography confirms the diagnosis, which should be suspected in any patient with a prothrombotic state. Management comprises anticoagulation and close observation for complications of increased intracranial pressure. Severe intractable increases in intracranial pressure usually requires surgical decompression.

Carotid or vertebral artery dissection

This condition occurs when the internal vessel lining ruptures, thereby precipitating acute thrombosis and infarction. An acute onset Horner's syndrome with headache or neck pain strongly suggests dissection. Urgent CT, MRI and stroke review are needed.

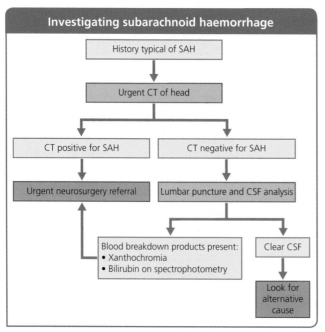

Figure 17.1 Investigation of suspected subarachnoid haemorrhage. CSF, cerebrospinal fluid; CT, computed tomography; SAH, subarachnoid haemorrhage.

Case 19 Sudden focal neurological deficit

Presentation

Joan Atkinson, aged 70 years, presents with acute onset weakness affecting her right face and arm, as well as slurred speech.

Initial interpretation

Sudden onset neurological symptoms strongly suggest an acute vascular event such as ischaemic or haemorrhagic stroke. Mrs Atkinson's presentation fits the FAST criteria for suspected acute stroke:

- Facial drooping
- Arm weakness
- Slurring of speech, necessitating
- Transfer to hospital urgently

History and examination

History and examination enable the stroke syndrome to be classified and its likely cause determined. Mrs Atkinson developed the symptoms 2 h ago. She has dense weakness in her right arm and face, along with expressive dysphasia. She has ischaemic heart disease and peripheral vascular disease, and is a smoker.

With any sudden onset focal neurological deficit, the history is critical in establishing diagnosis. Features that need to be determined include:

- speed of symptom onset (**Table 17.2**)
- level of consciousness
- associated symptoms (e.g. headache, seizures and other neurological deficits)

Immediate intervention

Rapid symptom onset, focal signs of dysfunction in a single arterial territory (in this case the left middle cerebral artery) and history of systemic atherosclerotic

Neurological deficit: causes	
Speed of symptom onset	Causes
Acute (minutes)	Vascular event (ischaemic or haemorrhagic)
	Seizure
	Acute metabolic abnormality [e.g. electrolyte (sodium, calcium, potassium) and glucose (hypo-/hyperglycaemia) abnormalities]
Subacute (minutes to hours)	Migraine
	Demyelination (multiple sclerosis)
Chronic (days to weeks)	Infection (e.g. encephalitis, cerebral abscess)
	Space-occupying pathologies (e.g. tumour, intracerebral abscess)

Table 17.2 Causes of focal neurological deficit

vascular disease all suggest an acute stroke. In ischaemic stroke, thrombolysis is offered if symptom onset was within 3.5 h. Immediate CT head scan is carried out to exclude haemorrhage.

Mrs Atkinson is assessed by the acute stroke team. She is deemed eligible for thrombolysis, given intravenous alteplase and transferred to the stroke ward for further treatment.

> **Stroke is the commonest cause of sudden onset focal neurological deficits.** Thrombolysis can rescue cerebral perfusion and limit the extent of ischaemic injury. It must be administered as soon as possible and is usually only given if the patient presents within 3.5 h of symptom onset.

Differential diagnoses

As with most neurological presentations, the timing of symptom onset is highly suggestive of the likely diagnosis. The acute nature usually is indicative of a vascular aetiology.

Stroke

Strokes arise because of ischaemic infarction or haemorrhage. Urgent CT excludes differential diagnoses contraindicating thrombolysis, i.e. intracranial haemorrhage, tumour and abscesses. However, thrombolysis must be considered when clinical assessment and imaging suggest ischaemic stroke.

It is crucial to establish the timing of symptom onset, because the benefits of thrombolysis are less reliable if administered after 3.5 h of symptom onset, and its risks may exceed benefits beyond this time interval. Mrs Atkinson is transferred to a stroke ward to monitor complications, such as post-reperfusion haemorrhage, and establish the cause, for example arrhythmias and hypertension. Secondary prevention follows, for example with antiplatelet therapy, antihypertensive agents and anticholesterol drugs, as well as rehabilitation.

Case 20 Injuries from a road traffic accident

Presentation

Air ambulance services alert the emergency department that a 25-year-old man is on his way after a road traffic accident. His Glasgow coma scale score is 8/15: E1 (eyes not opening) V2 (verbal response: making incomprehensible sounds) M5 (motor response: localised to pain). His other variables are stable.

Initial interpretation

This is a major trauma alert: acute head injury causing impaired consciousness. A trauma team comprising emergency physicians, trauma surgeons, anaesthetists, trauma nurses and a neurosurgeon are rapidly mobilised to systematically evaluate the patient.

History and examination

The patient is assessed systematically with Advanced Trauma and Life Support (ATLS) protocols. First, his airway, breathing and circulation are stabilised. He has bruising around the eyes and behind the left ear, from which clear fluid is leaking. His left pupil is dilated and unresponsive to light.

The Advanced Trauma Life Support protocol is a systematic evaluation whose use ensures that injuries are not missed during assessment of patients with major trauma. The primary survey is followed to assess and treat dysfunction of the airway, breathing, circulation, neurological system and other major organs, and thereby stabilise acute life-threatening injuries before imaging and definitive treatment.

Further interpretation

This patient has features of basal skull fracture: cerebrospinal fluid leakage from the ear (otorrhea), peri-orbital and retro-mastoid bruising. The dilated left pupil suggests left oculomotor nerve compression from tentorial herniation, probably secondary to severe traumatic brain injury and intracranial haemorrhage.

Immediate intervention

The patient is intubated, ventilated and transferred for trauma CT. The scan shows an extensive acute subdural haemorrhage affecting the left cerebral hemisphere,

Case 20 *continued*

with signs of increased intracranial pressure and herniation (see Figure 3.6). He is given mannitol and hyperventilated to reduce his carbon dioxide level and thereby decrease intracranial pressure. He is then transferred to theatre for emergency evacuation of the acute subdural haemorrhage.

Differential diagnoses

Patients suffering from traumatic injuries require urgent systematic assessment for rapid identification, resuscitation and stabilisation of their injuries. Principles of management of traumatic brain and spinal injury are described below.

Traumatic brain injury

The commonest causes of traumatic brain injury (TBI) are motor vehicle accidents, assaults and falls. It is critical to avoid any episodes of hypoxia and/or hypotension following traumatic brain injury as these can profoundly increase mortality.

The severity of traumatic brain injury is classified by initial Glasgow coma scale score (see Table 2.11):

- A score of 14–15 indicates mild injury
- 9–13 is moderate injury
- 3–8 is severe injury

Urgent neurosurgical treatment is essential in selected cases. Increased intracranial pressure can develop several days after the acute injury; various medical and surgical measures are used to decrease intracranial pressure in this setting (see Table 3.8). Long-term care focuses on neurological rehabilitation.

Acute spinal injury

This type of injury frequently accompanies head trauma. Initial management is immobilisation of the spine to prevent further damage, and urgent CT and MRI (**Figure 17.2**). Subsequent approaches are listed in **Table 17.3**.

Spinal cord compression by haematoma or bone fragments presents with different neurological deficits depending on the level affected. Neurogenic shock is the term for

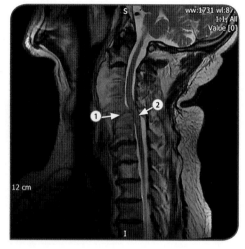

Figure 17.2 Sagittal magnetic resonance imaging of cervical spine, showing C5–6 vertebral body fracture with anterior movement and slip (anterolisthesis) of C5 on C6 ① with cord injury and prevertebral soft tissue swelling. The spinal cord is compressed and there is signal change within it ② representing spinal cord contusion and injury.

sympathetic chain disruption causing loss of blood vessel tone and unopposed parasympathetic activity. It occurs with upper thoracic or lower cervical cord injury. Differentiating this from the more common hypovolaemic shock (shock secondary to blood and circulatory volume loss resulting from haemorrhage), as outlined in **Figure 17.3**, is important as management strategies differ. Failure to recognise neurogenic shock will result in inappropriate treatment and a patient that is inadequately resuscitated with persistent hypotension and poor outcomes.

Spinal cord injuries lead to predictable complications requiring prolonged rehabilitation in specialist spinal injury units (see **Table 17.3**).

Management of acute spinal cord injury

Aim	Example(s)
Prevention of hypoxia and hypotension	Fluid resuscitation and drugs (usually vasopressor agents that increase sympathetic tone with vasoconstriction to offset the effects of neurogenic shock if indicated) to optimise cord perfusion
Decompression of spinal cord	Evacuation of haemorrhage, soft tissues and fragments compressing cord
Stabilisation of fracture	Fixation of spinal fracture to prevent further injury
Prevention of pressure sores	Regular turning and skin care
Prevention of venous thromboembolism	Compression stockings and low molecular weight heparin
Regulation of bowels	Laxatives and stool softeners
Provision of bladder and bowel care	Long-term catheterisation in some cases
Rehabilitation	Physiotherapy and occupational therapy to: decrease muscle contractures improve mobility and help patient adapt to their disability

Table 17.3 Management of acute spinal cord injury

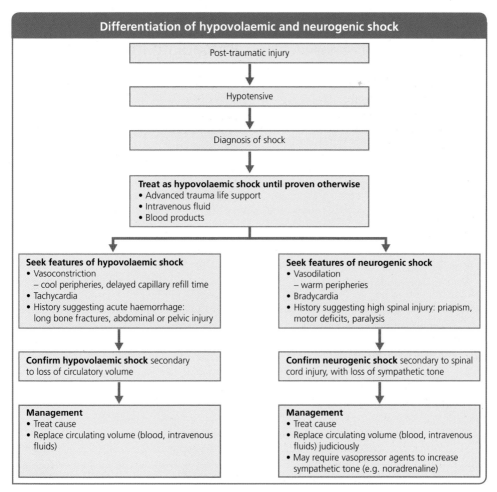

Figure 17.3 Differentiation of hypovolaemic and neurogenic shock.

Case 21 Status epilepticus

Presentation

Paramedics bring 21-year-old Jane Francis to the emergency department. She is having a persistent generalised tonic–clonic seizure. A friend found her convulsing, and the convulsions have not stopped in the 12 min before her arrival at the department.

Initial interpretation

Jane's prolonged seizure warrants rapid assessment and emergency treatment. Establishing the likely cause is crucial; an accurate witness account is urgently required.

> **Patients undergoing seizures must have their condition stabilised by Advanced Life Support protocols.** They need airway protection and/or suctioning as well as high-flow oxygen; also, intravenous access needs to be obtained and samples taken for blood tests, including glucose and electrolyte measurement. Simultaneously, a history should be taken from a witness.

History and examination

The friend states that Jane has generalised epilepsy, for which she takes carbamazepine. He adds that she mentioned having had diarrhoea and vomiting recently.

> **Status epilepticus is a seizure that continues for over 30 min, or over 30 min of recurrent seizures without return of consciousness between them.** Seizures lasting more than few minutes are usually treated in the same way as status epilepticus.

Further interpretation

Jane is having a prolonged generalised tonic–clonic seizure. It will progress to status epilepticus if untreated. Precipitants must be identified and treated along with the seizure:

- systemic or intracranial infection
- non-adherence with anticonvulsant medication
- impaired absorption or effectiveness of medication (in this case from recent diarrhoeal illness and vomiting)
- metabolic derangements
- any intracranial lesion
- drug overdose or withdrawal

Immediate intervention

Most hospitals have their own protocols; **Table 17.4** is a typical example.

Management of status epilepticus	
Principles of treatment	Example(s)
Immediate resuscitation	Advanced Life Support principles for resuscitation
	Recovery position
	Airway, breathing and circulation: assessment and treatment
First line	Intravenous lorazepam (0.5–2 mg over 2 min; repeat to 4–8 mg maximum)
	If no intravenous access, diazepam rectally (0.5 mg/kg, maximum 40 mg) is considered
Second line	Intravenous phenytoin (15–18 mg/kg loading dose at 50 mg/min)
Third line	General anaesthetic (requires intensive care unit support)

Table 17.4 Management of status epilepticus: a typical protocol

Case 21 *continued*

The seizures do not stop, despite the use of first- and second-line medications, so she undergoes general anaesthesia in intensive care. The results of blood tests, cerebrospinal fluid analysis and CT are normal. The event was probably triggered by impaired carbamazepine absorption during Jane's recent gastrointestinal illness. She makes a full recovery after 2 days in the intensive care unit, and is then discharged.

Eclampsia is a differential diagnosis for any pregnant or possibly pregnant woman presenting with seizures. A pregnancy test is required for any woman of child-bearing age whose pregnancy status is unknown. Magnesium infusion and delivery of the baby are required for eclampsia induced seizures in a pregnant patient.

Case 22 Acute neuromuscular paralysis

Presentation

Aisha Kapoor, aged 40 years, presents to the emergency department with progressive limb weakness. It started in her feet 3 days ago and ascended to involve her hips and hands. She cannot stand and has pins and needles in her legs.

Initial interpretation

Subacute progressive motor weakness over a few days suggests an acute neuromuscular syndrome. Acute spinal cord, peripheral nerve, neuromuscular junction and muscular diseases need to be considered. However, the sensory symptoms make a neuromuscular junction or muscular disease less likely.

History and examination

Aisha had diarrhoea 2 weeks ago, and 3 days ago she began tripping over both feet; her legs have since weakened progressively. Today she cannot stand and has developed weakness in both hands. The pins and needles started few days before the weakness and also 'crept up' her legs. She has no cranial nerve, bulbar or respiratory symptoms.

Examination reveals profound flaccid weakness in all four limbs, in multiple peripheral nerve territories, and loss of reflexes and sensation from the feet to the knees. Aisha's bladder and bowels are functioning normally.

Further interpretation and diagnosis

Table 17.5 shows the common causes of acute neuromuscular syndromes. Flaccid, areflexic weakness progressing over a few days along with sensory symptoms is almost certainly an acute polyneuropathy. Sensory involvement is unlikely with muscle and neuromuscular junction pathology. Lower motor neurone signs presenting after several days argue against spinal injury.

The clinical picture and preceding diarrhoea strongly suggest Guillain–Barré syndrome. Aisha has a lumbar puncture to exclude infective causes, and her respiratory function is closely monitored with 4-hourly forced vital capacity measurements. Nerve conduction studies confirm an acute demyelinating polyneuropathy.

Case 22 *continued*

Causes of acute neuromuscular syndromes

Compartment affected	Compartment-specific features	Example(s)
Spinal cord	LMN pattern of weakness initially	Acute spinal cord compression
	Sensory level and sphincter dysfunction (common)	Acute transverse myelitis
	UMN features develop after a few days	Anterior spinal artery syndrome
Anterior horn motor neurone	Flaccid weakness	Infection (e.g. polio virus)
	Wasting	Motor neurone disease
	Fasciculations	
Peripheral nerve	LMN pattern of weakness	Guillain–Barré syndrome
	Reflexes usually depressed or absent	Vasculitic neuropathy
	Autonomic features	Toxin- or drug-induced neuropathy
	Sensory symptoms and signs	
Neuromuscular junction	Fatiguable weakness	Myasthenia gravis
	Reflexes intact	Lambert–Eaton myasthenic syndrome
	Normal sensation	
Muscle	Reflexes intact	Inflammatory myopathy (e.g. polymyositis and dermatomyositis)
	Proximal weakness	
	Pain in muscle at rest	
	Sensation normal	

LMN, lower motor neurone; UMN, upper motor neurone.

Table 17.5 Common causes of acute neuromuscular syndromes

Immediate intervention

Aisha is started on intravenous immunoglobulin. Her condition initially deteriorates, and she requires intubation and ventilation for respiratory failure. However, she makes a full recovery over 4 months.

> **Neurophysiological studies are crucial in distinguishing between nerve, neuromuscular junction and muscle disorders.** The results of such studies help in diagnosis and monitoring response to treatment.

Differential diagnoses

Acute neuromuscular paralysis is a medical emergency. The differential is wide but systematically encompasses spinal cord, peripheral nerve, neuro-muscular junction and muscular pathologies.

The clinical symptoms/signs should aid localisation of the lesion (e.g. absence of sensory symptoms makes the site of pathology most likely to be muscular or neuro-muscular junction).

Spinal cord pathologies

In the acute phase, spinal cord pathologies present with lower motor neurone features: flaccid weakness and depressed reflexes. Acute spinal cord compression (see page 350) requires urgent MRI and is usually caused by metastases or other compressive lesions. Treatment is directed at the cause. Metastatic cord compression, for example, requires steroids and discussion with oncologists and neurosurgeons for radiotherapy and surgical decompression.

Acute transverse myelitis (see page 350) is spinal cord inflammation (**Figure 17.4**). It is another cause of acute (i.e. over hours) to subacute (i.e. days) spinal cord dysfunction. MRI and cerebrospinal fluid analysis confirm diagnosis. Steroids are often given to increase recovery rates.

Spinal cord stroke (see page 359) is rare (1% of strokes). Occlusion of the anterior spinal artery causes dysfunction of the descending motor tracts and ascending tracts carrying pain and temperature sensation, leaving the dorsal columns and therefore proprioception intact. Urgent spine MRI and standard stroke investigations are required.

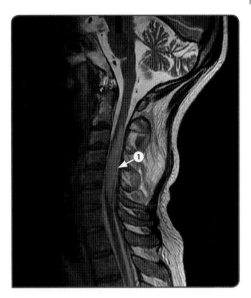

Figure 17.4 Sagittal T2W magnetic resonance image showing long segment cervical cord abnormality of increased signal intensity ①, which is consistent with transverse myelitis.

Anterior horn (motor) neurone pathologies

These pathologies (see page 378) are usually caused by either infection (e.g. poliovirus) or motor neurone disease, but they rarely present acutely. Wasting and fasciculations are typical. Dysphagia, dysarthria and dysphonia are common in motor neurone disease as a consequence of dysfunction of bulbar nuclei (lower cranial nerves IX, X and XII). Clinical assessment by a neurologist and neurophysiological studies confirm diagnosis.

Peripheral nerve pathologies

Guillain-Barré syndrome (see page 427) is the commonest cause of acute flaccid weakness. It is often preceded by respiratory or gastrointestinal infection and usually presents with bilateral motor neuropathy with some sensory involvement. Cerebrospinal fluid analysis after a lumbar puncture shows high protein and a normal cell count. Intravenous immunoglobulin halves the associated disability so is started as soon as possible. Respiratory and bulbar involvement is common, and 25% of patients require admission to an intensive care unit.

Neuromuscular junction pathologies

Myasthenia gravis (see page 438) is the commonest neuromuscular junction disorder; all others are very rare. It usually presents with ocular, ocular–bulbar or generalised (ocular, bulbar and limb) fatiguable weakness. Patients can present with an acute myasthenic crisis, which is often triggered by infection, interacting medications or medication nonadherence. Rarely, patients present with isolated or early respiratory involvement.

Muscle pathologies

Primary muscle disorders (see page 433) very rarely present with acute weakness. They tend to present with a subacute or chronic progressive weakness.

Case 23 Unconsciousness and coma

Presentation

A 42-year-old woman is bought to the emergency department after being discovered unconscious by the roadside. Her Glasgow coma scale score is 3/15: E1 (eyes not opening) V1 (no verbalisation) M1 (no movements).

Initial interpretation

Unconsciousness has numerous causes (**Table 17.6**). In the acute setting, especially in cases of profound coma, the priorities are resuscitation and stabilisation, with simultaneous identification and treatment of reversible causes.

History and examination

There are no witnesses to provide a history. The patient is hypertensive and bradycardic, with disordered breathing. She is unkempt, smells of alcohol and has no signs of trauma. Her pupils are normal sized and react to light. She is hypoglycaemic and jaundiced. Arterial blood gases show no electrolyte or acid–base disturbance.

Witnesses are not always available to provide a history for an unconscious patient. A meticulous head-to-toe assessment is needed. Arterial blood gases and glucose blood tests give vital clues regarding possible reversible causes such as hypoglycaemia and electrolyte or acid–base disturbances.

Immediate intervention and diagnosis

The patient is resuscitated and given intravenous thiamine and B vitamins, because the signs of alcohol abuse suggest nutritional depletion. She then receives intramuscular glucagon and glucose to reverse her hypoglycaemia. She is intubated and ventilated for airway protection. The jaundice suggests liver dysfunction, possibly from alcohol excess. Samples are taken for

Causes of coma	
Site of derangement	Causes
Systemic	Drugs and toxins (e.g. overdose of opiate, tricyclic antidepressant or barbiturate, or alcohol withdrawal)
	Metabolic derangement: high or low sodium, glucose, calcium and potassium (e.g. in renal failure, liver failure and thyroid dysfunction)
	Cardiovascular (e.g. myocardial infarction and aortic dissection)
	Respiratory (e.g. pulmonary embolism)
	Trauma (e.g. assault and road traffic accident)
	Infection (e.g. severe sepsis)
Neurological	Trauma (e.g. acute subdural haemorrhage and acute extradural haemorrhage)
	Vascular (e.g. stroke, subarachnoid haemorrhage and subdural haemorrhage)
	Infection (e.g. meningitis, encephalitis and cerebral abscess)
	Hydrocephalus (e.g. acute obstruction by a tumour)
	Seizures (e.g. status epilepticus and post-seizure drowsiness)

Table 17.6 Causes of coma

Case 23 *continued*

coagulation, infection and toxicology blood studies.

Urgent CT of the head is arranged, because the hypertension, bradycardia and altered breathing (Cushing's reflex) are signs of brain stem compression. The scan shows acute cerebellar haemorrhage with acute hydrocephalus (**Figure 17.5**).

The patient's coagulopathy is corrected. She undergoes emergency decompressive surgery and haematoma evacuation, with cerebrospinal fluid diversion to treat the hydrocephalus. After a prolonged stay in intensive care, she makes a slow recovery and is referred to the liver team to manage an underlying liver dysfunction from alcohol abuse.

> **A systemic examination is essential to identify all possible reversible causes of unconsciousness.** There may be multiple concomitant causes.

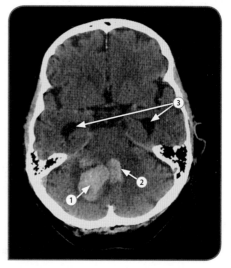

Figure 17.5 Computerised tomography scan of the brain, showing acute cerebellar haemorrhage ① with compressed 4th ventricle (not visible as almost completely effaced by haemorrhage) ② and dilated temporal horns of lateral ventricles ③. These findings suggest obstructive hydrocephalus with associated increased intracranial pressure.

Case 24 Fever and confusion

Presentation

Peter Kinkade, 65 years of age, attends the emergency department with a 1-week history of confusion, fever and possible seizures.

Initial interpretation

An intracranial or systemic illness can cause confusion and seizures. Fever and new seizures make central nervous system infection highly likely.

History and examination

Mr Kinkade is normally fit and well. However, 2 weeks ago he developed fever and swollen glands. He was behaving bizarrely for 7 days: forgetting where he was and not recognising family members. Today he had seizures, precipitating his hospital attendance.

On examination, he is awake but drowsy and confused. He has no focal neurological signs but does not follow commands. He has no rashes, neck stiffness or papilloedema.

Further interpretation

The differential diagnosis is wide and includes all possible causes of acute confusion. But the fever, confusion, new seizure and swollen lymph nodes make an intracranial infection such as encephalitis, cerebral abscess or meningitis highly likely.

Case 24 *continued*

Immediate intervention

Blood is drawn for infection screening: cultures, blood films, viral serology and inflammatory markers. Contrast-enhanced CT of the head shows changes in both temporal lobes. Viral encephalitis is suspected; he undergoes a lumbar puncture and is empirically started on intravenous aciclovir. The cerebrospinal fluid has increased lymphocyte count and protein, and the result of polymerase chain reaction analysis for herpes simplex virus is positive. Mr Kinkade is also started on anticonvulsants, given his previous seizure.

After 2 weeks of treatment, he undergoes a repeat lumbar puncture and cerebrospinal fluid analysis shows clearance of the virus. He makes a gradual recovery over the next 4 months.

Differential diagnoses

Intracranial infection can become rapidly life-threatening if not recognised early. On suspicion of any intracranial infection, empirical treatment with anti-microbials must be initiated rapidly.

Encephalitis

The cause of encephalitis is usually viral (e.g. herpes simplex type 1 and 2, and arboviruses) or non-viral (e.g. tuberculosis). It should be suspected in any patient with fever, confusion, altered behaviour and focal neurology. If the condition is untreated, mortality is nearly 80%. Therefore empirical treatment with intravenous aciclovir is given, pending the results of cerebrospinal fluid analysis.

Cerebral abscess

This is suspected in any patient with signs of increased intracranial pressure, focal neurological deficits and fever, especially in the presence of risk factors such as recent neurosurgical intervention; ear, nose or throat infection; endocarditis; and pulmonary bronchiectasis. Patients with immune suppression may have unusual organisms (e.g. *Toxoplasma* species, parasites and fungi), as well as very subtle symptoms and signs. Imaging shows ring-enhancing lesions (**Figure 17.6**). Urgent

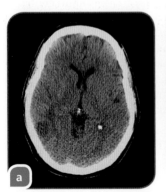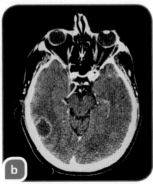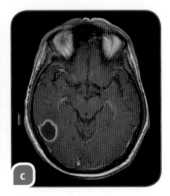

Figure 17.6 (a) Unenhanced and (b) contrast-enhanced computerised tomography scan showing an acute ring-enhancing lesion in the right temporal lobe. The clinical history of fever, confusion and increased inflammatory markers made abscess the most likely clinical and radiological diagnosis. (c) T1-weighted post-gadolinium contrast-enhanced magnetic resonance imaging scan showing the right ring-enhancing temporal lobe lesion.

neurosurgical assessment is mandated for definitive treatment.

Meningitis

Headache, fever and photophobia are considered bacterial meningitis until proven otherwise. Patients may have sepsis and a purpuric rash. Empirical treatment with antibiotics, for example benzylpenicillin or ceftriaxone, is started immediately when meningitis is suspected.

Cerebrospinal fluid analysis confirms the diagnosis. Imaging is often required first to exclude a mass lesion. Prophylaxis may be needed for close contacts.

Case 25 Increased intracranial pressure

Presentation

Gemma Ford, a 29-year-old woman, attends the emergency department with persistent early morning headaches, vomiting and blurred vision.

Initial interpretation

This triad of symptoms suggests increased intracranial pressure. Visual blurring suggests optic nerve compression, and the threat of visual loss warrants emergency admission and investigation.

History and examination

Gemma had been fit and well. Her headaches started 2 months ago. They are worse in the morning and with straining, bending and coughing. She feels nauseated intermittently. Vision in her right eye has become blurry over the past week.

On examination, she has no focal neurological deficits, is alert and oriented, and has bilateral papilloedema. There is nothing else of significance in her medical and drug history.

> **The optic nerve can be damaged by direct compression resulting from increased intracranial pressure.** The nerve may be compressed by:
>
> ■ an intracranial space-occupying lesion (e.g. pituitary tumour)
>
> ■ the generalised increase in intracranial pressure (e.g. from acute hydrocephalus)
>
> Compression causes ischaemia of the nerve by reducing arterial perfusion and impairing venous drainage.

Initial interpretation

The semiology of the headache together with blurring of vision suggests that Gemma's intracranial pressure is increased. Anything that increases intracranial volume can increase intracranial pressure (**Table 17.7**; see page 190) and all causes can have potentially grave sequelae if not diagnosed and appropriately treated.

Case 25 *continued*

Causes of increased intracranial pressure	
Aetiology	**Examples**
Increased cerebrospinal fluid	Hydrocephalus
	Impaired cerebrospinal fluid drainage (space-occupying lesion, meningitis and subarachnoid haemorrhage) or increased production (rare)
	Idiopathic intracranial hypertension
Space-occupying lesion	Tumours
	Cerebral abscess
	Cerebral oedema (e.g. trauma, stroke and infection)
	Vascular causes (e.g. aneurysm)
Increased cerebral blood volume	Intracranial haemorrhage
	Obstruction to venous outflow (e.g. cerebral venous sinus thrombosis)

Table 17.7 Causes of increased intracranial pressure (see Table 3.2)

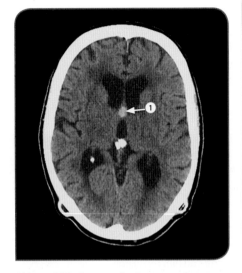

Figure 17.7 Computerised tomography scan showing acute hydrocephalus caused by colloid cyst (the hyperdense circular structure) in the roof of the 3rd ventricle ①.

Immediate intervention

An urgent CT scan shows acute hydrocephalus caused by a colloid cyst lying in the roof of the 3rd ventricle (**Figure 17.7**).

Urgent ophthalmological assessment is arranged to formally assess visual acuity and visual fields and to confirm the papilloedema. Gemma undergoes operative removal of the colloid cyst. The hydrocephalus resolves, and 2 weeks later a repeat ophthalmological assessment confirms improvement in her visual acuity and resolution of papilloedema.

> The level of symptoms of increased intracranial pressure depends on how well the body is compensating for it. Chronic causes give the body time to adapt. However, acute presentations, such as acute hydrocephalus, can cause rapid deterioration, loss of consciousness and Cushing's reflex (hypertension, bradycardia and altered respiration).

Case 26 Cauda equina syndrome

Presentation

Joshua Cook, aged 25 years, presents with back and bilateral lower limb pain along with difficulty passing urine and altered perineal sensation.

Initial interpretation

The main diagnosis to consider is cauda equina syndrome (see page 356), which can feature:

Case 26 *continued*

- low back pain or sciatica
- bladder or bowel dysfunction
- motor or sensory deficits in lower limbs
- sensory dysfunction in the perineal region

Not all are necessarily present, but the key features are sphincter disturbance and altered perineal sensation.

History and examination

Joshua was lifting weights in the gym 2 weeks ago when he developed acute onset severe back pain. This eventually settled with painkillers, but over the past 24 hours he noticed difficulty voiding urine and could not feel the toilet paper after defecating. He has no motor weakness but has pain in both S1 dermatomes. Sciatic stretch test is positive bilaterally at 30°. He has no perineal pain sensation. He has preserved anal tone and sphincter contraction. The clinical diagnosis is cauda equina syndrome.

Differential diagnosis

The most common cause of compression of the cauda equina is a posteriorly prolapsed lumbar intervertebral disc. The history of straining, back pain and examination findings make this likely. Other causes include vascular (e.g. post-operative haematoma), tumour, degenerative and traumatic aetiologies.

Immediate intervention

Cauda equina syndrome is an emergency. MRI is required to exclude a compressive lesion. Joshua's spine MRI showed a large disc prolapse compressing the cauda equina (see Figure 11.8). He had emergency decompressive spinal surgery to remove the disc and relieve the compression.

> **Imaging and surgery must be done as quickly as possible in cauda equina syndrome.** A delay in diagnosis or treatment leads to poor recovery, has devastating consequences for the patient and leads to litigation.

Chapter 18
Integrated care

Starter questions

Answers to the following questions are on page 466.

1. Why might patients with chronic conditions be frustrated with the continuity of their care?
2. Are long-term conditions managed better in hospitals or in the community?

Introduction

Many neurological conditions require regular support from physicians, specialist nurses, physiotherapists, occupational therapists, speech and language therapists, dieticians, psychologists and others. Much of this care occurs in the outpatient setting and helps patients remain as independent as possible.

For some conditions, such as multiple sclerosis, epilepsy and motor neurone disease, many hospitals have specialist nursing services which patients can contact directly.

Many patients who have chronic neurological conditions see their neurologists only infrequently. The bulk of their long-term 'hands on' care is provided by a combination of their family, friends, physiotherapists, occupational therapists, specialist nurses and general practitioner.

Case 27 Caring for a stroke patient

Presentation

Stanley Cuthbert, aged 80 years, was admitted to hospital 3 months ago with a large infarction in the non-dominant hemisphere middle cerebral artery territory. At first, he was hemiparetic, dyspraxic, dysphagic and disoriented. Hospital staff thought he might not survive the stroke. However, after a few weeks his condition began to improve, and he began to regain some speech and movement on his affected side.

Case 27 *continued*

Initial interpretation

Many elderly patients do not survive the acute period after a major stroke; pulmonary emboli, sepsis and myocardial infarction are common life-ending events. Mr Cuthbert had a major stroke, which left him initially very disabled and highly dependent on nursing care.

History

In the first few weeks after his stroke, Mr Cuthbert remained bedbound, with minimal ability to communicate. He required treatment for aspiration pneumonia. His attending physicians felt that he was likely to die. Therefore, after discussion with his family, the decisions were made not to resuscitate him if he experienced a cardiac arrest and not to start artificial feeding through a nasogastric tube. Antibiotics and fluids continued to be given.

Mr Cuthbert survived this period and began to communicate and make more movements with his affected side.

Interpretation of history

Large hemispheric strokes have a poor prognosis but it is difficult to predict which patients will survive. There are difficult decisions for patients, families and physicians to make about what level of intervention is appropriate for individual patients, especially if elderly and frail.

Mr Cuthbert was given simple supportive measures, including antibiotics, that were not invasive or distressing. On improving after the initial post-stroke period, further review of the treatment plan is required.

Further history

Because Mr Cuthbert has made some recovery, his family and physicians decide to involve physiotherapists, occupational therapists and dieticians in his care and start rehabilitation to maximise his recovery. As his stroke was non-dominant it is more likely that meaningful communication will be regained. Nasogastric feeding is initiated to provide nutritional support.

Progress

After spending several months working with his therapists, Mr Cuthbert regains good language function, his swallowing returns to normal and he resumes a normal diet. His mobility is slow to improve, but he is able to sit in a chair and take a few steps with a walking frame and some support from an assistant.

Further rehabilitation

In view of Mr Cuthbert's improvements, the team decides to offer an extended period of rehabilitation until his recovery plateaus. He remains on the ward for another month, becoming able to use the walking frame on his own. He remains dependent on some help for activities such as washing and toileting.

Long-term living

The physicians, nursing staff, physiotherapists, occupational therapists and speech and language therapists meet with Mr Cuthbert and his family. His daily needs are discussed and joint decisions are made on physical adjustments to his house and to allow him to go home for a trial period.

Mr Cuthbert's family arrange to have a downstairs bathroom installed. He will need carers to help him dress and bathe in the morning and go to bed, but his large family is available to provide support with most other tasks during the day.

Outcome

With adaptations to his house, family support and daily help from carers, Mr Cuthbert manages to live at home.

Case 27 *continued*

A week after after discharge, he attends the outpatient stroke clinic to review progress and identify and address any difficulties.

He receives outpatient physiotherapy for a few months until his therapists feel that no further progress is likely to be achieved.

Stroke

Patients have complex care needs, from urgent assessment and treatment through to rehabilitation and rehousing (**Figure 18.1**). Most stroke patients require frequent long-term multidisciplinary follow-up and care, including risk factor reduction to prevent future strokes (**Table 18.1**).

Public health campaigns

Public health campaigns, such as the UK's Act FAST campaign, highlights the core features of acute stroke and the importance of rapid treatment.

- Face: facial weakness
- Arm: limb weakness
- Speech: speech problems
- Time: call ambulance

The aim is to help the public recognise these symptoms and to seek medical attention immediately.

Immediate management

Chapter 6 outlines the immediate management of stroke.

Rehabilitation

Care from specialist nurses, physiotherapists, occupational therapists and other staff in dedicated stroke units reduces stroke mortality and morbidity.

Community stroke teams comprise stroke nurses, physiotherapists, occupational therapists and speech and language therapists who

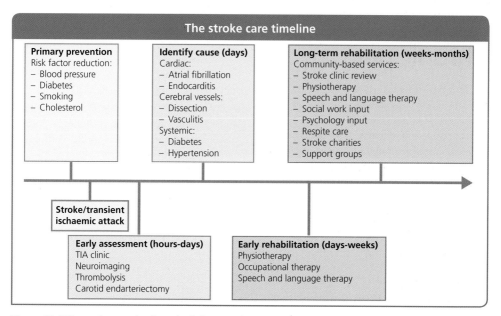

Figure 18.1 The stroke care timeline. The full range of stroke management begins and ends in the community.

Treatments for reducing risk factors for stroke		
Treatment target	Role	Intervention(s)
Blood pressure	Primary and secondary prevention	Lifestyle changes
		Medication
Blood glucose	Strict control of chronic hyperglycaemia in patients with diabetes	Lifestyle changes
		Oral medications
		Insulin
Atrial fibrillation	Reduction of embolic stroke risk	Oral anticoagulation
Cholesterol	Primary and secondary prevention	Lifestyle changes
		Statins
Platelets	Primary and secondary prevention of ischaemic stroke	Aspirin
		Clopidogrel
Acute thrombus	Restoration of arterial blood flow in acute setting	Thrombolysis
		Thrombectomy
Severely stenosed carotid artery	Prevention of further occlusion or embolism from unstable plaque	Carotid endarterectomy

Table 18.1 Established treatments for reducing risk factors for stroke

visit patients at home. They provide ongoing rehabilitation support and continuity of care.

Many charities, such as the Stroke Association, and Different Strokes in the UK, support people who have had a stroke. They provide practical advice, respite care, information and connections to networks of people who have experienced similar illnesses.

> **Stroke management is tailored to meet the needs of the individual patient.** Each stroke is different, with different consequences in the context of each patient's life.

Chronic pain

Chronic pain affects 8–10% of adults in the UK and up to 20% worldwide, and is associated with significant long-term disability, depression, anxiety and low quality of life. The condition has a wide range of causes, including bone pain from bony cancer metastases and neuropathic pain from diabetic neuropathy.

The focus in this chapter is neuropathic pain. This is chronic pain arising from damage to the nervous system. It affects up to 1 in 4 patients with diabetes and 1 in 5 with shingles.

Aetiology

Disease processes causing neuropathic pain can be split broadly into peripheral and central causes.

Peripheral neuropathic pain

Peripheral causes of neuropathic pain include any type of damage to peripheral nerves, cranial nerves and spinal roots. Commoner causes include:

- diabetes
- shingles
- traumatic or post-surgical neuropathies

Central neuropathic pain

Damage to the spinothalamic and cortical pathways anywhere from the spinal cord to the sensory cortex can cause central neuropathic pain. Central causes include:

- stroke

- traumatic spinal cord injury
- multiple sclerosis
- any other disease process that affects the central nervous system

Pathogenesis

Damage to peripheral fibres results in a host of pathological adaptations (**Figure 18.2**). These include the spontaneous discharge of pain fibres and the up-regulation of neurotransmitter release and receptor activation.

Central injury often disrupts descending inhibitory pathways, thereby increasing pain.

Clinical features

There is no gold standard test to diagnose neuropathic pain. In clinical practice, much information is gained from the history and description of the nature of the pain.

Neuropathic pain is often:

- spontaneous (occurring in the absence of stimuli)
- evoked (occurring with stimuli that are normally non-painful)
- shooting, stabbing, lancinating or burning

Management

Pain management is holistic: it addresses psychological, physiological, emotional, social and spiritual factors. A specialist pain service or palliative care service is the most effective way to manage long term neuropathic pain disorders.

The perception of pain may be heightened by unresolved personal problems. This aspect of pain is not intuitive to some patients. However, they can be helped by introducing this concept while also providing medical treatment. For other patients, pain perception is

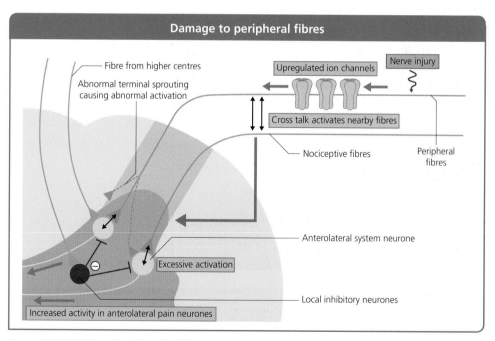

Figure 18.2 Multiple molecular and cellular changes mediate excess pain signalling into the spinal cord, within the spinal cord or by disinhibiting descending control of pain pathways. Peripheral nerve fibres carrying pain information synapse in the dorsal horn of the spinal cord. Local interneurones and descending fibres modulate the signalling and control the pain signals ascending in the anterolateral system. Injury to the nervous system results in upregulation of ion channels, excess activation and terminal sprouting of peripheral pain fibres. The excess electrical activity can trigger spontaneous activity in nearby 'normal' pain fibres and together lead to increased pain signalling in the dorsal horn of the spinal cord.

exacerbated by the fear and anticipation of pain, which leads to a vicious cycle. Educating patients about this psychological effect can empower them to control their own pain by dealing with their anxiety.

> Patients often misinterpret attempts to address non-physical aspects of their pain as dismissal of pain as purely psychological. Explanation of the pain–depression/anxiety–pain cycle is needed to help them engage in addressing this aspect.

Medication

Medication should be initiated with clear goals (**Figure 18.3**):

- reduction of pain but possibly not its elimination
- improvement in mobility or quality of life
- minimisation of adverse effects

Medications commonly used to treat neuropathic pain are listed in **Table 18.2**.

Neuropathic pain medications

Order	Medications	Adjuvant therapy or therapies
First line	Amitriptyline Gabapentin	Paracetamol (acetominophen) Transcutaneous electrical nerve stimulation Acupuncture
Second line	Capsaicin Lidocaine patch Duloxetine Opioids	Referral to pain clinic Multiple medications
Third line	Opioids Ketamine	Referral to palliative care team

Table 18.2 Medications commonly used to treat neuropathic pain

Tricyclic antidepressants

Amitriptyline is well-established as an effective first-line agent for neuropathic pain. It can cause sedation, but this effect can help

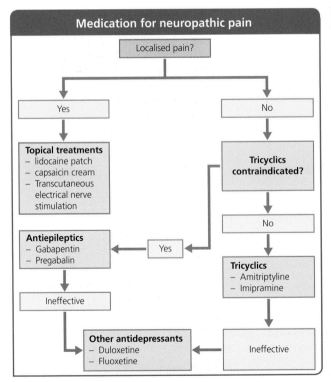

Figure 18.3 Approach to selecting medications for neuropathic pain.

Medication for neuropathic pain

Localised pain?

Yes — No

Topical treatments
- lidocaine patch
- capsaicin cream
- Transcutaneous electrical nerve stimulation

Tricyclics contraindicated?

No

Antiepileptics
- Gabapentin
- Pregabalin

Yes

Tricyclics
- Amitriptyline
- Imipramine

Ineffective

Ineffective

Other antidepressants
- Duloxetine
- Fluoxetine

patients with poor sleep. Amitriptyline commonly causes a dry mouth.

Antiepileptic drugs

Gabapentin or pregabalin is as effective as amitriptyline.

Opioid analgesics

Tramadol, morphine and oxycodone can be used as additional therapy. They have synergistic actions with amitriptyline and gabapentin, and therefore allow lower effective doses of these drugs.

Adjuvant therapy

Paracetamol (acetaminophen), acupuncture and transcutaneous electrical stimulation can be added to treatment at any stage. These adjuvant therapies often enable the use of lower doses of medications.

Long-term support for chronic neurological conditions

Many neurological conditions are lifelong, and some patients develop disability and other medical complications over time. These patients require:

- ready access to expert outpatient care
- support from community rehabilitation teams
- access to in-patient care or rehabilitation services

For patients in the terminal phase of an illness, sensitive planning and high-quality palliative care are essential.

There is no single long-term care pathway. Different conditions require a focus on different areas for different patients at different stages of their illness. The following sections outline key areas of long-term management.

Outpatient care

Regular clinic review by a neurologist or specialist nurse allows early identification of:

- any change in clinical condition (e.g. relapse, progression or indeed improvement)
- adverse effects of medication
- treatment failure

Specialist nurses often see patients in clinics, in parallel with consultants. These nurses also offer a readily accessible point of telephone or e-mail contact, and can explain common symptoms and address any patient concerns or problems.

Community teams

Specialist nurses also often act as a vital link between patients and community services. Many patients with a neurological condition require long-term support from:

- **speech and language therapists,** to manage dysphagia, dysarthria and dysphasia
- **occupational therapists,** to offer adaptations to home and work environments
- **physiotherapists,** to treat spasticity, improve balance and mobility, etc.
- **social workers,** to help with access to welfare benefits, funding for housing adaptations, etc.
- **psychologists,** to treat cognitive impairments, associated mood or psychiatric disturbances, etc.

Much of this can be provided without hospital admission, through home visits, day hospital facilities or charitable organisations.

In-patient care

Patients may have significant relapses (e.g. in MS), exacerbations (e.g. in myasthenia gravis and treatment-resistant epilepsy) or deteriorations (e.g. in motor neurone disease). In these cases, in-patient care is required.

Most neurology units have short stay wards to which patients are admitted for a few days for investigations or treatments such as:

- lumbar puncture

- intravenous immunoglobulin or plasma exchange (e.g. for chronic inflammatory demyelinating polyneuropathy and myasthenia gravis)
- natalizumab infusions (monthly infusions for patients with relapsing MS)
- intravenous caffeine, aspirin or dihydroergotamine (for certain types of treatment-resistant headache)

Only a small proportion of patients with a neurological condition require longer in-patient admission. They are usually severely ill, with rarer or undiagnosed conditions, or they require very urgent specialist treatment or investigations. Examples of conditions requiring in-patient admission are:

- autoimmune encephalitis
- Creutzfeldt–Jakob disease
- Guillain–Barré syndrome
- severe exacerbation of myasthenia gravis
- severely disabling functional illness

Rehabilitation

For patients with significant disability and the potential to regain function or to adapt to their disability, a period of in-patient admission to a specialist rehabilitation unit improves outcomes and the likelihood of functional independence. These patients typically have:

- extended and intensive help from physiotherapists and occupational therapists
- rehabilitation consultants with expertise in physical rehabilitation, spasticity, bladder and bowel problems, etc.
- support from clinical psychologists

Palliative care

For patients entering the terminal phase of illness, palliative care physicians and nurses help ease symptoms such as pain, vomiting, depression, anxiety and breathlessness.

For many neurological conditions, the terminal phase is predictable or becomes readily apparent, with plenty of time to discuss end-of-life care with patients and their families. Decisions about the type and extent of interventions, the place of death and other final wishes should be actively addressed and clarified with patients and their families.

Patients with chronic conditions often suffer from depression or anxiety. These may result directly from the illness, traumatic experiences or the loss of function and participation in life. Good psychological support is essential.

Answers to starter questions

1. Chronic conditions may require a range of types of specialist support. However, this entails having to deal with many different health care professionals, which can be overwhelming for patients and create a sense of being passed back and forth, without a focus to their care.

2. For most patients, long-term care requires management both in hospital and in the community. Specialised diagnostic services or consultations require attendance at outpatient clinics or admission to hospital. However, maximising the amount of care provided at home or at local centres is crucial to enable patients to remain as independent as possible.

Chapter 19
Self-assessment

SBA questions

Raised intracranial pressure and head injury

1. A 24-year-old man is hit by a car during a road traffic accident. He is unconscious with bleeding from an open scalp laceration. He has a compound open fracture in his left leg.
What is the single most appropriate next action?

A Call the on-call neurosurgeon for a review
B Immediate neurological examination, including GCS
C Perform primary assessment of the patient's ABCDE as per ATLS protocols
D Prescribe a dose of mannitol (0.5g/kg)
E Urgent CT brain scan

2. A 40-year-old woman is assaulted while walking home from work. She has a GCS of 8 (E1, V2, M5). Her right pupil is dilated and unresponsive to light. She is resuscitated, stabilised and transferred for an emergency CT brain scan. Her CT shows a right-sided, crescent-shaped hyper-dense collection.
What is the single most appropriate statement regarding her condition?

A Mild extradural haematoma
B Mild chronic subdural haematoma
C Severe acute subdural haematoma
D Severe chronic subdural haematoma
E Severe extradural haematoma

3. A 30-year-old woman has hit her head on the pavement following a fall. She has a short period of loss of consciousness after which she is well with GCS of 15. 2 hours later she starts vomiting and collapses.

What is the single most likely cause of these symptoms?

A Acute subdural haematoma
B Chronic subdural haematoma
C Intracerebral haematoma
D Extradural haematoma
E Hydrocephalus

4. A 56-year old man is in the intensive care unit following a road traffic accident. His brain CT scan shows some contusions in both frontal lobes. The on-call neurosurgeon is concerned about raised intracranial pressure.
What is the single next best step?

A Decrease CO_2 level by increasing ventilation rate
B Increase CO_2 level by decreasing ventilation rate
C Increase core body temperature with a warming device
D Place him in the 'head down' position
E Start corticosteroids infusion

5. A 78-year-old man is drowsy. His GCS is 10 (E3, V2, M5). He had a fall 3 weeks ago. He is on warfarin for atrial fibrillation. His brain CT scan shows a significant chronic subdural haematoma (CSDH). The neurosurgeon decides to operate.
What is the single best next step?

A Observe the patient
B Operate on the patient immediately
C Stop warfarin and observe the patient
D Stop warfarin, give 2 units of platelets and operate
E Stop warfarin, give vitamin K and clotting factors, and operate

Headache and pain syndromes

1. A 40-year-old man has developed unilateral retro-orbital stabbing pain. He has ipsilateral eye watering, nasal stuffiness and ptosis. The pain is very severe and he is restless and pacing around the ward.
What is the single best initial treatment plan?

A High flow oxygen and oral triptan
B High flow oxygen and subcutaneous triptan
C Paracetamol and NSAID
D Paracetamol, NSAID and antiemetic
E Paracetamol, NSAID and morphine

2. A 29-year-old woman has unilateral throbbing headaches associated with nausea and mild photophobia. They occur once per month around her period and she sleeps them off in a dark room. She has not tried any medications. She wants to get pregnant in the future.
Which is the single best initial treatment plan?

A 900 mg aspirin, 10 mg domperidone during acute attack, no prophylactic treatment
B 900 mg aspirin, 10 mg domperidone during acute attack, propranolol
C 900 mg aspirin, 10 mg domperidone during acute attack, topiramate
D 1000 mg paracetamol, 30 mg dihydrocodeine during acute attack, no prophylactic treatment
E 1000 mg paracetamol, 30 mg dihydrocodeine during acute attack, propranolol

3. A 32 year old woman has a severe left-sided headache that came on suddenly and reached its peak within 10 seconds. She is apyrexial, vomiting and photophobic.
What is the single best initial investigation?

A CT brain with contrast
B Lumbar puncture
C MRI brain
D MRI brain with contrast
E Plain CT brain

4. A 63-year-old woman has new persistent dull headaches, worse in the morning and on coughing, over the last 2 months. She has a history of breast cancer.
Which is the single best management option?

A Reassure her
B Refer to breast surgeon
C Routine referral to neurology outpatient clinic
D Urgent referral to neurology headache clinic
E Start treatment with high dose NSAIDs and Domperidone

5. A 21-year-old overweight woman has 2 months of increasing frontal throbbing headaches. They are worse on lying down and coughing. She has markedly reduced peripheral vision. A CT head and CT venogram are normal. Lumbar puncture shows a very high opening pressure of 42 cm of water.
What is the single best initial action?

A Analgesia and outpatient review
B Insert lumbar-peritoneal(LP)shunt
C MRI to identify any malignancy
D Repeat lumbar punctures to reduce intracranial pressure
E Start acetazolamide

6. A 34-year-old pregnant woman with a recent diagnosis of sinusitis has a fever and severe right-sided headache which is worse on straining. She is vomiting and has had a generalised tonic-clonic seizure.
What is the single most appropriate initial management plan?

A Check for proteinuria and hypertension
B CT venogram
C Lumbar puncture and antibiotics
D MRI head
E Observe and refer to first seizure clinic

Seizures

1. A 26-year-old woman is out shopping with her family when they notice her left arm and leg shaking. This continues for 2 minutes after which it stops spontaneously. She has no recollection of the event.
Which is the single best description of her seizure type?

A Complex partial
B Complex partial with secondary generalisation
C Generalised
D Simple partial
E Status epilepticus

2. A 44-year-old man is referred for investigation of his seizures. He describes suddenly waking up in the night with a sense of fear. He then has a funny 'metallic' taste in his mouth and hears unknown voices talking to him. The symptoms stop within a few minutes.
What is the single most likely site of origin for this seizure?

A Frontal lobe
B Occipital lobe
C Parietal lobe
D Pituitary gland
E Temporal lobe

3. A 19-year-old man has a recent diagnosis of epilepsy. He has several episodes during the day where he seems to 'lose focus and forget where he is', stopping talking and staring into space. He promptly recovers in 10–15 seconds. His EEG shows 3 Hz symmetrical spike-and-wave complexes in all leads.
What is the single best description of his seizure type?

A Complex partial
B Complex partial with secondary generalisation
C Generalised
D Simple partial
E Status epilepticus

4. A 30-year-old woman is newly diagnosed with epilepsy and her neurologist wants to start her on an anti-epileptic drug. She suffers from complex partial seizures. She is planning on becoming pregnant in the near future.
What is the single most appropriate antiepileptic medication?

A Carbamazepine
B Clobazam
C Lamotrigine
D Lamotrigine and levetiracetam
E Sodium valproate

5. A 21-year-old man is newly diagnosed with epilepsy. His neurologist is planning on starting an antiepileptic drug. He suffers from sudden shock-like involuntary jerking movements of his arms and legs.
What single drug is most likely to exacerbate this type of jerking and should be avoided?

A Carbamazepine
B Lamotrigine
C Levetiracetam
D Sodium valproate
E Topiramate

6. A 29-year old woman has been in seizure persistently for 10 minutes without regaining consciousness. She has no history of seizures. She is resuscitated and placed in the recovery position. No drugs have been administered. The seizures continue.
What is the single most appropriate next step?

A Give carbamazepine
B Give IV lorazepam
C Start magnesium sulphate infusion
D Start phenytoin infusion
E Transfer to the intensive care unit for intubation and ventilation

Neurovascular disease

1. A 58-year-old woman develops acute-onset weakness in the right side of her face and right arm with slurring of speech. She is assessed within 90 minutes of symptom onset and deemed a candidate for thrombolysis.
What is the single most appropriate next action?

A Alteplase infusion (0.9 mg/kg dose)
B Aspirin 300 mg immediately
C CT brain
D MRI brain
E Therapeutic dose LMWH infusion (1.5 mg/kg dose)

2. A 65-year-old man has left arm and face weakness with left-sided homonymous hemianopia. There are no other neurological deficits. The stroke physician diagnoses a stroke.
What is the single best description of his stroke according to the Oxford classification?

A Lacunar stroke
B Partial anterior circulation stroke (PACS)
C Posterior circulation stroke
D Total anterior circulation stroke (TACS)
E Weber's syndrome

3. A 49-year-old man has vertigo and difficulty swallowing. He is ataxic on the right side with right-sided Horner's syndrome. He has loss of pain and temperature sensation on the right side of his face and the left side of his body.
What is the single most likely vessel affected?

A Anterior cerebral artery
B Anterior communicating artery
C Middle cerebral artery
D Posterior cerebral artery
E Posterior inferior cerebellar artery

4. A 30-year-old woman had a sudden onset headache while having sexual intercourse 1 hour ago. She describes it as the worst headache of her life. She is GCS 15 with neck stiffness and photophobia. Her CT brain is normal.
What is the single next most appropriate course of action?

A Give analgesia, discharge and advise to return if symptoms worsen
B Perform cerebral angiography (digital subtraction angiogram)
C Perform lumbar puncture 6–12 hours after onset of symptoms
D Prescribe immediate IV antibiotics
E Repeat CT brain in 2 hours and discharge if normal

5. A 21-year-old man has a subarachnoid haemorrhage. His GCS is 13 (E3 V4 M6) with weakness in his left arm. A CT angiogram confirms the presence of a middle cerebral artery aneurysm with normal-sized ventricles and no haemorrhage within them. He suddenly becomes comatose (GCS 3, E1 V1 M1) with a fixed dilated right pupil What is the single most likely cause of his symptoms?

   A Hydrocephalus
   B Hyponatraemia
   C Repeat rupture of aneurysm with repeat haemorrhage
   D Seizures
   E Vasospasm and delayed ischaemic neurologic deficit (DIND)

6. A 29-year-old woman has developed a sudden onset seizure while at work. She is now clinically well with a GCS of 15 and no focal neurological deficit. A CT brain reveals haemorrhage suggesting an underlying arteriovenous malformation. What is the single most appropriate investigation to perform?

   A CT angiogram
   B Delayed MR angiogram
   C Formal cerebral (catheter) angiography with digital subtraction (DSA)
   D MR spectroscopy
   E MR venogram

7. A 75-year-old man's wife suddenly noticed his slurring of speech and right arm weakness which completely resolved within 30 minutes. He has a history of diabetes. His blood pressure is normal. Which single answer best represents his ABCD2 score?

   A 2
   B 3
   C 4
   D 5
   E 7

8. A 30-year-old woman has recently undergone cardiac surgery for rheumatic valve disease. She has a metallic mitral valve inserted and is started on warfarin for primary prevention of stroke. What is the single best INR range that should be aimed for?

   A < 1.2
   B 1.0–2.0
   C 2.0–3.0
   D 3.5–4.5
   E 5.0–6.0

Neurological tumours

1. A 20-year-old man has noticed a progressive decline in his hearing bilaterally over the past 2 years. He has numbness and weakness affecting his face, worse on the right. His MRI scan demonstrates bilateral vestibular schwannomas. What is the single most likely diagnosis?

   A Cowden syndrome
   B Neurofibromatosis type 1
   C Neurofibromatosis type 2
   D Tuberous sclerosis
   E Von Hippel–Lindau disease

2. A 50-year-old man has sudden onset headache, vomiting and impaired eye movements. Over the past 6 months he has noticed a progressive decline in his peripheral vision and his shoes, hat and wedding ring have become too small for him. An MRI confirms he has a brain tumour. What is the single most likely location of his lesion?

   A Brainstem
   B Cerebellum
   C Frontal lobe
   D Pituitary gland
   E Thalamus

3. A 68-year-old woman has worsening back pain and weakness in both legs that has worsened over the past 3 days. She has difficulty walking but her bowel and bladder function is normal. She has a past history of breast cancer. Which is the single most appropriate next step?

   A CT spine
   B Dexamethasone infusion
   C MRI of the lumbar spine
   D MRI of the whole spine
   E Refer to oncology and neurosurgery departments

Neurological infections

1. A 58-year-old woman has a fever and meningism. She has no focal neurological deficits. Meningitis is suspected and a lumbar puncture is performed which reveals a high white cell count (mainly polymorphs), low glucose in comparison to serum and turbidity. Gram-negative bacilli are seen. What is the single most likely causative pathogen?

   A *Haemophilus influenzae*
   B *Herpes simplex virus*
   C *Neisseria meningitidis*

D *Staphylococcus aureus*
E *Streptococcus pneumonia*

2. A 30-year-old man has a history of fever, memory impairment and behavioural change. There is no meningism. Shortly before an MRI scan of his brain he develops a seizure. His MRI demonstrates increased signal intensity and oedema affecting the temporal lobes, with some haemorrhagic regions.
What is the single most likely cause?

A Cytomegalovirus
B Herpes simplex virus type 1
C Herpes simplex virus type 2
D Human immune deficiency virus
E Varicella zoster virus

3. A 21-year-old man is a university student who has recently been unwell with flu-like symptoms. Since yesterday he has had nausea and vomiting, aversion to light and neck stiffness. He has a rash that is non-blanching on his arms and legs.
What is the single most appropriate next action?

A Immediate broad-spectrum IM/IV antibiotics
B Perform lumbar puncture
C Prescribe oral antibiotics and discharge
D Transfer immediately to emergency department
E Urgent CT brain scan

4. A 34-year-old man has progressively deteriorated with increasing confusion and agitation with a recent history of weight-loss and night sweats in the last 6 weeks. He recently arrived in the UK from abroad. A CT scan excludes a space-occupying lesion. CSF analysis reveals elevated white cell count (predominantly mononuclear), decreased glucose and elevated protein.
What is the single most likely causative pathogen?

A Echovirus
B HIV
C *Mycobacterium tuberculosis*
D *Streptococcus pneumoniae*
E *Toxoplasma gondii*

5. A 68-year-old man has seizures. He has become increasingly confused over the past week and now complains of headache and fever. It is difficult to confirm the presence of meningism. He has no other focal neurological deficits. Emergency CT brain is negative. A decision is made to treat him while awaiting CSF analysis.
What is the single most appropriate treatment?

A Ceftriaxone
B Ceftriaxone + Vancomycin + Ampicillin
C Ceftriaxone + Vancomycin + Ampicillin + Acyclovir

D Ethambutol + Isoniazid + Rifampicin + Pyrazinamide
E Ganciclovir + Pyrimethamine

6. A 51-year old man has lower lumbar back pain and fever. He had an operation 1 week ago to remove an intervertebral disc prolapse causing nerve root compression. He has no neurological deficit. A MRI scan confirms vertebral osteomyelitis following surgery.
What is the single most likely causative organism?

A Aspergillus
B Escherichia coli
C Salmonella
D Staphylococcus aureus
E Mycobacterium tuberculosis

Movement disorders

1. A 31-year-old woman's partner reveals that there has been a recent change in her personality. She has also started to develop irregular, rapid, jerking movements especially affecting her arms. She doesn't take any regular medication.
What single mutation is she most likely to have?

A Defect in *hamartin* gene on chromosome 9
B Defect in *merlin* gene on chromosome 22
C Defect in *tuberin* gene on chromosome 16
D Expansion in CAG trinucleotide repeats on chromosome 4
E Expansion in CTG trinucleotide repeats on chromosome 19

2. A 25-year old woman has been increasingly forgetful and complains of hearing voices. She appears to have bradykinesia and bilateral tremor, and is jaundiced. Her liver function tests are abnormal. She is referred for slit lamp examination of her eyes.
What is the single most likely diagnosis?

A Dementia with Lewy body formation
B Huntington's disease
C Idiopathic Parkinson's disease
D Progressive supranuclear palsy
E Wilson's disease

3. A 40-year-old man has worsening tremor in his right hand and a generalised slowing in motor function. He has noticed that his arm is becoming increasingly stiff. He also has difficulty sleeping due to bad dreams.
What is the single most appropriate treatment?

A Apomorphine
B Carbidopa
C Levodopa (L-Dopa)
D Ropinirole
E Sub-thalamic nucleus stimulation

4. A 27-year old man has developed a bilateral tremor and generalised rigidity in his arms and legs. He has recently been diagnosed with schizophrenia and takes chlorpromazine.
What is the single most likely diagnosis?

   A Anti-psychotic medication non-compliance
   B Dementia with Lewy bodies
   C Drug-induced parkinsonism
   D HSV encephalitis
   E Idiopathic Parkinson's disease

5. A 50-year-old woman has a history of bilateral progressive tremor and recent falls. She has difficulty swallowing and is very tearful. On examination she has severe stiffness in her neck and trunk. She has difficulty moving her eyes in a vertical direction.
What is the single most likely diagnosis?

   A Dementia with Lewy bodies
   B Idiopathic Parkinson's disease
   C Multiple systems atrophy
   D Progressive supranuclear palsy
   E Pseudo-bulbar palsy

6. A 69-year-old man has increasing stiffness and heaviness in his right arm and leg over the past 2 years with a general slowing in his movements. He has no tremor but has increased reflexes in his right upper and lower limbs. He has a history of ischaemic heart and peripheral vascular disease, hypertension and smoking. A trial of L-Dopa hasn't improved his symptoms.
What is the single most likely diagnosis?

   A Cortico-basal degeneration
   B Idiopathic Parkinson's disease
   C Multiple systems atrophy
   D Vascular Parkinsonism
   E Wilson's disease

Multiple sclerosis

1. A 40 year-old female has a MRI brain scan for episodic headaches that sound like migraines, which shows several lesions in the corpus callosum and cerebellar peduncles that have features of demyelination. She has no history of focal neurological symptoms.
What is the single most likely diagnosis?

   A Clinically isolated syndrome (CIS)
   B Devic's disease
   C Primary progressive multiple sclerosis (PPMS)
   D Radiologically-isolated syndrome (RIS)
   E Relapsing-remitting multiple sclerosis (RRMS)

2. A 34 year-old woman with a history of CIS 4 months ago develops new left leg weakness, ataxia and diplopia. MRI demonstrates new demyelinating lesions and she is prescribed steroids. After discussion of the risks and benefits she is keen to avoid further relapses.
What is the single most appropriate management?

   A Alemtuzumab therapy
   B Further steroids
   C Interferon injections
   D Regular natalizumab infusions
   E Vitamin D supplementation

3. A 42 year old man has relapsing remitting multiple sclerosis and has developed slowly progressive left arm weakness and numbness over 3 weeks. He has monthly natalizumab infusions.
What is the single most appropriate management?

   A Inform patient they have entered the progressive phase
   B MRI brain with contrast and lumbar puncture
   C Prescribe steroids
   D Prescribe steroids then give next natalizumab infusion
   E Switch to an alternative drug due to failure of natalizumab

Spinal disorders

1. A 21-year-old man has sudden onset back and leg pain. He was lifting weights in the gym when he developed acute pain radiating down his right leg. He has difficulty passing urine and cannot feel the toilet paper while using the bathroom.
What is the single most appropriate next step?

   A Analgesia and discharge with MRI scan in 6 weeks
   B Analgesia and discharge with outpatient referral to neurosurgery
   C CT spine
   D Dexamethasone infusion
   E MRI spine

2. A 40-year-old woman has neck pain and burning pain in her right arm radiating to her middle finger. She has weakness in elbow extension and absent triceps reflex. MRI spine demonstrates a cervical disc prolapse.
What is the single most likely combination of nerve root and disc to be affected?

   A C4 nerve root with C3–4 disc prolapse
   B C6 nerve root with C4–5 disc prolapse

C C6 nerve root with C5–6 disc prolapse
D C7 nerve root with C6–7 disc prolapse
E C7 nerve root with C7–T1 disc prolapse

3. A 56-year-old man has a history of leg weakness. He has no previous medical history. He has weakness in his left leg with loss of light touch and proprioception on the left side. He has loss of pain and temperature sensation on the right side. His MRI confirms a tumour affecting his spinal cord.
What is the single most likely location of the tumour?

A Anterior part of the spinal cord
B Central aspect of the spinal cord
C Left side of the spinal cord
D Posterior part of the spinal cord
E Right side of the spinal cord

4. A 78-year old man has neck pain following a fall. On examination he has weakness in both hands with loss of reflexes. Pain and temperature sensation is reduced in both arms. He has increased tone in his legs with hyper-reflexia and a positive Babinski sign. MRI demonstrates a C6 segmental cervical cord injury.
What is the single most likely diagnosis?

A Anterior cord syndrome
B Brown-Séquard syndrome
C Cauda equina syndrome
D Central cord syndrome
E Posterior cord syndrome

Systemic disease affecting the nervous system

1. A 21-year-old woman has a history of seizures and mood disturbance. On examination she has an erythematous rash over her nose and cheeks, arthritis within her finger and knee joints and oral ulceration. Urine analysis demonstrates a nephritic syndrome.
What single antibody is most likely to be positive in this woman?

A Anti acetyl choline receptor (ACH-R) antibody
B Anti double-stranded DNA (dsDNA) antibody
C Anti GQ-1B antibody
D Anti Hu antibody
E Anti mitochondrial antibody (AMA)

2. A 42-year-old woman has features of painful subacute sensory polyneuropathy affecting her lower limbs. She has a history of persistent nosebleeds with nasal crusting and on examination has a saddle-nose deformity. She develops haemoptysis and her renal function is deranged. She is ANCA +ve.
Which is the single most likely diagnosis?

A Churg–Strauss syndrome
B Dermatomyositis
C Giant cell (temporal) arteritis
D Lambert–Eaton myasthenic syndrome
E Wegener's granulomatosis

3. A 50-year old woman has subacute development of short-term memory deficits. She also complains of sleep dysfunction, generalised irritability and her family think she may be having visual hallucinations. Paraneoplastic limbic encephalitis is suspected and she is positive for anti Hu antibodies.
What is the single most likely associated malignancy?

A Breast
B Lymphoma
C Ovary
D Small cell lung cancer
E Thymoma

Neurodegenerative disease

1. A 68-year-old man has had dysarthria and dysphagia for 4 months and left arm weakness for 1 month but no sensory signs. He has a wasted left hand, brisk limb reflexes, brisk jaw jerk and a stiff, slow tongue.
What is the single most likely diagnosis?

A Bulbar onset motor neurone disease
B Cervical myelopathy
C Multifocal motor neuropathy
D Multiple sclerosis
E Primary lateral sclerosis

2. A 21-year-old woman has progressive dysarthria, dysphagia ataxia and diplopia. She has poor smooth pursuits, nystagmus, a slow, stiff tongue, slurred speech, wide based gait, reduced tone in her legs, reduced knee and ankle reflexes, and reduced pinprick and joint position sense to the shins.
What is the single most likely diagnosis?

A Bulbar onset motor neurone disease
B Friedreich ataxia
C Multiple sclerosis
D Spinocerebellar ataxia
E Spinal muscular atrophy

3. A 30-year-old man has had 6 months of proximal leg weakness, 3 months of bilateral hand intention tremor and now tongue fasciculations. He has no leg reflexes, flaccid weakness in his leg

which is worse proximally, and some past pointing with both hands. He has no upper motor neurone signs.
What is the single most likely diagnosis?

A Friedreich ataxia
B Limb onset motor neurone disease
C Multiple sclerosis
D Spinal muscular atrophy
E Spinocerebellar ataxia

4. A 20-year-old diabetic man has a history of difficulty walking since childhood. He has worsening stiffness, balance and co-ordination in his legs. His grandfather had a similar undiagnosed illness. He is kyphotic, has increased tone in his legs, no knee or ankle reflexes and loss of joint position sense in his legs.
What is the single most likely diagnosis?

A Friedreich ataxia
B Hereditary motor neurone disease
C Multiple sclerosis
D Spinal muscular atrophy
E Spinocerebellar ataxia

Dementia

1. An 84-year-old man with a history of ischaemic heart disease, hypertension and a previous minor stroke develops progressive memory problems and disinhibition over 8 months. He is diagnosed with dementia.
What is the single most likely underlying aetiology?

A Alzheimer's disease
B Delirium
C Dementia with Lewy bodies
D Parkinson's disease
E Vascular dementia

2. A 68-year-old man with a 2-year history of dementia develops frequent daytime visual hallucinations and increasing stiffness and slowness in his movements.
What is the single most likely diagnosis?

A Alzheimer's disease
B Delirium
C Dementia with Lewy bodies
D Parkinson's disease
E Vascular dementia

3. A 45-year-old man has an 8-month history of progressive change in personality, sexual disinhibition, aggression and lack of insight into these problems. An MRI of his brain shows significant frontal lobe atrophy, but nothing else.
What is the single most likely diagnosis?

A Depression

B Creutzfeld—Jakob disease
C Frontotemporal dementia
D Vascular dementia
E Young-onset Alzheimer's disease

Congenital and hereditary conditions

1. A 10-year-old boy has developmental delay in motor function. There is evidence of myotonia and muscle weakness in facial, ocular and shoulder girdle. He is to be referred for genetic testing. What single genetic abnormality is most likely to be found in this case?

A Defect in *hamartin* gene on chromosome 9
B Defect in *merlin* gene on chromosome 22
C Defect in *tuberin* gene on chromosome 16
D Expansion in CAG trinucleotide repeats on chromosome 4
E Expansion in CTG trinucleotide repeats on chromosome 19

2. A 1-day-old baby girl has a cystic membrane covered swelling over the lower part of her back that was noted immediately after birth. It does not transilluminate with light. She has a defect in the lower spine posteriorly and obvious deformities of her hips and ankles.
What is the single most likely diagnosis?

A Meningocele
B Myelomeningocele
C Spina bifida occulta
D Sturge–Weber syndrome
E Von Hippel–Lindau syndrome

3. A 12-year-old girl with 10 cafe-au-lait spots and several Lisch nodules develops resistant seizures.
What is the most likely diagnosis?

A Cerebral palsy
B Neurofibromatosis type 1
C Sturge–Weber syndrome
D Tuberous sclerosis complex
E Von Hippel–Lindau syndrome

4. A 9-year-old boy has a history of delay in speech, language development and seizures. On examination there are depigmented areas of skin on his back and patches of 'leathery' skin. A MRI brain demonstrates a subependymal tumour. ECHO demonstrates a cardiac muscle rhabdomyoma.
What is the single most likely diagnosis?

A Cerebral palsy
B Neurofibromatosis type 1
C Sturge–Weber syndrome
D Tuberous sclerosis complex
E Von Hippel–Lindau syndrome

Peripheral neurological disease

1. A 19-year-old man has fallen from his motorcycle in a road traffic incident. His wrist and finger extension are impaired as is the sensation on the dorsal aspect of the arm. Elbow extension is preserved.
   Which is the single most likely diagnosis?

   A Median nerve injury at carpal tunnel
   B Radial nerve injury at axilla
   C Radial nerve injury at elbow
   D Radial nerve injury at wrist
   E Ulnar nerve injury at elbow

2. A 50-year-old woman with diabetes has noticed weakness in her left leg in the last few weeks. She has a foot drop on the left side with weakness of great toe dorsiflexion and eversion. Inversion is preserved. There are no other clinical signs.
   What single nerve is most likely to be causing her symptoms?

   A Common peroneal nerve
   B Deep branch of peroneal nerve
   C Femoral nerve
   D Sciatic nerve
   E Tibial nerve

3. A 36-year-old woman has bilateral motor weakness affecting both legs that started distally and has spread proximally over a few days. She had a recent diarrhoeal illness 3 weeks previously but is otherwise well.
   What is the single most appropriate treatment?

   A Cylcophosphamide
   B Intravenous immunoglobulin
   C Intubation and ventilation
   D High dose steroids
   E Plasma exchange

4. A 46-year old man has a past medical history of alcohol use. He is unkempt and looks emaciated. On examination he is confused, has an ataxic gait and complains of diplopia especially on lateral gaze.

What is the single most likely diagnosis?

A Cobalamin deficiency
B Nicotinic acid deficiency
C Pyridoxine deficiency
D Riboflavin deficiency
E Thiamine deficiency

5. A 53-year-old woman has aching muscles. Both arms and legs are affected with the proximal muscles affected more than the distal. She has a violet discolouration around her eyelids and purple patches over her knuckles. Her EMG is myopathic.
   What is the single most likely diagnosis?

   A Becker muscular dystrophy
   B Dermatomyositis
   C Fascio-scapulo-humeral dystrophy
   D Inclusion body myositis
   E Mitochondrial disease

6. A 29-year-old woman has bilateral weakness and drooping of both eyelids. She also has fatigable weakness in both her arms and legs. She has a past medical history of pernicious anaemia.
   What single treatment will cause a catastrophic deterioration in her condition if given?

   A Anti-cholinergic
   B Anti-cholinesterase
   C Cyclophosphamide
   D Intravenous immunoglobulin
   E Steroids

7. A 68-year-old woman has weakness affecting her lower limbs initially. She doesn't have any ocular or bulbar symptoms. Her symptoms seem to improve following exercise. She is a lifelong smoker and has been newly diagnosed with small cell lung cancer.
   What is the single most appropriate investigation to perform?

   A Anti ACHR-antibody
   B Anti dsDNA-antibody
   C Anti Hu-antibody
   D Anti Ri-antibody
   E Anti VGCC-antibody

SBA answers

Raised intracranial pressure and head injury

1. C

Management via ATLS (Advanced Trauma and Life Support) protocols requires immediate assessment, resuscitation and treatment of life-threatening injuries before embarking on specialist intervention. (B) would happen as part of the 'D' in the ABCDE with an urgent CT brain scan (E) once the patient is initially stabilised. Alerting the on-call neurosurgeon (A) should follow the CT brain scan and (D) (mannitol) is indicated only if there are clinical signs of brain herniation (e.g. dilated pupil unreactive to light) after discussion with a neurosurgeon.

2. C

The GCS of 8 confirms a severe traumatic brain injury (TBI). Mild TBI is GCS 14–15 and moderate GCS 9–13. Crescent-shaped collections are subdural in origin. Extradural collections are bi-convex as they are restricted by skull sutures. The hyper-dense nature confirms an acute collection. Chronic collections are hypo-dense.

3. D

The history is typical of a lucid interval following traumatic injury, followed by sudden deterioration that is seen with an acute extradural haematoma. Acute subdural haematomas (B) can present like this, but are more commonly associated with impaired conscious level from outset, as are intra-cerebral haematomas (C). Chronic subdural haematomas present with progressive neurological deficits over a longer time period. Hydrocephalus (E) is unlikely given the clear history of trauma.

4. A

Decreasing CO_2 levels will vasoconstrict cerebral blood vessels, decrease cerebral blood flow and volume, and decrease intracranial pressure. Increasing CO_2 levels (B) will cause vasodilation, raising intracranial pressure. Hyperthermia (C) and placing the patient's head down (D) both increase intracranial pressure, the latter by impairing jugular venous outflow from the brain. Corticosteroids (E) are contraindicated in traumatic brain injury, as they are associated with poor outcomes and increased mortality.

5. E

The patient has a significant impairment in conscious level with a haemorrhage. Therefore he cannot be observed (D). He requires an operation (B). He is coagulopathic and needs this to be corrected before any surgical intervention (A). The warfarin must be stopped. Platelet transfusions do not reverse warfarin-induced coagulopathy (C) and are used to reverse aspirin-induced coagulopathy. Vitamin K and clotting factors help rapidly reverse warfarin-induced coagulopathy.

Headache and pain syndromes

1. B

The restlessness, ptosis, eye watering and nasal stuffiness are consistent with cluster headache. First-line treatment is with high flow oxygen and subcutaneous or intranasal triptans.

2. A

High-dose aspirin (or an NSAID) with a prokinetic antiemetic to speed up gastric emptying is first-line treatment for a migraine. She has infrequent attacks and wants to become pregnant, so prophylactic treatment is best avoided at present. Opioid medication should be avoided in migraine as they are ineffective.

3. E

The very short time from onset to peak makes this likely to be a thunderclap headache; migraines usually takes longer to peak. The photophobia and vomiting are potential red flag signs. Subarachnoid haemorrhage is the most serious cause to exclude initially and is best shown on plain CT.

4. D

New persistent headaches in this age group are potentially secondary to serious underlying causes. The persistence of symptoms and their postural nature are also warning signs for a mass lesion. The history of breast cancer raises suspicion of metastatic intracranial masses. An urgent outpatient neurology clinic is required to assess the headache and investigations are required.

5. D

This headache has postural features and the high opening pressure on lumbar puncture confirms raised intracranial pressure. Scans excluded mass lesions and venous thrombosis. Idiopathic intra-cranial hypertension is the most likely diagnosis and is most common in young obese women. Immediate treatment with repeat lumbar punctures to reduce the intracranial pressure is the only option which will address the immediate risk of visual loss, proceeding to LP shunt (B) if this is unsuccessful.

6. B
A septic venous sinus thrombosis is likely with the history of sinus infection, fever, severe headache and a new seizure. There is no confusion or meningism to suggest meningitis. An immediate CT venogram is required to confirm the diagnosis and exclude complications such as intracranial haemorrhage that would prohibit anti-coagulation.

Seizures

1. A
This is a seizure with a focal onset: a partial seizure. She has lost awareness during the seizure so it is a complex partial seizure not a simple partial seizure (D). It terminated after 2 minutes excluding (E). It is not (C) because the seizure focus is clearly localised to the right frontal lobe with no secondary generalisation (B).

2. E
Temporal lobe seizures produce a sense of fear and gustatory and auditory hallucinations. Frontal lobe seizures (A) usually have motor features whilst occipital lobe seizures (B) produce visual hallucinations. Parietal lobe seizures (C) usually produce sensory features (e.g. tingling). The pituitary gland (D) is not an anatomical site for seizures.

3. C
This seizure semiology and the neurophysiology findings are classical for absence seizures, which is a type of generalised seizure. Status epilepticus (E) is when seizures continue uninterrupted for at least 30 minutes or when there is no regaining of conscious level in between seizures. Absence seizures are not simple partial (D) where there is a focal seizure onset with preservation of awareness. Nor are they complex partial with loss of awareness (B) or complex partial with secondary generalisation (C).

4. C
Lamotrigine is very useful as first-line monotherapy for seizures especially if pregnancy is being considered as it is the least associated with teratogenic side effects. (D) is not indicated as monotherapy with a range of medications must be used first. Valproate (E) and carbamazepine (A) are both teratogenic. Clobazam (B) is usually second-line and an add-on therapy.

5. A
The clinical features are suggestive of myoclonic epilepsy. Carbamazepine is not recommended for myoclonic epilepsy as it may paradoxically worsen myoclonic seizures.

6. B
This patient is in status epilepticus and needs prompt intervention to stop her seizures. Intravenous lorazepam or rectal diazepam are first-line treatments for status epilepticus. Phenytoin infusion (D) is a second-line treatment for status epilepticus and (E) with barbiturate infusion for deep sedation is third-line. Carbamazepine (A) is not used in status epilepticus. Magnesium sulphate (C) is used in eclampsia-related seizures.

Neurovascular disease

1. C
A CT of the brain is needed to exclude haemorrhagic stroke first, which would contraindicate thrombolysis. (A) and (B) would usually follow if this is proven to be ischaemic not haemorrhagic stroke. Therapeutic dose heparin is not indicated in the treatment of acute ischaemic stroke (E). (D) is not performed to exclude haemorrhagic stroke acutely but has a role with diffusion weighted imaging (DWI) sequences in confirming ischaemic stroke.

2. B
This is a PACS with motor weakness and homonymous hemianopia without higher cognitive dysfunction. With higher cognitive dysfunction, it would be a TACS (D). Posterior circulation strokes (C) usually affect the brainstem or medial temporal or occipital lobes, and usually have isolated visual dysfunction, cranial nerve or extensive long tract signs. Lacunar strokes (A) have only isolated features (e.g. pure motor, pure sensory, ataxic hemiparesis). Weber's syndrome (E) is due to midbrain stroke following occlusion of posterior cerebral or basilar arteries with ipsilateral 3rd cranial nerve palsy and contralateral hemiparesis.

3. E
These are clinical features of the lateral medullary syndrome of Wallenberg (stroke affecting right lateral medulla) with dysfunction of the vestibular nuclei (vertigo), vagal nerve nuclei (swallowing), cerebellum and inferior peduncle (ataxia), sympathetic tracts (Horner's), trigeminal nuclei (loss of pain and temperature on face) and crossed spinothalamic tract (loss of pain and temperature contralateral body). The vessel involved is usually the posterior inferior cerebellar artery (PICA).

4. C
This is an acute subarachnoid haemorrhage (SAH). The initial CT of the brain may be normal

but xanthochromia following lumbar puncture can confirm the presence of acute SAH. (A) is unsafe and (E) will not alter management if repeat CT is normal. (B) is performed once SAH is confirmed and an aneurysmal cause is suspected. There is no indication for antibiotics with this clinical history, which is consistent with acute SAH and not infectious meningitis.

5. **C**
All of the options are known complications following a subarachnoid haemorrhage (SAH) and the patient will require close monitoring for them. Any drop in conscious level or neurological deterioration should prompt a search for and exclusion of all of them. However, the most important life-threatening complication following acute aneurysmal subarachnoid haemorrhage (especially in the first few days) is a repeat rupture of the aneurysm and recurrent haemorrhage. The presence of normal ventricles without haemorrhage makes hydrocephalus unlikely (A). Hyponatraemia does not occur in the acute phase in SAH or cause a fixed dilated pupil (B). Vasospasm and delayed ischaemic neurological deficits occur between days 4–9 (E). Seizures are unlikely to be the cause in the presence of features of uncal herniation (D).

6. **C**
DSA is the gold standard investigation to plan treatment for a vascular malformation (aneurysm or arteriovenous malformation). MR spectroscopy (D) evaluates the biometabolic parameters of brain tissue and so is more useful for neurological tumours. (A), (B) and (E) are non-invasive tests, which may be useful in diagnosis but only formal angiography can measure exact inflow and outflow to an AVM and plan treatment.

7. **D**
This patient scores 1 for his age, 2 for the presence of weakness, 1 for diabetes and 1 for resolution of symptoms within 60 minutes. The ABCD2 score assesses risk of subsequent stroke. A score of 6 confers an 8.1% risk of developing a stroke within 2 days and a 35.5% risk of stroke within 7 days. Patients scoring 4 or more should be seen by a specialist stroke physician within 24 hours.

8. **D**
Metallic valves (especially mitral) have a high risk of thrombus development so require anticoagulation with warfarin at high therapeutic ranges to prevent systemic and cranial thrombotic complications, and stroke. (A) is normal coagulation function. (B) is mildly deranged coagulation function. (C) is the range employed in patients with atrial fibrillation or following deep vein thrombosis or pulmonary embolism. (E) is excessively over anti-coagulated.

Neurological tumours

1. **C**
The presence of bilateral vestibular schwannomas is diagnostic of NF 2. There are no features to suggest NF1 (B) as a diagnosis, which requires at least 2 out of 7 features. TS (D) is classically associated with sub-ependymal giant cell astrocytomas. VHL (E) is classically associated with cerebellar haemangioblastomas. Cowden syndrome (A) is an inherited syndrome predisposing to development of meningiomas.

2. **D**
The patient is likely to be presenting with pituitary apoplexy, which is a sudden haemorrhagic infarction of usually a pituitary tumour. The history suggests the presence of bitemporal hemianopia (due to optic chiasm compression). The finding that the patient's hat, shoes and wedding ring have all become too small is typical of patients with pituitary adenomas with excessive secretion of growth hormone because it results in increased size of head, hands and feet. Given the history suggests a pituitary adenoma likely hyper-secreting growth hormone, the presentation is most likely due to a pituitary lesion.

3. **D**
The clinical features and history of malignancy suggest an acute spinal cord compression, so metastatic spinal cord compression must be excluded. (C) will not evaluate the whole spine. (A) is good for bone detail and fractures, but MRI is gold standard for evaluating spinal cord compression and evaluating soft tissue detail. (B) is only started once the diagnosis is confirmed radiologically and (E) follows imaging and confirmation of diagnosis.

Neurological infections

1. **A**
The CSF findings are consistent with bacterial meningitis. *Haemophilus influenzae* is the only Gram-negative bacillus listed. B is a virus, (D) and (E) are both Gram-positive cocci and (C) are Gram-negative cocci.

2. **B**
The history suggests encephalitis. HSV-1 is the commonest sporadic cause of viral encephalitis. The MRI changes affecting the temporal lobes are usually seen in HSV-1 encephalitis. (C) (HSV-2) can cause viral encephalitis in neonates especially. (A), (D) and (E) can all cause encephalitis but they are not the commonest causes of sporadic encephalitis. CMV in particular effects patients who are immuno-compromised such as patients with HIV infection and AIDS.

3. A

The most likely diagnosis is bacterial meningitis as the patient has photophobia and neck stiffness, and a non-blanching rash suggestive of meningococcal sepsis. Immediate treatment with broad-spectrum antibiotics is indicated by administering a dose of intramuscular antibiotics before admission. (D) should happen next followed by (E) to exclude any mass lesions and then lumbar puncture to obtain CSF. (C) would be dangerous given the suspicion of bacterial meningitis

4. C

The CSF picture and history is consistent with infectious meningitis of tuberculous origin. (A) and (B) are unlikely although with tuberculosis, a diagnosis of underlying immune-suppression with HIV should be considered. Bacterial meningitis is unlikely without a raised polymorphic white cell count. (E) is usually seen in immune-suppression and causes multiple space-occupying lesions in the brain.

5. C

Both bacterial meningitis and viral encephalitis must be considered, especially viral encephalitis given the seizures. Empirical antibiotics in an elderly patient must cover Gram-positive cocci (e.g. ceftriaxone and vancomycin), *Listeria monocytogenes* (ampicillin) and aciclovir to cover viral encephalitis. (A) and (B) are insufficient and (D) is treatment for tuberculosis. (E) is cover for CMV and toxoplasmosis (commonly used in patients with HIV).

6. D

The commonest cause of osteomyelitis due to iatrogenic surgery is *Staphylococcus aureus*. Empirical antimicrobials need to cover for both methicillin sensitive (MSSA) and methicillin-resistant (MRSA) strains. There are no features to suggest (E) (e.g. foreign travel, immune-suppression, long clinical history). (C) is common in patients with sickle cell anaemia and immune suppression. (A) is a rare cause of osteomyelitis and is common in immune-suppression. (B) can cause osteomyelitis but (D) is far more likely following recent surgery.

Movement disorders

1. D

The patient's young age, new psychiatric symptoms (change in personality), new abnormal movements (chorea) and lack of medicinal causes makes Huntington's disease the likely diagnosis. This is caused by a CAG trinucleotide expansion on chromosome 4. (E) is the genetic abnormality in myotonic dystrophy. (A) and (C)

are associated with tuberous sclerosis. (D) is the gene defect in neurofibromatosis type 2.

2. E

Neuropsychiatric manifestations together with features of parkinsonism and abnormal liver function in a young patient strongly raise the possibility of Wilson's disease, and slit lamp examination may reveal Kayser–Fleischer rings, a sign of Wilson's disease. (B) is an autosomal dominant condition with neuropsychiatric manifestations plus severe choreiform movements. (A) and (C) are unlikely in a young patient and (D) would include a vertical gaze palsy.

3. D

This patient, although young, has classical features of idiopathic Parkinson's disease (unilateral onset of tremor, bradykinesia and rigidity); non-REM sleep behaviour disorder may also be an early manifestation. Dopamine agonists are used first-line in young patients to delay the use of L-Dopa (C). (A) is also used at a later stage. (E) is reserved for selected patients after failure of medical therapy. (B) is used in combination with L-Dopa, not alone.

4. C

The patient's young age suggests a degenerative cause. His use of the dopamine-blocking agent chlorpromazine and the symmetrical nature of the symptoms make a drug-induced parkinsonism most likely.

5. D

Bilateral progressive tremor suggests atypical parkinsonian symptoms. Along with the difficulty swallowing, emotional lability, truncal axial rigidity and vertical gaze palsy, progressive supranuclear palsy is most likely. (A) causes atypical parkinsonian symptoms but presents with prominent visual hallucinations and no gaze paresis. (C) may present with predominantly cerebellar or autonomic symptoms. (B) presents with classical parkinsonism and no gaze paresis. (E) presents with difficulty swallowing and emotional lability but usually no gaze restriction.

6. D

Step-wise decline in function and multiple risk factors for atherosclerotic vascular disease suggest vascular parkinsonism. Upper motor neurone signs (hyperreflexia and lack of improvement with L-Dopa) also point to this. (B) would have parkinsonian symptoms and good initial response to L-Dopa. (C) is an atypical cause of parkinsonism with prominent cerebellar or autonomic symptoms. (E) presents with neuropsychiatric manifestations and features of liver disease. (A) usually presents with myoclonus, dementia and abnormal arm movements.

Multiple sclerosis

1. D

RIS is the incidental finding of MRI evidence of CNS demyelination in the absence of neurological symptoms. Around 50% will progress to clinical symptoms and signs (CIS or RRMS). (A) is a single episode of clinical symptoms potentially caused by CNS demyelination with insufficient radiological or clinical evidence of previous episodes. (C) is slow, progressive accumulation of neurological disability with radiological and CSF evidence of demyelination. (B) (neuromyelitis optica) is an antibody-mediated CNS demyelinating disorder characterised by bilateral optic neuritis and transverse myelitis. (E) requires multiple clinical episodes of neurological dysfunction with resolution between episodes and demyelination on MRI/CSF.

2. D

This patient has an aggressive form of multiple sclerosis (two disabling episodes in 12 months). She is eligible for natalizumab to significantly reduce the frequency of relapse. Alemtuzumab (A) is used for failed or contraindicated therapy with natalizumab. Steroids (B) do not reduce relapse frequency. Interferon (C) is used as first-line disease modifying therapy but with aggressive multiple sclerosis she is eligible for more potent therapies. Vitamin D (E) should be offered but has unknown effect on relapses or progression.

3. B

Suspected relapse or slowly progressive symptoms on natalizumab needs investigating to exclude progressive multifocal leukoencephalopathy (PML) which is caused by the JC virus. An MRI with contrast will show new lesions and if the patient has PML there will be JC viral DNA in the CSF. The progression over 3 weeks is quite long for a relapse and needs investigating rather than treating (C, D and E). (A) cannot be accepted without excluding PML in a patient taking natalizumab since this also causes progressive symptoms.

Spinal disorders

1. E

This is acute cauda equina syndrome (perianal numbness and saddle anaesthesia, urinary sphincter dysfunction), a medical emergency. The clinical history suggests acute lumbar disc prolapse. Urgent MRI of the spine will establish diagnosis. (A) and (B) are inappropriate as surgical decompression within 48 hours is essential to preserve neurological function. A CT spine (C) is useful for bony visualisation but will not identify compression of the cauda equina and disc prolapse. (D) is not indicated in cauda equina syndrome.

2. D

The patient has clinical features of a radiculopathy. The dermatomal and myotomal distributions of sensory and motor symptoms respectively determine the spinal nerve root affected and the level of disc prolapse. Elbow extension is controlled by triceps and C7 nerve root in particular, which includes sensory distribution of the middle finger.

3. C

The clinical features suggest Brown–Séquard syndrome. Therefore the tumour is compressing the left spinal cord. (D) would cause a right-sided Brown–Séquard syndrome with motor weakness and dorsal column impairment on the right side. (E) would cause features of central cord syndrome. (A) would cause anterior cord syndrome with preserved dorsal column function but loss of bilateral motor function and pain and temperature sensation. (B) would cause bilateral loss of dorsal column function but preserved motor function and pain and temperature sensation.

4. D

This is classical central cord syndrome (upper limbs affected more than lower, distal muscles affected more than proximal, loss of pain and temperature in a cape-like distribution, lower motor neurone signs in arms with upper motor neurone signs in lower limbs). Anterior cord syndrome (A) is bilateral motor weakness and loss of pain and temperature distribution with preservation of dorsal column function. (B) is ipsilateral loss of motor and dorsal column function with contralateral loss of pain and temperature. (C) is sphincter dysfunction, perianal numbness and cauda equina syndrome. (E) is isolated dorsal column dysfunction.

Systemic disease affecting the nervous system

1. B

This patient has systemic lupus erythematosus, confirmed by the presence of classical malar rash, arthropathy, oral ulceration, and renal and neurological complications. The classic auto-antibody is anti-dsDNA antibody. (A) is associated with myasthenia gravis. (C) is associated with the Miller Fisher variant of Guillain–Barré syndrome. (D) is associated with neurological paraneoplastic syndromes and (E) is associated with primary biliary cirrhosis.

2. E

Nasal discharge with saddle-nose deformity, renal complications (likely nephritic syndrome) and haemoptysis (as a result of pulmonary haemorrhage) suggests Wegener's granulomatosis. ANCA positivity confirms vasculitis. (D) is a paraneoplastic syndrome presenting with weakness improving with exercise and anti-voltage-gated calcium channel antibodies. (C) presents with headache, jaw claudication and visual dysfunction. (B) is associated with arthropathy, characteristic rashes (Gottron's papules, shawl rash) and anti-Jo/Mi2 antibodies. (A) presents asthma, eosinophilia and small-to-medium vessel vasculitis.

3. D

Anti-Hu antibodies are typically associated with small cell lung cancer. (E) is usually associated with anti-CV2 antibodies, (C) with anti-Yo antibodies, (B) with anti-Tr antibodies and (A) may be associated with anti-Yo, anti-Ri and anti amphiphysin antibodies.

Neurodegenerative disease

1. A

There are mixed upper and lower motor neurone signs, with upper motor neurone signs at a more rostral level of the nervous system than lower motor neurone signs (e.g. brisk jaw jerk, wasted hand muscles). Multifocal motor neuropathy (C) and cervical myelopathy (B) do not cause bulbar dysfunction. His age and progressive symptoms argue against multiple sclerosis. The lower motor neurone signs exclude primary lateral sclerosis.

2. D

Her sensory signs exclude motor neurone disease. Friedreich ataxia could account for loss or reflexes and altered joint position sense but would not cause eye movement abnormality, nystagmus or slurred speech. Multiple sclerosis is possible but the progressive nature argues against the common relapsing remitting form and it would not cause reduced tone and reflexes in the legs.

3. D

Spinal muscular atrophy causes slowly progressive lower motor neurone symptoms and signs in this manner.The lack of both upper and lower motor neurone signs at the same level argues against motor neurone disease. Spinocerebellar ataxia (E), Friedreich's ataxia (A) and multiple sclerosis (C) would not cause tongue fasciculation.

4. A

The long history of motor problems and physical deformity argue against motor neurone disease (B) and multiple sclerosis (C). Spinal muscular atrophy (D) does not cause increased muscle tone. The family history and diabetes are consistent with Freidreich's ataxia, as are the other symptoms and signs. There are no other cerebellar signs suggestive of spinocerebellar ataxia.

Dementia

1. E

The history of hypertension, ischaemic heart disease and previous stroke make vascular dementia the most likely cause. Alzheimer's disease is possible but these other risk factors make vascular dementia the most likely. There are no signs of parkinsonism to suggest Parkinson's disease or dementia with Lewy bodies.

2. C

The early visual hallucinations and symptoms of parkinsonism make dementia with Lewy bodies most likely. Alzheimer's doesn't usually cause the stiffness and slowness at such an early stage. Parkinson's disease can cause dementia but this usually occurs after the movement disorder and much later in the disease.

3. C

The symptoms point to frontal lobe dysfunction and the lengthy time course suggest a slowly progressive degenerative condition, making frontotemporal dementia most likely. Young-onset Alzheimer's usually presents with memory problems and Creutzfeld–Jakob disease would cause dysfunction in other cognitive domains and have characteristic findings on MRI. There are no risk factors for vascular dementia. Depression can sometimes cause an apathetic or withdrawn state causing some impairment in cognition but doesn't cause these types of personality change.

Congenital and hereditary conditions

1. D

The diagnosis is likely to be myotonic dystrophy. The genetic abnormality is in the *DM-PK* gene with a trinucleotide repeat expansion of >37 repeats (A) is associated with Huntington's disease. (C) and (E) are associated with tuberous sclerosis. (D) is associated with neurofibromatosis type 2.

2. B

The patient has a myelomeningocele as opposed to a pure meningocele (A). (D) is facial port-wine stain with abnormal cranial vascular calcification. (E) is a syndrome associated with cerebellar haemangioblastomas. (C) is a 'closed' posterior spinal defect with normal skin overlying the defect and no herniation of spinal cord tissue.

3. B

The presence of more than 6 café-au-lait spots and multiple Lisch nodules suggest a diagnosis of neurofibromatosis type 1. The resistant seizures suggest an associated structural lesion within the CNS and that requires further investigation.

4. D

The clinical features meet the diagnostic criteria for tuberous sclerosis (TS) complex. The depigmented areas of skin are known as ash-leaf macules. The patches of leathery skin describe shagreen patches. Shagreen patches, subependymal giant cell astrocytoma and cardiac rhabdomyoma are all major features. A definite diagnosis of TS occurs in the presence of two major features or one major and two minor (e.g. bone cysts, pitting of teeth) features.

Peripheral neurological disease

1. C

The extensors of the upper limb are supplied by the radial nerve. Preservation of elbow extension means the injury is at a lower level than the axilla, so it is not (B). Loss of wrist and finger extension with altered sensorium means the injury is at a higher level than the wrist, so it is not (A) or (D). The ulnar nerve supplies the flexor compartment with no involvement in the extensors, so it is not (E).

2. A

The patient has weakness in ankle dorsiflexion, great toe dorsiflexion and eversion indicating involvement of both branches of the peroneal nerve, so it is not (B). Preservation of inversion suggests that the tibial nerve is preserved, so it is not (E). The sciatic nerve divides into common peroneal and tibial nerves so it is not the sciatic nerve (D). The femoral nerve (C) supplies knee extensors, which are unaffected.

3. B

The patient has clinical features consistent with Guillain–Barré syndrome (GBS). Intravenous immunolobulin and plasma exchange are equally effective at improving symptoms, but intravenous immunoglobulin is easier to administer and so is the first-line treatment. Steroids and cyclophosphamide are not treatments for GBS. The patient has no signs of imminent respiratory failure requiring intubation and ventilation, but needs to be observed for this.

4. E

The clinical features are consistent with Wernicke's encephalopathy. (A) (B12) deficiency causes subacute combined degeneration of the spinal cord, (C) is vitamin B6, deficiency of which causes dermatitis, confusion and neuropathy; vitamin B3 deficiency causes pellagra, which is characterised by dementia, dermatitis and diarrhoea. (D) is vitamin B2 deficiency, which leads to anaemia, stomatitis and other skin changes.

5. B

The clinical features are consistent with a myopathy: the heliotrope rash (violet discolouration around the eyelids) and Gottron's papules (patches over the knuckles) suggest dermatomyositis, an inflammatory myositis. (D) commonly affects more elderly people, particularly males, with the distal muscles affected initially. (A) is an inherited muscular dystrophy affecting much younger patients. (C) affects specific muscle groups of the face, scapula and limb girdle. Mitochondrial disorders (E) frequently have slowly progressive myopathies but do not cause the skin changes described here.

6. A

The patient has myasthenia gravis, a disorder of cholinergic neurotransmission at the neuromuscular junction. Anticholinergic medication can acutely exacerbate the impaired neurotransmission in these patients and cause life-threatening respiratory and bulbar weakness. (C), (D) and (E) are all used in the treatment of myasthenia gravis.

7. E

This patient has features consistent with Lambert–Eaton myasthenic syndrome (LEMS), a paraneoplastic syndrome commonly associated with small cell lung cancer in particular. The autoantibody associated is the anti-voltage-gated calcium channel antibody. (C) and (D) are paraneoplastic autoantibodies but not associated with LEMS. (A) is associated with myasthenia gravis in which the symptoms of weakness do not paradoxically improve with exercise. (B) is associated with systemic lupus erythematosus.

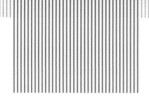

Index

Note: Page numbers in **bold** or *italic* refer to tables or figures, respectively.